Neural Regeneration and Transplantation

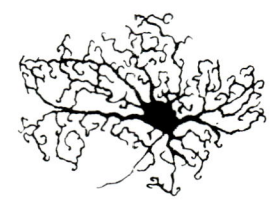

Frontiers of Clinical Neuroscience

Series Editors

Ivan Bodis-Wollner, M.D.
Mt. Sinai School of Medicine
New York

Earl A. Zimmerman, M.D.
Oregon Health Sciences University
Portland

Frontiers of Clinical Neuroscience
VOLUME 6

NEURAL REGENERATION AND TRANSPLANTATION

Edited by

FREDRICK J. SEIL, M.D.

Office of Regeneration Research Programs
Veterans Administration Medical Center
Department of Neurology
Oregon Health Sciences University
Portland, Oregon

ALAN R. LISS, INC.
New York

Address all Inquiries to the Publisher
Alan R. Liss, Inc., 41 East 11th Street, New York, NY 10003

Copyright © 1989 Alan R. Liss, Inc.

Printed in the United States of America

While the authors, editors, and publisher believe that drug selection and dosage and the specifications and usage of equipment and devices, as set forth in this book, are in accord with current recommendations and practice at the time of publication, they accept no legal responsibility for any errors or omissions, and make no warranty, express or implied, with respect to material contained herein. In view of ongoing research, equipment modifications, changes in governmental regulations and the constant flow of information relating to drug therapy, drug reactions and the use of equipment and devices, the reader is urged to review and evaluate the information provided in the package insert or instructions for each drug, piece of equipment or device for, among other things, any changes in the instructions or indications of dosage or usage and for added warnings and precautions.

Library of Congress Cataloging-in-Publication Data

Neural regeneration and transplantation / edited by Fredrick J. Seil.
    p.   cm. — (Frontiers of clinical neuroscience ; v.6)
    Includes bibliographies and index.
    ISBN 0-8451-4505-3
    1. Nervous system—Regeneration. 2. Central nervous system—Transplantation.   I. Seil, Fredrick J. II. Series.
    [DNLM: 1. Nerve Regeneration. 2. Nerve Tissue—transplantation.
    W1 FR946DM v. 6 / WL 102 N4938]
    QP363.5.N468 1988
    591.1'88--dc19
    DNLM/DLC   88-13602
    for Library of Congress   CIP

Contents

Contributors

Albert J. Aguayo, M.D., Neurosciences Unit, The Montreal General Hospital and McGill University, Montreal, Quebec H3G 1A4, Canada **[67]**

Barry G.W. Arnason, M.D., Department of Neurology and The Brain Research Institute, University of Chicago, Chicago, IL 60637 **[239]**

Kevin D. Barron, M.D., Research Service, Veterans Administration Medical Center and Department of Neurology, Albany Medical College, Albany, NY 12208 **[79]**

Garth M. Bray, M.D., Neurosciences Unit, The Montreal General Hospital and McGill University, Montreal, Quebec H3G 1A4, Canada **[67]**

György Buzsáki, M.D., Department of Neurosciences, University of California at San Diego, La Jolla, CA 92093 **[211]**

Bruce M. Carlson, M.D., Ph.D., Department of Anatomy and Biology, University of Michigan, Ann Arbor, MI 48109 **[1]**

Lawrence F. Eng, Ph.D., Department of Pathology, Veterans Administration Medical Center and Stanford University School of Medicine, Palo Alto, CA 94304 **[183]**

Fred H. Gage, Ph.D., Department of Neurosciences, University of California at San Diego, La Jolla, CA 92093 **[211]**

G.A. Gerhardt, Ph.D., Departments of Pharmacology and Psychiatry, University of Colorado Health Sciences Center, Denver, CO 80262 **[227]**

A.-C. Granholm, Ph.D., Department of Pharmacology, University of Colorado Health Sciences Center, Denver, CO 80262 **[227]**

Barth A. Green, M.D., Department of Neurological Surgery, University of Miami School of Medicine and Veterans Administration Medical Center, Miami, FL 33136 **[171]**

T. Hagg, M.D., Department of Biology, School of Medicine, University of California at San Diego, La Jolla, CA 92093 **[101]**

B.J. Hoffer, M.D., Ph.D., Department of Pharmacology, University of Colorado Health Sciences Center, Denver, CO 80262 **[227]**

Lyn Jakeman, Departments of Neurological Surgery and Neuroscience, University of Florida College of Medicine, Gainesville, FL 32610 **[183]**

K. John Klose, Ph.D., Department of Neurological Surgery, University of Miami School of Medicine and Veterans Administration Medical Center, Miami, FL 33136 **[171]**

M. Manthorpe, Ph.D., Department of Biology, School of Medicine, University of California at San Diego, La Jolla, CA 92093 **[101]**

Irvine G. McQuarrie, M.D., Ph.D., Division of Neurosurgery and Department of Developmental Genetics, School of Medicine, Case Western Reserve University and Neural Regeneration Center, Veterans Administration Medical Center, Cleveland, OH 44106 **[29]**

The number in brackets is the opening page number of the contributor's article.

Martin K. Nicholas, Ph.D., Department of Neurology and The Brain Research Institute, University of Chicago, Chicago, IL 60637 **[239]**

L. Olson, M.D., Ph.D., Department of Histology and Neurobiology, Karolinska Institute, Stockholm, Sweden **[227]**

Paul J. Reier, Ph.D., Departments of Neurological Surgery and Neuroscience, University of Florida College of Medicine, Gainesville, FL 32610 **[183]**

Stephen W. Scheff, Ph.D., Department of Anatomy and Neurobiology, Sanders-Brown Research Center on Aging, University of Kentucky College of Medicine, Lexington, KY 40536 **[137]**

Å. Seiger, M.D., Ph.D., Department of Neurological Surgery, Research Laboratories, University of Miami School of Medicine, Miami, FL 33101 **[227]**

Fredrick J. Seil, M.D., Office of Regeneration Research Programs, Veterans Administration Medical Center, Department of Neurology, Oregon Health Sciences University, Portland, OR 97201 **[ix,123]**

I. Strömberg, Ph.D., Department of Histology and Neurobiology, Karolinska Institute, Stockholm, Sweden **[227]**

D. Stephen Snyder, Ph.D., V.A. Medical Center, and Departments of Pathology and Neurology, University of Tennessee at Memphis, Memphis, TN 38104 **[15]**

Betty G. Uzman, M.D., V.A. Medical Center and Departments of Pathology and Neurology, University of Tennessee at Memphis, Memphis, TN 38104 **[15]**

S. Varon, M.D., Department of Biology, School of Medicine, University of California at San Diego, La Jolla, CA 92093 **[101]**

Gloria M. Villegas, M.D., Ph.D., V.A. Medical Center, and Departments of Pathology and Neurology, University of Tennessee at Memphis, Memphis, TN 38104; present address: Instituto Internacional de Estudios Avanzados, Caracas, Venezuela **[15]**

Stephen G. Waxman, M.D., Ph.D., Department of Neurology, Yale University School of Medicine, New Haven, CT 06510; PVA/EPVA Neuroscience and Regeneration Research Center, V.A. Medical Center, West Haven, CT 06516 **[43]**

Wise Young, M.D., Ph.D., Department of Neurosurgery, New York University Medical Center, New York, NY 10016 **[157]**

Preface

The purpose of this volume is to present an overview of neural regeneration research in language understandable to those who are not presently investigators in the field, but who have an interest in the current status of this work. The book is thus aimed at clinicians who deal with neural injuries and at students who plan to or have already begun to pursue a career in regeneration research.

The fifteen chapters cover the nervous system from muscle to peripheral nerve to spinal cord to brain. Aspects of regeneration reviewed include axonal transport, axon-glia interactions, neuronal survival and rescue, neuronal growth factors, axonal sprouting, synaptic reorganization, and the still debated role of glia as a help or hindrance to central nervous system regeneration. Two chapters are devoted to spinal cord injury, as this remains a most difficult area in regeneration research, and another two to the burgeoning field of central nervous system transplantation, including both animal and human studies. The book concludes with a chapter on immunologic considerations in transplantation to the central nervous system, a subject too often neglected in the rush toward clinical application of the results of some promising basic research.

The chapters have been written by or under the direction of leading neural regeneration research investigators, many of whom are physicians as well as basic scientists. The task that they were given, that of communicating to an audience less familiar with the subject than the usual audience of scientific peers, was a difficult one. The authors have, for the most part, succeeded admirably in accomplishing this task, without qualitative or quantitative changes in their usual standards of communication. For this reason, perhaps even some of their scientific peers might find the volume of use.

In addition to thanking the chapter authors for their superb efforts, I would like to express my gratitude to the Medical Research Service of the Veterans Administration for support of the Office of Regeneration Research Programs. The creation and support of this unique office by the Veterans Administration has made this volume possible.

FREDRICK J. SEIL, M.D.

1

Neuromuscular Regeneration in Mammals

BRUCE M. CARLSON, MD, PhD

Department of Anatomy and Biology, University of Michigan, Ann Arbor, Michigan 48109

Skeletal muscle can be looked upon as one of the major end organs of the nervous system. Our muscles are responsible for translating a continuous barrage of motor nerve output into the mechanical forces that control our breathing, movements of joints, and resting posture. In order to do this, muscles must be able to receive a modulated neural stimulus and respond by either contracting or relaxing to the appropriate extent. A break in continuity anywhere between the motor centers of the brain and the muscle fibers themselves can seriously impair muscle function in the affected individual. The extent to which damage along this pathway can be repaired and function restored varies considerably and depends upon the level of the lesion. This chapter will describe the ability of skeletal muscle to regenerate after damage. It will also cover inter-relationships between regenerating muscle fibers and their associated nerve terminals.

NORMAL ADULT STRUCTURE
Skeletal Muscle

From the standpoint of development and regeneration, the functional unit of skeletal muscle is a complex, consisting of: 1) the multinucleated skeletal muscle fiber itself; 2) its enveloping basal lamina; and 3) the muscle satellite cell, an undistinguished-appearing mononuclear cell located between the muscle fiber and its basal lamina (Fig. 1–1). In mature muscle, roughly 1 out of 20 nuclei within a muscle fiber complex belongs to a satellite cell.

Unfortunately, satellite cells can be identified with certainty only with the electron microscope. Satellite cells are significantly involved in both the growth and regeneration of muscle fibers. These functions will be described later in the text.

Neuromuscular Junction

In typical mammalian muscle, there is one discrete site on each muscle fiber where the motor nerve terminates. This region is called the neuromuscular junction, or sometimes the motor endplate (Fig. 1–2). The three fundamental components of the neuromuscular junction are: 1) the nerve terminal, 2) the specialized postsynaptic apparatus of the muscle fiber, and 3) an intervening basal lamina.

The terminal branches of the motor nerve trace a roughly oval outline on the surface of the muscle fibers. At the ultrastructural level, accumulations of synaptic vesicles containing packets of acetylcholine molecules are concentrated in the region of the nerve terminal closest to the muscle fiber. The terminal branches of the motor nerve are unmyelinated, but they are covered by a Schwann cell sheath in all areas except where they interface with the muscle fiber.

The nerve terminal rests in a synaptic furrow, which indents the surface of the muscle fiber. Along the surface of the synaptic furrow, the plasma membrane (sarcolemma) of the muscle fiber is thrown into a series of postsynaptic folds, separated from one another by postsynaptic clefts. Closely associated with the surface of the folds are acetylcholine receptor molecules.

The basal lamina that surrounds the muscle

Neural Regeneration and Transplantation, pages 1–14
© 1989 Alan R. Liss, Inc.

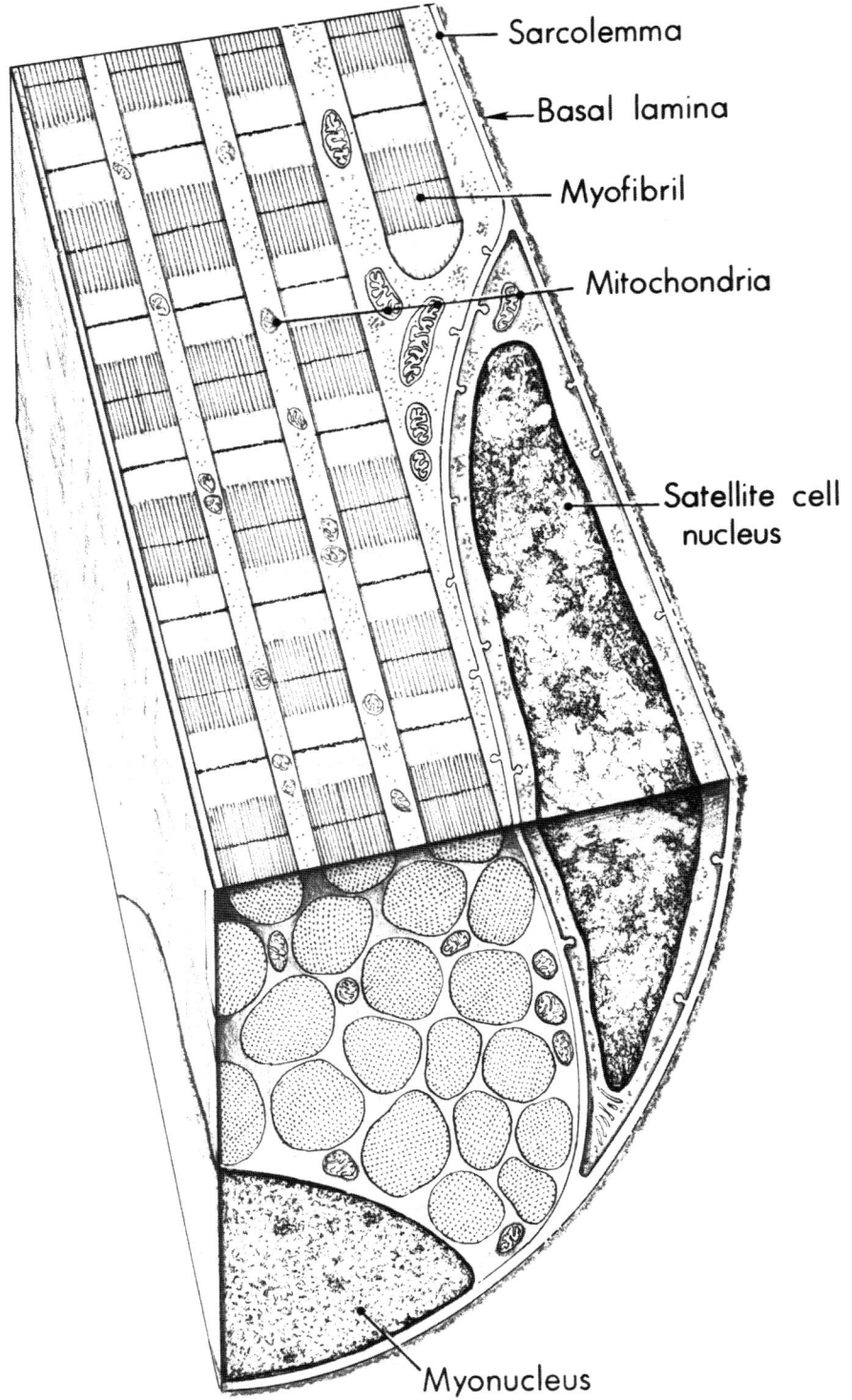

Figure 1–1. Schematic drawing of a muscle fiber complex, including the muscle fiber, a satellite cell, and surrounding basal lamina.

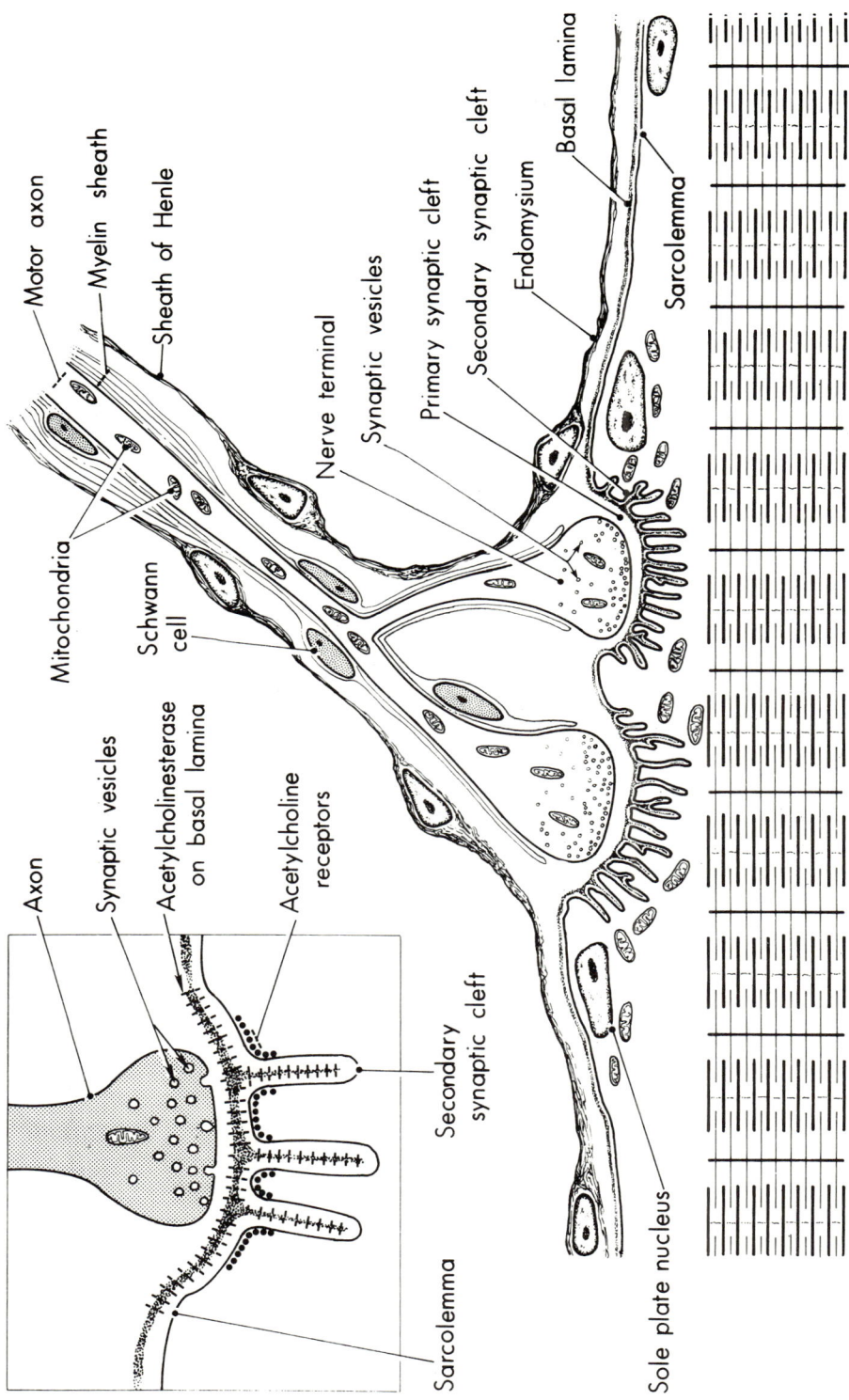

Figure 1–2. Schematic drawing of a neuromuscular junction. The inset shows the structural and molecular components involved in the release and uptake of acetylcholine from the nerve terminal to the muscle fiber.

Motor axon

Myelin sheath

Sheath of Henle

Nerve terminal

Synaptic vesicles

Primary synaptic cleft

Secondary synaptic cleft

Endomysium

Basal lamina

Sarcolemma

Mitochondria

Schwann cell

Sole plate nucleus

Axon

Synaptic vesicles

Acetylcholinesterase on basal lamina

Acetylcholine receptors

Secondary synaptic cleft

Sarcolemma

fiber is continuous through the neuromuscular junction; it separates the nerve terminals from the postsynaptic apparatus of the muscle fiber. Small branches of the basal lamina penetrate the postsynaptic clefts. A prominent molecular constituent of the synaptic basal lamina is the acetylcholinesterase molecule, which is adherent to the basal lamina and which persists for long periods after the nerve has been separated from the motor endplate region. Investigators in several laboratories have recently demonstrated the existence of a number of unique molecular components in the synaptic basal lamina. Some of these cause the aggregation of acetylcholine receptors in developing muscle, whereas the function of others is less well defined (Barald et al., 1987; Magill et al., 1987).

Associated with the neuromuscular junction is a loose aggregate of myonuclei. There is increasing evidence that these nuclei differ from other myonuclei by synthesizing macromolecules related to motor endplate function.

Under normal conditions the neuromuscular junction is the site where the electrical signal that rapidly passes along the length of a nerve fiber is briefly converted to a chemical signal (acetylcholine), which, in turn, stimulates the genesis of another rapidly moving electrical signal that passes along the length of the muscle fiber and causes the muscle fiber to contract. The essence of the chemical signal is the release of packets of acetylcholine from the synaptic vesicles. The acetylcholine molecules pass through the basal lamina that intervenes between the nerve terminal and the muscle fiber, and they then bind to the acetylcholine receptors on the surface of the postsynaptic folds. The interaction between acetylcholine and its receptor results in a change in configuration of the receptor, which permits the influx of cations into the muscle fiber and stimulates the action potential that travels along the plasma membrane (sarcolemma) of the muscle fiber.

EMBRYOGENESIS AND REGENERATION OF THE SKELETAL MUSCLE FIBER
Embryogenesis

Most skeletal muscle is derived from mononuclear cells that arise in the somites (blocklike structures that lie along the precursor of the spinal cord in the early embryo). As the limb buds are first taking shape, the myogenic (muscle-forming) cells migrate out from the somites and into the developing limb. There they form dorsal and ventral masses, which soon split up into smaller units that represent the precursors of individual muscles. Within these masses, the myogenic cells begin to line up side by side, and they fuse to form multinucleated bands called myotubes (Fig. 1–3). Within the myotubes, the active synthesis of contractile proteins and their organization into sarcomeres (the fundamental units of muscle contraction) are taking place. The nuclei of myotubes are arranged as central chains. Up to this point, all of the processes involved in myogenesis can take place in the absence of nerves. Embryonic nerve fibers enter the primordia of the muscles and begin to make contact with the developing myotubes. As the myotubes mature, the nuclei break away from the central chains and move toward the periphery. At this point the myotube has matured into a muscle fiber. Individual mononucleated myogenic cells remain scattered alongside the muscle fiber as satellite cells.

Figure 1–3. Major steps in the embryonic differentiation of a skeletal muscle. **A:** Unspecialized mesenchymal cell. **B:** Myoblast. This spindle shaped cell possesses large numbers of free ribosomes, including helical polyribosomes upon which the myosin molecules are formed. Cytoplasmic filaments and microtubules are present, but identifiable contractile proteins are not found. **C:** Myotube. This is a long multinucleated cell formed by the fusion of mononucleated myoblasts. The nuclei are arranged in long central chains. Myofilamentogenesis is actively occurring, and bundles of well-ordered contractile filaments are present in the periphery. The large numbers of ribosomes attest to the continued protein synthetic activity. The small mononucleated cell alongside the myotube will eventually fuse with the myotube during further maturation. **D:** Cross-striated muscle fiber. The nuclei have moved to a peripheral location, and the bulk of the cytoplasm (sarcoplasm) is filled with bundles of contractile filaments demonstrating the characteristic banding pattern of skeletal muscle. (Reproduced from Carlson, 1981, with permission of the publisher.)

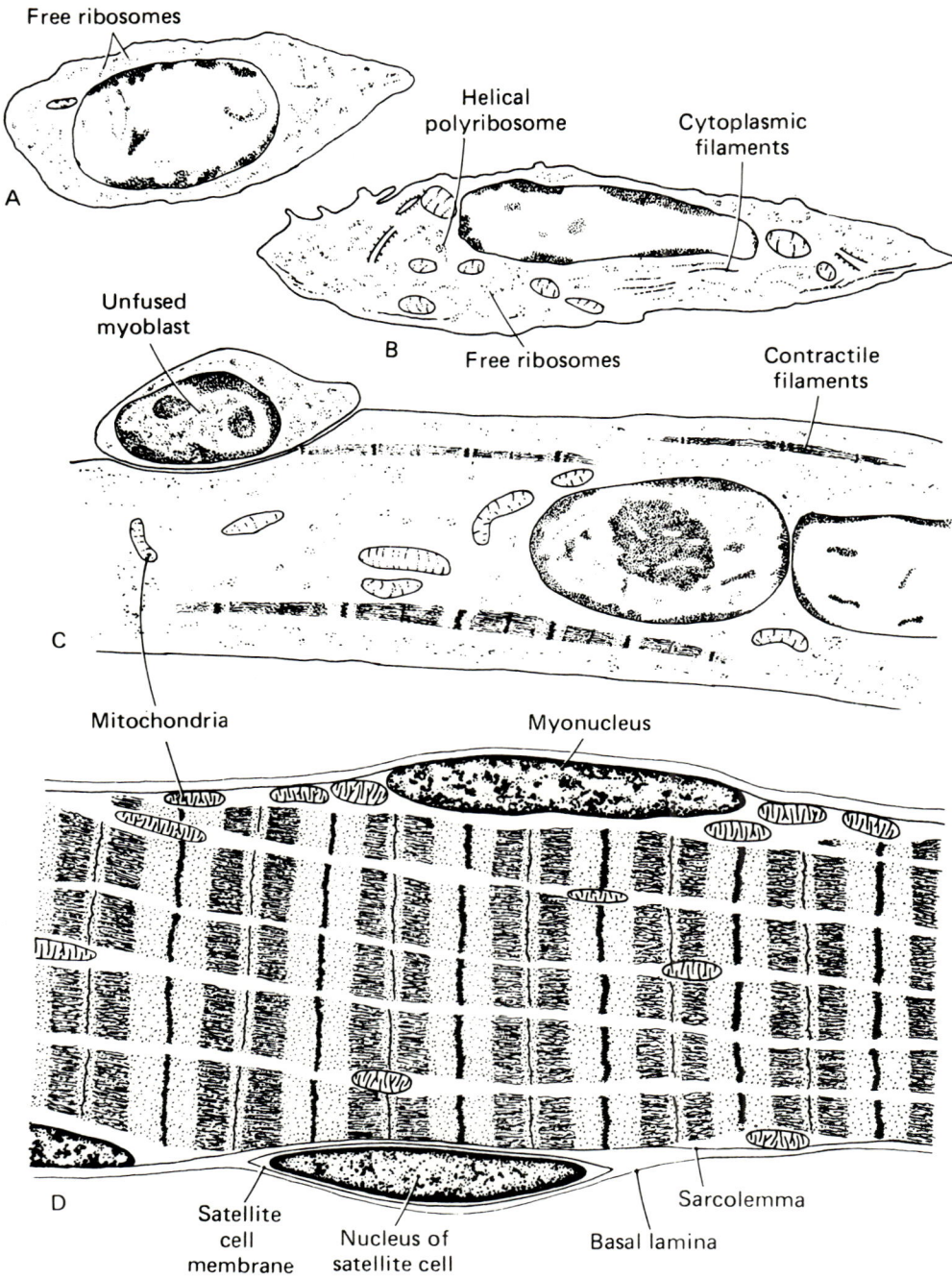

Free ribosomes

A

Helical
polyribosome

Cytoplasmic
filaments

B   Free ribosomes

Unfused
myoblast

Contractile
filaments

C

Mitochondria   Myonucleus

D

Satellite
cell
membrane

Nucleus of
satellite cell

Sarcolemma

Basal lamina

Regeneration

Mature muscle fibers subjected to a variety of insults undergo a sequence of degeneration, followed by regeneration (Fig. 1–4). Among the external factors that precipitate muscle fiber degeneration are direct mechanical trauma, extremes of heat and cold, ischemia, certain forms of exercise, and exposure to many of the commonly used local anesthetics (Carlson and Faulkner, 1983).

There are typically two phases in the degeneration of an injured muscle fiber. The first is an intrinsic degeneration, manifested by the breaking up of the myofilaments into individual sarcomeric units (often at the expense of the integrity of the Z-line). This is accompanied by disturbances in the integrity of the mitochondria, swelling of the internal membrane systems, and breakdown of the nuclei. Surprisingly little attention has been paid to the processes that lead to internal breakdown, but common factors are an increase in intracellular calcium ions and activation of the few lysosomal enzymes that have been studied. After a certain point, internal degeneration seems to come to a halt, and further degenerative changes do not occur until the damaged muscle fiber is invaded by blood-borne phagocytic cells. The duration of the intrinsic phase of muscle fiber degeneration can be as little as 1 day in well-vascularized muscle or as long as 6 or 7 weeks in ischemic areas of transplanted or otherwise devascularized muscles.

The phase of cell-mediated degeneration begins with the penetration of macrophages (mostly blood-borne) through the basal lamina that surrounds the damaged muscle fiber. The macrophages actively engulf bundles of myofilaments and other cytoplasmic debris and gradually retreat, leaving a largely empty basal lamina with a population of activated satellite cells inside.

Muscle fiber regeneration begins with the activation of satellite cells. The exact cause(s) of satellite cell activation is not known, but there is some evidence for a stimulation of satellite cell activity by products of damaged or degenerating muscle (Bischoff, 1986). Initial activation of satellite cells occurs while macrophages are still removing the debris of the damaged muscle fiber. They become aligned along the inner surface of the original muscle fiber basement membrane, although they can also escape through tears in the basement membrane into the extracellular space. The nuclei enlarge, a nucleolus becomes prominent, and the amount of cytoplasm increases. Within a day or two, as a rule, the activated satellite cells fuse to form myotubes (Snow, 1977). The maturation of regenerating myotubes follows a morphological and biochemical course similar to that of embryonic myotubes. Similarly, the regenerating myotubes mature into muscle fibers by the breaking up of the central chains of nuclei, although not infrequently some nuclei remain in central positions in regenerated muscle fibers. As in embryogenesis, some myogenic cells fail to fuse with the regenerating muscle fiber, and a new population of satellite cells becomes associated with the regenerated muscle fiber.

The last phase in the maturation of a regenerating muscle fiber is its differentiation into a fast or a slow type of muscle fiber as a result of the kinds of myosin that are synthesized in the regenerating muscle fiber. As in the normal ontogenesis of muscle, this step is nerve-mediated, and in the absence of the motor nerve it does not occur.

Figure 1–4.   Summary drawings of major phases of the degeneration and regeneration of a single muscle fiber. **A:** Early ischemic damage. The nucleus is becoming pyknotic, with chromatin clumping inside the nuclear membrane. The mitochondria are swollen, and the bundles of contractile filaments are breaking apart throughout the muscle fiber. **B:** Fragmentation phase. Macrophages (M) associated with ingrowing vasculature enter the degenerating muscle fiber and remove bundles of contractile filaments and other cytoplasmic debris. Beneath the basal lamina (arrow), spindle-shaped myoblasts (Mb) line up in preparation for the formation of new muscle fibers. **C:** Myotube. Beneath the original basal lamina, myoblasts have fused to form a multinucleated fiber with bundles of newly forming contractile filaments at the periphery. **D:** Muscle fiber. The mature regenerated muscle fiber is in most respects indistinguishable from a normal muscle fiber. (Reproduced from Foster and Carlson, 1980, with permission of the publisher.)

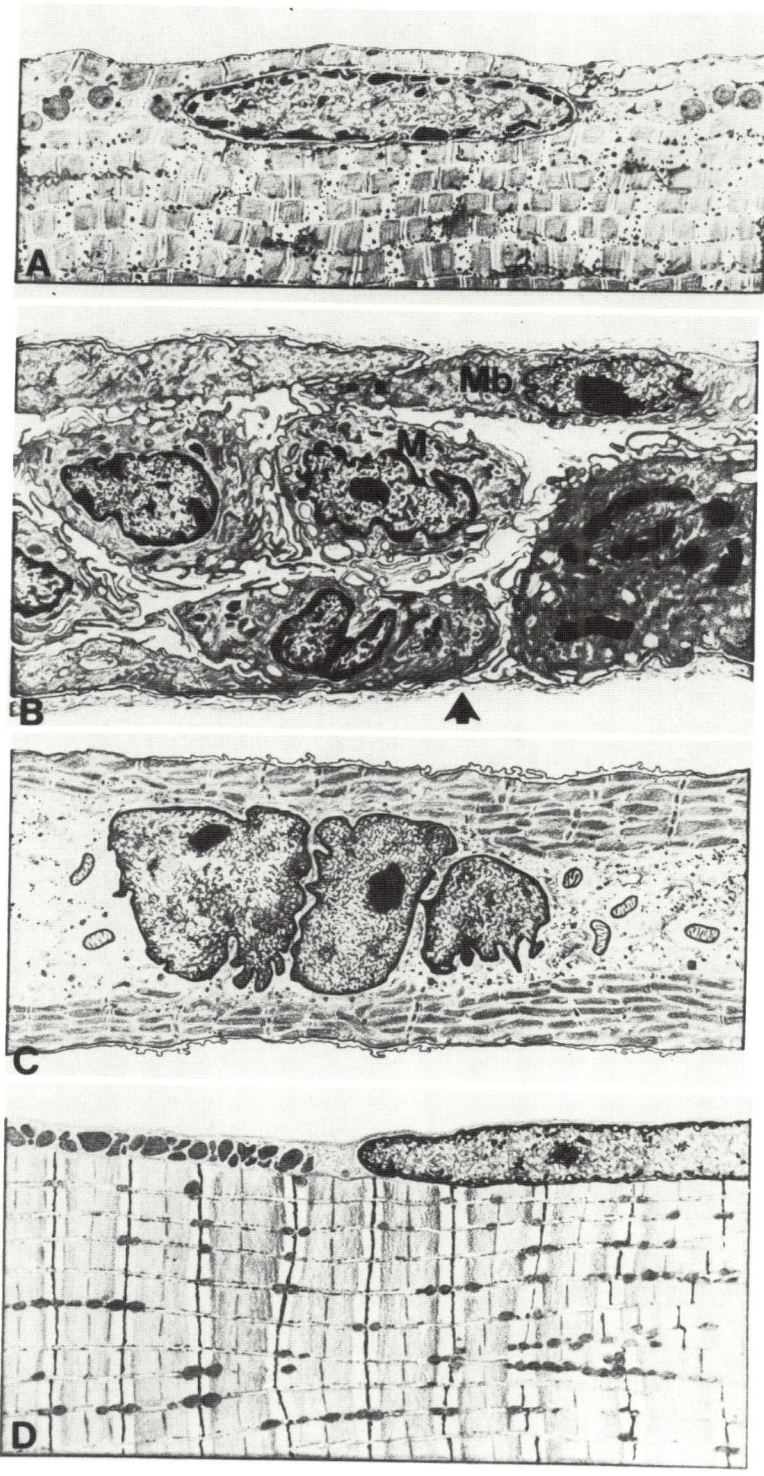

REGENERATION AND TRANSPLANTATION OF ENTIRE MUSCLES

Muscle regeneration takes place not only at the level of individual muscle fibers, but at the level of muscle as a tissue and an organ. In laboratory rodents, entire muscles can be regenerated by several experimental means. The two most commonly used methods have been mincing (Studitsky, 1959; Carlson, 1972) and the free transplantation of muscle (Studitsky, 1977; Carlson, 1978).

Minced Muscle Regeneration

An entire muscle is removed from its bed and chopped into small pieces (about 1 mm³) with scissors. Then the mince is replaced either into the bed from which the muscle was taken or into another site. In this experimental model, the mince has been completely separated from its blood supply, its nerve supply, and the proximal and distal tendon connections. Reintegration with the body of the host is of prime importance for regeneration of the muscle.

The first reintegrative process is revascularization of the mince. Within minutes after being replaced into the body, the fragments of the mince fall into a state of ischemic necrosis, and the phase of intrinsic degeneration of the muscle fibers in the fragments begins. Little further happens until a few days later, when the first vascular sprouts grow from the blood vessels of the host onto the surface of the mince. The sprouts then penetrate into the mince, much like an ingrowing root system. With vascular ingrowth, an important cellular relationship is set up. The tips of the vascular sprouts are spatially and temporally associated with large numbers of activated macrophages, which appear in both the intercellular spaces and within the damaged fragments of muscle fibers. At this point, the phase of cell-mediated degeneration begins, and shortly thereafter the activation of satellite cells is evident. As the regenerating blood vessels penetrate toward the center of the graft, three zones of cellular activity may be seen.

1. An outer zone in which muscle regeneration is well underway. This zone is well vascularized, and myotubes are closely associated with the vessels.

2. An intermediate zone in which macrophage-mediated cell fragmentation and the early activation of satellite cells are prominent. The zone represents the furthest inward penetration of new blood vessels.

3. A central zone of ischemic necrosis, where the original muscle fibers remain in a stable state of intrinsic degeneration. No blood vessels have yet penetrated into this region.

Usually within a week, in rodents, blood vessels have penetrated into the center of the mince, and muscle fiber regeneration is seen throughout the mince. During the next month, the regenerating muscle fibers undergo structural and functional maturation.

While early revascularization is taking place, the process of mechanical reintegration also begins. When they are first replaced into the muscle bed, the minced muscle fragments are chaotically arranged, without any dominant orientation. At first, starting within minutes, the muscle fragments are held in place by a meshwork of fibrin, and their overall shape is molded by mechanical pressures of the surrounding tissues. Toward the end of the first week, tenuous connections begin to form between the tendon stumps of the host and the proximal and distal ends of the mince. As the tendon connections become strengthened, they mediate the transmission of mechanical tension into the mince. The result of this process is the alignment of the formerly randomly organized myotubes into roughly parallel rows and the reconstruction of the internal architecture of the regenerating mince into a form appropriate for the mechanical environment imposed upon it.

The last major reintegrative process is reinnervation. Nerve fibers must grow into the regenerating muscle from the stumps of the nerves that were cut when the muscle was removed. The process of reinnervation is relatively lengthy, and in rats, functional neuromuscular junctions are not made until late in the third week. Details of the process of reinnervation will be provided later in this review.

Minced muscle regeneration is an excellent system for studying the overall biological possibilities of muscle regeneration, but as a model it also has certain disadvantages. One is that the size of the muscle that can be regenerated by mincing is limited. As a rule, it is best to start with no more than 1 or 2 gm of muscle. The main limitation appears to be the total cross-sectional area in relation to the speed of revascularization. Another major limitation in minced muscle regeneration in rats (to a lesser degree in mice) is the formation of large amounts of connective tissue adhesions. Mincing appears to stimulate both the proliferation of fibroblasts and the production of collagen fibers by them. From the functional standpoint, the adhesions probably limit to a considerable extent the ability of the regenerated muscles to provide useful contractions. Total contractile forces of only 15–20% of control levels are not uncommon in regenerated minced muscles.

Free Muscle Transplants

For those interested in studying the function of regenerating muscles or for clinical application, free muscle transplantation is a more suitable model. As used in this article and in the muscle regeneration literature, a free graft is a muscle that has been completely removed from its bed and then replaced into its own bed or that of another muscle with no attempt to reconnect the vascular supplies of graft and host. In the recent clinical literature, grafts that have been connected with vessels of the host by surgical anastomosis are commonly called free muscle transplants or grafts. It is important to recognize that the postoperative course of a vascular-anastomosed graft is quite different from that of a nonanastomosed free muscle graft. In this chapter, only nonanastomosed grafts will be discussed.

In most respects the dynamics of the development of a free muscle graft are remarkably similar to those of a minced muscle. The main difference is that the original architecture of the muscle is preserved in a free graft. The basic pattern of degeneration and regeneration within a free muscle graft is illustrated in Figure 1–5. One characteristic of a free muscle graft is the survival of a thin rim of original muscle fibers around the periphery of the graft. Even though the early graft is completely devascularized, apparently the diffusion of oxygen and nutrients is sufficient for these peripheral muscle fibers to survive. Despite the lack of mechanical disruption of the vascular chan-

nels within the muscle, the pattern of revascularization of a free muscle graft is almost identical to that seen in a mince. The tendon stumps of a free muscle graft are normally sutured to the corresponding stumps of the host. Therefore, functional reintegration is achieved earlier in a free graft than in a mince. A free graft differs from a mince in that the topography of the original band(s) of the motor endplates and also the capsules of the muscle spindles are not mechanically destroyed. As a rule, free muscle grafts are not characterized by the excessive production of collagen, either in the form of adhesions or as deposits within the muscle.

Development of Function in Regenerating Muscles

Regenerating muscle fibers are first capable of contraction when they are in the late myotube stage. Since the muscle fibers are not yet innervated, they respond only to direct stimulation. At first, regenerating muscle fibers contract very slowly, but their speed of contraction steadily increases up to the end of the third week, when functional reinnervation begins to occur (Carlson and Gutmann, 1972). It is only after reinnervation has occurred that the final stages of differentiation of contractile properties into those of a fast or a slow muscle occur. The overall pattern of development of contractile speeds is quite similar to that of a normal muscle during ontogenesis (Gutmann and Melichna, 1972). The total strength of contraction (tetantic tension) is usually considerably less in a regenerated muscle than in its normal counterpart (e.g., typically 35–50% in a free graft), but in at least one model of whole muscle regeneration, close to 90% of normal tetanic tension can be achieved.

MOTOR NERVE RELATIONS DURING REGENERATION

Many aspects of muscle regeneration are intimately bound to the pattern and type of reinnervation. Basically, as in normal development, the motor innervation appears to determine the final phenotype and contractile properties of the regenerating muscle fibers.

Normal Pattern of Reinnervation of a Regenerating Muscle

As mentioned previously, the earliest stages of muscle fiber regeneration within a free graft

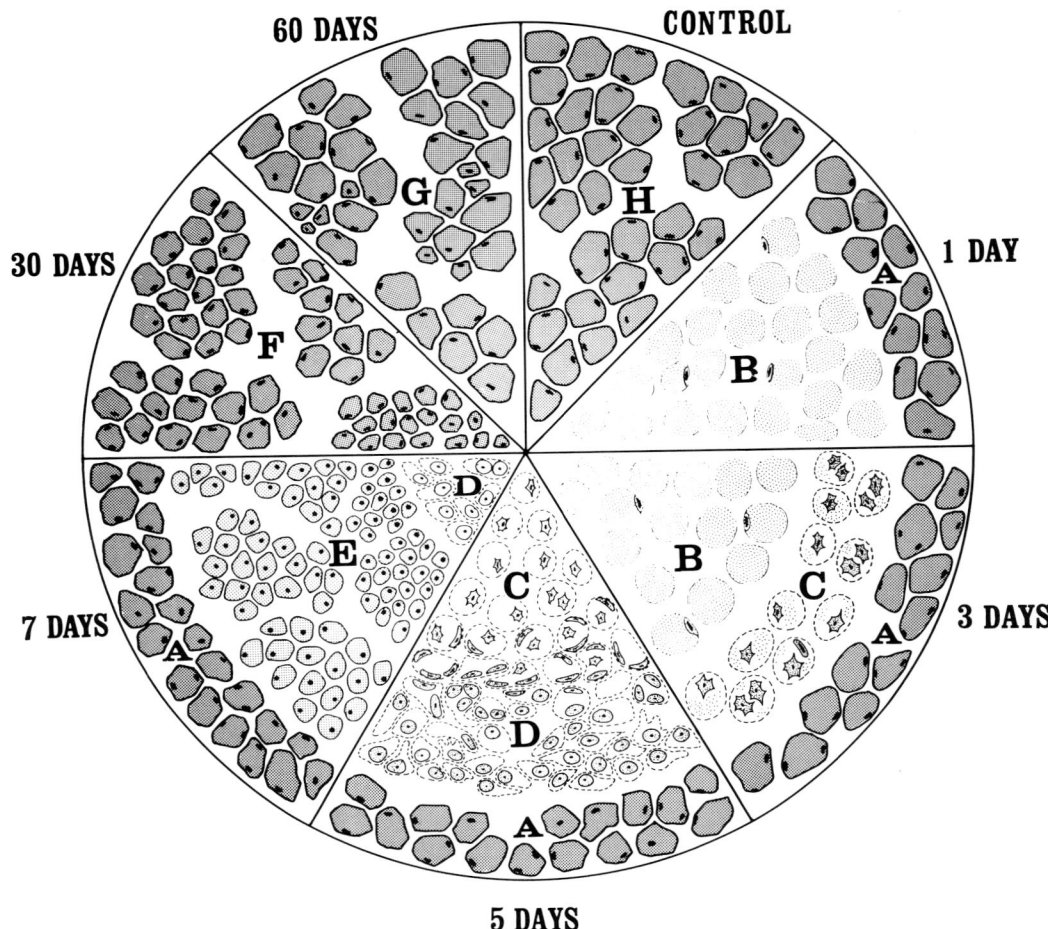

Figure 1–5. Schematic diagram showing major stages in the development of a free muscle graft. The days refer to times after grafting of extensor digitorum longus muscles in rats and cats. The diagram is divided into segments that represent the histological appearance of the grafts in cross section. The letters refer to groups of cells showing similar histological reactions. **A:** Surviving muscle fibers. **B:** Original muscle fibers in a state of ischemic necrosis. **C:** Muscle fibers invaded by macrophages, which are phagocytizing the necrotic cytoplasm. **D:** Myoblasts and early myotubes within the basal laminae of the original muscle fibers. **E:** Early cross-striated muscle fibers. **F:** Maturation of regenerating muscle fibers. **G:** Mature regenerated muscle fibers. **H:** Normal control muscle fibers. (Reproduced from Carlson et al., 1979a, with permission of the publisher.)

or a mince occur in the absence of nerve fibers. In rat muscles undergoing spontaneous reinnervation, the first regenerating nerve fibers enter the muscle early during the second week (Carlson et al., 1979b). Typically, the earliest neuromuscular contacts are tenuous connections in proximal ectopic sites, and aggrega-tions of acetylcholine receptors are associated with the earliest sites of contact (Womble, 1986). Gross contraction of the muscle after stimulation of the nerve can usually be first elicited late during the third week of regeneration in rats. In free grafts there is a tendency for the nerve terminals to move from ectopic sites to sites of previous neuromuscular junctions, but typically substantial numbers of ectopic junctions remain. The morphology of regenerated neuromuscular junctions varies considerably, with some motor endplates closely resembling those of control muscles and others showing varying degrees of abnormality on both the presynaptic and postsynaptic sides (Hansen-Smith, 1983).

A typical free muscle graft in the rat is hypoinnervated, with only about 50% of the regenerated muscle fibers having direct neural connections (Bader, 1980). Whether the myomyous junctions that have been shown to connect regenerating muscle fibers are capable of transmitting a contractile signal to noninnervated muscle fibers within a graft remains to be determined.

At the histochemical level, a normal muscle demonstrates a checkerboard pattern of staining fast vs. slow muscle fibers with reactions for myosin ATPase activity. Regenerated muscles, however, show the "type grouping" of fast vs. slow muscle fibers. This is manifest as patches of all fast or all slow muscle fibers and is a phenomenon commonly seen in reinnervated muscles, whether regenerated or not. The number of motor units in mature muscle grafts is only slightly greater than half of that found in control muscles, and the mean tetanic tension generated per motor unit is about 80% of normal (Côté and Faulkner, 1984).

Muscle Regeneration in the Absence of the Nerve

Early muscle regeneration normally takes place in the absence of direct innervation. How far muscle regeneration will proceed in the absence of nerves varies from one species to the next. For example, noninnervated muscle fibers in mice and frogs degenerate and disappear within 3 weeks, whereas in the rat the regenerating muscle fibers reach the cross-striated stage of development before undergoing a long period of atrophy. However, histochemical fast and slow muscle fiber types never appear, and the gross contractile properties of the transplant do not mature (Carlson and Gutmann, 1976).

Despite the absence of direct innervation, the postsynaptic apparatus on the regenerating muscle fiber is restored to a remarkable degree

beneath the synaptic site on the original basal lamina, a finding first demonstrated in amphibian muscle (Burden et al., 1979) and later in rat muscle (Bader, 1981; Hansen-Smith, 1986; Womble, 1986). This process is reflected in the presence of postsynaptic folds and the aggregation of acetylcholine receptors on them, which is not surprising considering that even in normal regeneration the postsynaptic apparatus takes shape before the regeneration of nerves into the muscle. It appears that the persisting basal lamina is able to direct the differentiation of the postsynaptic component of the neuromuscular junction, and currently considerable effort is being directed toward identifying the specific molecular properties of the junctional basal lamina responsible for inducing the aggregation of acetylcholine receptor molecules (Barald et al., 1987; Magill et al., 1987).

Role of Acetylcholine Receptors and the Junctional Basal Lamina in Reinnervation of Regenerating Muscle

Reports from McMahan's laboratory on neuromuscular regeneration in frogs suggested that the region of the basal lamina associated with the original motor endplate is important in determining both the site of newly regenerated neuromuscular junctions and the site and character of the postsynaptic specializations (Sanes et al., 1978; Rubin and McMahan, 1982). The latter phenomenon has already been discussed in this review.

The question of the old junctional basal lamina as a factor determining the ability of regenerating nerve terminals to settle down and form neuromuscular junctions has been examined by two types of experimentation. The first was a careful descriptive study of the normal pattern of reinnervation in free muscle grafts. The second consisted of examining the reinnervation of grafted muscles from which the original zone of motor endplates was surgically removed (motor endplate-less [MEP-less] grafts). As discussed above, Womble (1986) found that in the normal reinnervation of a free muscle graft the typical pattern was the formation of mostly ectopic neuromuscular junctions during the early stages of the reinnervation of grafts. Only at later periods did some new neuromuscular junctions form in the area of the old motor endplate zone.

It has been more difficult to interpret the results of experiments involving the reinnervation of MEP-less grafts. In an early study, Bader (1980) found numerous nerve fibers in early MEP-less grafts of the rat soleus muscle, but by 40 days only 1–2% of the muscle fibers possessed regenerated neuromuscular junctions. He concluded that nerve fibers could enter MEP-less grafts, but were unable to settle down in the absence of cues provided by the original motor endplate regions. Womble (1986), on the other hand, used the same surgical model and found large numbers (over 40%) of new motor endplates in 15 MEP-less grafts. The reason for the variation in these two studies still remains unexplained, although variations in the initial surgical procedure and the time of sampling (40 vs. 60 days) are possibilities. However, there is little doubt that in regenerating muscle new neuromuscular junctions can form in areas other than that of the original motor endplates, but the basal lamina of the old neuromuscular junction can, without the nerve itself, determine the postsynaptic characteristics of the muscle fiber.

Nerve-Intact Model of Muscle Grafting

As has already been mentioned, a muscle graft that has to rely upon spontaneous reinnervation becomes typically hypoinnervated, with only about one-half of the muscle fibers receiving direct innervation. On the more practical side, both the mass and the maximum tetanic tension produced by spontaneously reinnervated grafts are typically less than 50% of control levels. In an attempt to determine the extent to which these deficiencies are due to the process of reinnervation itself, the nerve-intact model of muscle grafting was devised (Carlson et al., 1981). In essence, this model consists of cutting the tendons and all vascular connections to a muscle, but not mechanically disrupting the motor nerve supply. Because of the limitations imposed by the length of the nerve, it is normally necessary to graft the muscle back into its own bed. Due to devascularization, the muscle fibers break down and regenerate like those of a standard free muscle graft, and the distal portions of the nerve fibers also die back as a result of the ischemic conditions. However, nerve fibers grow back into the graft much more quickly and in greater numbers than in standard grafts. Mature nerve-intact grafts in rats return to normal weights, and the tetanic tension is restored to about 90% of control value (Faulkner and Carlson, 1985). In larger animals, nerve-intact grafts, although significantly larger than spontaneously innervated grafts, are not restored to normal mass or contractile strength (Faulkner and Côté, 1986). It has been shown (Carlson et al., 1983) that the earlier return of nerve fibers to the graft was not the critical factor in determining the success of nerve-intact grafts. Rather, the critical factor seems to be the better distribution of regenerating nerve fibers throughout the graft, presumably through the channels of the original nerve fibers.

REGENERATION OF MUSCLE SPINDLES

Neuromuscular relations during muscle regeneration are not only confined to the motor component of the nervous system. Muscle spindles are important stretch receptors of skeletal muscles. Their complex structure, including several specialized intrafusal muscle fibers, an array of both sensory and motor nerve terminals, and a specialized capsule surrounding them, is determined as the result of an interaction between sensory nerve fibers and muscle fibers during the late days of embryonic development in the rat (Zelená, 1957). Muscle spindles break down and regenerate in free muscle grafts, but they do not form in minced muscle regenerates. However, regenerated muscle spindles are typically poorly differentiated (Rogers, 1982), and their function is not normal (Quick and Rogers, 1983). Despite the requirement for sensory nerve-muscle fiber interactions in the embryogenesis of muscle spindles, muscle spindles do regenerate in denervated muscles (Rogers and Carlson, 1981). Like extrafusal muscle fibers, regenerating intrafusal muscle fibers do not undergo histochemical differentiation in the absence of nerves.

MUSCULAR NEUROTIZATION

Many of the early muscle grafting models in humans relied heavily upon "muscular neurotization" as a means of getting nerve fibers into the graft (Thompson, 1974). The idea behind muscular neurotization is that a grafted or denervated muscle, placed alongside a normally innervated muscle, stimulates the sprouting of motor nerve fibers in the normally innervated "feeder" muscle and the growth of the sprouting nerve fibers into the denervated muscle (Holle, 1976). It is common clinical practice to "freshen" the feeder muscle by scraping its surface ajoining the denervated or grafted muscle. Recent research by Must (1987), however, has provided evidence that muscular neurotization is due to the regeneration of damaged nerve fibers near the surface of the feeder muscle rather than the sprouting of mechanically undamaged motor nerve fibers.

CONCLUSIONS

From the clinical standpoint, the fundamental problem in neuromuscular regeneration is how to increase the functional mass of regenerating muscle and how to decrease variability from one case to the next. The two fundamental variables that at present seem most important in determining functional mass are revascularization and reinnervation. Revascularization is the prime determinant of the initial mass of muscle that can be regenerated. With spontaneous revascularization, it is rarely possible to regenerate over 3 gm of muscle. This imposes a strong limitation on the types of muscles that can be freely grafted in humans; facial muscles or muscles of the anal or urethral sphincter are the most commonly grafted. With the advent of microvascular surgery, size of the grafted muscle is in many respects no longer a limiting factor. Because of the vascular anastomosis, the bulk of muscle fibers in an anastomosed graft survive intact, but there seems to be a price for this. Evidence from a number of different types of muscle transplants suggests that vascularized grafts tend to retain the original architecture of the grafted muscle, rather than adapting to the mechanical environment of the new site. In contrast, free muscle grafts, while showing more severe limitations on the total mass of transplantable muscle, become better adapted to the sites in which they are placed. Therefore it seems that for cases such as facial or sphincter muscles, in which delicacy of function may be more important than total strength of contraction, free muscle grafting may be the preferred procedure, whereas for cases in which overall bulk and strength are more important, vascularized grafts are more effective.

Regardless of the initial mass of muscle that is regenerated, the final functional mass depends upon the efficacy of innervation. From the experimental observations to date, it appears that the most important factor in determining the overall success of reinnervation of a regenerating muscle is the topographical distribution of the regenerating nerve fibers. To date, the best way of ensuring a good distribution of nerves is to allow the nerve fibers to grow through channels occupied by previous nerve fibers. Whether a mass of devascularized muscle is allowed to become revascularized spontaneously, or whether a blood supply is provided immediately through vascular anastomosis, reinnervation is probably facilitated best by neural anastomosis between graft and host. In the clinical treatment of facial paralysis, where denervation is the initial cause of a neuromuscular deficit, nerve fibers are allowed to regenerate from the healthy side of the face to the denervated side of the face through grafts of segments of sensory nerves (Freilinger, 1975). When the nerve fibers have regenerated across the face to the denervated side, then a muscle graft is put in place. Such a two step procedure reduces the delay between the regeneration of muscle fibers and their innervation.

How well regenerated muscles can function in the absence of a fully functional proprioceptive apparatus also remains to be seen. The problem of directing regenerating sensory nerve fibers to muscle spindles would appear to be considerably more difficult than that of restoring the motor innervation. The restoration of functional Golgi tendon organs, the other major sensory receptors of muscle, has received minimal attention. Other problems, such as the influence of age on the efficiency of reinnervation have received scant attention.

At the level of the individual muscle fiber, much yet remains to be learned about the molecular nature of the influences of the endplate basal lamina on the process of reinnervation and the response of the muscle fiber to it. It is important to know if there are several available ways for nerve fibers to interact with and form connections regenerating muscle fibers.

ACKNOWLEDGMENTS

Original research cited in this review was supported by NIH grants PO1 DE 07687 and EY 05813.

REFERENCES

Bader D (1980): Reinnervation of motor end-plate-containing and motor endplate-less muscle grafts. Dev Biol 77:315–327.

Bader D (1981): Density and distribution of alpha-bungarotoxin-binding sites in postsynaptic structures of regenerated and skeletal muscle. J Cell Biol 88:338–345.

Barald KF, Phillips, GD, Jay JC, Mizukami IF (1987): A component of mammalian muscle synaptic basal lamina induces clustering of acetylcholine receptors. In Seil FJ, Herbert E, Carlson BM (eds): "Neural Regeneration Progress in Brain Research" vol 71. Amsterdam: Elsevier, pp 397–408.

Bischoff R (1986): A satellite cell mitogen from crushed adult muscle. Dev Biol 115:140–147.

Burden SJ, Marshall LM, McMahan UJ (1979): Acetylcholine receptors in regenerating muscle accumulate at original synaptic sites in the absence of the nerve. J Cell Biol 82:412–425.

Carlson BM (1972): The regeneration of minced muscles. In: "Monographs in Developmental Biology." Basel: S. Karger Ag.

Carlson BM (1978): A review of muscle transplantation in mammals. Physiol Bohemoslov 27:387–400.

Carlson BM (1981): "Patten's Foundations of Embryology," 4th Ed. New York: McGraw-Hill.

Carlson BM, Gutmann E (1972): Development of contractile properties of minced muscle regenerates in rats. Exp Neurol 36:239–249.

Carlson BM, Gutmann E (1976): Contractile and histochemical properties of sliced muscle grafts regenerating in normal and denervated rat limbs. Exp Neurol 50:319–329.

Carlson BM, Faulkner JA (1983): The regeneration of skeletal muscle fibers following injury. Med Sci Sports Exerc 15:187–198.

Carlson BM, Hansen-Smith FM, Magon DK (1979a): The life history of a free muscle graft. In Mauro A (ed): "Muscle Regeneration." New York: Raven Press, pp 393–407.

Carlson BM, Wagner KR, Max SR (1979b): Reinnervation of rat extensor digitorum longus muscles after free grafting. Muscle Nerve 2:304–307.

Carlson BM, Hník P, Tuček S, Vejsada R, Bader DM, Faulkner JA (1981): Comparison between grafts with intact nerves and standard free grafts of the rat extensor digitorum longus muscle. Physiol Bohemoslov 30:505–513.

Carlson BM, Foster AH, Bader DM, Hník P, Vejsada R (1983): Restoration of full mass nerve-intact muscle grafts after delayed reinnervation. Experientia 39:171–172.

Faulkner JA, Carlson BM (1985): Contractile properties of standard and nerve-intact muscle grafts in the rat. Muscle Nerve 8:413–418.

Foster AF, Carlson BM (1980): Myotoxicity of local anesthetics and regeneration of the damaged muscle fibers. Anesth Analg 58:727–736.

Freilinger G (1975): A new technique to correct facial paralysis. Plastic Reconstr Surg 56:44–48.

Gutmann E, Melichna J (1972): Contractile properties of different skeletal muscles of the rat during development. Physiol Bohemoslov 21:1–8.

Hansen-Smith FM (1983): Development and innervation of soleplates in the freely grafted extensor digitorum longus (EDL) muscle in the rat. Anat Rec 207:55–67.

Hansen-Smith FM (1986): Formation of acetylcholine receptor clusters in mammalian sternohyoid muscle regenerating in the absence of nerves. Dev Biol 118:129–140.

Holle J (1976): Die musculäre Neurotisation in der rekonstruktiven Chirurgie. Wien Klin Wochenschr [Suppl] 88:1–21.

Magill C, Reist NE, Fallon JR, Nitkin RM, Wallace BG, McMahan UJ (1987): Agrin. In Seil FJ, Herbert E, Carlson BM (ed): "Neural Regeneration Progress in Brain Research," vol 71. Amsterdam: Elsevier, pp 391–396.

Must R (1987): Experimental investigation of muscular neurotization in the rat. Muscle Nerve 10:530–536.

Quick DC, Rogers SL (1983): Stretch receptors in regenerated rat muscle. Neuroscience 10:851–859.

Rogers SL (1982): Muscle spindle formation and differentiation in regenerating rat muscle grafts. Dev Biol 94:265–283.

Rogers SL, Carlson BM (1981): A quantitative assessment of muscle spindle formation in reinnervated and non-reinnervated grafts of the rat extensor digitorum longus muscle. Neuroscience 6:87–94.

Rubin LL, McMahan UJ (1982): Regeneration of the neuromuscular junction: Steps toward defining the molecular basis of the interaction between nerve and muscle. In Schotland DL (ed): "Disorders of the Motor Unit." New York: J. Wiley, pp 187–196.

Sanes JR, Marshall LM, McMahan UJ (1978): Reinnervation of muscle fiber basal lamina after removal of muscle fibers. J Cell Biol 78:176–198.

Snow MH (1977): Myogenic cell formation in regenerating rat skeletal muscle injured by mincing. II. An autoradiographic study. Anat Rec 188:200–218.

Studitsky AN (1959): "The Experimental Surgery of Muscle" (in Russian). Moscow: Izdatel Akad Nauk, SSSR.

Studitsky AN (1977): "Transplantation of Muscles in Animals" (in Russian). Moscow: Meditsina.

Thompson N (1974): A review of autogenous skeletal muscle grafts and their clinical applications. Clin Plast Surg 1:349–403.

Womble MD (1986): The clustering of acetylcholine receptors and formation of neuromuscular junctions in regenerating mammalian muscle grafts. Am J Anat 176:191–205.

Zelená J (1957): The morphogenetic influence of innervation on the ontogenetic development of muscle-spindles. J Embryol Exp Morphol 5:283–292.

2

Status of Peripheral Nerve Regeneration

BETTY G. UZMAN, MD, D. STEPHEN SNYDER, PhD, AND GLORIA M. VILLEGAS, MD, PhD

V. A. Medical Center and Departments of Pathology and Neurology, University of Tennessee-Memphis, Memphis, Tennessee 38104, and the Instituto Internacional de Estudios Avanzados, Caracas, Venezuela

Ramón y Cajal's early descriptions (1905, 1913) of successful and thwarted regeneration of peripheral nerve fibers in animals have formed the base for all subsequent studies. During each of two World Wars, the numerous opportunities to study (and attempt repairs of) peripheral nerve injuries and traumatic nerve defects gave impetus to experiment. The importance of detailed anatomic, histologic, and physiologic knowledge of experimental systems was heightened when analogous structures and the same progression of events were found in patients. Any encouraging experimental manipulation of the wounded nerve or its environment met immediate clinical application and testing. Still, not all regenerating nerves reached their proper targets, and scarring at the injury site was often uncontrollable. The resulting functional disabilities, especially after injury or loss of long nerve segments, still occur in patients today.

Since the time of Ramón y Cajal's early work, the phenomena of nerve injury and regeneration have been studied in experimental animals and in tissue cultures; young, old, and embryonic tissues have been used; new stains and higher resolution electron microscopes have allowed refinements of Ramón y Cajal's descriptions; and clinical research and application have employed every promising avenue—microsurgery, antibiotics, protective envelopment of approximated nerve ends, funicular (fascicular) repair, guidance of outgrowing fibers, and replacement of large deficits with grafts. Today, major efforts stem from the opportunities to reexplore each facet of peripheral nervous system (PNS) regeneration with the penetrating tools of molecular biology and molecular genetics. To seek clarification of the histologic changes in regenerating nerves, it is no longer sufficient to determine whether or not the amounts of categorical components such as nucleoproteins, proteins, lipids, or carbohydrate-containing compounds are affected at specified times after nerve injury; it is now possible and necessary to demonstrate how changes are related to altered gene expression, to seek ways of modulating or controlling such alterations, and to locate the products of such genes in temporal and spatial relation to the degenerative/regenerative events.

The outcome of studies directed toward molecular controls and interactions in regeneration of the PNS is expected to have wider implications by specifying opportunities for effective encouragement of central nervous system (CNS) regeneration. This hope has come from the laboratories of Aguayo and Bray (Aguayo et al., 1981, 1985; David and Aguayo, 1981; Aguayo and Bray, 1984; Bray and Aguayo, Chapter 5, this volume), where rodent peripheral nerve autografts have proved to be favorable conduits for spinal cord and optic nerve regeneration, with long conducting trajectories accomplished and synapses on central targets established.

This status report emphasizes examples of current research in which the tools of molecular biology and genetics significantly deepen understanding of the events in PNS degeneration and regeneration. Changes in the neuron, i.e., the nerve cell body, underlie the successive stages of sprouting, outgrowth, and maturation of the regenerating axon. Such changes, as well as each of these stages, are subjects of

Neural Regeneration and Transplantation, pages 15–28

intense experimental scrutiny today, and directions of significant progress can now be ascertained. However, appropriate functional reinnervation of a distal stump by regenerated axons that reconnect with their original targets remains an elusive goal. Recent experiments in rodents indicating some progress will be described (de Medinaceli et al., 1982, 1983a,b, 1984; de Medinaceli and Freed, 1983; de Medinaceli and Church, 1984). For more extensive discussion of clinical problems arising from nerve injuries, Lundborg (1987) in a recent review considers techniques of nerve repair in light of current experimental studies.

HISTORICAL PERSPECTIVE

Waller (1850) gave the first detailed account of peripheral nerve degeneration following separation of the axon from its trophic center, the body of the neuron. In Waller's account, a succession of changes occurs in the severed nerve fiber. Beginning the second day, retraction of myelin and widening of Schmidt-Lantermann clefts are followed by fragmentation of myelin, and later of axons. Successive changes in Schwann cells are initiated early, with nuclear thickening, mitotic divisions, and increase in cytoplasm. By 15 days after transection, axons are no longer seen, and within the endoneurium solid, granular, or vacuolated Schwann cell bands (of Büngner) with occasional leucocytes appear. By one month, the "bands" wither and Schwann cell nuclei diminish and are located peripherally, leaving a central "channel" to receive new nerves. In his original description, Waller also noted degenerative changes in the central stump (retrograde degeneration) that did not involve its entire trajectory and that were attributed to trauma or inflammation. From enlargements of the preterminal portion of central axon stumps, fine unmyelinated regenerating fibers directed themselves toward the distal stump and could be found within this stump in 12–28 days. These early observations are still a valid summary of the events that have become embellished for a century with more details of timing and cellular substructure in a variety of species.

Ramón y Cajal (1905, 1913) studied degeneration and regeneration to strengthen his monogenic hypothesis that nerves originate only from the body of the neuron, and not from a reticulum in the degenerated nerve stump. He concluded that regeneration proceeded by the sprouting of numerous branches from each central axon stump within a few days. Only after 3–4 days did new axon sprouts appear to become associated with Schwann cells. (Hence the sprouts could not arise from them.) New sprouts followed a tortuous path. If they formed a large encapsulated tangled mass at the terminus of the central stump (neuroma), they did not reinnervate the distal stump. After 10–12 days, a few "nonlost" fibers, some ramified into several branches, reached the distal stump, where they invaded the "bands of Büngner," pushed away myelin debris, and grew distally.

Sunderland (1978), in a massive compilation on nerves and nerve injuries, has provided an overview and details of the phenomenological studies of peripheral nerve regeneration and evaluated many therapeutic maneuvers stemming from their findings. He defined five degrees of nerve injury, in order of increasing severity: 1) conduction block; 2) transection of the axon, leaving the endoneurium and all other outer layers intact; 3) transection of nerve fiber(s) inside an intact perineurium; 4) transection of one or more of the nerve funiculi within an unlesioned surrounding epineurium; and 5) transection of the entire nerve (see Fig. 2–1). Recovery of function is dependent on restoration of structure, and hence is directly related to these anatomically defined degrees of injury.

NEURONAL CHANGES AFTER AXON INJURY

As summarized by Sunderland (1978), the chromatolysis or loss of Nissl body staining in the neuronal cytoplasm begins as early as 6 hr after axon section; at the electron microscope level it is seen as a loss of endoplasmic reticulum (membrane enclosed cisternae in the cytoplasm) with liberation of associated ribonucleoprotein particles (ribosomes, the sites of protein synthesis in the cell). Also evident very early are decreases in the cytoskeletal elements—actin, microtubules (neurotubules), and intermediate size filaments (neurofilaments)—of the neuron cell body and later of the axon.

Regeneration requires synthesis of new pro-

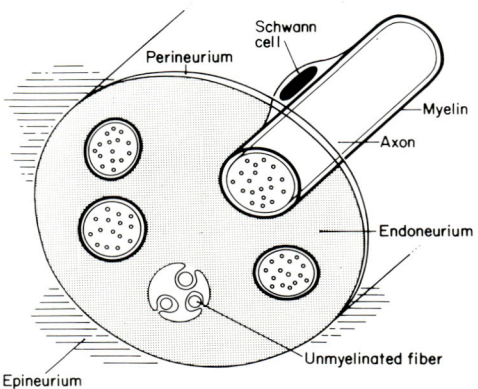

Figure 2–1. Diagram of a peripheral nerve funiculus (fasciculus) showing four myelinated axons and a group of three unmyelinated axons within the supporting connective tissue framework, the endoneurium. The funiculus is surrounded by a cellular and collagenous sheath, the perineurium. A small nerve may consist of only a single funiculus, but a large nerve or nerve trunk contains multiple funiculi held together by layers of connective tissue, the epineurium.

teins by the neuron cell body or "factory" for transport down the axon and assembly at the regenerating tip or "construction site." Parts of the genetic material, DNA, in the neuronal nucleus must be selectively opened up and *transcribed* into smaller molecules of coded messenger RNA (mRNA) that go from the nucleus to the cytoplasm, where they link up with ribosomes. Here, each amino acid, specified by *translation* of a sequence of three nucleic acid units (nucleotide triplet codon) in the mRNA, is selected from the amino acids in the cytoplasm by a complementary anticodon on transfer RNA. This tRNA can bind to ribosomes and covalently to one end (the carboxyl-terminal) of a forming protein molecule to add the next amino acid. This process can be studied in cultures or in vivo by the binding of radioactive labeled compounds. Bound labeled complementary nucleoprotein sequences (cDNA or cRNA) locate "opened up" or actively transcribing DNA (gene) or RNA sequences; labeled amino acids, by their incorporation, tag proteins being synthesized.

It has been shown that Nissl bodies do not

reform completely if the regenerating axon cannot progress beyond the site of injury to its target organ, but after "reversible axotomy" (second degree crush injury), full reconstitution of the Nissl body stacks of ribosome studded lamellar endoplasmic reticulum is found (Sears, 1987). These same workers have evidence of a signal(s) from the target (in this case, muscle) that appears to be responsible and necessary for the synthesis of Nissl substance, that is, the endoplasmic reticulum with its ribosome binding proteins and associated messenger RNAs, and its stabilizing cytoskeletal elements.

Bisby et al. (1988) found that as early as 12 hr after rat facial nerve section, an embryonic-type messenger RNA for tubulin $\delta 1$ (microtubule protein) is reinduced in neurons, rather than glia; that axotomy increases, or upregulates, the synthesis of actin and tubulin and simultaneously decreases, or downregulates, neurofilament synthesis. After a second injury closely following the first, or "conditioning," lesion, the rate of regeneration of a new axon can accelerate without greater actin or tubulin synthesis but with a further decrease in neurofilament synthesis. Presumably the new tubulin building blocks can be transported along the axon to the "construction site" (injury site) faster when reassembly of new filaments is slowed and they are less dense.

Although most axonal proteins are synthesized in the neuronal soma, with its Nissl substance providing the ribosomal machinery, Zanakis et al. (1984), as well as others, have provided evidence that tRNAs are transported along the axon, where they modify proteins originally synthesized in the cell body; this activity is increased 15–150 times in segments of rat sciatic nerve regenerating after crush. Synthetic activity also occurs at a great distance from the cell body. Tedeschi and Wilson (1983) have demonstrated modification (labeled methionine incorporation) of a rapidly transported axon protein after its arrival at the regenerating axon tip, from which it was then transported in a retrograde fashion.

Accelerated regeneration is observed following a second nerve injury inflicted 2 weeks or less after the first, which has therefore been termed a "conditioning" lesion (McQuarrie and Grafstein, 1973). The above evidence that altered gene expression and initiation of protein synthesis begins only hours after nerve transection to provide building blocks for neurite reconstruction means that a second injury one or two weeks later is inflicted on an already regenerating nerve.

FACTORS THAT PROMOTE NEURAL GROWTH AND ADHESION

Earlier in this century Ramón y Cajal (1905, 1913) suggested that distal degenerating stumps provided a diffusible substance responsible for attracting outgrowing axons and that Schwann cell multiplication in the distal stump is aimed at the secretion of stimulating substances that attract and guide wandering axons from the scar toward their motor and sensory endings. He used the terms "chemotropism" and "neurotropism" for this favorable influence of the distal stump on axon outgrowth from the proximal stump. Such *tropic factors* can be said to attract nerve fibers. To be distinguished are *trophic factors*, which are concerned with cell maintenance and general growth; neuronotrophic factors promote the survival and differentiation of neurons. The sprouting of axons is encouraged by *neuritogenic factors;* some affect metabolic events or cytoskeletal scaffolding at the cell surface. Some neuronotrophic factors, such as nerve growth factor, are also neuritogenic. *Cell adhesion molecules* (CAMs) exist on the surface of cells. Most are glycoproteins and have carbohydrate antigenic determinants (epitopes) for which specific monoclonal antibodies are available. When labeled, these antibodies can be used to determine the presence and distribution of CAMs. Substrates on which axons or axon-Schwann cell units prefer to grow can be demonstrated by selective outgrowth in cultures, and, with the use of labeled antibodies, the pathways formed by these *substrate adherence molecules* (SAMs) can be traced in experimental animals.

All of these factors and molecules are currently under intense scrutiny (see also Varon et al., Chapter 7, this volume). Relevant to each factor are complementary cDNAs, amino acid sequences, presence or absence of antigenic carbohydrates on proteins, migration patterns and distributions of proteins on two-dimensional polyacrylamide gel electrophoresis (PAGE), with estimation of molecular weight (M_r), and more specific identification by immunoblotting. Many of these characteristics change and may be compared during development, at maturity, and in degenerating and regenerating nerve segments. Not all such factors are proteins—gangliosides can exert both neuronotrophic and neuritogenic effects (Ledeen, 1984). The following examples relate to areas currently of particular interest.

Tropic Factors

Seldom quoted but antedating Ramón y Cajal's hypothesis of chemotropism is the work of Forssman (1898), in which he describes the tendency of regenerating nerves to grow toward distal stumps even if misplaced. Straw tubes and chambers were used as conduits for regenerating nerves. Negating tropism from his own large body of experimental evidence, Weiss (1941) espoused random axonal outgrowth and mechanical guidance of axons by submicroscopic linear aggregates of fibrin or by pre-existing fibers. The effect of the distal stump was to offer conditions for maturation to the subset of randomly regenerating neurites that came its way.

In large part due to carefully executed experiments in Peter Spencer's laboratory, the evidence for distal stump tropic activity is now unequivocal. Politis et al. (1982) used Y-shaped silastic tubes with alternative "lures" placed in the Y-branches opposite an inserted rat sciatic proximal stump. Distal stumps of rat sciatic nerve and extracts therefrom, and even degenerating optic nerves (Politis, 1985b), were preferred lures, compared with a number of other tissues and extracts; the activity in the distal stump was shown to be diffusible (Politis and Spencer, 1983). The specificity of tropic activity has been similarly demonstrated with motor nerve outgrowth favoring motor over sensory distal stumps (Brushart and Seiler, 1987), and tibial nerve axons favoring tibial over peroneal distal stumps (Politis et al., 1982; Politis, 1985a).

Trophic Factors

The trophic factors that appear to have a direct effect on nerve regeneration are: nerve growth factor (NGF); glial growth factor (GGF); glia derived neurite promoting factor (GdNPF);

basic fibroblast growth factor (bFGF); and ciliary neuronotrophic factor (CNTF).

Best characterized and of demonstrated physiologic importance is NGF, a molecular complex with alpha, beta, and gamma subunits, two each. The beta-NGF dimer has the activity needed for the survival and development of sympathetic and some (neural crest derived) sensory neurons (Levi-Montalcini, 1987). It is a paracrine ligand, i.e., it is bound to the surface of one cell and acts on a neighboring cell, but does not enter the circulation. After synthesis by a target cell, NGF binds to the nerve terminal at NGF-specific receptors (NGF^{rec}), is internalized, and then reaches the neuron cell body by retrograde transport.

The activity of NGF in the neuron soma has been studied in cultures of rat pheochromocytoma (PC) cells (Greene and Tischler, 1976) derived from adrenal medullary cells of neural crest origin. In this PC-12 cell system, NGF promotes the following: differentiation and neurite outgrowth (Greene and Tischler, 1976); induction of enzymes involved in neurotransmitter synthesis (Honneger and Lenoir, 1982); synthesis of a neuron-specific protein kinase substrate B50, also called F1 or growth-associated protein (GAP)-43 (Snipes et al., 1987a,b; van Hooff et al., 1986); induction of cell adhesion molecules (McGuire et al., 1978; Friedlander et al., 1986) synthesis and phosphorylation of neurofilament proteins (Lindenbaum et al., 1987); and expression of the c-fos oncogene (Curran and Morgan, 1985).

In animals, NGF-responsive cells include: autonomic ganglion neurons and satellite cells (Levi-Montalcini and Angeletti, 1968); neural crest-derived cells of sensory ganglia (Levi-Montalcini and Angeletti, 1963; Johnson et al., 1980); PNS Schwann cells by re-expression of NGF^{rec} (Heumann et al., 1987b); and in the CNS the cholinergic neurons of basal forebrain nuclei and magnocellular neurons in the nucleus basalis region (Korsching et al., 1985; Whittemore et al., 1986). NGF detected by immunoreactivity is widespread in embryonic mouse CNS (Finn et al., 1987).

That NGF exerts both sustaining trophic metabolic influences and guiding tropic effects in vivo and in vitro has been amply documented (Thoenen and Barde, 1980; Varon and Adler, 1980; Levi-Montalcini, 1987; Sandrock and Matthew, 1987). Apparently contradictory evidence is contained in reports that fibers from sensory ganglia are not attracted to cutaneous targets by NGF (Davies et al., 1987), and that immunoreactive NGF in denervated iris is detected in Schwann cells, but not in the target smooth muscle cells (Finn et al., 1986).

NGF receptors have been directly studied in sensory ganglia (Buck et al., 1987), developing peripheral nerve (Heumann, et al., 1987b), Schwann cells during regeneration (Taniuchi et al., 1986a, 1988), Schwann cells in culture (Zimmerman and Sutter, 1983; Rohrer, 1985; DiStefano and Johnson, 1988), CNS cholinergic neurons (Taniuchi et al., 1986b), and PC12 cells (Landreth and Shooter, 1980). Two types of cell surface NGF^{rec} molecules are recognized: type I, a high-affinity (10^{-11} M), slow dissociating form, and type II, a low-affinity (10^{-9} M), fast dissociating form (Buxser et al., 1985). Schwann cells have low-affinity type II receptors, PC12 cells have both types, and cultured neonatal rat brain astrocytes have neither (DiStefano and Johnson, 1988). NGF^{rec} immunoprecipitated from Schwann cells yields two polypeptides of M_r 95 and 220 kD (kiloDalton), and slightly smaller components from PC12 cells (DiStefano and Johnson, 1988).

NGF mRNA has been demonstrated in epithelial and smooth muscle target cells of sensory/sympathetic fibers, as well as in their Schwann cells and fibroblasts (Bandtlow et al., 1987). All Schwann cells in newborn rat sciatic nerve express NGF (Bandtlow et al., 1987). Schwann cells neither internalize NGF (DiStefano and Johnson, 1988) nor have detectable responses to NGF (Green et al., 1985). After transection, Schwann cells re-express NGF^{rec} (Heumann et al., 1987b). In sensory neurons, NGF functions as a target-controlled neuronotrophic factor without neuritogenic effect (Davies et al., 1987).

The regulation of mRNAs encoding NGF and NGF^{rec} proteins has been examined in developing and regenerating rat sciatic nerve. Both ligand and receptor mRNAs are downregulated (decreased) during development (Heumann et al., 1987b), with the NGF^{rec} mRNA decreasing steadily through 21 postnatal days and the mRNA for NGF declining during the second postnatal week. By contrast, the NGF mRNA in rat forebrain remains upregulated at least until

13 weeks of age (Buck et al., 1987). After transection (without regeneration) and after crush injury (with regeneration), Heumann et al. (1987a) found upregulated mRNA levels for both NGF and NGF^{rec} in the distal nerve segment. However, the elevated levels in crushed nerve were not maintained; as regenerating axons entered the distal segments, both NGF and NGF^{rec} mRNAs were downregulated. Further analysis of distal segments located mRNAs for NGF and NGF^{rec} in Schwann cells and endoneurial fibroblasts associated with axons of both sensory and motor neurones (Heumann et al., 1987a; Raivich and Kreutzberg, 1987).

The other trophic factors have received less attention. GGF, found in bovine pituitary and brain by Brockes et al. (1980), is a mitogen for Schwann cells, astrocytes, and muscle fibroblasts, but not oligodendroglia. It has been used with cholera toxin or forskolin to amplify the Schwann cell population in primary cultures (Porter et al., 1986). GdNPF, found by Monard et al. (1973) in serum-free C6 glioma cell-conditioned media, induces neurite outgrowth in cultured neuroblastoma cells (Monard et al., 1973; Guenther et al., 1985), is a potent inhibitor of serine proteases (Monard et al., 1973; Stone et al., 1987), is thought to affect migratory movements of the growth cone, since the purified factor inhibits cerebellar neuroblast migration (Lindner et al., 1986; Monard, 1987), and has an aminoterminal sequence similarity to protease-nexin I, thus perhaps allying it with this family of inhibitors (Gloor et al., 1986). Basic FGF, found in bovine pituitary by Gospodarowicz (1974, 1978), promotes neurite outgrowth and survival of rat cortical neurons (Morrison et al., 1986) and survival of chick ciliary ganglion neurons (Unsicker et al., 1987); it is closely related to astroglial growth factor 2, which enhances choline acetyltransferase activity (Unsicker et al., 1987). CNTF, found in chick embryo intraocular tissues and rat PNS nerves and spinal roots (Barbin et al., 1984; Williams et al., 1984), is required for the maintenance of cultured ciliary ganglion neurons and supports the survival of embryonic chick and rodent sensory and sympathetic ganglia neurons (Barbin et al., 1984; Unsicker et al., 1987). Additional trophic factors are discussed in recent reviews (Dekker et al., 1987; Lundborg, 1987).

Cell Adhesion Molecules (CAMs)

These cell surface molecules, usually glycoproteins, function by binding to other such molecules of the same (homotypic) or similar (heterotypic) type, thereby influencing cell aggregation, tissue pattern formation, and histogenesis in general. In the PNS they have a role in neurite outgrowth and fasciculation, and in pattern development. Five of the six major types of CAMs (Table 2.1) appear to be closely related, based on their distribution, similar molecular weights, and the cross reactivity of monoclonal and polyclonal antibodies prepared to representative examples of each type. Three CAMs (N-CAM; myelin-associated glycoprotein (MAG); and P$_o$, a PNS myelin protein) are coded by genes that structurally resemble the immunoglobulin gene superfamily (Lemke and Axel, 1985; Williams et al., 1985; Cunningham et al., 1987; Salzer et al., 1987).

CAMs are identified by surface carbohydrate antigenic loci called epitopes, some of which are shared by several CAMs, and by surface markers on lymphocytes. The lymphocyte marker HNK-1 of human natural killer cells (Abo and Balch, 1981), also termed Leu-7, is a sulfated glucuronyl glycolipid epitope (Chou et al., 1986) equivalent to the CAM epitope, L2 (Chou et al., 1985). Its presence on a molecule implies its role in adhesion (Kruse et al., 1984); HNK-1 can be detected on a large subset of CAMs, as shown in Table 2.2. The presence of a different epitope, L3, on the CAM, AMOG (adhesion molecule on glia), together with the absence of HNK-1/L2 reactivity, suggests that other HNK-1/L2 negative adhesion molecules may be identified.

The role of CAMs in morphogenesis of defined structures has been examined using antibodies, or active Fab fragments, to specific CAMS. Fab fragments of anti-L1, anti-N-CAM, and anti-NILE affect external granular cell migration and, in vitro, the extent of axon fasciculation (Fischer et al., 1986, Lindner et al., 1986). The latter action could be evoked only if tissues were explanted at particular developmental stages (Stallcup and Beasley, 1985), suggesting developmental regulation of these CAMs. Antibodies to CAMs variably affect neurite elongation, depending on the substrate

TABLE 2.1. Nervous System Cell Adhesion Molecules*

	Cell adhesion Molecules	M_r (kD)	Association	Reference no.
I.	N-CAM (chicken)	120, 140, 180	My/unmy axons, muscle	(1)
II.	Cognin (chicken)	50	Cell-cell aggregation in retina	(2)
III.	N-cadherin (chicken)	127	Separation/sealing in morphogenesis	(3)
IV.	NILE (rat)	140, 180, >200	Migratory granule cells; N-N contact	(4)
	L1 (mouse)	140, 180, >200	Migratory granule cells; N-N contact	(5)
	Ng-CAM (chicken)	80, 135, 200	My/unmy axons; N-N and N-G contact	(6)
	G4/F11 (chicken)	135	Neurite fasciculation	(7)
	8D9 (chicken)	85, 135, >200	Neurite fasciculation	(8)
	J1 (mouse)	160, 200, 220	Neurite/astrocyte adhesion	(9)
	MAG/1B236 (rat)	100	Maintains periaxonal spacing	(10)
V.	AMOG: L3 epitope (mouse)	45–50	Granule cell migration; macroglia loci	(11)
	P_o (rat)	28–30	Myelin lamellae compaction	(12)
VI.	Chondroitin sulfate proteoglycan[a] or CTBP (chicken)	280 (core)	Neuron surface and extracellular matrix cytotactin binding; nodes of Ranvier	(13)

*CAM, cell adhesion molecule; NILE, nerve growth factor—inducible large external glycoprotein; MAG, myelin associated glycoprotein; my, myelinated; unmy, unmyelinated; CTBP, cytotactin binding proteoglycan; AMOG, adhesion molecule on glia; L1, G4, F11, 8D9, J1, and 1B236 are the laboratory designations for specific epitopes; M_r, molecular weight.
[a]Provisional inclusion as a CAM.

References: (1) Hoffman et al., 1982; (2) Hausman and Moscona, 1975; Schubert et al., 1983; (3) Takeichi et al., 1985; (4) McGuire et al., 1978, Bock et al., 1985, Sajovic et al., 1986; (5) Faissner et al., 1984, Fischer et al., 1986; (6) Grumet et al., 1984; (7) Rathjen et al., 1987; (8) Lagenaur and Lemmon, 1987; (9) Kruse et al., 1985; (10) Quarles et al., 1972, Salzer et al., 1987, Lai et al., 1987; (11) Antonicek et al., 1987, Kücherer et al., 1987; (12) Greenfield et al., 1973, Bollensen and Schachner, 1987; (13) Hoffman and Edelman, 1987; Hoffman et al., 1988.

and the particular CAM (Chang et al., 1987; Lagenaur and Lemmon, 1987).

Regenerating mouse and chick nerves exhibited transient elevations of N-CAM and Ng-CAM 10 days after crush or transection; by 50–150 days, only slight elevations of both CAMs were found (Daniloff et al., 1986). In regenerating nerves, labeled antibodies stained both N-CAM and Ng-CAM in Schwann cells; however, only N-CAM was demonstrated in unmyelinated fibers and connective tissue elements (Daniloff et al., 1986). L1, as well as N-CAM, is re-expressed by Schwann cells after axotomy of adult mouse sciatic nerve (Nieke and Schachner, 1985; Martini and Schachner, 1986). Immunoblots of nerve homogenates

TABLE 2.2. Immunologic Cross-reactivity of CAMs

Cell adhesion molecules	CAM mAb epitopes L2/HNK-1	L3[a]
N-CAM	+	−
CTBP	+ (HNK-1)	ND
Ng-CAM	+	ND
NILE:L1	+	+
G4/F11/8D9	+	ND
J1	+	−
MAG	+	+
AMOG	−	+
P_o	+	+

[a]ND, not determined.

also demonstrated elevations of N-CAM and Ng-CAM 50–60 days after crush or transection, with N-CAM present in polydispersed high molecular weight embryonic form (Daniloff et al., 1986). The hypothesis that reinnervation regulates N-CAM and L1 (or Ng-CAM) expression by Schwann cells is suggested by these studies.

In vitro, growth factors have been shown to regulate Schwann cell expression of CAMs (Seilheimer and Schachner, 1987). Upregulation of L1 by NGF could be abolished by anti-NGF antibodies. GdNPF simultaneously upregulated L1 expression and downregulated surface N-CAM. J1, produced by CNS macroglia and associated with neuron-astrocyte adhesion (Kruse et al., 1985), is also present on Schwann cells in polydispersed 160–220kD forms but is unaffected by either NGF or GdNPF.

Substrate Adherence Molecules (SAMs)

It has been known for some time that the enveloping or supporting substrate influences neurite outgrowth (Rogers et al., 1983; Kromer and Cornbrooks, 1987). The precise mechanisms by which CAMs interact with SAMs continue to be actively investigated. Laminin and fibronectin, two well-characterized extracellular matrix proteins (Baron-Van Evercooren et al., 1982; Rogers et al., 1983), are widely present in nerve and exhibit neurite-promoting activity. Laminin decreases in atrophied Schwann cell columns (bands of Büngner) with chronic denervation (Salonen et al., 1987). A third matrix protein, cytotactin, mediates neuron-glia interactions (Grumet et al., 1985) and, along with N-CAM and Ng-CAM, is concentrated at nodes of Ranvier (Rieger et al., 1986). It was not found around unmyelinated fibers.

The strength of neurite attachment can vary with the substrate. It is found less on a base of laminin than on laminin absorbed to collagen, and is still stronger on type IV collagen with or without fibronectin (Gundersen, 1987). Laminin upregulation of catecholamine biosynthesis enzymes in cultured calf adrenal chromaffin cells is blocked by antibodies to its heparin-binding domain (Acheson et al., 1986), suggesting control of cellular gene expression by matrix interactions at the cell surface. The interactions of CAMs and SAMs have been studied with respect to the epitopes involved (Kruse et al., 1985), neural crest cell localization (Tan et al., 1987), and ligand-coated particle aggregation (Hoffman and Edelman, 1987). The results suggest that particular conformations of CAMs, SAMs, and neuronotrophic factors can favor neurite extension and successful reinnervation.

CRITICAL ROLE OF SCHWANN CELLS

Schwann cells envelop unmyelinated fibers and form myelin sheaths around larger axons. They are neural crest derivatives. Along its entire length each myelinated nerve or unmyelinated bundle is enclosed by a basal lamina continuous from around one enveloping Schwann cell to the next (Raine, 1984). Maintenance of basal lamina continuity is critical for guidance of axon sprouts during reinnervation, just as a ready supply of Schwann cells is for axon maturation. These cells have been studied extensively in vivo and in vitro.

In the animal, Schwann cells proliferate during development (Peters and Muir, 1959; Asbury, 1967; Terry et al., 1974; Aguayo and Bray, 1984), and during degeneration and regeneration (Bradley and Asbury, 1970; Romine et al., 1976; Pellegrino et al., 1982; Pellegrino and Spencer, 1985). In vitro, Schwann cells lack response to many factors or agents that elicit mitoses in other cells (Ratner et al., 1986a), but they do proliferate when contacted by neurites from explanted dorsal root ganglia (Wood and Bunge, 1975). Their proliferation can be stimulated by axolemma-enriched fractions, myelin, and some components of basement membrane (DeVries et al., 1982, 1983; McGarvey et al., 1984; Baron- Van Evercooren et al., 1986).

The mitogenic factor in the neurite and in axolemma is located on the membrane surface (Salzer et al., 1980a,b), but unlike many CAMs is not an N-linked glycoprotein (Ratner et al., 1986b). The mitogenic response of the Schwann cell can be inhibited by preventing surface glycosaminoglycan chain extension; this inhibition does not affect Schwann cell adhesion to axons (Ratner et al., 1986a). The mitogenic response is related to a surface heparan sulfate moiety (Ratner et al., 1986b), and is selectively elicited by at least one mitogen, myelin (Yoshino et al., 1987), which also requires endocytosis and lysosomal processing (Meador-Woodruff et al., 1985). Myelin is a more effective mitogen for Schwann cells of 6-day-old rats than for those from 2-day-old rats, when myelination has barely begun (Yoshino et al., 1987). Perhaps related is the fact that 6-day-old rat Schwann cells induced by gamma interferon to present antigens will activate rat T cell lines specific for myelin basic protein in the absence of this antigen (Wekerle et al., 1986). In some Schwann cell cultures, however, the presence of macrophages may imply that an interleukin-mediated pathway is involved in proliferation of the cells (Lindholm et al., 1987), particularly since activated macrophages can upregulate NGF mRNA in cultures of sciatic nerve (Heumann et al., 1987b). Finally, laminin, in a concentration much higher than that required for cell attachment, stimulates Schwann cell proliferation (McGarvey et al., 1984).

Schwann cell proliferation, both in vivo and in vitro, may be under the control of NGF and one or more components of the extracellular matrix.

ANATOMIC RESTORATION AND RECOVERY OF FUNCTION

PNS regeneration with recovery of appropriate function remains an elusive goal, or, as noted by Mark (1969), "In . . . mammals and man, the easy coordinated use of muscles reinnervated by the cut nerve is lost forever." Restoration of effective function after severance of a nerve, like mending a cut 10,000 wire electrical cable, would seem to require exact matching of the severed ends of every conducting unit. Claims and counterclaims about the effectiveness of repair techniques often reflect the uncertainty of measuring the recovery of coordinated muscle functions, or other modalities, as well as variability in the application of a particular repair technique, be it fastidious microsurgical fascicular repair or simple gluing with plasma.

In a series of experiments, de Medinaceli and coworkers (de Medinaceli et al., 1982, 1983a,b, 1984; de Medinaceli and Freed, 1983; de Medinaceli and Church, 1984) have reported significantly improved recovery of function with use of a reliably quantifiable

measure of coordinated function and novel conditions for nerve transection and repair. The sciatic functional index (SFI) used is based on measurements of footprints made on X-ray film by the developer-coated hind paws of walking rats. Seventeen favorable conditions for transection and repair were identified. Features of the technique included the use of a vibrating (150-Hz) razor blade to transect the rapidly cooled and frozen rat sciatic nerves attached to anti-retraction rubber cuffs. Best results were obtained (de Medinaceli et al., 1983a) if the nerves were soaked during the cooling cycle in calcium-free Ringer's solution and then in phosphate-buffered saline containing a chelator. The latter was added to reduce calcium entry into exposed axoplasm in order to stabilize cytoskeletal tubules and filaments and minimize outflow of axoplasm; lysophosphatidyl choline was added during thawing to minimize the perceived tendency of myelin to slip and cover the cut nerve ends. Functional recovery from complete nerve transection (Sunderland degree 5 injury) in these rats was shown to be optimal when all the above precautions were used. Recovery was assessed by determining sciatic functional indices and was comparable to, if slightly slower than, that following nerve crush (a degree 2 injury). Terzis and Smith (1986) have corroborated the initial results in a larger series of animals.

Experimental Paradigms

Tubular prostheses of novel permeable, semipermeable, and bioresorbable materials that enclose both ends of the transected nerve have become popular again with experimentalists, primarily because nerve regeneration in small experimental animals is not only rapid but predictable when they are used (Lundborg et al., 1981; Varon and Williams, 1986; Ashur et al., 1987). Some tubes permit sampling and alteration of the environment of the nerve stumps; in this way some trophic factors have been obtained and identified (see Varon et al., Chapter 7 this volume). In addition, cellular construction of a new nerve bridge between stumps follows a well-documented pattern and time frame, permitting quantitative comparisons of substances and manipulations under test (Uzman and Villegas, 1983). However, none of the tubes has shown particular promise for patients. Sunderland (1978) summarized most of the early clinical attempts to use tubes in repairing nerves or bridging gaps; one of the more promising prostheses, Millipore filters fashioned into enclosures, led to scarring that eventually constricted and reinjured regenerated nerve segments. Prospects for clinical use of bioresorbable tubes seem uncertain, in part because of swelling and deformation of the tube, effectively reducing luminal size and population of regenerated axons (Henry et al., 1985).

CONCLUSIONS

To understand the state of regeneration research today is to appreciate the possibility and practicality of applying molecular genetics and molecular biology strategies and techniques to every important and unsolved biomedical problem and question. Nowhere is there brighter hope for a deeper level of understanding than in the neurosciences. Progress in regeneration research, with enormous potential for relieving human disabilities, is proceeding apace, relying heavily on the entire scientific research support base.

Hope for the discovery of effective therapeutic measures seems justified. With continuing progress in understanding changes and controls of gene expression, an ideal scenario for treatment can be visualized. In such a scheme, fibroblasts and collagen production will be downregulated, angiogenesis turned on and modulated, injured neurons instructed to synthesize and sprout; Schwann cells and pathways will be specifically decorated or induced to bristle with attracting receptors and guidepost epitopes, and target end organs ordered to display inviting and uniquely appropriate ligands.

REFERENCES

Abo T, Balch CM (1981): A differentiation antigen of human NK and K cells identified by a monoclonal antibody (HNK-1). J Immunol 127:1024–1029.

Acheson A, Edgar D, Timpl R, Thoenen H (1986): Laminin increases both levels and activity of tyrosine hydroxylase in calf adrenal chromaffin cells. J Cell Biol 102:151–159.

Aguayo AJ, Bray GM (1984): Cell interactions studied in the peripheral nerves of experimental animals. In Dyck PS, Thomas PK, Lambert EH, Bunge R (eds): "Peripheral Neuropathy." Philadelphia: WB Saunders Co, pp 360–377.

Aguayo AJ, David S, Bray GM (1981): Influences of the glial environment on the elongation of axons after injury: Transplantation studies in adult rodents. J Exp Biol 95:231–240.

Aguayo AJ, Vidal-Sanz M, Villegas-Perez MP, Bray GM (1985): Growth and connectivity of axotomized retinal neurons in adult rats with optic nerves substituted by PNS grafts linking the eye and the midbrain. Ann NY Acad Sci 495:1–9.

Antonicek H, Persohn E, Schachner M (1987): Biochemical and functional characterization of a novel neuronglia adhesion molecule that is involved in neuronal migration. J Cell Biol 104:1587–1595.

Asbury AK (1967): Schwann cell proliferation in developing mouse sciatic nerve. J Cell Biol 34:735–743.

Ashur H, Vilner Y, Finsterbush A, Rousso M, Weinberg H, Devor M (1987): Extent of fiber regeneration after peripheral nerve repair: Silicone splint vs. suture, gap repair vs. graft. Exp Neurol 97:365–374.

Bandtlow CE, Heumann R, Schwaub ME, Thoenen H (1987): Cellular localization of nerve growth factor synthesis in in situ hybridization. EMBO J 6:891–899.

Barbin G, Manthorpe M, Varon S (1984): Purification of the chick eye ciliary neuronotropic factor. J Neurochem 43:1468–1478.

Baron-Van Evercooren AB, Kleinman HK, Ohno S, Marangos P, Schwartz JP, Dubois-Dalcq ME (1982): Nerve growth factor, laminin, and fibronectin promote neurite growth in human fetal sensory ganglia cultures. J Neurosci Res 8:179–193.

Baron-Van Evercooren A, Gansmüller A, Gumpel M, Baumann N, Kleinman HK (1986): Schwann cell differentiation in vitro: Extracellular matrix deposition and interaction. Dev Neurosci 8:182–196.

Bisby MA (1988): Synthesis of cytoskeletal proteins by axotomized and regenerating motoneurones. In Reier PJ, Bunge RP, Seil FJ (eds): "Current Issues in Neural Regeneration." New York: Alan R. Liss, in press.

Bock E, Richter-Landsberg C, Faissner A, Schachner M (1985): Demonstration of immunochemical identity between the nerve growth factor inducible large external (NILE) glycoprotein and the cell adhesion molecule L1. EMBO J 4:2765–2768.

Bollensen E, Schachner M (1987): The peripheral myelin glycoprotein P_o expresses the L2/HNK-1 and L3 carbohydrate structures shared by neural adhesion molecules. Neurosci Lett 82:77–82.

Bradley WG, Asbury AK (1970): Duration of synthesis phase in neurilemma cells in mouse sciatic nerve during degeneration. Exp Neurol 26:275–282.

Brockes JP, Lemke GE, Balzer DR (1980): Purification and preliminary characterization of glial growth factor from the bovine pituitary. J Biol Chem 255:8374–8377.

Brushart TME, Seiler WA IV (1987): Selective innervation of distal motor stumps by peripheral motor axons. Exp Neurol 97:289–300.

Buck CR, Marinez HJ, Black IB, Chao MV (1987): Developmentally regulated expression of the nerve growth factor receptor gene in the periphery and brain. Proc Natl Acad Sci USA 84:3060–3063.

Buxser S, Puma P, Johnson GL (1985): Properties of the nerve growth factor receptor. J Biol Chem 260:1917–1926.

Chang S, Rathjen FG, Raper JA (1987): Extension of neurites on axons is impaired by antibodies against specific neural cell surface glycoproteins. J Cell Biol 104: 355–362.

Chou KH, Ilyas AA, Evans JE, Quarles RH, Jungalwala FB (1985): Structure of a glycolipid reacting with monoclonal IgM in neuropathy and with HNK-1. Biochem Biophys Res Commun 218:383–388.

Chou DKH, Ilyas AA, Evans JE, Costello C, Quarles RH, Jungalwala FB (1986): Structure of sulfated glucuronyl glycolipids in the nervous system reacting with HNK-1 antibody and some IgM paraproteins in neuropathy. J Biol Chem 261:11717–11725.

Cunningham BA, Hemperly JJ, Murray BA, Prediger EA, Brackenbury R, Edelman GM (1987): Neural cell adhesion molecule: Structure, immunoglobulin-like domains, cell surface modulation, and alternative RNA splicing. Science 236:799–806.

Curran T, Morgan JI (1985): Superinduction of c-fos by nerve growth factor in the presence of peripherally active benzodiazepines. Science 229:1265–1268.

Daniloff JK, Levi G, Grumet M, Rieger F, Edelman GM (1986): Altered expression of neuronal cell adhesion molecules induced by nerve injury and repair. J Cell Biol 103:929–945.

David S, Aguayo AJ (1981): Axonal elongation into peripheral nervous system "bridges" after central nervous system injury in adult rats. Science 214:931–933.

Davies AM, Bandtlow C, Heumann R, Korsching S, Roher H, Thoenen H (1987): Timing and site of nerve growth factor synthesis in developing skin in relation to innervation and expression of the receptor. Nature (London) 326:353–358.

Dekker A, Gispen WH, de Wied D (1987): Axonal regeneration, growth factors and neuropeptides. Life Sci 41: 1667–1678.

de Medinaceli L, Church AC (1984): Peripheral nerve reconnection: Inhibition of early degenerative processes through the use of a novel fluid medium. Exp Neurol 84:396–408.

de Medinaceli L, Freed WJ (1983): Peripheral nerve reconnection: Immediate histologic consequences of distributed mechanical support. Exp Neurol 81:459–468.

de Medinaceli L, Freed WJ, Wyatt RJ (1982): An index of the functional condition of rat sciatic nerve based on measurements from walking tracks. Exp Neurol 77: 634–643.

de Medinaceli L, Wyatt RJ, Freed WJ (1983a): Peripheral nerve reconnection: Mechanical, thermal, and ionic conditions that promote the return of function. Exp Neurol 81:469–487.

de Medinaceli L, Freed WJ, Wyatt RJ (1983b): Peripheral nerve reconnection: Improvement of long-term functional effects under simulated clinical conditions in the rat. Exp Neurol 81:488–496.

de Medinaceli L, de Renzo E, Wyatt RJ (1984): Rat sciatic functional index data management system with digitized input. Comput Biomed Res 17:185–192.

DeVries GH, Salzer JL, Bunge RP (1982): Axolemma-enriched fractions isolated from PNS and CNS are mitogenic for cultured Schwann cells. Dev Brain Res 3:295–299.

DeVries GH, Minier LN, Lewis BL (1983): Further studies on the mitogenic response of cultured Schwann cells to rat CNS axolemma-enriched fraction. Dev Brain Res 9:87–93.

DiStefano PS, Johnson EM Jr (1988): Nerve growth factor receptors on cultured rat Schwann cells. J Neurosci 8:231–241.

Faissner A, Kruse J, Goridis C, Bock E, Schachner M (1984): The neural cell adhesion molecule L1 is distinct from the N-CAM related group of surface antigens BSP-2 and D2. EMBO J 3:733–737.

Finn PJ, Ferguson IA, Renton FJ, Rush RA (1986): Nerve growth factor immunohistochemistry and biological activity in the rat iris. J Neurocytol 15:169–176.

Finn PJ, Ferguson IA, Wilson PA, Vahaviolos J, Rush RA (1987): Immunohistochemical evidence for the distribution of nerve growth factor in embryonic mouse. J Neurocytol 16:639–647.

Fischer G, Künemund V, Schachner M (1986): Neurite outgrowth patterns in cerebellar microexplant cultures are affected by antibodies to the cell surface glycoprotein L1. J Neurosci 6:605–612.

Forssman J (1898): Über dis ursachen welche die Wachstumrichtung der peripheren nervenfasern bei der regeneration bestimmen. Beitr Pathol Anat 24:56. Cited, Editorial (1987) Acta Orthop Scand 58:91–92.

Friedlander DR, Grumet M, Edelman GM (1986): Nerve growth factor enhances expression of neuron-glia cell adhesion molecule in PC12 cells. J Cell Biol 102:413–419.

Gloor S, Odink K, Guenther J, Nick H, Monard D (1986): A glia-derived neurite promoting factor with protease inhibitory activity belongs to the protease nexins. Cell 47:687–693.

Gospodarowicz D (1974): Localisation of a fibroblast growth factor and its effect alone and with hydrocortisone in 3T3 cell growth. Nature 249:123–127.

Gospodarowicz D (1978): Purification of fibroblast growth factor from bovine pituitary. J Biol Chem 250: 2515–2520.

Green SH, Rydel RE, Connolly JL, Greene LA (1985): PC12 cell mutants that possess low- but not high-affinity nerve growth factor receptors neither respond to nor internalize nerve growth factor. J Cell Biol 102:830–843.

Greene LA, Tischler AS (1976): Establishment of a noradrenergic clonal line of rat adrenal pheochromocytoma cells which respond to nerve growth factor. Proc Natl Acad Sci USA 73:2424–2428.

Greenfield S, Brostoff S, Eylar EH, Morell P (1973): Protein composition of myelin of the peripheral nervous system. J Neurochem 20:1207–1216.

Grumet M, Hoffman S, Edelman GM (1984): Two antigenically related neuronal cell adhesion molecules of different specificities mediate neuron-neuron and neuron-glia adhesion. Proc Natl Acad Sci USA 81:267–271.

Grumet M, Hoffman S, Crissub KL, Edelman GM (1985): Cytotactin, an extracellular matrix protein of neural and non-neural tissues that mediates glia-neuron interaction. Proc Natl Acad Sci USA 82:8075–8079.

Guenther J, Nick H, Monard D (1985): A glia-derived neurite-promoting factor with protease inhibitory activity. EMBO J 4:1963–1966.

Gundersen RW (1987): Response of sensory neurites and growth cones to patterned substrata of laminin and fibronectin in vitro. Dev Biol 121:423–431.

Hausman RE, Moscona AA (1975): Purification and characterization of the retina-specific cell-aggregating factor. Proc Natl Acad Sci USA 72:916–920.

Henry EW, Chiu T-H, Nyilas E, Brushart TM, Dikkes P, Sidman RL (1985): Nerve regeneration through biodegradable polyester tubes. Exp Neurol 90:652–676.

Heumann RJ (1987): Regulation of the synthesis of nerve growth factor. J Exp Biol 132:133–150.

Heumann R, Korsching S, Bandtlow C, Thoenen H (1987a): Changes of nerve growth factor synthesis in nonneuronal cells in response to sciatic nerve transection. J Cell Biol 104:1623–1631.

Heumann R, Lindholm D, Bandtlow C, Meyer M, Radeke MJ, Misko TP, Shooter E, Thoenen H (1987b): Differential regulation of mRNA encoding nerve growth factor and its receptor in rat sciatic nerve during development, degeneration, and regeneration: Role of macrophages. Proc Natl Acad Sci USA 84:8735–8739.

Hoffman S, Edelman GM (1987): A proteoglycan with HNK-1 antigenic determinants is a neuron-associated ligand for cytotactin. Proc Natl Acad Sci USA 84:2523–2527.

Hoffman S, Sorkin BC, White PC, Brackenbury R, Mailhammer R, Rutishauser U, Cunningham BA, Edelman GM (1982): Chemical characterization of a neural cell adhesion molecule purified from embryonic brain membranes. J Biol Chem 257:7720–7729.

Hoffman S, Crossin KL, Edelman GM (1988): Molecular forms, binding functions, and developmental expression patterns of cytotactin and cytotactin-binding proteoglycan, an interactive pair of extracellular matrix molecules. J Cell Biol 106:519–532.

Honegger P, Lenoir D (1982): Nerve growth factor (NGF) stimulation of cholinergic telencephalic neurons in aggregating cell cultures. Brain Res 255:229–238.

Johnson EM Jr, Gorin PD, Brandeis LD, Pearson J (1980): Dorsal root ganglion neurons are destroyed by exposure in utero to maternal antibody to nerve growth factor. Science 210:916–918.

Korsching S, Auburger G, Heumann R, Scott J, Thoenen H (1985): Levels of nerve growth factor and its mRNA in the central nervous system of the rat correlate with cholinergic innervation. EMBO J 4:1389–1393.

Kromer LF, Cornbrooks DJ (1987): Identification of trophic factors and transplanted cellular environments that promote CNS axonal regeneration. Ann NY Acad Sci 495:207–225.

Kruse J, Mailhammer R, Wernecke H, Faissner A, Sommer I, Goridis C, Schachner M (1984): Neural cell adhesion molecules and myelin-associated glycoprotein share a common carbohydrate moiety recognized by monoclonal antibodies L2 and HNK-1. Nature 311:153–155.

Kruse J, Keilhauer G, Faissner A, Timpl R, Schachner M (1985): The J1 glycoprotein—a novel nervous system cell adhesion molecule of the L2/HNK-1 family. Nature 316:146–148.

Kücherer A, Faissner A, Schachner M (1987): The novel carbohydrate epitope L3 is shared by some neural cell adhesion molecules. J Cell Biol 104:1597–1602.

Lagenaur C, Lemmon V (1987): An L1-like molecule, the 8D9 antigen, is a potent substrate for neurite extension. Proc Natl Acad Sci USA 84:7753–7757.

Lai C, Brow MA, Klaus-Armin N, Noronha AB, Quarles RH, Bloom FE, Milner RJ, Sutcliffe JG (1987): Two forms of 1B236/myelin-associated glycoprotein, a cell adhesion molecule for postnatal neural development, are produced by alternative splicing. Proc Natl Acad Sci USA 84:4337–4341.

Landreth GE, Shooter EM (1980): Nerve growth factor receptor on PC12 cells: ligand-induced conversion from low- to high-affinity states. Proc Natl Acad Sci USA 77:4751–4755.

Ledeen RW (1984): Biology of gangliosides: Neuritogenic and neuronotrophic factors. J Neurosci Res 12:147–159.

Lemke G, Axel R (1985): Isolation and sequence of a cDNA encoding the major structural protein of peripheral myelin. Cell 40:501–508.

Levi-Montalcini R (1987): The nerve growth factor 35 years later. Science 237:1154–1162.

Levi-Montalcini R, Angeletti PU (1963): Essential role of the nerve growth factor on the survival and maintenance of dissociated sensory and sympathetic embryonic nerve cells in vitro. Dev Biol 7:653–659.

Levi-Montalcini R, Angeletti PU (1968): Nerve growth factor. Physiol Rev 48:534–569.

Lindenbaum MH, Carbonetto S, Mushynski WE (1987): Nerve growth factor enhances the synthesis, phosphorylation, and metabolic stability of neurofilament proteins in PC12 cells. J Biol Chem 262:605–610.

Lindholm D, Heumann R, Meyer M, Thoenen H (1987): Interleukin-1 regulates synthesis of nerve growth factor in non-neuronal cells of rat sciatic nerve. Nature 330:658–659.

Lindner J, Guenther J, Nick H, Zinser G, Antonicek H, Schachner M, Monard D (1986): Modulation of granule cell migration by a glia derived protein. Proc Natl Acad Sci USA 83:4568–4571.

Lundborg G (1987): Nerve regeneration and repair. Acta Orthop Scand 58:145–169.

Lundborg G, Dahlin LB, Danielsen NP, Hansson HA, Larsson K (1981): Reorganization and orientation of regenerating nerve fibers, perineurium and epineurium in preformed mesothelial tubes. An experimental study on the sciatic nerve of rats. J Neurosci Res 6:265–281.

Mark RF (1969): Matching muscles and motoneurons. A review of some experiments on motor nerve regeneration. Brain Res 14:245–254.

Martini R, Schachner M (1986): Immunoelectron microscopic localization of neural cell adhesion molecules (L1, N-CAM, and MAG) and their shared carbohydrate epitope and myelin basic protein (MBP) in developing sciatic nerve. J Cell Biol 103:2439–2448.

McGarvey ML, Baron-Van Evercooren A, Kleinman HK, Dubois-Dalcq M (1984): Synthesis and effects of basement membrane components in cultured rat Schwann cells. Dev Biol 105:18–28.

McGuire J, Greene L, Furano A (1978): NGF stimulates incorporation of fucose or glucosamine into an external glycoprotein in cultured rat PC12 pheochromocytoma cells. Cell 15:357–365.

McQuarrie IG, Grafstein B (1973): Axon outgrowth enhanced by a previous nerve injury. Arch Neurol 29:53–55.

Meador-Woodruff JH, Yoshino JE, Bigbee JW, Lewis BL, DeVries GH (1985): Differential proliferative responses of cultured Schwann cells to axolemma and myelin-enriched fractions. II. Morphological studies. J Neurocytol 14:619–635.

Monard D (1987): Role of protease inhibition in cellular migration and neuritic growth. Biochem Pharmacol 36:1389–1392.

Monard D, Solomen F, Rentsch M, Gysin R (1973): Glia-induced morphological differentiation in neuroblastoma cells. Proc Natl Acad Sci USA 70:1894–1897.

Morrison RS, Sharma A, de Vellis J, Bradshaw RA (1986): Basic fibroblast growth factor supports the survival of cerebral cortical neurons in primary culture. Proc Natl Acad Sci USA 83:7537–7541.

Moya F, Bunge MB, Bunge RP (1980): Schwann cells proliferate but fail to differentiate in defined medium. Proc Natl Acad Sci USA 77:6902–6906.

Nieke J, Schachner M (1985): Expression of the neural cell adhesion molecules L1 and N-CAM and their common carbohydrate epitope L2/HNK-1 during development and after transection of the mouse sciatic nerve. Differentiation 30:141–151.

Peters A, Muir AR (1959): The relationship between axons and Schwann cells during development of peripheral nerves in the rat. Q J Exp Physiol 64:117–130.

Pellegrino RG, Spencer PS (1985): Schwann cell mitosis in response to regenerating peripheral axons in vivo. Brain Res 341:16–25.

Pellegrino RG, Ritchie JM, Spencer PS (1982): The role of Schwann cell division in the clearance of nodal axolemma following nerve section in the cat. J Physiol (Lond) 334:68P.

Politis MJ (1985a): Specificity in mammalian peripheral nerve regeneration at the level of the nerve trunk. Brain Res 328:271–276.

Politis MJ (1985b): Tropic factors in reactive mammalian central nervous system tissue. Brain Res 328:277–281.

Politis MJ, Spencer PS (1983): An in vivo assay of neurotropic activity. Brain Res 278:229–231.

Politis MJ, Ederle K, Spencer PS (1982): Tropism in nerve regeneration in vivo. Attraction of regenerating axons by diffusible factors derived from cells in distal nerve stumps of transected peripheral nerve. Brain Res 253:1–12.

Porter S, Clark MB, Glaser L, Bunge RP (1986): Schwann cells stimulated to proliferate in the absence of neurons retain full functional capability. J Neurosci 6:3070–3078.

Quarles RH, Everly JL, Brady RO (1972): Demonstration of a glycoprotein which is associated with a purified myelin fraction from rat brain. Biochim Biophys Res Commun 47:491–497.

Raine CS (1984): Morphology of myelin and myelination. In Morell P (ed): "Myelin." New York: Plenum Press, pp 1–50.

Raivich G, Kreutzberg GW (1987): Expression of growth factor receptors in injured nervous tissue. I. Axotomy leads to a shift in the cellular distribution of specific β-nerve growth factor binding in the injured and regenerating PNS. J Neurocytol 16:689–700.

Ramón y Cajal S (1905): Méchanisme de la régénéresence des nerves. Trav Lab Rech Biol Univ Madrid 3–4:123–218.

Ramón y Cajal S (1913): "Estudios Sobre la Degeneración y Regeneración del Sistema Nervioso." Madrid: Imprenta Hijos de Nicolás Moya.

Rathjen FG, Wolff SM, Frank R, Bonhoeffer F, Rutishauser U (1987): Membrane glycoproteins involved in neurite fasciculation. J Cell Biol 104:343–353.

Ratner N, Bunge RP, Glaser L (1986a): Schwann cell proliferation in vitro: An overview. Ann NY Acad Sci 486:170–181.

Ratner N, Elbein A, Bunge MB, Porter S, Bunge RP (1986b): Specific asparagine-linked oligosaccharides are not required for certain neuron-neuron and neuron-Schwann cell interactions. J Cell Biol 103:159–170.

Rieger F, Daniloff JK, Pincon-Raymond M, Crossin KL, Grumet M, Edelman GM (1986): Neuronal cell adhesion molecules and cytotactin are colocalized at the node of Ranvier. J Cell Biol 103:379–391.

Rogers SL, Letourneau PC, Palm SL, McCarthy J, Furcht LT (1983): Neurite extension by peripheral and central nervous system neurons in response to substratum-bound fibronectin and laminin. Dev Biol 98:212–220.

Rohrer H (1985): Nonneuronal cells from chick sympathetic and dorsal root sensory ganglia express catecholamine uptake and receptors for nerve growth factor during development. Dev Biol 111:95–107.

Romine JS, Bray GM, Aguayo AJ (1976): Schwann cell multiplication after crush injury of unmyelinated fibers. Arch Neurol 33:49–54.

Sajovic P, Kouvelas E, Trenkner E (1986): Probable identity of NILE glycoprotein and the high-molecular-weight component of L1 antigen. J Neurochem 47:541–546.

Salonen V, Peltonen J, Röyttä M, Virtanen I (1987): Laminin in traumatized nerve: Basement membrane changes during degeneration and regeneration. J Neurocytol 16:713–720.

Salzer JL, Williams AK, Glaser L, Bunge RP (1980a): Studies of Schwann cell proliferation. II. Characterization of the stimulation and specificity of the response to a neurite membrane fraction. J Cell Biol 84:753–766.

Salzer JL, Bunge RP, Glaser L (1980b): Studies of Schwann cell proliferation. III. Evidence for the surface localization of the neurite mitogen. J Cell Biol 84:767–778.

Salzer JL, Holmes WP, Colman DR (1987): The amino acid sequences of the myelin-associated glycoproteins: Homology to the immunoglobulin gene superfamily. J Cell Biol 104:957–965.

Sandrock AW, Matthew WD (1987): Substrate-bound nerve growth factor promotes neurite growth in peripheral nerve. Brain Res 425:360–363.

Schubert D, LaCorbiere M, Klier G, Bridwell C (1983): A role for adherons in neural retina cell adhesion. J Cell Biol 96:990–998.

Sears TA (1987): Structural changes in motoneurones following axotomy. J Exp Biol 132:93–109.

Seilheimer B, Schachner M (1987): Regulation of neural cell adhesion molecule expression on cultured mouse Schwann cells by nerve growth factor. EMBO J 6:1611–1616.

Snipes GJ, Chan SY, McGuire CB, Costello BR, Norden JJ, Freeman JA, Routtenberg A (1987a): Evidence for the coidentification of GAP-43, a growth-associated protein, and F1, a plasticity-associated protein. J Neurosci 7:4066–4075.

Snipes GJ, Costello B, McGuire CB, Mayes BN, Bock SS, Norden JJ, Freeman JA (1987b): Regulation of specific neuronal and nonneuronal proteins during development and following injury in the rat central nervous system. In Seil FJ, Herbert E, Carlson BM (ed): "Neural Regeneration. Progress in Brain Research," Vol 71. Amsterdam: Elsevier, pp 155–175.

Stallcup WB, Beasley L (1985): Involvement of the nerve growth factor-inducible large external glycoprotein (NILE) in neurite fasciculation in primary cultures of rat brain. Proc Natl Acad Sci USA 82:1276–1280.

Stone S, Nick H, Hofsteenge J, Monard D (1987): Glia-derived neurite-promoting factor is a slow-binding inhibitor of trypsin, thrombin and urokinase. Arch Biochem Biophys 252:237–244.

Sunderland S (1978): "Nerves and Nerve Injuries." Edinburgh: Churchill Livingston.

Takeichi M, Hatta K, Nagafuchi A (1985): Selective cell adhesion mechanism: Role of the calcium-dependent cell adhesion system. In Edelman GM (ed): "Molecular Determinants of Animal Form." New York: Alan R. Liss, pp 223–233.

Tan S-S, Crossin KL, Hoffman S, Edelman GM (1987): Asymmetric expression in somites of cytotactin and its proteoglycan ligand is correlated with neural crest cell distribution. Proc Natl Acad Sci USA 84:7977–7981.

Taniuchi M, Clark HB, Johnson EM Jr (1986a): Induction of nerve growth factor receptor in Schwann cells after axotomy. Proc Natl Acad Sci USA 83:4094–4098.

Taniuchi M, Schweitzer JB, Johnson EM Jr (1986b): Nerve growth factor receptor molecules in rat brain. Proc Natl Acad Sci USA 83:1950–1954.

Taniuchi M, Clark HB, Schweitzer JB, Johnson EM Jr (1988): Expression of nerve growth factor receptors by Schwann cells of axotomized peripheral nerves: Ultrastructural location, suppression by axonal contact, and binding properties. J Neurosci 8:664–681.

Tedeschi B, Wilson DL (1983): Modification of a rapidly transported protein in regenerating nerve. J Neurosci 3:1728–1734.

Terry LC, Bray GM, Aguayo AJ (1974): Schwann cell multiplication in developing rat unmyelinated nerves. A radioautographic study. Brain Res 69:144–148.

Terzis J, Smith KJ (1986): "De Medinaceli" versus microsuture: A critical appraisal of nerve repair. Periph Nerve Repair Regen 2:63–67.

Thoenen H, Barde Y-A (1980): Physiology of nerve growth factor. Physiol Rev 60:1284–1335.

Unsicker K, Reichert-Preibsh H, Schmidt R, Pettmann B, Labourdette G, Sensenbrenner M (1987): Astroglial and fibroblast growth factors have neuronotrophic functions for cultured peripheral and central nervous system neurons. Proc Natl Acad Sci USA 84:5459–5463.

Uzman BG, Villegas GM (1983): Mouse sciatic nerve regeneration through semipermeable tubes: A quantitative model. J Neurosci Res 9:325–338.

Van Hooff COM, De Graan PNE, Boonstra J, Oestreicher AB, Schmidt-Michels MH, Gispen WH (1986): Nerve growth factor enhances the level of the protein kinase C substrate B-50 in the pheochromocytoma PC12 cells. Biochim Biophys Res Commun 139:644–651.

Varon S, Adler R (1980): Nerve growth factors and control of nerve growth. Curr Top Dev Biol 16:207–252.

Varon S, Williams LR (1986): Peripheral nerve regeneration in a silicone model chamber: Cellular and molecular aspects. Periph Nerve Repair Regen 1:9–25.

Waller A (1850): Experiments on the section of the glossopharyngeal and hypoglossal nerves of the frog, and observations of the alterations produced thereby in the structure of their primitive fibers. Philos Trans R Soc Lond 140:423–429.

Weiss P (1941): Nerve patterns: The mechanisms of nerve growth. Third Growth Symposium. Growth 5:163–203.

Wekerle H, Schwab M, Linington C, Meyermann R (1986): Antigen presentation in the peripheral nervous system: Schwann cells present endogenous myelin autoantigens to lymphocytes. Eur J Immunol 16:1551–1557.

Whittemore SR, Ebendal T, Larkfors L, Olson L, Seiger A, Stomberg I, Persson H (1986): Developmental and regional expression of β-nerve growth factor messenger RNA and protein in the central nervous system. Proc Natl Acad Sci USA 83:817–821.

Williams AF, Barclay AN, Clark MJ, Gagnon J (1985): Cell surface glycoproteins and origins of immunity. In Anderson LC, Gahmberg CG, Ekblom P (eds): "Gene Expression During Normal and Malignant Differentiation." New York: Academic Press, pp 125–138.

Williams LR, Manthorpe M, Barbin G, Nieto-Sampedro M, Cotman C, Varon S (1984): High ciliary neuronotrophic specific activity in rat peripheral nerve. Int J Dev Neurosci 2:177–180.

Wood PM, Bunge RP (1975): Evidence that sensory axons are mitogenic for Schwann cells. Nature 256:662–664.

Yoshino JE, Mason PW, DeVries GH (1987): Developmental changes in myelin-induced proliferation of cultured Schwann cells. J Cell Biol 104:655–660.

Zanakis MF, Chakraborty G, Sturman JA, Ingoglia NA (1984): Posttranslational protein modification by amino acid addition in intact and regenerating axons of the rat sciatic nerve. J Neurochem 43:1286–1294.

Zimmerman A, Sutter A (1983): β-nerve growth factor receptors on glial cells. Cell-cell interaction between neurons and Schwann cells in cultures of chick sensory ganglia. EMBO J 2:879–885.

3

Axonal Transport and the Regenerating Nerve

IRVINE G. McQUARRIE, MD, PhD

Division of Neurosurgery and Department of Developmental Genetics, School of Medicine, Case Western Reserve University and Neural Regeneration Center, Veterans Administration Medical Center, Cleveland, Ohio 44106

The term "axonal transport" refers to the movement of macromolecules and organelles through thin extensions of nerve cell cytoplasm called axons. The same types of movement apparently occur in all nucleated cells. Accordingly, "intracellular transport in neurons" is perhaps a more accurate term than "axonal transport" (Grafstein and Forman, 1980). Specifically, these terms denote the movement of materials through the "expressional" cytoplasm, as distinct from analogous movements within the "translational" cytoplasm, where protein synthesis can occur (Lasek and Brady, 1982). In mature neurons, the expressional cytoplasm has evolved into a specialized extension, the axoplasm, which is quite distinct from the translational cytoplasm of the perikaryon and dendrites. This distinction is also evident at the ultrastructural level, since ribosomes are excluded from the axon (Zelena, 1972).

Although neurons have the longest and most highly developed extensions of expressional cytoplasm, many nonneuronal cells can produce similar extensions that exclude translational cytoplasm. Examples include the flagella of protozoa and the pseudopods of cultured fibroblasts. These regenerate following amputation in a manner similar to axonal regeneration—through a reorganization of both translational and expressional cytoplasm that mimics developmental growth (McQuarrie, 1984; Baas and Heidemann, 1986). Thus the amputation of a cell extension presents a problem for intracellular transport that is not unique to neurons, and a variety of cell types appear to solve the problem by making similar adjustments.

MECHANISM OF TRANSPORT
Axonal Transport in Normal Neurons

Protein synthesis does not occur in axons, yet axons typically contain 90–99% of neuronal cytoplasm and terminate at great distances from the perikaryon—distances that exceed the diameter of the nerve cell body by several orders of magnitude. To maintain subcellular structures at loci far removed from the source of "replacement parts" requires a major investment of neuronal resources in the axonal transport system. The capacity, energy requirements, and complexity of this system must exceed those needed to simply transport neurotransmitter-related molecules to the axon terminal. Transport mechanisms can be ordered into subcategories that relate to turnover rates for all of the structural and membrane proteins, in addition to replacing losses due to exocytosis at the axon terminal.

Most materials are transported anterogradely through the axon at two rates, fast and slow, which differ by two orders of magnitude. Some materials are also transported retrogradely (from the axon terminal to the perikaryon) at rates similar to the corresponding anterograde rates. Fast retrograde transport represents an important route for communicating information from the environment of the axon terminal to the nerve cell body, particularly during axonal regeneration (Bisby, 1984). The fast com-

Neural Regeneration and Transplantation, pages 29–42
© 1989 Alan R. Liss, Inc.

ponent (FC) of anterograde transport carries neurotransmitter-related materials for export and tubulovesicular elements for membrane replacement, whereas the slow component (SC) carries the cytoskeletal elements responsible for the extreme asymmetry of the axon plus the enzymes of intermediary metabolism that provide energy for axonal transport (Grafstein and Forman, 1980; Tytell et al., 1981; Lasek et al., 1984; McQuarrie et al., 1986). Approximately 80% of the anterograde protein traffic is carried by SC, and less than 10% by FC (McEwen and Grafstein, 1968; Karlsson and Sjostrand, 1971; Grafstein and Forman, 1980).

The slow component consists of two subcomponents, SCa and SCb (Lasek et al., 1984). The slower of these, SCa, carries all of the moving neurofilaments and a variable fraction of the moving microtubules, whereas the faster subcomponent (SCb) represents the moving cytoplasmic matrix and carries the remaining microtubules (Tashiro et al., 1984; Brady and Black, 1986; McQuarrie et al., 1986; Oblinger et al., 1987). None of the FC proteins are carried by SC (Tytell et al., 1981). The triplet of neurofilament polypeptides is specifically transported by SCa, whereas identified SCb proteins include aldolase, pyruvate kinase, creatine kinase, neuron-specific enolase, choline acetyltransferase, clathrin, and synapsin I (Grafstein and Forman, 1980; Lasek et al., 1984; Baitinger and Willard, 1987). Actin, spectrin, calmodulin, and tubulin are carried by both SCa and SCb in many neurons, though some neurons exclude calmodulin from SCa and tubulin from SCb (McQuarrie et al., 1986; Oblinger et al., 1987).

The principal method for studying the rate, amount, and composition of the rate components of axonal transport is to label newly synthesized proteins by microinjecting a radioactive amino acid near the corresponding nerve cell bodies that send axons to the nerve under study. Following an appropriate delay, labeled polypeptides characteristic of that rate component are found in the nerve. These are typically separated by homogenizing serial nerve segments in a buffered high-salt solution (8 M urea) that contains a compound to break disulfide bonds (beta-mercaptoethanol) plus the anionic detergent SDS (sodium dodecyl sulfate). Each polypeptide molecule is thereby de-

natured, without disrupting the primary structure, and surrounded with negatively charged lipid molecules that make it soluble in aqueous solution. When forced through a porous polymer of acrylamide by the application of an electric field (polyacrylamide gel electrophoresis, PAGE), the SDS polypeptides are arrested after traveling a distance that is inversely proportional to the logarithm of the SDS molecular mass. Polypeptides are detected in a gel lane by staining with brilliant Coomassie blue; the radiolabeled polypeptides among these are located by treating the destained gel with a fluor and incubating it under X-ray film in a frozen state. The exposed film (fluorogram) can be used as a template for removing proteins of interest from the gel, and these can be solubilized for quantitation of radioactivity by liquid scintillation spectrometry (McQuarrie et al., 1986). Figure 3–1 shows the fluorograms and plotted distributions of radioactivity for SCa tubulin and the neurofilament triplet (NFT) at 28 d after labeling motor neurons in the rat spinal cord with [^{35}S]methionine. For greater specificity of protein identification, nerve segments can be solubilized in a neutral detergent so that natural charge characteristics are retained. This permits an initial electrophoretic separation based on differences in isoelectric point (pI), which is followed by SDS-PAGE to separate polypeptides with similar pI on the basis of differences in SDS molecular mass, a method termed two-dimensional (2D) PAGE (Oblinger et al., 1987; Perry et al., 1987).

In mammalian neurons, FC advances at 200–400 mm/d and SC at 0.2–6 mm/d; mitochondria, transfer RNA, some of the spectrin, and a nonmuscle myosin are transported at intermediate rates of 6–100 mm/d (Lasek et al., 1984; McQuarrie et al., 1986). In fish and amphibia, the corresponding rates are tenfold slower because of the difference in body temperature (McEwen and Grafstein, 1968; Cancalon, 1985). In retinal ganglion cells of goldfish, the rate for FC is 40–100 mm/d, and the rate for SC is 0.02–0.4 mm/d (McQuarrie and Grafstein, 1982a,b; McQuarrie, 1984; McQuarrie et al., 1985).

The mechanisms underlying fast and slow transport have been partially dissected. The fast transport of tubulovesicular structures in

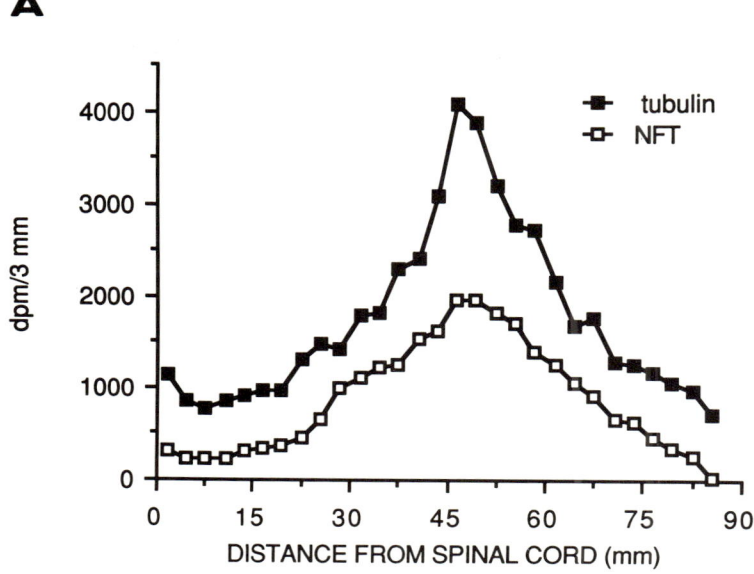

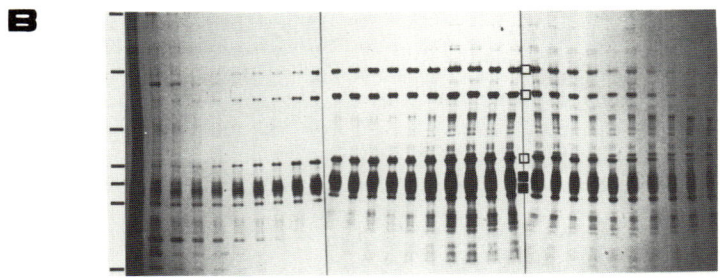

Figure 3–1. The distribution of mean amounts of labeled tubulin and NFT polypeptides in motor axons of the rat sciatic nerve at 28 d after microinjection of the lumbar spinal cord with 750 μCi [^{35}S]methionine (**A**). The rat weighed 160 gm at the time of injection. Quantitation of radioactivity in these polypeptides is obtained by using fluorograms of the SDS-PAGE gels (**B**) as templates to remove appropriate gel segments for solubilization with hydrogen peroxide and liquid scintillation spectrometry (McQuarrie et al., 1986). In the fluorogram, closed squares denote alpha- and beta-tubulin; open squares the 200-kD, 145-kD, and 68-kD neurofilament triplet (NFT) polypeptides. SDS-molecular mass standards are in the first lane on the left (335, 200, 94, 68, 57, 43, and 14 kD reading top to bottom); the spinal cord is in the second lane. Each lane to the right of the second denotes labeled polypeptides in serial 3-mm nerve segments: L5 ventral root to L5 spinal nerve to sciatic nerve (beginning at 45 mm from the spinal cord; 30% of the radioactivity beyond this point is contributed by the L4 spinal nerve). Radioactivity levels for tubulin and NFT are plotted in A directly above the corresponding gel lane in the fluorogram (B).

either direction depends on proteins in the cytoplasm that can hydrolyze adenosine triphosphate (ATP) and attach to both membranous organelles and microtubules. Kinesin and dynein are two such proteins (Brady, 1985; Vale et al., 1985; Cheng et al., 1987; Paschal et al., 1987; Paschal and Vallee, 1987). These act to briefly attach a vesicle to a microtubule and propel it either anterogradely (kinesin) or retrogradely (dynein) by extending a bend in the kinesin or dynein molecule. Each of these is an ATPase and accordingly provides the energy needed for this motile event.

Slow transport may be based on the movement of a membrane system within the axon, the endoplasmic reticulum (ER). Recent findings suggest that the ER can move anterogradely through the axon at an intermediate rate, by an interaction between an ATPase (nonmuscle myosin) on the outer surface of the ER and an actin microfilament in the subaxolemmal zone (Hirokawa, 1982; Sheetz et al., 1984; Kachar and Reese, 1985; Terazaki et al., 1987). The microtubules and neurofilaments that form the axonal cytoskeleton may attach to this "motor" indirectly, perhaps through linking polymers of spectrin, and be towed through the axon at the SCa rate (Hirokawa, 1982; Schnapp and Reese, 1982; McQuarrie et al., 1986; Weisenberg et al., 1987).

Axonal Transport in Regenerating Neurons

Regeneration often implies cell division or replacement. However, neuronal division or replacement (from a stem cell) is rarely observed following morphogenesis of either the central nervous system (CNS) or peripheral nervous system (PNS). Accordingly, "axonal regeneration" refers to the regrowth and reconnection of an axon, beginning at the proximal axon stump that remains following a break in the axon (axotomy). The distal axon stump undergoes "Wallerian" degeneration because it has been cut off from its nutrient source, the perikaryon.

In response to axotomy, the translational cytoplasm typically increases the production of structural proteins and membrane constituents and decreases the production of neurotransmitter-related proteins (Grafstein and McQuarrie, 1978). These changes are reflected in axonal transport by a reduction in the transport of FC materials that support synaptic transmission, and an increase in the transport of SC materials that contribute to the cytoskeleton and FC materials that contribute to the axolemma (Skene and Willard, 1981b; Gould et al., 1982; Alberghina et al., 1983; McQuarrie, 1983, 1988a). Another change is an increase in

the transport of tRNA at an intermediate rate. Transfer RNA apparently is utilized at the growth cone to shorten the half-lives of certain unidentified proteins by adding a single amino acid to an exposed amino group (Bachmair et al., 1986; Chakraborty et al., 1986; Shyne-Athwal et al., 1986).

There is also a robust increase in the transport of certain "growth associated proteins" (GAPs) carried by FC (Skene and Willard, 1981a,c). GAP-43 shows the most pronounced increase, the time course of which coincides with axonal regrowth. It is a neuron-specific axolemmal protein that appears to have internal polar groups, suggesting a capability for interaction with the cytoskeleton (Skene and Willard, 1981a; McGuire et al., 1987). Electron microscopic (EM) immunocytochemistry of normal and regenerating neural tissues, using monoclonal antibodies raised against GAP-43, show it to be localized in axon terminals, growth cones, and Schwann cells that have been contacted by growth cones (Bisby et al., 1987). These findings suggest that GAP-43 is secreted by growth cones to become incorporated into the plasmalemma of Schwann cells.

GAP-43 can be phosphorylated by protein kinase C, and this posttranslational modification appears to increase the capacity of growth cones to both buffer free calcium and phosphorylate certain proteins (Benowitz, 1984; Burgess et al., 1986; Jacobson et al., 1986; Meiri et al., 1986; Akers and Routtenberg, 1987; Perry et al., 1987; Snipes et al., 1987). While there is some evidence that these changes can facilitate axonal outgrowth, outgrowth can proceed in the absence of GAPs (Perry et al., 1983; Lozano et al., 1987; Bisby et al., 1988).

To analyze axonal transport changes during nerve regeneration, it is important to appreciate that these are influenced by the *phases of regeneration,* which are sprouting, elongation, and maturation (Fig. 3–2), and the *metabolic differences* between neuronal types (Bisby, 1982; McQuarrie, 1983, 1988a; Benowitz, 1984; Willard et al., 1984). Accordingly, the changes during regeneration have been documented below for two neuronal types, one in the CNS and one in the PNS, taking care to correlate these changes with the phase of regeneration. Retinal ganglion cells of goldfish and sciatic motor neurons of rats have been

NORMAL NEURON

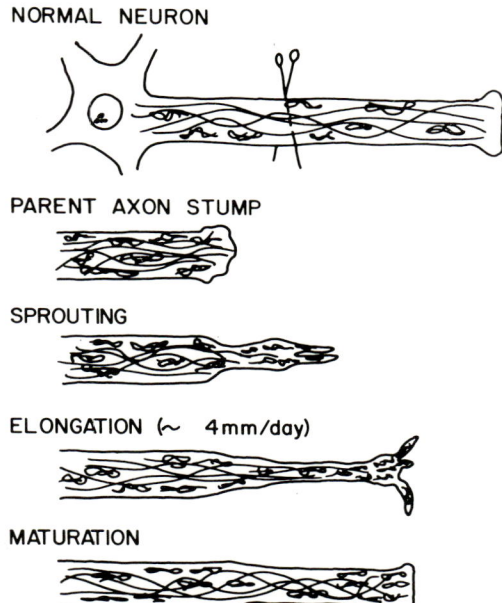

PARENT AXON STUMP

SPROUTING

ELONGATION (~ 4mm/day)

MATURATION

Figure 3–2. The three phases of axonal regeneration in a mammalian peripheral motor axon. Phase one is sprout formation, an activity that depends on growth cone function and requires the ability to rapidly polymerize monomeric actin (G-actin) into actin microfilaments (F-actin), and to rapidly disassemble F-actin to G-actin. Phase two is sprout elongation and depends on the ability to assemble microtubules from dimers of tubulin plus microtubule associated proteins such as tau factors. Phase three is radial growth, which largely depends on the axonal transport of assembled neurofilaments into sprouts after these have reconnected with an appropriate end organ. Reproduced from McQuarrie, 1983, with permission of the publisher.

chosen because these exhibit robust axonal regeneration and as a result have been well studied. The changes in protein transport have been examined most closely, so these will be reviewed in some detail.

CHANGES IN FAST COMPONENT
Optic Nerve Regeneration in Goldfish

CHANGES IN RATE AND AMOUNT OF PROTEIN TRANSPORT

The maximum rate for FC in unoperated goldfish optic nerves is 40–100 mm/d; the rate doubles between the second and tenth day af-

ter the optic tract has been cut (McEwen and Grafstein, 1968; McQuarrie and Grafstein, 1982a). The amount of protein being transported also appears to increase, beginning within 18–24 hr after axotomy; by 2 weeks there is a 5–20-fold increase in the amount of pulse-labeled protein being carried by FC (Grafstein and McQuarrie, 1978; McQuarrie and Grafstein, 1982a; Perry et al., 1987).

These changes correlate mainly with the elongation phase of axonal regeneration. Sprout formation begins 2–3 d after axotomy (Lanners and Grafstein, 1980), and leading axons begin to cross the lesion by 5 d (McQuarrie and Grafstein, 1981; McQuarrie, 1985a). These elongate at approximately 0.4 mm/d and begin to reach the contralateral tectum in large numbers 12–16 d after a crush or cut of the optic nerve (Ingoglia et al., 1973; McQuarrie and Grafstein, 1981; Heacock and Agranoff, 1982; Stuermer and Easter, 1984). Synapse formation begins by the end of the third week, coincident with the return of primitive visual reflexes to near-normal thresholds (Edwards et al., 1981; Murray and Edwards, 1982; Stuermer and Easter, 1984).

CHANGES IN PROTEIN COMPOSITION

To evaluate the composition of FC after optic nerve crush, the eye is injected with a radiolabeled amino acid 6–24 h before retrieving the optic nerve and tract (Perry et al., 1987). The nerve and tract are separately homogenized, following which the proteins are separated by SDS-PAGE. A fluorogram is used for locating labeled proteins in the gel; these are removed for radioactivity determination by liquid scintillation spectrometry. Ideally, proteins are separated by 2D-PAGE. This approach has been used after optic nerve crush by Perry et al. (1987), who find that no new FC proteins appear in either the "parent axons" of the optic nerve segment or the newly formed sprouts ("daughter axons") of the optic tract segment. However, each of the 30 most heavily labeled proteins show increased labeling, with GAP-43 having the greatest increase in both parent and daughter axons. Of the four proteins that are most heavily labeled in daughter axons, the three other than GAP-43 are all glycoproteins, as judged by the incorporation of labeled glucosamine (Perry et al., 1987). This is not surprising, since studies using the protein glycosylation inhibitor tunicamycin indicate that glycoprotein transport is essential for the regrowth of goldfish optic axons (Heacock, 1982).

Motor Neuron Regeneration in Rats

CHANGES IN RATE AND AMOUNT OF PROTEIN TRANSPORT

Axonal regeneration is a more orderly process in motor neurons than sensory neurons, apparently because the growth cones of motor neurons sprout with a more uniform latency and advance at a narrower range of rates (Bisby, 1979, 1985). Possibly this is because there are many types and sizes of sensory neurons but only two types of motor neurons, alpha and gamma, and only the alpha motor neurons appear to regenerate during the first month after axotomy (Brown and Butler, 1976; Takano, 1976).

The normal rate of FC in mammalian PNS axons is close to 400 mm/d, regardless of differences in taxonomic class, axon diameter, degree of myelination, physiological function (motor, sensory, autonomic), or frequency of action potentials (Ochs and Worth, 1978). The only physiological event that appears to affect the rate of FC is embryonic and neonatal development, during which the rate is slower than in adult animals (Grafstein and Forman, 1980). There is practically no delay in the onset of fast transport following the injection of labeled amino acids: incorporation is complete within 10–15 min, and labeled proteins enter the axon immediately thereafter (Ochs and Worth, 1978).

To examine FC in the newly formed axons of regenerating motor neurons, Griffin et al. (1976) have injected the spinal cord with tritiated leucine at various intervals after freezing the L4-L6 spinal nerves. They find no change of rate (compared with contralateral control axons) in parent axons, no accumulation of label or slowing at the level of axotomy, and no slowing in daughter axons. The only differences from normal are that the amount of labeled material carried by FC doubles during axonal elongation, and labeled tubulovesicular structures are seen to accumulate in growth cones. When glycoproteins are labeled (by injecting tritiated fucose into the spinal cord),

this accumulation is more pronounced, and EM autoradiography shows that tubulovesicular structures are incorporated into the new axolemma as it is laid down behind the advancing growth cone (Griffin et al., 1981).

CHANGES IN PROTEIN COMPOSITION

Motor axons are rich in acetylcholine esterase (AChE), a protein carried by FC. During axonal regeneration, a decrease in AChE transport begins at 1 d, falls to its lowest level at 5–11 d, and recovers by 21–29 d after axotomy (Heiwall et al., 1979). When FC proteins are labeled with [^{35}S]methionine and separated by SDS-PAGE, fluorograms show increases in labeling for two bands at 18 and 66 kD, and a decrease in one band at 13 kD (Bisby, 1980). In each case, the change begins after 1–3 d, reaches maximum at 7–14 d, and recovers by 21–42 d. This time course corresponds to the elongation and maturation phases of axonal regeneration. Sprouting begins at 1–2 d after crush, following which the leading axons advance at approximately 4 mm/d (Griffin et al., 1976; Forman and Berenberg, 1978; Bisby, 1985). The withdrawal reflex recovers in 50% of animals by 19–20 d (Bijlsma, 1981). The sciatic functional index (calculated from an assessment of walking pattern and footprints) reflects a more advanced stage of motor function; it begins to recover at 12 d and exhibits full recovery by 25–30 d (Bisby, 1985).

In the only study of FC composition in regenerating sciatic motor neurons of the rat, Bisby (1980) reports no change for polypeptides in the SDS molecular mass range of GAP-43. Since GAP proteins had not been described at the time of this report, and special attention must be given to buffer conditions to dissolve GAP-43 in aqueous solutions, the absence of a change does not mean that one did not occur. It is likely that GAP-43 does increase during axonal outgrowth in rodents, since an increase has been found in motor neurons of the rabbit (Skene and Willard, 1981c).

CHANGES IN SLOW COMPONENT
Optic Nerve Regeneration in Goldfish

CHANGES IN RATE AND AMOUNT OF PROTEIN TRANSPORT

In both normal and regenerating optic axons, the peak of labeling for SCa advances in parent axons at 0.02 mm/d and the leading edge at 0.1 mm/d (McQuarrie, 1984; McQuarrie et al., 1985). Preliminary studies suggest that the amount of SCa labeling is reduced in parent axons by 2 weeks after axotomy (McQuarrie, 1984).

The peak of labeling for SCb normally advances at approximately 0.4 mm/d (Grafstein and Murray, 1969; Grafstein et al., 1971; Heacock and Agranoff, 1982; McQuarrie and Grafstein, 1982b). During regeneration, it accelerates to approximately 1.0 mm/d, a change that begins 6–8 d after axotomy and is maximal at 14–17 d (Grafstein and Murray, 1969; McQuarrie and Grafstein, 1982b; Grafstein, 1986). Thus the increase in transport rate specifically coincides with the elongation phase of axonal regeneration, as first demonstrated by Grafstein (1971).

The amount of labeled SCb proteins being conveyed in the 3-mm segment of nerve on the eye side of the crush begins to increase at 1 d and reaches a maximum of 7 times normal at 15 d (McQuarrie and Grafstein, 1982b). Since the increase begins before the onset of increased protein synthesis at the nerve cell body (at 4–5 d), it is presumably due to the diversion of perikaryal proteins to the injured axon (Grafstein and McQuarrie, 1978). A similar diversion is seen for FC beginning 18–24 h after axotomy (Grafstein and McQuarrie, 1978).

CHANGES IN PROTEIN COMPOSITION

For SCa, preliminary studies suggest that there is a decrease in the labeling of neurofilament polypeptides by 2 weeks after nerve crush (McQuarrie, 1984). SCb normally carries most of the actin and tubulin, and during regeneration there are increases in the transport of both to reach maximum amounts that are approximately tenfold greater than the overall three-to-tenfold increase in SCb labeling (Giulian et al., 1980; Heacock and Agranoff, 1982; McQuarrie, 1984). The same compositional change is seen in the regenerating toad optic nerve (Skene and Willard, 1981b). These prompt and large-scale increases are supported by a fivefold increase in protein synthesis that is associated with a tripling of both perikaryal cross-sectional area and nucleoli per cell (McQuarrie and Grafstein, 1982b).

The importance of SCb changes for regeneration can be recognized when a second nerve lesion is made after the changes are maximal at 2 weeks (McQuarrie, 1984). The first lesion then "conditions" the neuron for growth; after a 2-week "conditioning interval," the second lesion tests the effect on outgrowth of waiting until the vast increase in SCb transport has reached the site of the testing lesion. The effect is dramatic: the initial delay before sprouts start to elongate is halved, and the rate of elongation is doubled. Associated with this acceleration of outgrowth are a further 60% increase in protein synthesis and a doubling of both the rate and amount of SCb transport; FC is unchanged (McQuarrie and Grafstein, 1982b; McQuarrie, 1984). The inescapable conclusion is that the delivery of cytomatrix proteins via SCb is rate-limiting for outgrowth.

Motor Neuron Regeneration in Rats

CHANGES IN RATE AND AMOUNT OF PROTEIN TRANSPORT

The transport rates for the peaks of labeling of SCa and SCb are normal, in both parent and daughter axons (Hoffman and Lasek, 1980; McQuarrie and Lasek, 1988). However, there are changes in the overall amounts of transport that reflect protein synthesis changes at the nerve cell body in response to axotomy (Hoffman and Lasek, 1980). By the end of elongation phase (20 d after crush), such changes have produced a 30% decrease in SCa labeling and a 75% increase in SCb labeling in parent axons. With respect to daughter axons, SCb-labeled materials evidently enter sprouts without difficulty (McQuarrie and Lasek, 1989). However, SCa-labeled materials are retained in the parent axon stump, presumably because the thin sprouts cannot accept the large numbers of microtubules and neurofilaments that continue to advance through parent axons (Friede and Bischhausen, 1980; McQuarrie and Lasek, 1989).

CHANGES IN PROTEIN COMPOSITION

The principal change in SCa composition is a 60–70% reduction in neurofilament labeling (relative to tubulin labeling), which begins 3 d after axotomy and is maximal at 2–3 weeks (Hoffman et al., 1985). This decrease is reflected morphologically by a reduction in the caliber of parent axons, which advances distally at the SCa rate. After the elongation phase of axonal regeneration is complete, neurofilament transport and axonal caliber begin to return to normal. In a different study of SCa in parent axons at 20 d after axotomy, Hoffman and Lasek (1980) have found that the labeling of neurofilament polypeptides is reduced 30–40% in association with a 20–25% reduction in tubulin labeling. In daughter axons, SCa is reduced overall, and the amount of labeled neurofilament proteins relative to tubulin is only 30% of that seen in parent axons (McQuarrie and Lasek, 1989). For SCb in parent axons, with labeling at 20 d after axotomy, the amounts of actin are normal, but the amounts of tubulin are more than twofold greater than normal (Hoffman and Lasek, 1980). These changes are ultimately reflected in daughter axons, since SCb-labeled proteins enter daughter axons with ease (McQuarrie and Lasek, 1989).

BASIS OF INCREASED PROTEIN TRANSPORT INTO DAUGHTER AXONS
Reorganization of Structures Within Parent Axon Stumps

In their study of changes in the rate, amount and composition of SC in parent axons of regenerating motor neurons, Hoffman and Lasek (1980) have concluded that "new outgrowth appears to be a fundamental property of the axon by virtue of the continuous movement of the cytoskeletal networks [and] this potential for cytoskeletal elongation during outgrowth results from organizational changes within the axon terminals and does not appear to require changes in transcription or translation in the cell body." Now that 8 years have passed, there is an increasing fund of knowledge to support this hypothesis (McQuarrie, 1988a). It almost follows intuitively from the fact that growing axons advance at approximately the same velocity as SCb, even when SCb advances at rates that are unusually fast or slow (McQuarrie and Grafstein, 1982b; Wujek and Lasek, 1983; McQuarrie, 1984).

The mechanism for partially preventing SCa neurofilaments and microtubules from entering sprouts (while allowing the entry of SCb proteins) is not yet understood. However, there are several types of posttranslational protein

modification that could be responsible, in addition to the physical constraint suggested above. Examples include activation of proteins by phosphorylation, and degradation of polymers by calcium-activated proteases, perhaps aided by N-terminal acylation (Shyne-Athwal et al., 1986; Larrivee and Grafstein, 1987; Liuzzi and Lasek, 1987).

Diversion of Existing Perikaryal Proteins to Axons

The initiation of fast transport in normal neurons requires ionic calcium; in its absence, proteins cannot be loaded onto the transport system (Hammerschlag et al., 1977; Grafstein and Forman, 1980). This calcium-dependent, cobalt-sensitive initiation step follows glycosylation and differs from the calcium requirement for ongoing fast transport. In regenerating neurons, there is evidence to suggest that the neuron can divert unusually large amounts of perikaryal proteins to both FC and SC, beginning within 24 h and lasting less than 1 week (Grafstein and McQuarrie, 1978; McQuarrie and Grafstein, 1982b). Diversion may be an important regulatory step because the increases are most dramatic in settings where sprout initiation is unusually rapid and robust. It has been suggested that the initiation of sprout formation is facilitated by these diversions (McQuarrie, 1985b), and that the resulting depletion of protein resources may potentiate (or even initiate) the changes in protein synthesis that occur in response to axotomy (McQuarrie and Grafstein, 1982b; McQuarrie, 1984).

Increased Perikaryal Protein Synthesis

It is now accepted that changes in perikaryal protein synthesis occur within days after axotomy, and that these mimic the program of synthesis seen in developing neurons (McQuarrie, 1984). The patterns of increased and decreased synthesis appear to be tailored to support the elongation phase of axonal regeneration (Grafstein and McQuarrie, 1978). In particular, the well-described increase in the fast transport of GAP-43 can be considered to facilitate regeneration (Bisby et al., 1988).

However, for axons that have been injured at loci more than a few centimeters from the perikaryon, only FC changes are likely to have an influence on outgrowth. Slow component changes would not have time to reach the growing axon tip, since daughter axons elongate at approximately the same rate as any increased amounts of structural proteins travel toward them (Hoffman and Lasek, 1980; McQuarrie, 1988a). However, if a second crush is made more proximally, at a locus where advantage can be taken of these changes, the axonal outgrowth that occurs following the second lesion is accelerated (McQuarrie and Grafstein, 1981; McQuarrie, 1984, 1985a, 1986, 1988a). This is called the "conditioning lesion effect" (McQuarrie et al., 1977).

Regulation of Axonal Transport Changes

The diversion of perikaryal protein resources to FC and SC soon after axotomy appears to be a reflexive and transient affair. As in the case of the more slowly developing changes in perikaryal protein synthesis, it may be initiated by a signal carried via retrograde fast transport (Bisby, 1984). This apparently happens through the nonarrival of trophic factors that are transferred to axons from Schwann cells located along the distal axon (Richardson and Verge, 1986; McQuarrie, 1988b). In addition, there is a correspondence between the magnitude of diversion and the magnitude of changes in protein synthesis, suggesting that the depletion of perikaryal resources acts to stimulate synthesis through a negative feedback mechanism (McQuarrie and Grafstein, 1982b).

Finally, there is evidence that the nerve cell body receives accurate and timely information on the status of the growing axon tip via retrograde fast transport, since different GAPs are synthesized and transported during successive phases of regeneration (Benowitz et al., 1984; Bisby, 1984; Willard et al., 1984). While the mechanism of regulation is not yet understood in detail, it is becoming clear that both increases and decreases in the transfer of trophic factors from nonneuronal cells to the axon have a direct and ongoing influence on the program of protein synthesis at the nerve cell body, as well as having a local effect on growth cones (Gunderson, 1985; Hammerback et al., 1985; Richardson and Verge, 1986; McQuarrie, 1988b).

The rate of axonal outgrowth is influenced by the availability of neuronotrophic factors arising from nonneuronal cells in the nerve. This can be readily demonstrated by using the conditioning lesion effect (McQuarrie, 1984; Richardson and Verge, 1986). When a testing lesion of the sciatic nerve is made 2 weeks after a conditioning lesion of its distal branches, axonal outgrowth is accelerated (McQuarrie et al., 1977; McQuarrie, 1984). However, when both lesions are made at the same locus on the nerve, thereby forcing the second crop of sprouts to enter a predegenerated distal nerve stump, the acceleration is significantly greater than when the conditioning and testing lesions are separated both spatially and temporally (Bisby and Pollock, 1983; Bisby, 1985). The additional acceleration of outgrowth (from 5.7 mm/d to 6.8 mm/d) can only be attributed to the different environment being traversed by the growth cone, whereas the basic acceleration (from 4.0 mm/d to 5.7 mm/d), which is seen when the second crop of axons enters a freshly degenerating distal nerve stump, can be attributed to an intrinsic response of the neuron to the loss of trophic input and the loss of cytoplasm (McQuarrie, 1988b). The predegenerated nerve presumably has a more stimulatory effect on outgrowth because it produces less of the trophic material that prevents the program of neuronal protein synthesis from reverting to the growth (embryonic) mode.

The acceleration of outgrowth appears to be a result of increases in SCb transport that are initiated by the conditioning axotomy. In part, this is a "diagnosis of exclusion," brought about by an inability to account for the increase in outgrowth rate by any of the changes in FC or SCa (McQuarrie and Grafstein, 1982b; Redshaw and Bisby, 1987; McQuarrie, 1988b). If there were an increase in the amount or composition of FC following a testing lesion, this could help explain accelerated outgrowth. However, there is no alteration in the changes that had been caused by the conditioning lesion, except that the transport of GAP-43 may have decreased (Redshaw and Bisby, 1987). With regard to SCa, there is a reduction in neurofilament protein transport that begins within 3 d and does not recover until outgrowth is complete and the daughter axons begin to exhibit radial growth (Hoffman et al., 1985). Since the ongoing transport of normal numbers

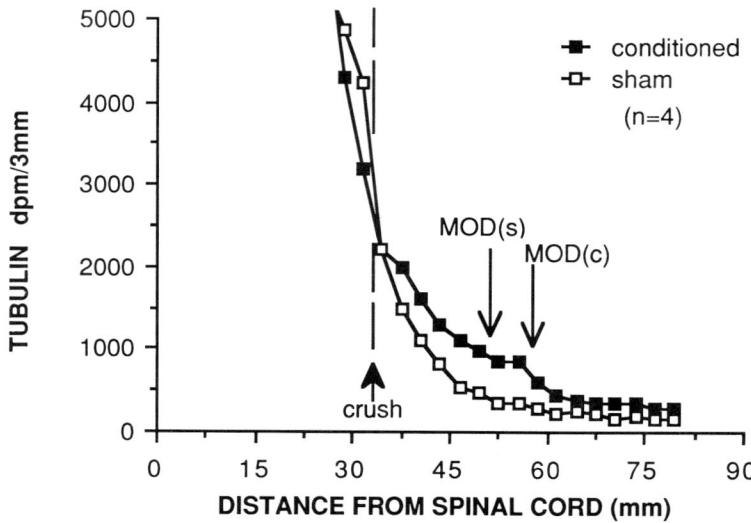

Figure 3–3. The distribution of mean amounts of labeled tubulin in motor axons of the rat sciatic nerve at 11 d after microinjection of the lumbar spinal cord with [^{35}S]methionine. Animals were killed for retrieval of tissues at 4 d after the testing lesion (crush). In four animals, a conditioning crush lesion was made at 90 mm from the spinal cord 7 d prior to isotope injection; four paired control animals received sham conditioning lesions. Rats weighed 170–200 gm at the time of injection. Conditioned animals received 769 ± 97 μCi of [^{35}S]methionine, and sham-conditioned animals received 806 ± 103 μCi. A testing lesion was made at the junction of the L4 and L5 spinal nerves 7 d after isotope injection (14 d after the conditioning lesion). Consecutive 3-mm nerve segments of the L4 and L5 ventral roots, L4 and L5 spinal nerves, and sciatic nerve were processed for SDS-PAGE, fluorography, and protein solubilization for liquid scintillation counting (McQuarrie et al., 1986). For plotted points, the standard error of the mean was less than 20% of the mean in over 90% of nerve segments. The mean maximum outgrowth distances (MOD) for conditioned (c) and sham-conditioned (s) nerves are indicated by arrows. The MOD in each nerve is the most distal nerve segment carrying a peak of actin labeling colocated with a peak of labeling for polypeptides at 58–76 kD, a zone enriched in MAPs identified as tau factors and chartins; the MOD located by this method corresponds to the location of growth cones identified by labeling FC (McQuarrie, 1986; McQuarrie and Lasek, 1989). The same MOD points are marked in Figure 3–4, which plots the distribution of actin labeling in the same nerves.

of neurofilaments may conceivably frustrate outgrowth, a reduction in neurofilament transport could facilitate outgrowth. The conditioning lesion paradigm would take advantage of this, if the testing lesion were placed where axonal thinning had occurred because of reduced neurofilament transport. However, the wave of thinning moves distally at the SCa rate of approximately 1 mm/d, and there is not sufficient time for it to reach the testing lesion site in most models of the conditioning lesion effect.

To demonstrate that the conditioning lesion effect is a result of an augmentation of SCb, this augmentation must be shown to reach the testing lesion (and the accelerated daughter axons) in greater amounts after a conditioning lesion than after a sham conditioning lesion. This has been shown to occur in motor axons of the rat sciatic nerve. The conditioning lesion of sciatic nerve branches is made 90 mm from the spinal cord and followed 2 weeks later by a testing crush made 33 mm from the spinal cord (McQuarrie, 1986). The outgrowth rate after the testing lesion is 5.3 mm/d in conditioned axons vs. 4.6 mm/d in sham-conditioned axons. When newly synthesized proteins are labeled with [^{35}S]methionine 7 d before the

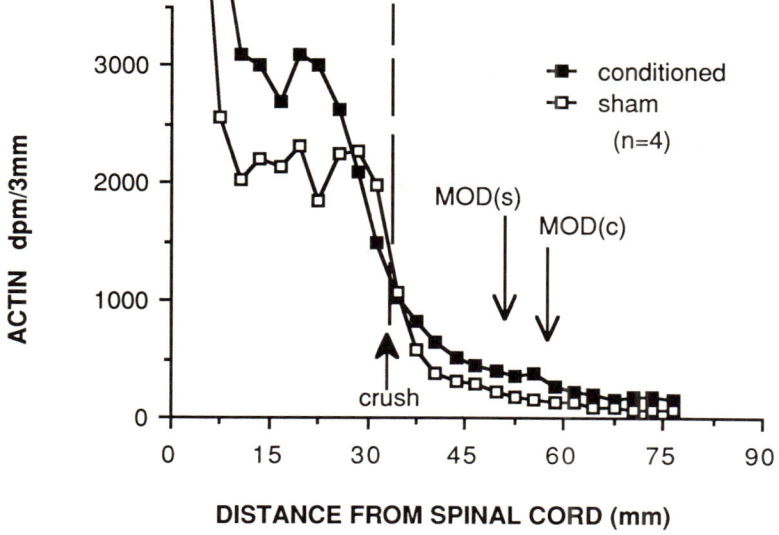

Figure 3–4. The distribution of mean amounts of labeled actin in motor axons of the rat sciatic nerve in 11 d after microinjection of the lumbar spinal cord with [^{35}S]methionine and 4 d after a testing lesion (same nerves and legend as Fig. 3–3).

testing lesion, the leading foot of SCb labeling reaches the testing crush as it is being made, since the peak of SCb labeling advances at 3 mm/d and the leading foot advances at 5–6 mm/d, in both lesioned and unlesioned nerves (McQuarrie et al. 1986; McQuarrie and Lasek, 1988). In Figs. 3–3 and 3–4, the distributions of labeling for tubulin and actin in motor axons of the rat sciatic nerve are shown at 4 d after the testing lesion, by which time SCb would have passed into the daughter axons but SCa would still be confined to parent axons. Daughter axons responding to a conditioning lesion show increases in labeling for actin and tubulin. (While there is no difference in SCa tubulin levels in parent axons, levels for SCa actin are almost twofold higher in response to the conditioning lesion.) When the interval after the testing crush is lengthened to 8 d, increases for tubulin and actin labeling in conditioned daughter axons are seen to persist (McQuarrie, 1986). These findings indicate that increased amounts of SCb tubulin and actin have reached daughter axons, and that these increases are associated with a sustained acceleration of outgrowth.

CONCLUSIONS

All the principal rate components of axonal transport (FC, SCa, SCb, and retrograde FC) appear to support nerve regeneration. The fast component carries additional membrane packets and a growth-associated protein that facilitates new membrane formation while carrying a reduced amount of neurotransmitter-related proteins—apparently for reasons of metabolic economy, since these proteins are unnecessary until the final phase of regeneration (Grafstein and McQuarrie, 1978). SCa carries a reduced number of neurofilaments, perhaps for the same reason. SCb has key structural elements that are already in transit within parent axons; the rate of sprout elongation appears to depend on them. Retrograde FC signals the perikaryon that an axotomy has occurred and provides it with a continuous flow of information concerning the status of the growth cone and its surroundings. This information is used to regulate the cell body response to axotomy, and to fine tune support for regenerating axons.

One interesting change that occurs in response to axotomy is an augmentation in the transport of tubulin and actin via SCb, even though this support is unlikely to reach distant sprouts (which elongate at approximately the SCb rate) in time to speed outgrowth. This augmentation can accelerate outgrowth and increase the frequency of elongating sprouts (McQuarrie, 1985b). It is a change that may have evolved when organisms were small enough to benefit from it. This hypothesis seems reasonable, since there are many parallels between regenerative axonal growth and regenerative flagellar growth (McQuarrie, 1984). Finally, the conditioning lesion effect has important implications for understanding the mechanism of axonal growth, since it highlights the role played by the cytomatrix in laying down a structural framework behind the advancing growth cone.

REFERENCES

Akers RF, Routtenberg A (1987): Calcium-promoted translocation of protein kinase C to synaptic membranes: Relation to phosphorylation of an endogenous substrate (protein F1) involved in synaptic plasticity. J Neurosci 7:3976–3983.

Alberghina M, Moschella F, Viola M, Brancati V, Micali G, Guiffrida AM (1983): Changes in rapid transport of phospholipids in the rat sciatic nerve during axonal regeneration. J Neurochem 40:32–38.

Baas PW, Heidemann SR (1986): Microtubule reassembly from nucleating fragments during the regrowth of amputated neurites. J Cell Biol 103:917–927.

Bachmair A, Finley D, Varshavsky A (1986): In vivo half-life of a protein is a function of its amino-terminal residue. Science 234:179–186.

Baitinger C, Willard M (1987): Axonal transport of synapsin I-like proteins in rabbit retinal ganglion cells. J Neurosci 7:3723–3735.

Benowitz LI (1984): Target-dependent and target-independent changes in rapid axonal transport during regeneration of the goldfish retinotectal pathway. In Elam JS, Cancalon P (eds): "Axonal Transport in Neuronal Growth and Regeneration. Advances in Neurochemistry," vol 6. New York: Plenum Press, pp 145–169.

Bijlsma WA, Jennekens FGI, Schotman P, Gispen WH (1981): Effects of corticotrophin (ACTH) on recovery of sensorimotor function in the rat: Structure-activity study. Eur J Pharmacol 76:73–79.

Bisby MA (1979): Differences in incorporation of axonally transported protein in regenerating motor and sensory axons. Exp Neurol 65:680–684.

Bisby MA (1980): Changes in the composition of labeled protein transported in motor axons during their regeneration. J Neurobiol 5:435–445.

Bisby MA (1982): Prolonged alteration in composition of fast transported protein in axons prevented from regenerating after injury. J Neurobiol 13:377–381.

Bisby MA (1984): Retrograde axonal transport and nerve regeneration. In Elam JS, Cancalon P (eds): "Axonal Transport in Neuronal Growth and Regeneration. Advances in Neurochemistry," vol 6. New York: Plenum Press, pp 45–67.

Bisby MA (1985): Enhancement of the conditioning lesion effect in rat sciatic motor axons after superimposition of conditioning and test lesions. Exp Neurol 90:385–394.

Bisby MA, Pollock B (1983): Increased regeneration rate in peripheral nerve axons following double lesions: Enhancement of the conditioning lesion phenomenon. J Neurobiol 14:467–472.

Bisby MA, Zweirs H, Tetzlaff W (1987): Localization and axonal transport of B50 (GAP43) in regenerating rat peripheral nerves: Association with outgrowing axons and Schwann cells. Soc Neurosci Abstr 13:1206.

Bisby MA, Redshaw JD, Carlsen RC, Reh TA, Zweirs H (1988): Growth associated proteins (GAPS) and axonal regeneration. In Gordon T, Stein RB, Smith PA (eds): "The Current Status of Peripheral Nerve Regeneration." Neurology and Neurobiology, vol 38. New York: Alan R. Liss, pp 35–52.

Brady ST (1985): A novel brain ATPase with properties expected for the fast axonal transport motor. Nature 317:73–75.

Brady ST, Black MM (1986): Axonal transport of microtubule proteins: Cytotypic variations of tubulin and MAPs in neurons. Ann NY Acad Sci USA 466:199–217.

Brown MC, Butler RG (1976): Regeneration of afferent and efferent fibres to muscle spindles after nerve injury in adult cats. J Physiol (Lond) 260:253–266.

Burgess SK, Sahyoun N, Blanchard SG, Levine H, Chang K-J, Cuatrecasas P (1986): Phorbol ester receptors and protein kinase C in primary neuronal cultures: Development and stimulation of endogenous phosphorylation. J Cell Biol 102:312–319.

Cancalon P (1985): Influence of temperature on various mechanisms associated with neuronal growth and nerve regeneration. Prog Neurobiol 25:27–92.

Chakraborty G, Leach T, Zanakis MF, Ingoglia NA (1986): Posttranslational protein modification by amino acid addition in regenerating optic nerves of goldfish. J Neurochem 46:726–732.

Cheng TPO, Schnapp BJ, Sheetz MP, Reese TS (1987): Immunocytochemical localization of kinesin in the squid giant axon. Soc Neurosci Abstr 13:122.

Edwards DL, Alpert RM, Grafstein B (1981): Recovery of vision in regeneration of goldfish optic axons: Enhancement of axonal outgrowth by a conditioning lesion. Exp Neurol 72:672–686.

Forman DS, Berenberg RA (1978): Regeneration of motor axons in the rat sciatic nerve studied by labeling with axonally transported radioactive proteins. Brain Res 156:213–225.

Friede RL, Bischhausen R (1980): The fine structure of stumps of transected nerve fibers in subserial sections. J Neurol Sci 44:181–203.

Giulian D, DesRuisseaux H, Cowburn D (1980): Biosynthesis and intra-axonal transport of proteins during neuronal regeneration. J Biol Chem 255:6494–6501.

Gould RM, Spivack WD, Sinatra RS, Lindquist TD, Ingoglia NA (1982): Axonal transport of choline lipids in normal and regenerating rat sciatic nerve. J Neurochem 39:1569–1578.

Grafstein B (1971): Role of slow axonal transport in nerve regeneration. Acta Neuropath (Berl) Suppl V: 144–152.

Grafstein B (1986): The retina as a regenerating organ. In Adler R, Farber DB (eds): "The Retina: A Model for Cell Biology Studies, Part II." New York: Academic Press, pp 275–335.

Grafstein B, Murray M (1969): Transport of protein in goldfish optic nerve during regeneration. Exp Neurol 25:494–508.

Grafstein B, McQuarrie IG (1978): Role of the nerve cell body in axonal regeneration. In Cotman CW (ed): "Neuronal Plasticity." New York: Raven Press, pp 155–195.

Grafstein B, Forman DS (1980): Intracellular transport in neurons. Physiol Rev 60:1167–1283.

Grafstein B, McEwen BS, Shelanski M (1971): Axonal transport of neurotubule protein. Nature 227:289–290.

Griffin JW, Drachman DB, Price DL (1976): Fast axonal transport in motor nerve regeneration. J Neurobiol 7: 355–370.

Griffin JW, Price DL, Drachman DB, Morris J (1981): Incorporation of axonally transported glycoproteins into axolemma during nerve regeneration. J Cell Biol 88: 205–214.

Gundersen RW (1985): Sensory neurite growth cone guidance by substrate adsorbed nerve growth factor. J Neurosci Res 13:199–212.

Hammerback JA, Palm SL, Furcht LT, Letourneau PC (1985): Guidance of neurite outgrowth by pathways of substratum-adsorbed laminin. J Neurosci Res 13:213–220.

Hammerschlag R, Bakhit C, Chiu AY (1977): Role of calcium in the initiation of fast axonal transport of protein: Effects of divalent cations. J Neurobiol 8:439–451.

Heacock AM (1982): Glycoprotein requirement for neurite outgrowth in goldfish retinal explants: Effect of tunicamycin. Brain Res 241:307–315.

Heacock AM, Agranoff BW (1982): Protein synthesis and transport in the regenerating goldfish visual system. Neurochem Res 7:771–788.

Heiwall PO, Dahlstrom A, Larsson PA, Booj S (1979): The intra-axonal transport of acetylcholine and cholinergic enzymes in rat sciatic nerve during regeneration after various types of trauma. J Neurobiol 10:119–136.

Hirokawa N (1982): Cross-linker system between neurofilaments, microtubules, and membranous organelles in frog axons revealed by the quick-freeze, deep-etching method. J Cell Biol 94:129–142.

Hoffman PN, Lasek RJ (1980): Axonal transport of the cytoskeleton in regenerating motor neurons: Constancy and change. Brain Res 202:317–333.

Hoffman PN, Thompson GW, Griffin JW, Price DL (1985): Changes in neurofilament transport coincide temporally with alterations in the caliber of axons in regenerating motor fibers. J Cell Biol 101:1332–1340.

Ingoglia NA, Grafstein B, McEwen BS, McQuarrie IG (1973): Axonal transport of radioactivity in the goldfish optic system following intraocular injection of labelled RNA precursors. J Neurochem 20:1605–1615.

Jacobson RD, Virag I, Skene JHP (1986): A protein associated with axon growth, GAP-43, is widely distributed and developmentally regulated in rat CNS. J Neurosci 6:1843–1855.

Kachar B, Reese TS (1985): Mechanism of cytoplasmic streaming in giant characean algae cells: Possible relationship to slow axonal transport. Soc Neurosci Abstr 11:1134.

Karlsson J-O, Sjostrand J (1971): Synthesis, migration and turnover of protein in axons of retinal ganglion cells. J Neurochem 18:749–767.

Lanners HN, Grafstein B (1980): Early stages of axonal regeneration in the goldfish optic tract: An electron microscopic study. J Neurocytol 9:733–751.

Larrivee DC, Grafstein B (1987): In vivo phosphorylation of axonal proteins in goldfish optic nerve during regeneration. J Neurochem 48:279–283.

Lasek RJ, Brady ST (1982): The axon: A prototype for studying expressional cytoplasm. Cold Spring Harbor Symp Quant Biol 46:113–124.

Lasek RJ, Garner JA, Brady ST (1984): Axonal transport of the cytoplasmic matrix. J Cell Biol 99:212s–221s.

Liuzzi FJ, Lasek RJ (1987): Astrocytes block axonal regeneration in mammals by activating the physiological stop pathway. Science 237:642–645.

Lozano AM, Doster SK, Aquayo AJ, Willard MB (1987): Immunoreactivity to GAP-43 in axotomized and regenerating retinal ganglion cells of adult rats. Soc Neurosci Abstr 13:1389.

McEwen BS, Grafstein B (1968): Fast and slow components in axonal transport of protein. J Cell Biol 38:494–508.

McGuire CB, Snipes GJ, Norden JJ (1987): Immunochemical evidence that a growth-associated protein (GAP-43) is localized specifically to developing neuronal processes and mature presynaptic terminals. Soc Neurosci Abstr 13:1481.

McQuarrie IG (1983): Role of the axonal cytoskeleton in the regenerating nervous system. In Seil FJ (ed): "Nerve, Organ, and Tissue Regeneration: Research Perspectives." New York: Academic Press, pp 51–88.

McQuarrie IG (1984): Effect of a conditioning lesion on axonal transport during regeneration. The role of slow transport. In Elam JS, Cancalon P (eds): "Axonal Transport in Neuronal Growth and Regeneration. Advances in Neurochemistry," vol 6. New York: Plenum Publishing Corp., pp 185–209.

McQuarrie IG (1985a): Stages of axonal regeneration following optic nerve crush in goldfish: Contrasting effects of conditioning nerve lesions and intraocular acetoxycycloheximide injections. Brain Res 333:247–253.

McQuarrie IG (1985b): Effect of a conditioning lesion on axonal sprout formation at nodes of Ranvier. J Comp Neurol 231:239–249.

McQuarrie IG (1986): Structural protein transport in elongating motor axons after sciatic nerve crush. Neurochem Pathol 5:153–164.

McQuarrie IG (1988a): Transport of cytoskeletal proteins

into axonal sprouts during nerve regeneration. In Gordon T, Stein RB, Smith PA (eds): "The Current Status of Peripheral Nerve Regeneration." Neurology and Neurobiology, vol 38. New York: Alan R. Liss, pp 25–34.

McQuarrie IG (1988b): Neuronal metabolic basis of the conditioning lesion effect. In Flohr H (ed): "Post-Lesion Neural Plasticity." Berlin: Springer-Verlag, in press.

McQuarrie IG, Grafstein B (1981): Effect of a conditioning lesion on optic nerve regeneration in goldfish. Brain Res 216:253–264.

McQuarrie IG, Grafstein B (1982a): Protein synthesis and fast axonal transport in regenerating goldfish retinal ganglion cells. Brain Res 235:213–223.

McQuarrie IG, Grafstein B (1982b): Protein synthesis and axonal transport in goldfish retinal ganglion cells during regeneration accelerated by a conditioning lesion. Brain Res 251:25–37.

McQuarrie IG, Lasek RJ (1989): Transport of cytoskeletal elements from parent axons into regenerating daughter axons. J Neurosci: In press.

McQuarrie IG, Grafstein B, Gershon, MD (1977): Axonal regeneration in the rat sciatic nerve: Effect of a conditioning lesion and of dbcAMP. Brain Res 132:443–453.

McQuarrie IG, Phillips LL, Autilio-Gambetti L (1985): Neurofilament proteins in goldfish optic axons. Ann NY Acad Sci 455:792–793.

McQuarrie IG, Brady ST, Lasek RJ (1986): Diversity in the axonal transport of structural proteins: Major differences between optic and spinal axons in the rat. J Neurosci 6:1593–1605.

Meiri KF, Pfenninger KH, Willard M (1986): Growth-associated protein, GAP-43, a polypeptide that is induced when neurons extend axons, is a component of growth cones and corresponds to pp46, a major polypeptide of a subcellular fraction enriched in growth cones. Proc Natl Acad Sci USA 83:3537–3541.

Murray M, Edwards MA (1982): A quantitative study of the reinnervation of the goldfish optic tectum following nerve crush. J Comp Neurol 209:363–373.

Oblinger MM, Brady ST, McQuarrie IG, Lasek RJ (1987): Cytotypic differences in the protein composition of the axonally transported cytoskeleton in mammalian neurons. J Neurosci 7:453–462.

Ochs S, Worth RM (1978): Axoplasmic transport in normal and pathological systems. In Waxman SG (ed): "Physiology and Pathophysiology of Axons." New York: Raven Press, pp 251–264.

Paschal BM, Vallee RB (1987): Retrograde transport by the microtubule-associated protein MAP 1C. Nature 330:181–183.

Paschal BM, Shpetner HS, Vallee RB (1987): MAP 1C is a microtubule-activated ATPase which translocates microtubules in vitro and has dynein-like properties. J Cell Biol 105:1273–1282.

Perry GW, Krayanek SR, Wilson DL (1983): Protein synthesis and rapid axonal transport during regrowth of dorsal root axons. J Neurochem 40:1590–1598.

Perry GW, Burmeister DW, Grafstein G (1987): Fast axonally transported proteins in regenerating goldfish optic axons. J Neurosci 7:792–806.

Redshaw JD, Bisby MA (1987): Proteins of fast axonal transport in regenerating rat sciatio sensory axons: A conditioning lesion does not amplify the characteristic response to axotomy. Exp Neurol 98:212–221.

Richardson PM, Verge VMK (1986): The induction of a regenerative propensity in sensory neurons following peripheral axonal injury. J Neurocytol 15:585–594.

Schnapp BJ, Reese TS (1982): Cytoplasmic structure in rapid-frozen axons. J Cell Biol 94:667–679.

Skene JHP, Willard M (1981a): Characteristics of growth-associated polypeptides in regenerating toad retinal ganglion cell axons. J Neurosci 1:419–426.

Skene JHP, Willard M (1981b): Changes in axonally transported proteins during axon regeneration in toad retinal ganglion cells. J Cell Biol 89:86–95.

Skene JHP, Willard M (1981c): Axonally transported proteins associated with axon growth in rabbit central and peripheral nervous systems. J Cell Biol 89:96–103.

Sheetz MP, Chasan R, Spudich JA (1984): ATP-dependent movement of myosin in vitro: Characterization of a quantitative assay. J Cell Biol 99:1867–1871.

Shyne-Athwal S, Riccio RV, Chakraborty G, Ingoglia NA (1986): Protein modification by amino acid addition is increased in crushed sciatic but not optic nerves. Science 231:603–606.

Snipes GJ, Chan SY, McGuire CB, Costello BR, Norden JJ, Freeman JA, Routtenberg A (1987): Evidence for the coidentification of GAP-43, a growth-associated protein, and F1, a plasticity-associated protein. J Neurosci 7:4066–4075.

Stuermer CAO, Easter SS (1984): A comparison of the normal and regenerated retinotectal pathways of goldfish. J Comp Neurol 223:57–76.

Takano K (1976): Absence of the gamma-spindle loop in the reinnervated hind leg muscles of the cat: "Alpha-muscle." Exp Brain Res 26:200–211.

Tashiro T, Kurokawa M, Komiya Y (1984): Two populations of axonally transported tubulin differentiated by their interactions with neurofilaments. J Neurochem 43:1220–1225.

Terazaki M, Gallant P, Reese TS (1987): Separation of endoplasmic reticulum from squid giant axon: Relationships to cytoskeletal elements and related proteins. J Cell Biol 105:128a.

Tytell M, Black MM, Garner J, Lasek RJ (1981): Axonal transport: Each rate component reflects the movement of distinct macromolecular complexes. Science 214:179–181.

Vale RD, Reese TS, Sheetz MP (1985): Identification of a novel force-generating protein, kinesin, involved in microtubule-based motility. Cell 42:39–50.

Weisenberg RC, Flynn J, Gao B, Awodi S, Skee F, Goodman SR, Riederer BM (1987): Microtubule gelation-contraction: Essential components and relation to slow axonal transport. Science 238:1119–1122.

Willard M, Skene JMP, Simon C, Mieri K, Hirokawa N, Glicksman M (1984): Regulation of axonal growth and cytoskeletal development. In Elam JS, Cancalon P (eds): "Axonal Transport in Neuronal Growth and Regeneration" (Advances in Neurochemistry, Vol. 6). New York: Plenum, pp 171–193.

Wujek JR, Lasek RJ (1983): Correlation of axonal regeneration and slow component B in two branches of a single axon. J Neurosci 3:243–251.

Zelena J (1972): Ribosomes in myelinated axons of dorsal root ganglia. Z Zellforsch 124:217–229.

4

Axon-Glial Interactions in Regeneration

STEPHEN G. WAXMAN, MD, PhD

Department of Neurology, Yale University School of Medicine, New Haven, Connecticut 06510; and PVA/EPVA Neuroscience and Regeneration Research Center, VA Medical Center, West Haven, Connecticut 06516

In order for regeneration to produce functional recovery following damage to the nervous system, a number of reparative events must occur. The regenerative response must include regrowth of axons from the injured neurons, guidance of these regrowing axons to appropriate regions, and formation of synapses with the correct target cells. Since the function of axons is to carry action potentials from one site to another in the nervous system, it is also necessary for growing axons to establish the capability for electrogenesis (the generation of nerve impulses) and reliable action potential transmission. In this respect, regeneration of axons involves not only regrowth of the fiber from the cell body, but also a recapitulation of active and passive electrical properties. Given the crucial importance of this problem in regeneration research, the purpose of the present chapter is to explore the available data concerning the development of electrical excitability in mammalian nerve fibers, and the role of glial or supporting cells in modulating the development of axonal excitability. As will be described below, the development of electrogenic mechanisms in axons does not occur in isolation, but rather reflects a complex set of interactions with nearby glial cells.

Myelinated fibers are surrounded by a myelin sheath, which consists of a nearly compact spiral of closely apposed glial cell membranes. The myelin sheath is produced by the Schwann cell in the peripheral nervous system (PNS) and by the oligodendrocyte in the central nervous system (CNS). These cells wrap around the axon in a spiral or "jelly-roll" configuration to form the myelin sheath. Following wrapping of the axon, most of the cytoplasm and extracellular space are extruded from the spiral of membranes, so that a relatively compact membranous structure, the myelin sheath, is formed around the axon. This compact structure imparts to the myelin a high electrical resistance and a low capacitance, characteristics that permit the myelin to function as an electrical insulator. The myelin sheath is interrupted at nodes of Ranvier (small zones devoid of myelin, which extend approximately 1 μm along the length of the fiber), located with a periodic spacing along the fiber. Nodes of Ranvier are separated by distances of approximately 100 μm in small-diameter fibers, and by more than 1 mm in large-diameter fibers; there is an approximately linear relationship between fiber diameter and internode distance. The region between nodes of Ranvier is referred to as the internode.

In mammalian axons, electrical excitability depends on the presence of voltage-dependent sodium channels. At the normal resting potential (approximately -70 mV), the sodium channels tend to be closed. As an action potential approaches a given axonal region, there is depolarization of this part of the membrane by the oncoming action potential, and, as a result, voltage-sensitive channels open. The difference in concentration of sodium ions on the two sides of the neuronal membrane (higher sodium ion concentration outside the axon than inside) provides an electrochemical gradient which depolarizes the axon by allowing sodium ions to enter. This depolarization results in an increased probability for the opening of sodium channels. If a threshold of depo-

Neural Regeneration and Transplantation, pages 43–66

larization is reached, the response becomes regenerative or self-reinforcing. This results in the production of an all-or-none action potential, which propagates along the axon.

The myelin sheath functions as an insulator, so that when the action potential is present at a given node of Ranvier, the majority of the action current is shunted to the next node. As a result, myelinated fibers conduct action potentials in a discontinuous or saltatory manner, with the impulse "jumping" from node to node (Huxley and Stämpfli, 1949). This saltatory mode of conduction in myelinated fibers is in sharp contrast to the continuous mode of conduction that is assumed to occur in most nonmyelinated fibers.

Recent studies have begun to elucidate the architecture of the myelinated fiber in terms of ion channel organization. In particular, it has become clear that the axon membrane in myelinated fibers is not a homogeneous structure. On the contrary, the axon membrane displays a nonuniform distribution of ion channels, with sodium channels present in high density in the axon membrane at the node of Ranvier, but present in very low density, if at all, in the internodal axon membrane under the myelin sheath (Ritchie and Rogart, 1977; Waxman, 1977). Voltage-sensitive potassium channels exhibit a complementary distribution, being present in the internodal axon membrane beneath the myelin (Waxman and Foster, 1980; Chiu and Ritchie, 1981). The potassium channels appear to play a role in modulating impulse firing patterns (Kocsis et al., 1982; Kocsis and Waxman, 1987).

By 1985, this complex pattern of organization of the axon membrane, as illustrated in Fig. 4–1, had been clearly demonstrated (Waxman and Ritchie, 1985). The organization of the myelinated fiber, as shown in Fig. 1, involves a highly coordinated differentiation of the axon and the surrounding myelin-forming cells. How this complex structure develops is not yet fully understood.

In order to understand how nerve fibers develop the capability for electrogenesis as they grow or regenerate, we must study the developmental mechanisms by which the axon and neighboring glial cells recognize each other and interact during development, so as to differentiate in this highly coordinated manner. It

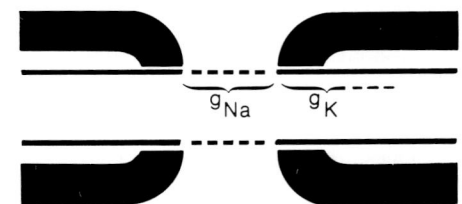

Figure 4–1. Ion channel organization of the mammalian myelinated fiber. Sodium channels (g_{Na}) are located in high density at the node of Ranvier, but are absent or present at very low density in the internodal axon membrane under the myelin sheath. Potassium channels (g_K) are present in the internodal axon membrane.

appears highly likely that cell recognition molecules, located on or near the surfaces of the axon and glial cells, provide specific signatures for these cells during their development. In an effort to understand the characteristics of these recognition molecules, our research group has carried out a series of studies that examine the macromolecular structure of the axon membrane during development and regeneration, as the axon and nearby glial cells recognize each other and interact to differentiate into the mature myelinated fiber.

Several lines of evidence suggest that axon-glial interactions during development and myelination involve cell recognition molecules located on the surfaces of the participating cells. Salzer et al. (1980) have demonstrated that a mitogenic signal for Schwann cells is located on, or near, the axon membrane. Moreover, it has been demonstrated that Schwann cells are pluripotential, with the axon determining whether or not myelination will take place (Aguayo et al., 1976; Weinberg and Spencer, 1976). The regulation of myelination, however, is highly specific, involving more than a simple yes/no decision as to whether or not to produce myelin around a given fiber. Thus, for example, patterns of myelin-formation, in both the PNS and the CNS, are highly specific. Myelin thickness (Williams and Wendell-Smith, 1971; Waxman and Bennett, 1972), internode distance (Gutrecht and Dyck, 1970; McDonald and Ohlrich, 1971), and nodal size (Waxman et al. 1972) vary in a systematic manner along certain fibers, and display a specific relationship to axonal size and type. Patterns of myelination, moreover, are not necessarily invariant along a given axon, but can change in a systematic manner along the axis of the fiber. An example is provided by reductions in internode distances, in regions proximal to axon branch points, and in the transition zone between myelinated and nonmyelinated parts of the axon (Ito and Takahashi, 1960; Waxman, 1970; Quick et al., 1979). This specialized arrangement has functional significance in providing increased current density that serves to ensure reliable impulse invasion (Revenko et al., 1973; Waxman and Brill, 1978). In these examples as well as others (Waxman et al., 1972), the axon serves as a spatial frame of reference with respect to myelin-formation.

In the CNS, a single oligodendrocyte forms myelin sheaths around a family of axons in its vicinity (containing up to several hundred axons). Notably, when a single oligodendrocyte myelinates several axons of different diameter, it forms thicker myelin sheaths around the larger axons (Waxman and Sims, 1984). Myelin thickness thus appears to be specified independently for each fiber by local axonal signals.

MACROMOLECULAR ORGANIZATION OF THE AXON MEMBRANE

As part of an effort to study the development of the axon membrane, our research group has, over the past 5 years, used quantitative freeze-fracture to examine the macromolecular structure of the axon membrane. The freeze-fracture method provides a powerful tool for such an analysis, because it permits large expanses of cell membranes to be studied quantitatively at submicron resolution (Sandri et al., 1977).

For freeze-fracture analysis, cells are rapidly frozen in liquid nitrogen, and their membranes are then cleaved using a special fracture device. Electron microscopy is then used to study the membrane en face at high magnification. The freeze-fracture method cleaves the lipid layer along the plane of the membrane and exposes the membrane face adhering either to the protoplasm (termed the "P-face" of the membrane) or the membrane face next to the extracellular matrix ("E-face") (Fig. 4–2). Within the bilayer, intramembranous particles (IMPs)

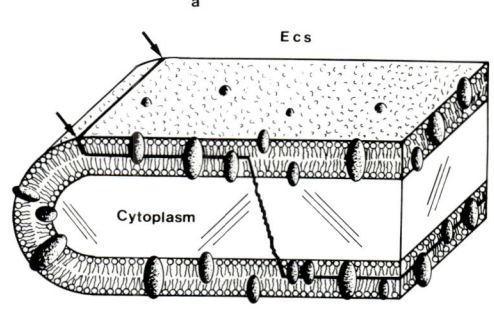

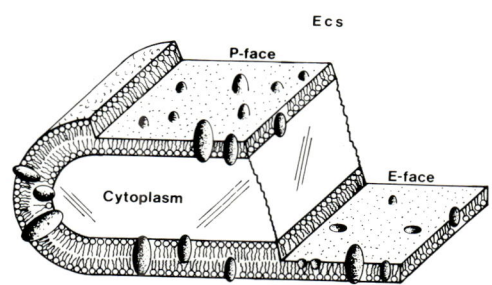

Figure 4–2. Diagrammatic representation of the freeze-fracture method. **a:** Following rapid freezing, tissue is fractured using a specialized device. The cleavage plain is represented by a heavy line entering the cell membrane at the arrows, traversing between the lipid bilayer, cross fracturing through the cytoplasm, and again traversing between the lipid bilayer. Intramembranous particles (IMPs) are intercalated in the lipid bilayer. **b:** Tissue above the fracture plane is removed by the fracturing process, and IMPs are observed as particles within the smooth lipid membrane framework. The P-face is the membrane half adherent to the cytoplasm, while the E-face is the membrane half immediately adjacent to the extracellular space (Ecs). (Reproduced from Waxman et al., 1983, by permission of the publisher.)

of various sizes are observed. It is now well established that IMPs represent protein or glycoprotein molecules interpolated within the membrane (Pinto da Silva and Miller, 1975; Bullivant, 1977). The distribution of IMPs, as well as their size, can be precisely determined by using electron microscopy. Freeze-fracture thus permits a mapping of the macromolecular structure of the axon membrane at the ultrastructural level.

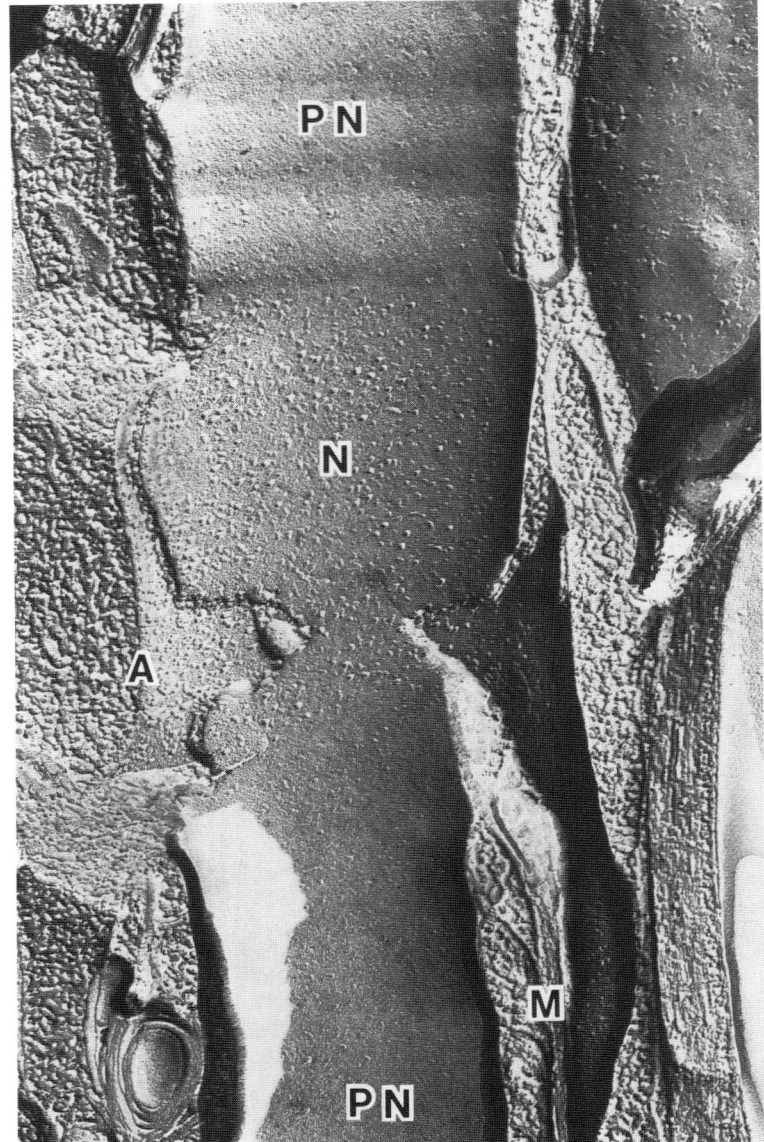

Figure 4–3. Electron micrograph showing a node of Ranvier, from CNS, as shown by freeze-fracture. The E-face of the axon membrane is displayed. Note the low density of IMPs in paranodal regions (PN), in contrast to the high density of IMPs at the node of Ranvier. M, terminating myelin loops; A, perinodal astrocyte. ×60,000. (Modified from Waxman, 1987 and reproduced by permission of the publisher.)

In mature myelinated axons from mammalian PNS or CNS, the axon membrane exhibits a highly nonuniform structure (Fig. 4–3). In internodal regions, the axon membrane displays an asymmetric distribution of IMPs, with an IMP density on the P-face of approximately $1,500/\mu m^2$, whereas the E-face displays a much lower IMP density ($100-200/\mu m^2$). In contrast, a distinct structure is exhibited by the axon membrane at the node of Ranvier. E-face and P-face of the nodal axon membrane each contain approximately 1,500 IMPs/μm^2. Within the nodal axon membrane, there is a significantly greater percentage of large (> 9.6 nm) IMPs (Rosenbluth, 1976; Kristol et al., 1978; Black et al., 1982). Thus nodal and internodal domains of the axon membrane display a different E-face structure. The nodal membrane forms a well-circumscribed annulus encircling the axon at the gap between adjacent myelin sheaths; this annulus of specialized nodal membrane extends approximately 1 μm along the fiber.

It has been suggested that large IMPs represent an ultrastructural correlate for voltage-sensitive ion channels at the node of Ranvier (Rosenbluth, 1976; Kristol et al., 1978; Black and Waxman, 1987). While some studies suggest that there is a specific relationship of large E-face IMPs to sodium channels, other studies suggest that both E-face and P-face IMPs are related to these channels. Definitive identification of sodium channels by freeze-fracture will require fracture-labeling using monoclonal antibodies or other ligands that bind specifically with sodium channels; techniques for fracture-labeling are currently being developed and will represent a major advance in our ability to study axonal development and regeneration. Irrespective of whether a definitive ultrastructural correlate for the sodium channel can be established at the present, freeze-fracture provides a clear morphological marker for nodal membrane.

Several model systems, including optic nerve and spinal cord, have been used to study the development of the myelinated axon. The rat optic nerve provides an especially tractable model system for these studies. At birth and for several days thereafter, the axons in this tract are totally devoid of myelin, while in the adult, all of the optic nerve fibers are myelinated. Thus, in terms of the end point of myelination, this tract presents a uniform population of axons. Moreover, studies on glial proliferation in this system indicate that, for several days after birth, premyelinated axons (axons prior to myelination) can be examined in the absence of contact with glial cells (Skoff et al., 1976; Foster et al., 1982). In addition,

optic nerve axons have been well studied from a physiological point of view. Electrophysiological and pharmacological studies indicate that there is reorganization of the axon membrane during development of the optic nerve (Foster et al., 1982).

AXON MEMBRANE REORGANIZATION FROM UNIFORM PRECURSOR INTO NODAL/INTERNODAL DOMAINS

Our studies indicate that the highly differentiated membrane of the mature myelinated fiber arises from a uniform premyelinated axon membrane precursor. When premyelinated axons are examined using freeze-fracture, it is seen that IMPs are distributed at random along the fiber and are not aggregated or grouped (Black et al., 1982). In this respect, the premyelinated fibers exhibit a uniform membrane structure similar to that observed in nonmyelinated axons (Black et al., 1981). This observation suggests that, in both premyelinated and nonmyelinated fibers, impulse conduction occurs in a uniform (rather than saltatory) manner. Interestingly, in both premyelinated and nonmyelinated fibers, potassium conductance mediates repolarization of the action potential.

How does the axon membrane of the myelinated fiber develop? Initially, while the axon continues to grow in terms of both surface area and length prior to ensheathment by glial cells, the macromolecular structure of the premyelinated axon membrane remains relatively constant prior to glial contact. IMP densities in the axon membrane thus remain stable over the first 4 weeks in premyelinated fibers (Table 4.1).

During the postnatal period, axon length increases more than twofold (Hildebrand and Waxman, 1984), and diameter increases by 50–100% (Foster et al., 1982). Although the membrane does not show changes in macromolecular composition during this phase of development, membrane surface area increases substantially, and there is thus a need for membrane biosynthesis.

AXON MEMBRANE SYNTHESIS IS A SEQUENTIAL PROCESS

This postnatal membrane assembly appears to occur in a sequential and spatially distributed manner. Initial stages of membrane syn-

TABLE 4.1. Particle Density per μm^2 of Developing Rat Optic Nerve Axolemma (Mean ± SEM)

Age (days)	Strain	Condition	P-face	E-face
2	Long Evans	Premyelinated	512 ± 50.7	125 ± 16.8
	Wistar	Premyelinated	553 ± 51.8	124 ± 14.3
8	Long Evans	Premyelinated	398 ± 31.0	117 ± 13.2
	Wistar	Premyelinated	564 ± 63.5	159 ± 24.9
12	Long Evans*	Premyelinated	661 ± 77.8	193 ± 20.8 [a]
		Ensheathed	1206 ± 105.5	
14	Wistar	Premyelinated	588 ± 95.4	104 ± 23.4 [a]
		Ensheathed	730 ± 56.3	
16	Long Evans*	Premyelinated	431 ± 17.4	104 ± 13.9 [a]
		Ensheathed	929 ± 96.4	
16	Wistar**	Premyelinated	629 ± 29.2	128 ± 8.9 [a]
		Ensheathed	924 ± 83.6	
28	Long Evans	Premyelinated	599 ± 29.2	67
14–16	Long Evans/ Wistar	Myelinated (internode)	1010 ± 74.1	90 ± 21.3
		Myelinated (node)	1175 ± 62.6	1312 ± 132.3
Adult	Long Evans	Myelinated (internode)	1709 ± 203.1	104 ± 23.6
		Myelinated (node)	1406 ± 152.2	1316 ± 104.2

*Difference between premyelinated and ensheathed significant at $P < 0.005$.
**Difference between premyelinated and ensheathed significant at $P < 0.01$.
[a]E-face not characterized as to premyelinated vs. ensheathed.
(Modified from Black et al. 1982, and reproduced by permission of the publisher.)

thesis involve the production, in the cell body, of a lipid bilayer framework that is relatively poor in terms of intramembranous particles. Pieces of the newly formed membrane framework are moved, in the form of intracytoplasmic vesicles that lack IMPs, to the axon via axoplasmic transport, and are then incorporated by fusion into the axon membrane. Axon membrane differentiation subsequently occurs in situ, via the insertion of IMPs into the membrane at specific locations, suggesting that ion channels and other intramembranous proteins are inserted, after formation of the lipid bilayer framework, into specific membrane domains (Griffin et al., 1981; Pfenninger and Johnson, 1983; Waxman and Black, 1985).

This distributed mode of membrane assembly is economical in terms of the genetic cost of neuronal differentiation. The large number of membrane types (possibly a continuum in some cell types; Waxman, 1984) required for neuronal differentiation does not have to be encoded within the nucleus, but is rather produced from a lipid bilayer precursor and a limited number of component proteins whose density and distribution in the membrane are modulated via local regulation. This permits the deployment of ion channels in highly specific patterns. It has been shown that changes in ion channel distribution within relatively small membrane domains can have important effects on axonal conduction properties (Waxman and Wood, 1984). Therefore in situ modification of the axon membrane also provides a mechanism for the modulation of physiological properties. Moreover, since electrical field effects can alter channel distribution (Orida and Poo, 1978), it is possible that impulse activity in the axon can lead to in situ modification of the membrane.

AXON MEMBRANE MODIFICATION IN ASSOCIATION WITH GLIAL ENSHEATHMENT

Observations on the optic nerve and spinal cord have been highly informative in terms of delineating the axon-glial interactions that accompany myelination. At the time of glial ensheathment (postnatal day 6 in rat optic nerve), two dramatic changes in axon membrane structure are observed. These changes indicate that there is a marked alteration in composi-

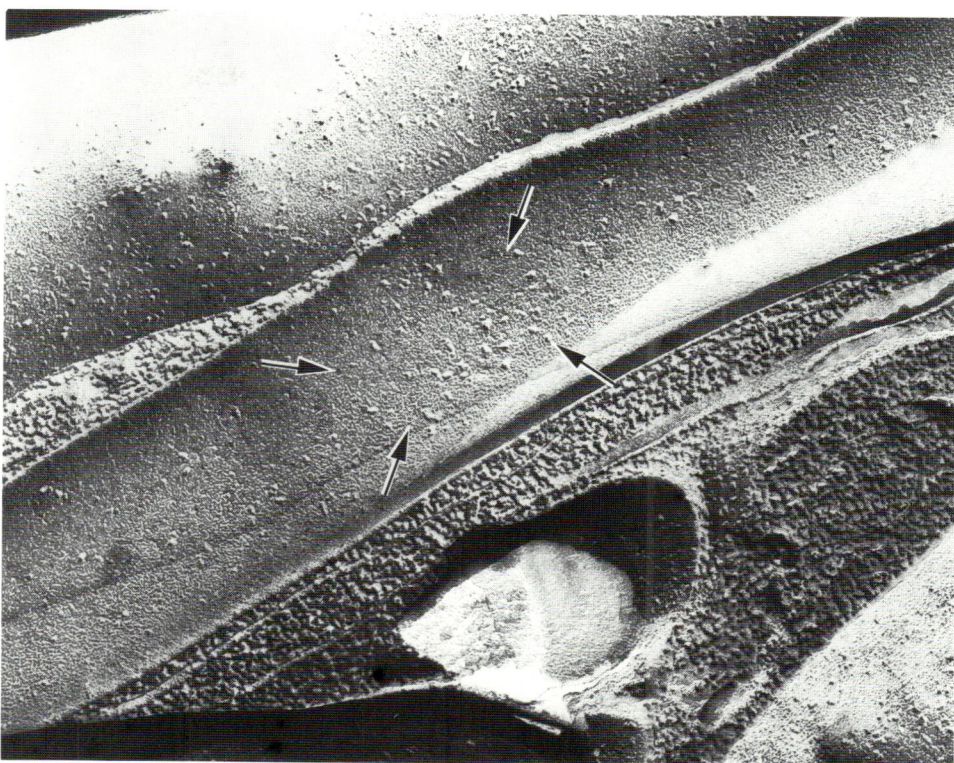

Figure 4–4. Precursor of node of Ranvier, from developing axon in optic nerve of 16-d-old rat. There is a cluster of large E-face IMPs (between arrowheads), which extends approximately 2 μm along the axis of the fiber. These nodal precursors appear prior to formation of myelin. ×85,800.

tion of the axon membrane in association with glial ensheathment:

1. As shown in Fig. 4–4, at the time of early glial contact prior to myelin formation, aggregates of IMPs develop on the axolemmal E-face. These membrane alterations, which occur in small domains extending less than several microns along the axis of the fiber, represent the precursors of nodes of Ranvier. These nodal precursors have been observed in developing CNS (Black et al., 1982; Waxman et al., 1982) and PNS axons (Wiley-Livingston and Ellisman, 1980; Tao-Cheng and Rosenbluth, 1982).

2. In addition, significant changes in ultrastructure of the axon membrane P-face occur in association with glial ensheathment. An example is shown in Fig. 4–5, which displays a premyelinated axon located adjacent to an en-

sheathed axon. As seen in this electron micrograph, P-face IMP density is greatly increased in ensheathed, compared with bare (premyelinated), axons (Black et al., 1982). Quantitative studies indicate that P-face IMP density increases by > 50% with glial ensheathment (Table 4.1). Thus, at the time of glial ensheathment, the axon membrane displays a significant change in structure, characterized by incorporation of a new population of protein molecules into the membrane.

GLIAL CELL-DEPRIVED AXONS

Having demonstrated that there are changes in axon membrane structure at the time of glial contact, an important question is whether the axonal changes are a result of association with glial cells, or on the other hand represent an alteration in axon membrane structure that

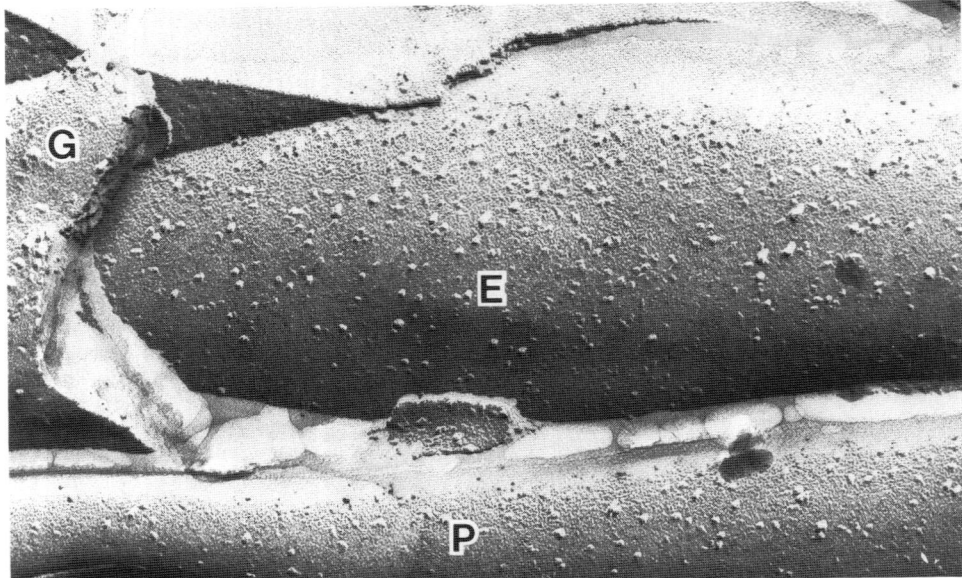

Figure 4–5. Alterations in axon membrane structure during development of rat optic nerve. This electron micrograph shows freeze-fractured axons from the optic nerve of 14-d-old rat. The fracture plane passes through a glial cell (G), which has ensheathed an axon (E); note the relatively high P-face IMP density on the ensheathed axon. A neighboring axon (P) remains premyelinated, and P-face IMP density on this fiber is relatively low. × 107,000. (Reproduced from Black et al., 1982, by permission of the publisher.)

serves to modulate glial cell behavior. To examine this question, we have carried out a number of studies on glial cell-deficient systems, including rat dorsal funiculus (Black et al., 1985a) and optic nerve (Black et al., 1985c). In these systems, axonal development can be studied in isolation from glial contact. In order to produce axonal tracts that have been experimentally deprived of glial cells, young rats are exposed to X-irradiation (Gilmore, 1963, 1966) or mitotic inhibitors such as 5-azacytidine (Ransom et al., 1985) during gliogenesis. Since these treatments interfere with the production of glial cells, they result in a marked reduction in the glial cell population.

Fig. 4–6 and Table 4.2 show the IMP densities in axons in glial-deprived CNS axons. Results are similar for spinal cord (Black et al., 1985a) and optic nerve (Black and Waxman, 1986); only the optic nerve is described here. As demonstrated in Fig. 4–6, treatment of neonatal rats with 5-azacytidine interferes with gliogenesis, so that the number of glial cells is

markedly reduced, which permits axons to be studied as they develop in the absence of glial ensheathment.

Axons in the optic nerve of neonatal rats, where oligodendroglia have not differentiated or contacted the fibers, exhibit a P-face IMP density of approximately $550/\mu m^2$. In the normal optic nerve at 14–16 postnatal d, approximately 25% of the fibers are myelinated; myelinated, ensheathed, and premyelinated fibers can be studied. In the normal optic nerve, myelinated axons and ensheathed axons display larger diameters than premyelinated axons (Fig. 4–5). Myelinated axons exhibit diameters of approximately 0.7 μm, while ensheathed fibers are approximately 0.4 μm in diameter, and most premyelinated fibers are approximately 0.3 μm. The axon membrane in internodal regions, beneath the myelin sheath, exhibits a high P-face density ($\sim 1100/\mu m^2$). The P-face IMP density for ensheathed axons at 14–16 d is approximately $900/\mu m^2$. In contrast, IMP density for premyelinated axons is

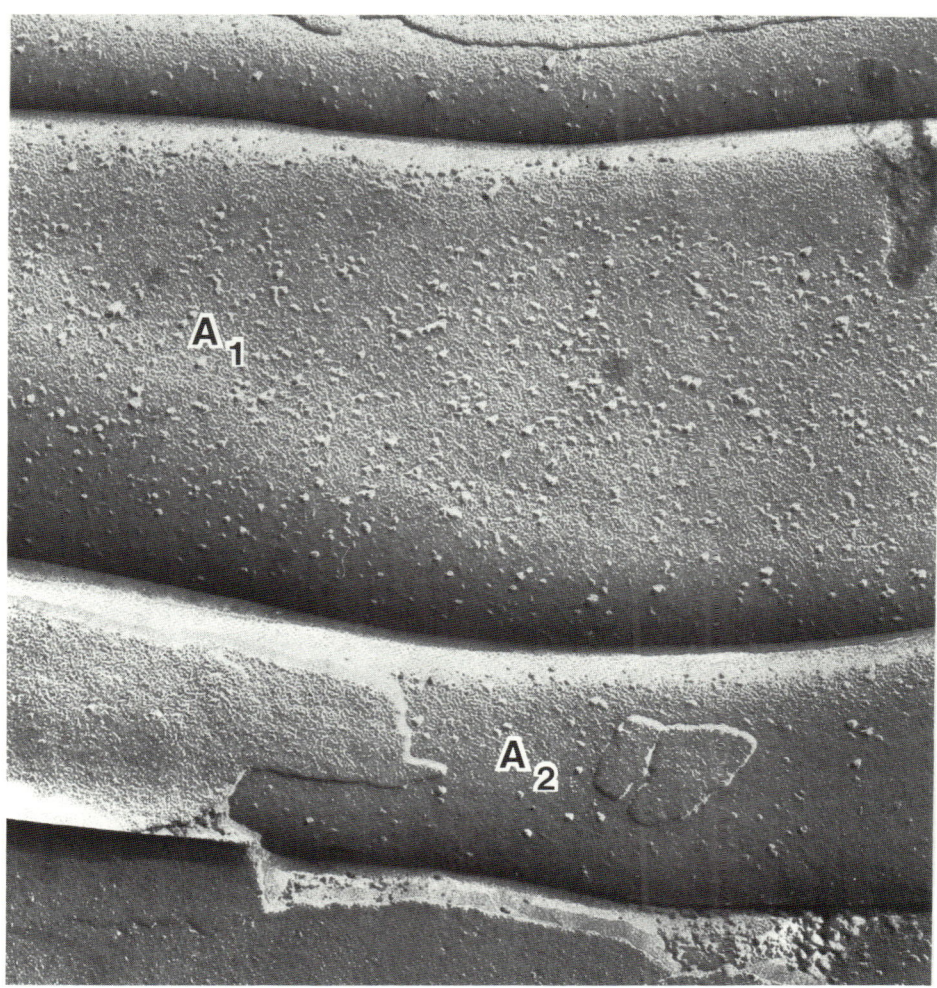

Figure 4–6. Freeze-fracture electron micrograph showing development of the axon membrane in glial cell-deprived optic nerve following treatment with 5-azacytidine, from 14-d-old rat. Note the increased P-face IMP density in the large diameter axon (A_1), which, on the basis of its size, would normally have been myelinated (compare with smaller axon, A_2). As shown in this figure, axon membrane structure is altered even in the absence of glial ensheathment. $\times 111,000$. (Reproduced from Black and Waxman, 1985, by permission of the publisher.)

lower and remains at approximately $600/\mu m^2$. Thus ensheathment by glial cells and myelination are associated with an increase in the number of P-face IMPs within the axon membrane.

As shown in Fig. 4–6 and Table 4.2, these changes in axon membrane P-face structure occur even in the absence of glial ensheathment (Black and Waxman, 1986). In the 14-d glial cell-deprived optic nerve, large ($> 0.6\ \mu m$) axons display a high P-face IMP density ($\sim 1024/\mu m^2$), similar to that for control internodal axolemma. On the basis of their diameter, these fibers would normally be expected to have acquired myelin sheaths. In contrast, small-diameter fibers ($< 0.3\ \mu m$; a diameter at which myelin is not normally seen) exhibit P-face IMP densities of $<\ 600/\mu m^2$. The

TABLE 4.2. Intramembranous Particle Densities in Control and Glial Cell-Deprived Dorsal Funiculus Axons (Means ± SE)

Condition	P-face	E-face
3 day Control		
Unmyelinated	868 ± 41.0	297 ± 25.8
19 day Control		
Unmyelinated	1098 ± 93.9**	452 ± 51.3*,**
Myelinated (internode)	2126 ± 135.2*	183 ± 27.5*
19 day Irradiated		
Unmyelinated (all)	1531 ± 78.9*,**	324 ± 34.0**
> 1.0 μm diameter	1988 ± 72.3*	439 ± 93.8**
< 0.5 μm diameter	1120 ± 92.0**	282 ± 37.4

*Significantly different ($P < 0.005$) compared with 3-d unmyelinated.
**Significantly different ($P < 0.005$) compared with 19-d myelinated internode.
(Modified from Black et al., 1985a, and reproduced by permission of the publisher.)

changes in P-face IMP density are similar to those that occur in normal axons as they become ensheathed by glial cells and acquire myelin. Thus, in the glial cell deprived system, the axon membrane P-face shows changes in structure similar to those that occur with myelination, irrespective of whether glial cells are actually present. Similar results are obtained in spinal cord (Black et al., 1985a).

These results indicate that incorporation of new P-face IMPs into the axon membrane does not represent a response to glial contact, but rather reflects an inherent change in membrane composition, which occurs on schedule even in the glial cell-deficient environment. Interestingly, in those instances in which, after several additional weeks, glial cells differentiate within the 5-azacytidine-treated optic nerve or irradiated spinal cord, axons elicit myelination (Black et al., 1985a,c).

INSERTION OF NEW MOLECULES INTO THE NODAL MEMBRANE DOES NOT DEPEND ON MYELIN FORMATION

Interestingly, the axon membrane begins to differentiate into zones that represent the precursors of nodes, even in the absence of glial cell ensheathment. An example is provided by glial cell-deprived axons in dorsal funiculus, where loose clusters of large E-face IMPs develop within the axon membrane of glial-deprived axons (Fig. 4–7). These islands of increased IMP density extend 1–2 μm along the axis of some axons, and up to 5 μm in other

axons (i.e., several times the length of a normal node of Ranvier). Within these specialized membrane zones, there is an increased number of large IMPs, similar to those seen at nodes of Ranvier. Although these specialized membrane regions can extend over an axonal area that is severalfold greater than that of a normal mature node, the total number of IMPs within these zones is similar to that at mature nodes. On the basis of these findings, it has been suggested that, even in the absence of ensheathment by myelin-forming cells, molecules destined for the node are inserted in loose clusters within the axolemma (Wiley-Livingston and Ellisman, 1980; Waxman et al., 1982; Black et al., 1985a).

Assuming that large E-face IMPs are related to sodium channels, as suggested by some workers (Rosenbluth, 1976; Kristol et al., 1978; Black and Waxman, 1987), these results can be interpreted as suggesting that sodium channels are inserted in relatively normal numbers into glial cell-deprived axon membrane at sites destined to develop into nodes of Ranvier. This conclusion extends the results of pharmacological studies (Oaklander et al., 1984) in which the binding of saxitoxin (a ligand that provides a marker for sodium channels) was examined in amyelinated axons of the myelin-deficient (md) rat. In this study, it was noted that binding of saxitoxin was similar in amyelinated and normally myelinated axons, suggesting that, during development, sodium channels are deployed within the axon mem-

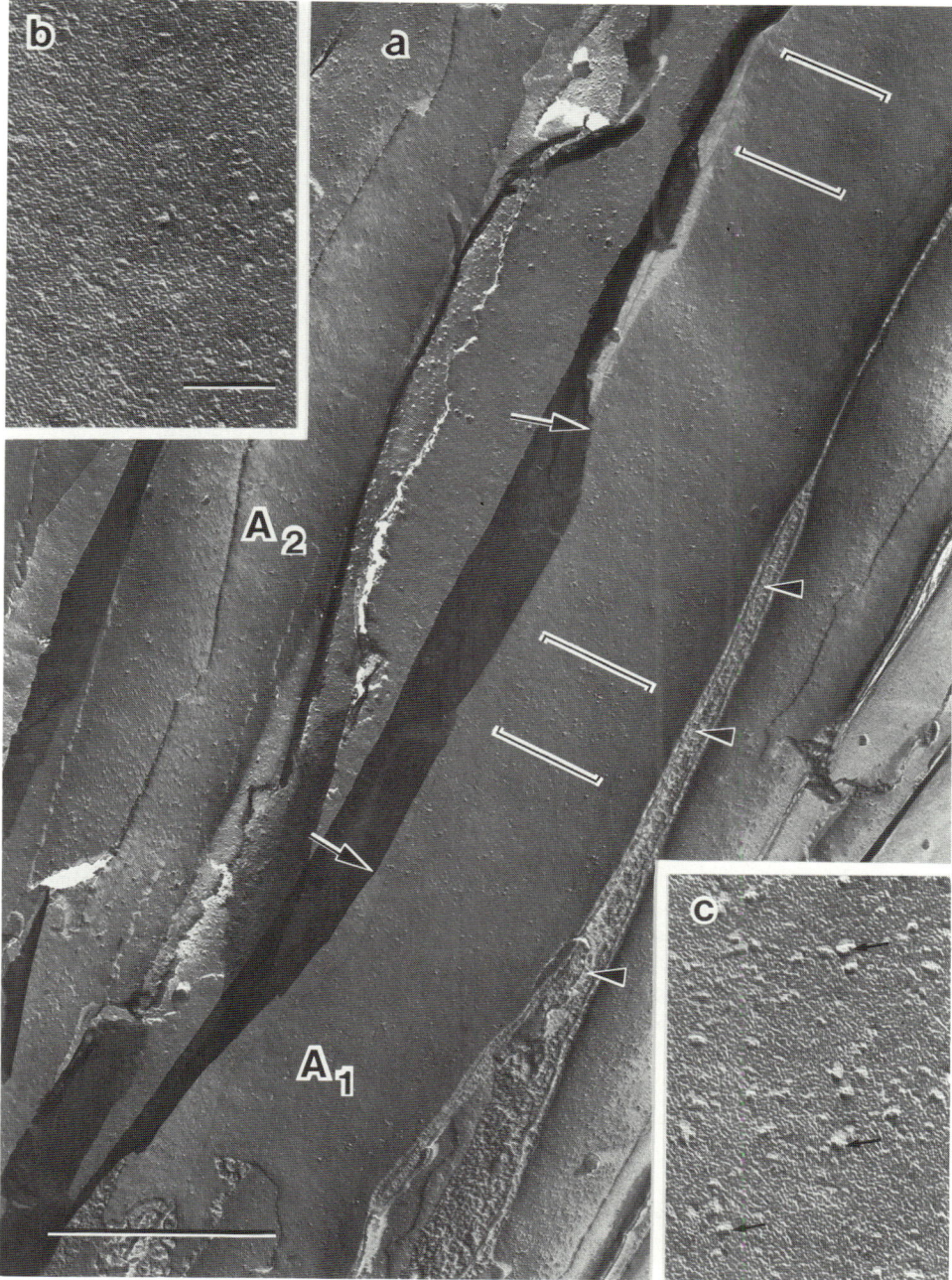

Figure 4–7. Unmyelinated axon from 19-d-old irradiated spinal cord. **a:** The E-face of an axon (A₁) is exposed to show a region of increased IMP density (between arrows) that is bounded proximally and distally by areas of lower particle density. A glial process (arrowheads) is present adjacent to the zone of increased IMP density. The E-face of an adjacent axon (A₂) has a lower density of IMPs. ×30,000. **b:** The upper right bracketed area of axon A₁ is shown at increased magnificiation. Note that few IMPs are apparent in this region. **c:** The lower area in brackets in axon A₁ is shown at increased magnification. Note the increased density of IMPs. b and c, ×125,000. (Modified from Black et al., 1985a and reproduced by permission of the publisher.)

brane irrespective of whether or not myelination actually occurs.

It is interesting, in this regard, that isolated patches of node-type membrane can develop in the absence of oligodendroglial wrapping or myelination within the normal central nervous system (Hildebrand and Waxman, 1983; Black et al., 1984). For example, the nonmyelinated axons of retinal ganglion cells within the retina exhibit islands of node-like membrane, with a surface area similar to that of the circumferential annuli of specialized membrane that occur at normal nodes (Hildebrand and Waxman, 1983). These specialized membrane foci, when examined by freeze-fracture, exhibit an increased density of large E-face particles, similar to those observed at normal nodes of Ranvier (Black et al., 1984). Foci of node-like membrane are also present in dysmyelinated (Bray et al., 1979; Rosenbluth, 1979) and demyelinated (Blakemore and Smith, 1983) axons. Smith et al. (1982) have demonstrated, in demyelinated (lysolecithin-treated) ventral root fibers, that foci of inward membrane current (termed "phi-nodes"), which presumably represent clusters of sodium channels, develop prior to the formation of new myelin sheaths. They represent the physiological correlate of nodal precursors that appear prior to the formation of myelin. Notably, phi nodes can support nonuniform conduction through demyelinated regions in some fibers.

On the basis of these findings, we conclude that the deployment of nodal membrane components is not dependent on myelin-formation. Specialized molecules destined for the node of Ranvier (possibly including voltage-sensitive sodium channels) are deployed in anticipation of myelination and are inserted into loose clusters in the axon membrane at the sites where nodes are destined to develop.

LOCALIZATION OF NODAL MEMBRANE MOLECULES BY GLIAL CELLS

As described above, specialized molecules that are normally destined for nodes of Ranvier are inserted, independently of myelin-formation, in loose clusters within the axon membrane. Their condensation into discrete annuli (as observed at normal nodes), however, is mediated by interactions between the axon and the myelin-forming glial cell. A possible role of the paranodal axon-glial junction is in limiting diffusion of IMPs within the plane of the membrane and confining large IMPs to the node of Ranvier, as suggested by Rosenbluth (1976). Observations on developing nodes provide some support for this suggestion and demonstrate that the nodal IMP population acquires a well demarcated boundary as the paranodal axon-glial junctions are established (Black et al., 1982; Tao-Cheng and Rosenbluth, 1982). Thus observations on the development of normal nodes suggest that paranodal junctions, formed by closely apposed axons and myelin-forming glial cells, function as a barrier that localizes certain membrane components within the axon membrane at the node.

Further evidence for a role of glial cells in modulating axon membrane structure is provided by the following observations. In some fibers there are ectopic extensions from the terminal loop of myelin-forming oligodendrocytes, which extend over the node of Ranvier (Hildebrand et al., 1985b). At the sites where these ectopic oligodendroglial processes contact the axon membrane at the node, there is a focal alteration in axon membrane structure. For example, as shown in Fig. 8, there is absence of E-face IMPs in the region of contact between oligodendrocyte processes and the axon membrane. This modification in axon membrane structure is spatially discrete, and corresponds to the area that is contacted by the oligodendrocyte (Black et al., 1985b). These observations demonstrate a focal modulation of axon membrane structure at sites of contact by myelin-forming cells.

On the basis of these findings, we conclude that, while specialized components are inserted into the axon membrane independent of myelin-formation, the precise location of nodal molecules reflects axon-glial interactions at the node of Ranvier.

SUPPRESSION OF INTERNODAL EXCITABILITY FOLLOWS AXONAL ENSHEATHMENT BY MYELIN-FORMING CELLS

In mature myelinated fibers, the internodal axon membrane is not electrically excitable (Ritchie and Rogart, 1977; Waxman, 1977), in contrast to the premyelinated axon membrane

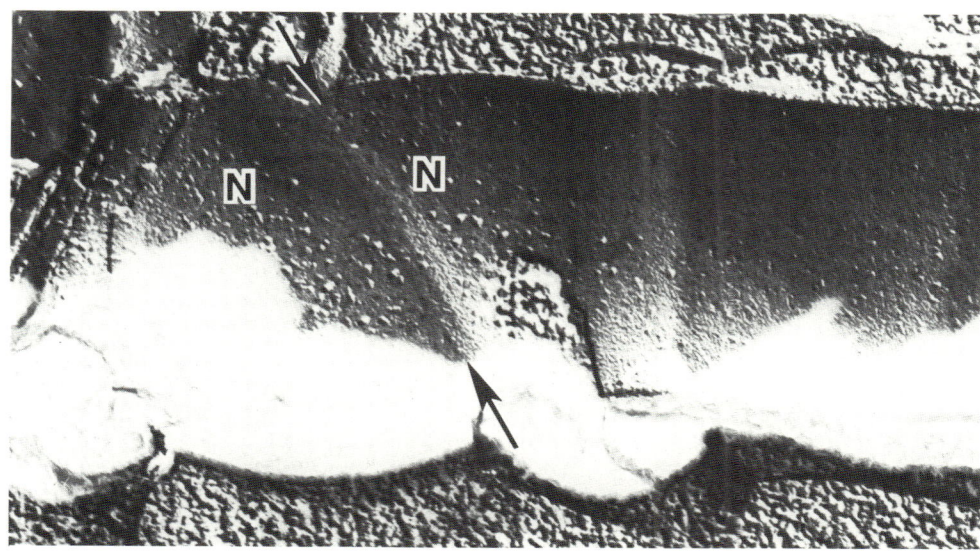

Figure 4–8. Modulation of axon membrane structure by overlying glial process. This electron micrograph shows a node of Ranvier (N) from the retina-optic nerve junction of the adult rat. An oligodendrocyte process (between arrows) crosses over the axon membrane. At the region where the nodal axon is contacted by the oligodendrocyte, there is a focal reduction in E-face IMP density. ×68,750. (Reproduced from Black et al., 1986, by permission of the publisher.)

(which exhibits widely distributed excitability, including electrogenesis in regions destined to develop into internodal membrane; Foster et al., 1982; Kocsis and Waxman, 1987). Thus differentiation of the myelinated fiber involves the loss of electrical excitability in the internodal axon membrane. Recent studies suggest that electrogenesis is lost following ensheathment of the axon by myelin-forming cells.

In glial cell-deprived dorsal funiculi, axons retain premyelinated characteristics in terms of E-face structure (in regions destined to develop under normal circumstances into internodes) until glial ensheathment has occurred (Black et al., 1986; Waxman, 1987). Control premyelinated axons, at 3 d of age, display E-face IMP densities of approximately 300/μm^2. Following myelination in the normal spinal cord, internodal E-face IMP density is reduced to approximately 180/μm^2 at 19 d. The reduction in E-face particle density occurs in the normal optic nerve and spinal cord following ensheathment by myelin-forming cells and appears to be correlated with the development,

from excitable premyelinated fibers (Foster et al., 1982), of inexcitability of the mature internodal membrane.

The density of E-face IMPs is higher in glial cell-deprived axons in the irradiated dorsal funiculus than in age-matched control myelinated (internodal) axon membrane. In the irradiated spinal cord, where ensheathment by glial cells does not occur at 19 d, E-face IMP density of the axon membrane is not reduced. On the contrary, a relatively high density of E-face IMPs (440/μm^2) is maintained in the glial cell deprived axons. This IMP density in glial cell-deprived axons is similar to that observed in control unmyelinated axons of similar age (approximately 450/μm^2). Thus, in the glial cell-deficient spinal cord where myelination does not occur, the axons retain the characteristics of premyelinated fibers (Black et al., 1986; Waxman 1987).

Action potential conduction through axons in the glial-deficient spinal cord is suggested by behavioral observations of locomotor activity in glial cell-deficient animals. Similarly, amyelinated PNS axons in the dy/dy mouse (in which myelin is absent on the basis of a genetic defect) display electrical excitability (Rasminsky et al., 1978). These observations suggest that normal maturation involves a reduction in excitability of the internodal axon membrane, which occurs consequent to ensheathment by myelin-forming cells. When myelination is prevented or delayed, the axon membrane retains structural characteristics that support the conduction of action potentials. This mode of development is a logical one from an ontogenetic point of view. If presumptive internodes were to become inexcitable prior to myelin-formation, development might include a transient period of conduction failure prior to myelination. The retention of internodal excitability until myelin-formation ensures the presence of a shield against capacitative current loss prior to reduction of internodal excitability.

This mode of axon membrane development also has important implications with respect to demyelination (Waxman, 1977). Following demyelination of ventral root axons with diphtheria toxin, continous conduction, reflecting the development of increased sodium channel densities within the former internodal membrane, occurs in some demyelinated fibers (Bostock and Sears, 1976, 1978). Electron microscopic studies have demonstrated structural reorganization of the demyelinated membrane, with the acquisition of nodal characteristics following demyelination (Foster et al., 1980; Coria et al., 1985; Meiri et al., 1985). The resumption of continuous conduction, following loss of the myelin sheath, may reflect derepression of an inherent capability for electrogenesis by the axon membrane.

NODE FORMATION INVOLVES ASTROCYTES AND SCHWANN CELLS

It has recently become clear that in the CNS, in addition to the axon and oligodendrocyte, the astrocyte plays a role in formation of the node of Ranvier. Astrocytic processes are present at nodes of Ranvier at a number of sites within the CNS (Hildebrand, 1971; Waxman and Swadlow, 1976; Raine, 1984; Waxman and Black, 1984). These astrocytic processes often extend through the neuropil or arc along trajectories of 5 or more μm to enter the nodal gap, where they exhibit a configuration similar to that of finger-like perinodal Schwann cell processes.

Within the irradiated spinal cord, glial cell-deprived axons exhibit occasional sites of node-like membrane specialization These zones of axon membrane specialization are always apposed by astrocyte processes (Black et al., 1985a). Moreover, when myelination occurs around occasional axons following protracted postirradiation intervals, astrocyte processes are observed in specific association with the nodes, in some cases extending for distances of several μm through the neuropil to contact the nodal part of the axon (Fig. 4–9) (Sims et al., 1985). Since random neuro-glial interactions are minimized as a result of the lower density of glial cells in the irradiated spinal cord (Waxman and Sims, 1984), these observations provide further evidence for a specific relationship of the astrocyte to the node.

Similar perinodal processes, originating from Schwann cells (Fig. 4–10), are observed at nodes of Ranvier in the normal PNS (Landon, 1981; Rydmarck and Berthold, 1983; Waxman and Black, 1987). The relationship of Schwann cell processes to zones of nodal membrane specialization is, however, not confined to the normal PNS. In the dystrophic mouse, ventral root fibers are amyelinated; at sites where these fibers exhibit patches of node-like membrane, finger-like Schwann cell processes are observed (Rosenbluth, 1979).

These observations suggest a specific role of the astrocyte and Schwann cell in formation of nodes of Ranvier. In studies on the optic nerve, ffrench-Constant et al. (1985) demonstrated the J-1 glycoprotein, which has been shown to mediate axon-astrocyte adhesion (Kruze et al., 1985), at sites of apposition between perinodal astrocytes and nodes of Ranvier. Both Schwann cells (Bunge, 1986) and astrocytes (Liesi et al., 1983) secrete extracellular matrix. One hypothesis is that molecules in the extracellular matrix participate in instructing sodium channels to cluster at the node. According to this hypothesis, formation of nodes of Ranvier would depend on mechanisms similar to those at the neuromuscular junction, where postsynaptic clustering of acetylcholine receptors reflects contact with a second cell process (in the case of the neuromuscular junction, the presynaptic terminal) or with basal lamina

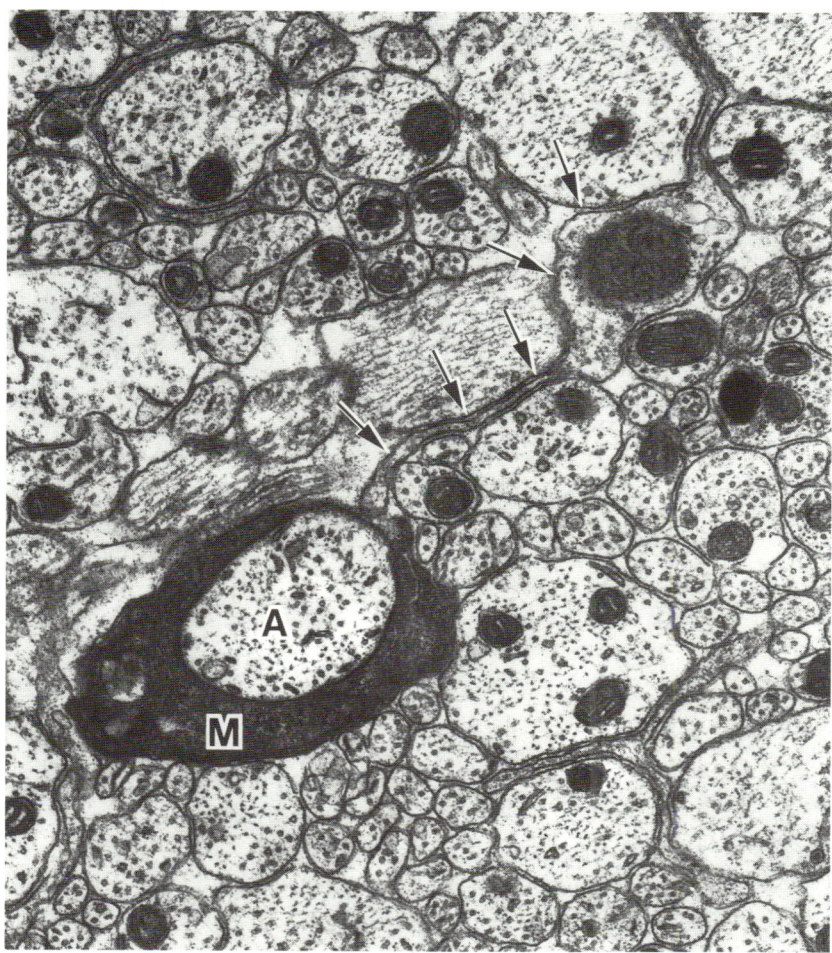

Figure 4–9. Perinodal astrocyte process from glial cell-deprived spinal cord of 18-d-old rat. As a result of the reduction in glial cell population following X-irradiation, random axon-glial interactions are minimized in this preparation. Despite the small number of astrocytes, an astrocyte process is present at the node of Ranvier. A, myelinated axon; M, myelin sheath. Note the small gap in the myelin sheath at this node of Ranvier, which is sectioned in an oblique plane. An astrocyte process (arrows) runs through the neuropil for more than 5 μm, to contact the axon at the site of myelin interruption at the node. ×52,900. (Reproduced from Sims et al., 1985, by permission of the publisher.)

(Rubin and McMahan, 1982). Alternatively, development of nodal membrane may provide a trophic signal to Schwann cells or astrocytes, instructing them to approach the axon and contact the nodal membrane. In either event, node formation appears to involve a closely coordinated sequence of events involving both the axon and glial cells. Axon-glial interactions are not confined to the internodal areas

that are myelinated, but also occur at the node of Ranvier, where they involve perinodal Schwann cell fingers in PNS, and perinodal astrocytes in CNS.

The participation of astrocytes in node formation has important implications for CNS injury. While the concept of the glial scar (Reier and Houle, 1987) is well established, it is clear that astrocytes play facilitory/modulatory, as

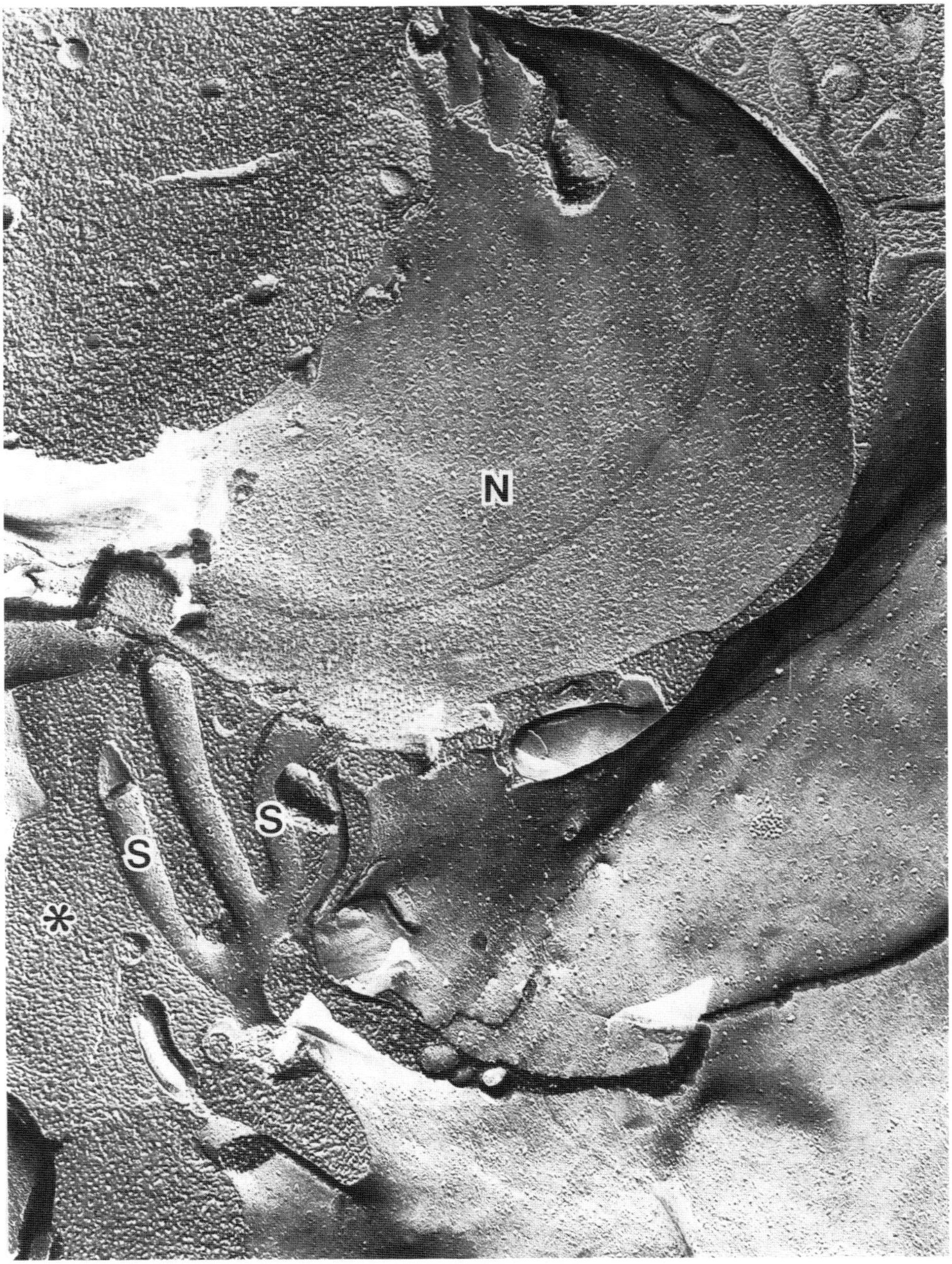

Figure 4–10.   Freeze-fracture electron micrograph showing node of Ranvier from rat sciatic nerve. A cuff of Schwann cell finger-like processes (S) surrounds the axon at the node. N, E-face of nodal axon membrane, containing high density of E-face IMPs. Asterisk, extracellular space. ×52,900. (Reproduced from Waxman and Black, 1987, by permission of the publisher.)

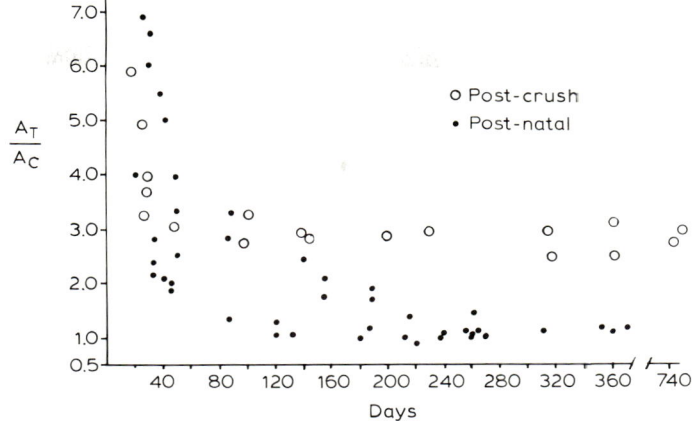

Figure 4–11. Graph showing the ratio A_T/A_C, which provides a measure of burst activity after potassium channel blockade. This bursting index is plotted vs. days postnatal or postcrush. While the A_T/A_C ratio decreases to approach 1.0 during normal maturation, it remains higher in long-term regenerated fibers. This result indicates that there are physiological differences between ion channel organization in regenerated, as compared with normal, myelinated fibers. (Reproduced from Kocsis and Waxman, 1987, by permission of the publisher.)

well as inhibitory, roles in axon development. Given the highly polarized structure of the astrocyte (Black and Waxman, 1985; Newman, 1986), it is even possible that a single astrocyte can have several effects on axonal growth or regeneration, one astrocyte process acting as a barrier while others play a facilitory role.

PHYSIOLOGY OF REGENERATING PNS AXONS

Intraaxonal and sucrose gap recording methods provide an important probe of electrogenesis and permit an examination of impulse conduction in regenerating axons. An important set of observations has emerged from studies that examine the response of axons to the potassium blocking agent 4-aminopyridine (4-AP). During normal development, sensitivity to 4-AP is considerably attenuated; thus, while immature myelinated fibers exhibit stimulus-evoked burst activity following exposure to 4-AP, this bursting is attenuated during normal development as the 4-AP sensitive channels are masked by the overlying myelin (Kocsis et al., 1982). Surprisingly, in contrast to normal mature sciatic nerve fibers, long-term regenerated axons retain their sensitivity to 4-AP (Kocsis and Waxman, 1983) (Fig. 4–11).

Fig. 4–12A2 shows compound action potentials recorded before and after (arrow) application of 4-AP to the sciatic nerve of a 47-d-old control rat; the late rippled activity following 4-AP application reflects stimulus-evoked bursting after 4-AP-sensitive channels are blocked with this drug. Recordings from a 12-week-old normal rat, however, show only slight alteration in spike wave form after 4-AP application, illustrating the attenuation of sensitivity to 4-AP during normal development.

In contrast to this normal developmental sequence, 4-AP sensitivity is retained in long-term regenerated axons (Kocsis and Waxman, 1983). Figure 4–12B1 shows the effects of 4-AP on the compound action potential in a regenerated sciatic nerve studied 1 year following crush. As in immature nerves from control rats, stimulus-evoked burst activity (arrow) is present following exposure to 4-AP in regenerated fibers. Figure 4–12B2 shows an intraaxonal recording from the same regenerated nerve shown in Figure 4–12B1. Note the burst of action potentials elicited by a single stimulus. These observations indicate that long-term regenerated fibers exhibit a response to potassium channel blockade similar to that of immature myelinated fibers.

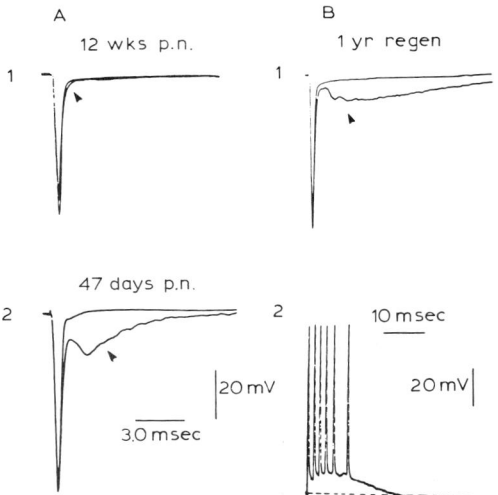

Figure 4–12. Effects of the potassium channel blocking agent 4-AP (arrowheads) on the compound action potential of normal mature (A1), immature (A2), and long-term regenerating (B1) sciatic nerves. B2 shows intraaxonal recordings, obtained from the same long-term regenerating nerve shown in B1 in the presence of 4-AP. Following potassium channel blockade with 4-AP, spike burst activity is elicited by single stimuli. (Reproduced from Kocsis and Waxman, 1987, by permission of the publisher.)

SCHWANN CELL REMODELING IN REGENERATING PNS AXONS

What is the morphological correlate for this persistence of immature physiological properties in regenerated nerve fibers? Long-term regenerated axons display conduction velocities close to normal and have established functional synaptic connections. In what ways do they differ from normal mature myelinated fibers?

During normal development, it is well established that there is a lengthening of internodes (Hess and Young, 1949). Newly formed myelin segments are approximately 150 μm long, whereas in the adult, internode lengths can be as great as 1 mm, being approximately 200 × the diameter for any given fiber. The increases in internode distance occur during the period of increase in limb length. Careful morphological studies (Berthold and Skoglund, 1968; Berthold, 1978; Fried and Hildebrand, 1982) show that during normal development, there is

a transient period of Schwann cell remodeling that includes degeneration of some internodes along the length of the fiber. This occurs as the myelin sheaths increase in length, with Schwann cells competing for territory along the fiber, and with some Schwann cells lengthening at the expense of others.

Since, in regenerated axons, internode distances remain relatively short compared with those in normal mature fibers (Sanders and Whitteridge, 1946), we examined Schwann cells along both short-term and long-term regenerating fibers in an effort to determine the time course of Schwann cell remodeling during regeneration. Plots of internode distance vs. fiber diameter, for both normal and regenerating fibers from rat sciatic nerve, are shown in Fig. 4–13. In normal sciatic nerve (upper right-hand graph), there is a nearly linear relationship between internode distance and fiber diameter, with internode distance reaching nearly 1.6 mm for large-diameter fibers. In contrast, in regenerating fibers following sciatic nerve crush, there is a reduction in internode distance of the regenerated segments, with abnormally short internodes present at even 11 months postcrush. In this respect, regenerated fibers display an axon-glial organization similar to that of immature fibers in the normal sciatic nerve.

Teased fiber (Hildebrand et al., 1985a) and electron microscopic (Hildebrand et al., 1986) studies demonstrate persistent Schwann cell remodeling in regenerating fibers (Fig. 4–14). This remodeling is seen even in long-term (> 1 year) regenerated fibers. Thus, in regenerating fibers, there is ongoing remodeling of Schwann cells and myelin sheaths, similar to that seen as a transient phenomena during normal development. Loosening of paranodal junctions, as a result of this remodeling, provides a morphological substrate for exposure of internodal potassium channels to extracellularly applied agents such as 4-AP.

Why does this remodeling persist in regenerating fibers? One possibility is that, in the absence of increasing length of the full-grown limb, Schwann cells along the regenerating nerve continue to compete for space, with some internodes lengthening at the expense of others. Since regeneration following nerve crush in the adult occurs in the absence of

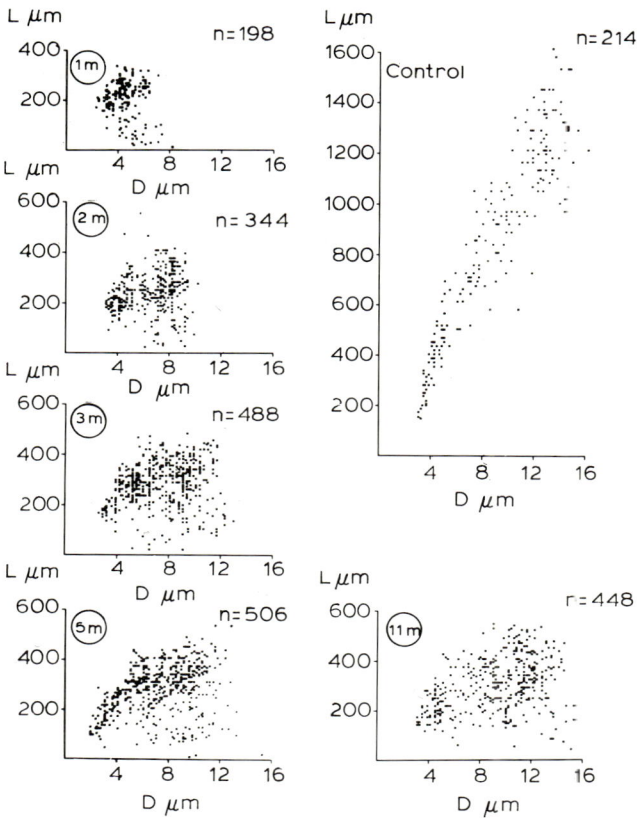

Figure 4–13. Graph showing internodal length, plotted as a function of fiber diameter, for normal (control) sciatic nerve, and for regenerating sciatic nerves at various intervals (months indicated in circles) following crush. During normal development, axons achieve an approximately linear relationship between fiber diameter (D) and internode distance (L), and short internodes are not present in mature control fibers (upper right-hand panel, control). In contrast, in regenerated fibers, short internodes are retained. (Modified from Hildebrand et al., 1985a, and reproduced by permission of the publisher.)

growth of the limb, Schwann cells cannot achieve stable internodal domains (as they do during normal development when increasing limb length permits expansion in internodal length). In support of this suggestion, Bowe et al. (1987) have shown that, when sciatic nerve regeneration is studied following crush lesions performed in immature (1–4 week-old) rats, there is less 4-AP-elicited bursting than in fibers lesioned at older ages. This result suggests that when regeneration occurs during the period of normal maturation, Schwann cells and myelinated internodes achieve stability, possibly as a result of remodeling during the period

of increasing limb length. Axon-glial interactions during regeneration thus cannot be examined in isolation, but must be considered in the context of the maturational state of the nerve under study.

AXON-GLIAL INTERACTIONS DURING DEVELOPMENT AND REGENERATION

As outlined above, the development of myelinated axons includes a sequence of steps, involving both the axon and nearby glial cells. In peripheral nerve, the neuron and Schwann cell comprise the myelinated fiber. In the central nervous system, three cell types are in-

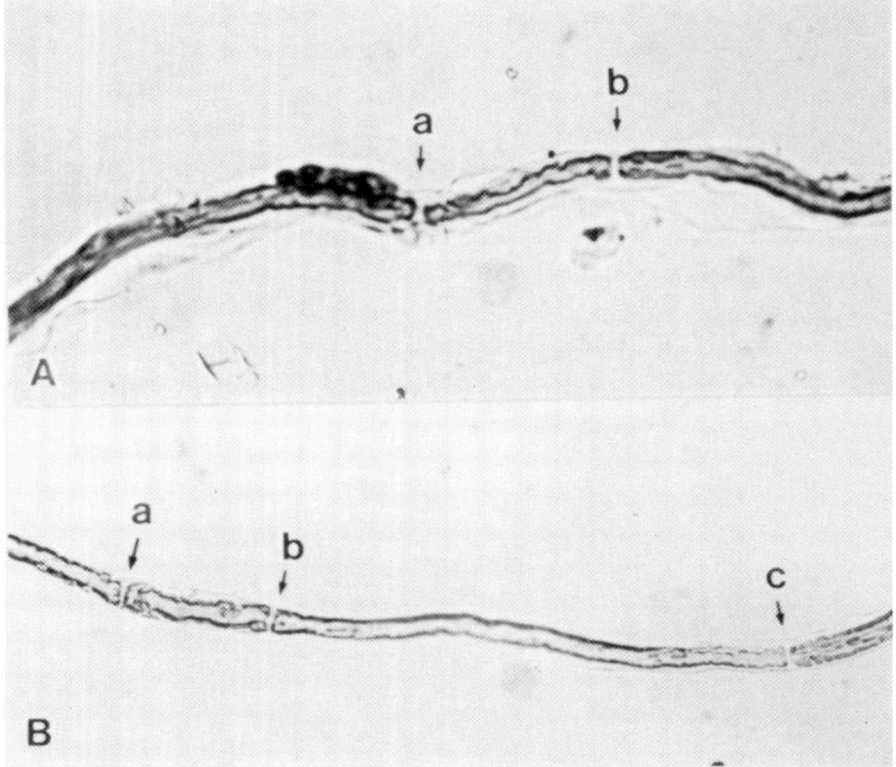

Figure 4–14.   These light micrographs show teased fibers from regenerating sciatic nerve, following crush 3 months **(A)** and eleven months **(B)** previously. Short internodes (a–b) are present in both fibers. A longer internode (b–c) in the 11-month regenerated fiber is also significantly shorter than normal. Note the dense and retracted myelin (to left of a) in the paranodal region in A. A, ×400; B, ×350. (Modified from Hildebrand et al., 1985a, and reproduced by permission of the publisher.)

cluded: axon, oligodendrocyte, and astrocyte; the participation of two glial cell types (oligodendrocyte and astrocyte) may reflect the common origin of these cells from a single progenitor, the O-2A cell (Raff and Miller, 1984), with the oligodendrocyte and astrocyte fulfilling the role that a single cell type (the Schwann cell) fulfills in the PNS.

The results of freeze-fracture studies strongly suggest that the development of myelinated axons involves cell membrane-associated instructional molecules (Fig. 4–15). Thus, our current working model of the myelinated fiber incorporates highly specific molecules on the axonal and glial surfaces, which provide complementary "signatures" for cell-cell recognition. The presence of such molecules at specific parts of the neuronal surface provides a mechanism that can guide neural development with a high degree of spatial specificity. Freeze-fracture permits the distribution of membrane-related molecules to be precisely mapped. Visualization of IMPs inserted into the axon membrane in anticipation of myelination provides a candidate for these instructional molecules. Similarly, the development of the nodes of Ranvier and nodal precursors provides a morphological correlate (with a high degree of spatial resolution) for pharmacological studies that show the insertion of sodium channels in anticipation of myelination and suggests that it may be possible to localize sodium channels, as they are deployed into the axon membrane, by electron microscopy.

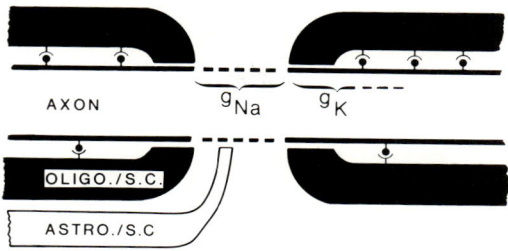

Figure 4–15. Model of the myelinated fiber that includes a mechanism for cell-cell recognition between the axon and surrounding glial cells. "Instructional molecules," associated with the axon surface, provide a specific signature for nodal and/or internodal parts of the axon membrane. Complementary molecules, on the glial cell (oligo) or Schwann cell (S.C.), form a template that recognizes the axonal signal. Note that even at the node of Ranvier, where myelin is absent and sodium channels cluster in the axon membrane, there is a specific association of the axon with Schwann cell (S.C.) finger-like processes (PNS) or astrocyte (astro) processes (CNS). (Modified from Waxman, 1987, and reproduced by permission of the publisher.)

CONCLUSIONS

Studies such as the ones outlined above permit the delineation of a number of rules governing membrane organization and axon-glial interactions during development and regeneration of myelinated fibers. These include the following:

1. New protein molecules are incorporated into the axon membrane P-face in association with glial ensheathment.

2. This reorganization of the axolemmal P-face does not depend on glial ensheathment, but can occur in a glial cell-deprived environment.

3. Loose clusters of large E-face IMPs (presumably the precursors of sodium channels) are inserted into the axon membrane at sites of developing nodes of Ranvier, independently of myelination or the formation of paranodal axon-glial junctions.

4. Interactions between the axon and the myelin-forming cell serve to locally modulate the structure of the axon membrane at the node, with condensation of loose clusters of E-face IMPs into discrete high-density annuli of nodal axolemma.

5. The density of large E-face IMPs does not decrease in the internodal membrane (suggesting that electrical excitability is not suppressed) until myelination has provided a shield against internodal current loss.

6. In the CNS, the astrocyte plays a role in the differentiation of the node of Ranvier.

7. In normally developing fibers, there is a transient period of myelin remodeling.

8. Regenerating fibers exhibit persistent myelin remodeling.

Now that these rules have been delineated, it will be important to understand the underlying mechanisms that mediate axon-glial interactions. One powerful approach to this problem would be the development of techniques for specifically labeling instructional molecules, i.e., immunocytochemical or fracture-labeling methods. The development of such methods will not only permit identification of the molecules involved, but will also provide information about localization of these molecules at the submicron domain. Alternatively, physiological blockade of these molecules might provide important insights into their function. Isolation and characterization of these molecules should provide important new information. Finally a molecular biological approach will permit an understanding of the transcriptional and translational events that underly axon-glial interactions. Studies such as those outlined in this chapter are beginning to delineate the mechanisms that regulate axonal growth and development.

As we understand these mechanisms in increasing detail, and as we isolate and characterize the molecules involved, it is not unlikely that new approaches to neurological disease will be developed. Thus we can begin to consider the development of interventions that would enhance axonal growth and regeneration, provide more accurate guidance of axons as they regenerate toward target cells, promote formation of synaptic connections, and accelerate the development of normal or near-normal impulse conduction properties in previously damaged nerve fibers.

ACKNOWLEDGMENTS

Work in the author's laboratory has been supported in part by grants from the National Institutes of Health and the National Multiple

Sclerosis Society, and by the Medical Research Service, Veterans Administration.

REFERENCES

Aguayo AJ, Charron L, Bray GM (1976): Potential of Schwann cells from unmyelinated nerves to form myelin: A quantitative ultrastuctural study. J Neurocytol 5:565–573.

Berthold CN (1978): Morphology of normal peripheral axons. In Waxman SG (ed): "Physiology and Pathobiology of Axons." New York: Raven Press, pp 3–63.

Berthold CN, Skoglund S (1968): Postnatal development of feline paranodal myelin segments. II. Electron microscopy. Acta Soc Med Upsaliensis 73:127–144.

Black JA, Waxman SG (1985): Specialization of astrocytic membrane at glia limitans in rat optic nerve: Freeze-fracture observations. Neurosci Lett 55:371–378.

Black JA, Waxman SG (1986): Molecular structure of the axon membrane in developing axons following altered gliogenesis in rat optic nerve. Dev Biol 115:301–312.

Black JA, Waxman SG (1988): Freeze-fracture studies on unmyelinated axolemma in cervical sympathetic trunk: Correlation with saxitoxin binding. Proc R Soc Lond 233:45–54.

Black JA, Foster RE, Waxman SG (1981): Freeze-fracture ultrastructure of rat CNS and PNS nonmyelinated axolemma. J Neurocytol 10:981–993.

Black JA, Foster RE, Waxman SG (1982): Rat optic nerve: Freeze-fracture studies during development of myelinated axons. Brain Res 250:1–10.

Black JA, Waxman SG, Hildebrand C (1984): Membrane specialization and axo-glial association in the rat retinal nerve fiber layer: Freeze-fracture observations. J Neurocytol 13:417–430.

Black JA, Sims TA, Waxman SG, Gilmore SA (1985a): Membrane ultrastructure of developing axons in glial cell deficient rat spinal cord. J Neurocytol 13:79–104.

Black JA, Waxman SG, Hildebrand C (1985b): Axo-glial relations in the retina-optic nerve junction of the adult rat: Freeze-fracture observations on axon membrane structure. J Neurocytol 14:887–907.

Black JA, Waxman SG, Ransom BR, Feliciano MD (1985c): A quantitative study of developing axons and glia following altered gliogenesis in rat optic nerve. Brain Res 380:122–136.

Black JA, Waxman SG, Sims TG, Gilmore SA (1986): Effects of delayed myelination by oligodendrocytes and Schwann cells on the macromolecular structure of axonal membrane in rat spinal cord. J Neurocytol 15:745–762.

Blakemore WF, Smith KJ (1983): Node-like axonal specializations along demyelinated central nerve fibers: ultrastructural observations. Acta Neuropathol 60:291–297.

Bostock N, Sears TA (1976): Continuous conduction in demyelinated mammalian nerve fibers. Nature 263:786–787.

Bostock N, Sears TA (1978): The internodal axon membrane: Electrical excitability and continuous conduction after segmental demyelination. J Physiol (Lond) 280:273–303.

Bowe CM, Kocsis JD, Waxman SG, Hildebrand C (1987): Physiological properties of regenerated rat sciatic nerve following lesions at different postnatal ages. Dev Brain Res 34:123–134.

Bray GM, Cullen MJ, Aguayo AJ, Rasminsky M (1979): Node-like areas of intramembranous particles in the unensheathed axons of dystrophic mice. Neurosci Lett 13:203–208.

Bullivant S (1977): Evaluation of membrane structure: Facts and artifacts produced by freeze-fracture. J Microsc 111:101–110.

Bunge RP (1986): The cell of Schwann. In Asbury AK, McKhann G, McDonald WI (eds): "Diseases of the Nervous System: Clinical Neurobiology." Philadelphia: W.B. Saunders Co, pp 153–161.

Chiu SY, Ritchie JM (1981): Evidence for the presence of potassium channels in the internodal region of acutely demyelinated mammalian nerves. J Physiol (Lond) 313:415–437.

Coria F, Silos I, Fernandez R, Morton R, La Farga M (1985): Demyelination-induced plasticity in the axon membrane: An ultrastructural cytochemical study of lead neuropathy. Neurosci Lett 58:359–364.

ffrench-Constant C, Miller RN, Kruze J, Schachner M, Raff MC (1985): Molecular specialization of astrocyte processes at nodes of Ranvier in rat optic nerve. J Cell Biol 102:844–852.

Foster RE, Whalen CC, Waxman SG (1980): Reorganization of the axonal membrane of demyelinated nerve fibers: Morphological evidence. Science 210:661–663.

Foster RE, Connors B, Waxman SG (1982): Rat optic nerve: Electrophysiological, pharmacological and anatomical studies during development. Dev Brain Res 3:361–376.

Fried K, Hildebrand C (1982): Qualitative structural development of feline alveolar nerve. J Anat 134:517–531.

Gilmore SA (1963): The effects of x-irradiation on the spinal cords of neonatal rats. J Neuropathol Exp Neurol 22:294–301.

Gilmore SA (1966): Delayed myelination of neonatal spinal cord induced by x-irradiation. Neurol 16:745–753.

Griffin JW, Price DL, Drachman DB, Morris J (1981): Incorporation of axonally transported glycoproteins into axolemma during nerve regeneration. J Cell Biol 88:205–214.

Gutrecht JA, Dyck PJ (1970): Quantitative teased-fiber and histologic studies of human sural nerve. J Comp Neurol 138:117–130.

Hess A, Young JZ (1949): Correlations of internodal length and fiber diameter in CNS. Nature 164:450–451.

Hildebrand C (1971): Ultrastructural and light-microscopic studies on developing feline spinal cord white matter. Acta Physiol Scand [Suppl] 364:81–101.

Hildebrand C, Waxman SG (1983): Regional node-like membrane specializations in non-myelinated axons of rat retinal nerve fiber layer. Brain Res 258:23–32.

Hildebrand C, Waxman SG (1984): Postnatal differentiation of rat optic nerve fibers: Electron microscopic observations on the development of nodes of Ranvier and axo-glial relations. J Comp Neurol 224:25–37.

Hildebrand C, Kocsis JD, Berglund S, Waxman SG (1985a): Myelin sheath remodelling in regenerated rat sciatic nerve. Brain Res 358:163–170.

Hildebrand C, Remahl S, Waxman SG (1985b): Axo-glial relations in the retina-optic nerve junction of the adult rat: Electron microscopic observations. J Neurocytol 14:597–617.

Hildebrand C, Mustafa GY, Waxman SG (1986): Remodeling of internodes in regenerated rat sciatic nerve: Electron microscopic observations. J. Neurocytol 15:681–692.

Huxley AF, Stämpfli R (1949): Evidence for saltatory conduction in myelinated nerve fibers. J Physiol (Lond) 108:315–339.

Ito M, Takahashi I (1960): Impulse transmission through spinal ganglia. In Katsuko Y (ed): "Electrical Activity of Single Cells." Tokyo: Ikago Shoin Ltd, pp 159–179.

Kocsis JD, Waxman SG (1983): Long-term regenerated nerve fibres retain sensitivity to potassium channel blocking agents. Nature 304:640–642.

Kocsis JD, Waxman SG (1987): Ionic channel organization of normal and regenerating mammalian axons. In Seil FJ, Herbert E, Carlson BM (eds): "Neural Regeneration Progress in Brain Research," vol 71. Amsterdam: Elsevier, pp 89–102.

Kocsis JD, Waxman SG, Hildebrand C, Ruiz JA (1982): Regenerating mammalian nerve fibres: Changes in action potential waveform and firing characteristics following blockage of potassium conductance. Proc R Soc Lond [Biol] 217:277–287.

Kristol C, Sandri C, Akert K (1978): Intramembranous particles at nodes of Ranvier in rat spinal cord. Brain Res 142:391–399.

Kruze J, Keilhaver C, Faissner A, Timpl R, Schachner M (1985): The J1 glycoprotein: A novel nervous system cell adhesion molecule of the L2/HNK-1 family. Nature (Lond) 315:146–148.

Landon DN (1981): Structure of normal peripheral myelinated fibers. In Waxman SG, Ritchie JM (eds): "Demyelinating Diseases: Basic and Clinical Electrophysiology." New York: Raven Press, pp 25–49.

Leisi P, Dahl D, Vaheri JA (1983): Laminin is produced by early rat astrocytes in primary culture. J Cell Biol 96:920–924.

McDonald WJ, Ohlrich G (1971): Quantitative anatomical measurements on single isolated fibers from cat spinal cord. J Anat 110:191–202.

Meiri H, Pre-Chen S, Koczya AD (1985): Sodium channel localization in sciatic nerve following lead-induced demyelination. Brain Res 359:326–331.

Newman EA (1986): The Muller cell. In Federoff S, Vernadakis A (eds): "Astrocytes," vol 1. New York: Academic Press, pp 149–171.

Oaklander AL, Pellegrino R, Ritchie JM (1984): Saxitoxin binding to central and peripheral nervous tissue of the myelin deficient (md) mutant rat. Brain Res 307:393–397.

Orida N, Poo M (1978): Electrophoretic movement and localization of acetylcholine receptors in embryonic muscle cell membrane. Nature (Lond) 275:31–35.

Pfenninger KN, Johnson MP (1983): Membrane biogenesis in the sprouting neuron: I. Selective transfer of newly synthesized phospholipid into the growing neurite. J Cell Biol 97:1038–1052.

Pinto Da Silva P, Miller RG (1975): Membrane particles on fracture faces of frozen myelin. Proc Natl Acad Sci USA 72:4046–4050.

Quick OC, Kennedy WR, Donaldson L (1979): Dimensions of myelinated fibers near the motor and sensory terminals of rat tenuissimus muscle. Neuroscience 4:1089–1096.

Raff MC, Miller RN (1984): Glial cell development in rat optic nerve. Trends Neurosci 7:469–472.

Raine CS (1984): On the association between perinodal astrocyte processes and nodes of Ranvier in the CNS. J Neurocytol 13:21–47.

Ransom BR, Yamate C., Black JA, Waxman SG (1985): Rat optic nerve: disruption of gliogenesis by 5-azacytidine. Brain Res. 337:41–51.

Rasminsky M, Kearny RE, Aguayo A, Bray GM (1978): Conduction of nerve impulses in spinal roots of dystrophic mice. Brain Res 143:71–85.

Reier PJ, Houlé JD (1987): The glial scar: Its bearing on axonal elongation and transplantation approaches to CNS repair. In Waxman SG (ed): "Functional Recovery in Neurological Disease." New York: Raven Press, pp 87–138.

Revenko S-V, Timin YN, Khodorov BI (1973): Special features of the conduction of nerve impulses from the myelinized part of the axon into the non-myelinated terminal. Biophysics 18:1140–1145.

Ritchie JM, Rogart RB (1977): The density of sodium channels in mammalian myelinated fibers and the nature of the axonal membrane under the myelin sheath. Proc Natl Acad Sci USA 74:211–215.

Rosenbluth J (1976): Intramembranous particle distribution at the node of Ranvier and adjacent axolemma in myelinated axons of frog brain. J Neurocytol 5:731–745.

Rosenbluth J (1979): Aberrant axon-Schwann cell junctions in dystrophic mouse nerves. J Neurocytol 5:731–744.

Rubin LL, McMahan UJ (1982): Regeneration of the neuromuscular junction: Steps toward defining the molecular basis for interaction between nerve and muscle. In Schotland DL (ed): "Diseases of the Motor Unit." New York: John Wiley and Sons, pp 187–196.

Rydmark M, Berthold CM (1983): Electron microscopic serial section analysis of nodes of Ranvier in lumbar spinal roots of cat. J Neurocytol 12:537–565.

Salzer JL, Bunge RP, Glaser L (1980): Studies of Schwann cell proliferation. III. Evidence for the surface localization of neurite mitogen. J Cell Biol 84:767–778.

Sanders FK, Whitteridge, D (1946): Conduction velocity and myelin thickness in regenerating nerve fibers. J. Physiol. 105:152–174.

Sandri C, Van Buren JM, Akert K (1977): Membrane morphology of the vertebrate nervous system: A study with freeze-etch technique. Progr Brain Res 46:1–380.

Sims TJ, Waxman SG, Black JA, Gilmore SA (1985): Perinodal astrocytic processes at nodes of Ranvier in developing normal and glial cell deficient rat spinal cord. Brain Res 337:321–333.

Skoff RP, Price DL, Stocks D (1976): Electron microscopic studies on gliogenesis in rat optic nerve. I. Glial cell proliferation. J Comp Neurol 169:291–312.

Smith KJ, Bostock N, Hall SM (1982): Saltatory conduction precedes remyelination in axons demyelinated with lysophosphatidyl choline. J Neurol Sci 54:13–31.

Tao-Cheng JN, Rosenbluth J (1982): Development of nodal and paranodal membrane specializations in amphibian peripheral nerve. Dev Brain Res 3:577–594.

Waxman SG (1970): Closely spaced nodes of Ranvier in the teleost brain. Nature 227:283–284.

Waxman SG (1977): Conduction in myelinated, unmyelinated, and demyelinated fibers. Arch Neurol 34:585–590.

Waxman SG (1984): Node-like membrane at extranodal sites: Comparative morphology and physiology. In Zagoren JC, Federoff S (eds): "Advances in Cellular Neurobiology," vol 6. New York: Academic Press, pp 311–351.

Waxman SG (1987): Rules governing membrane reorganization and axon-glial interactions during the development of myelinated fibers. In Seil FJ, Herbert E, Carlson BM (eds): "Neural Regeneration Progress in Brain Research," vol 71. Amsterdam: Elsevier, pp 121–142.

Waxman SG, Bennett MVL (1972): Relative conduction velocities of small myelinated and non-myelinated fibres in the central nervous system. Nature New Biol 238:217–219.

Waxman SG, Swadlow HA (1976): Ultrastructure of visual callosal axons in the rabbit. Exp Neurol 53:115–127.

Waxman SG, Black JA, Foster RE (1983): Ontogenesis of the axolemma and axo-glial relationships in myelinated fibers. Internat Rev Neurobiol 24:433–485.

Waxman SG, Brill MH (1978): Conduction through demyelinated plaques in multiple sclerosis: Computer simulations of facilitation by short internodes. J Neurol Neurosurg Psychiat 41:408–417.

Waxman SG, Foster RE (1980): Development of the axon membrane during differentiation of myelinated fibres in spinal nerve roots. Proc R Soc Lond [Biol] 209:441–446.

Waxman SG, Wood S (1984): Impulse induction in inhomogeneous axons: Effects of variation in voltage-sensitive ionic conductance on invasion of demyelinated axon segments and preterminal fibers. Brain Res 294:111–122.

Waxman SG, Black JA (1984): Freeze-fracture ultrastructure of the perinodal astrocyte and associated glial junctions. Brain Res 308:77–87.

Waxman SG, Sims TJ (1984): Specificity in central myelination: evidence for local regulation of myelin thickness. Brain Res 292:179–185.

Waxman SG, Black JA (1985): Membrane structure of vesiculotubular complexes in developing axons in rat optic nerve: Freeze-fracture evidence for sequential membrane assembly. Proc R Soc Lond [Biol] 225:357–363.

Waxman SG, Ritchie JM (1985): Organization of ion channels in the myelinated nerve fiber. Science 228:1502–1507.

Waxman SG, Black JA (1987): Macromolecular structure of the Schwann cell membrane: perinodal microvilli. J Neurol Sci 77:23–34.

Waxman SG, Pappas GD, Bennett MVL (1972): Morphological correlates of functional differentiation of nodes of Ranvier along single fibers in the neurogenic electric organ of the knife fish Sternarchus. J Cell Biol 53:210–224.

Waxman SG, Black JA, Foster RE (1982): Freeze-fracture heterogeneity of the axolemma of premyelinated fibers in the CNS. Neurology 32:418–421.

Weinberg MS, Spencer PS (1976): Studies on the control of myelinogenesis: II. Evidence for neuronal regulation of myelination. Brain Res 113:363–378.

Wiley-Livingston CA, Ellisman M (1980): Development of axonal membrane specializations defines nodes of Ranvier and precedes Schwann cell myelin elaboration. Dev Biol 79:334–354.

Williams PL, Wendell-Smith CP (1971): Some additional parametric variations between peripheral nerve populations. J Anat 109:505–526.

5

Exploring the Capacity of CNS Neurons to Survive Injury, Regrow Axons, and Form New Synapses in Adult Mammals

GARTH M. BRAY, MD, AND **ALBERT J. AGUAYO,** MD

Neurosciences Unit, The Montreal General Hospital and McGill University, Montréal, Québec, Canada H3G 1A4

Following the interruption of nerve fiber tracts by trauma or disease in the brain or spinal cord of adult mammals, including humans, the failure of central nervous system (CNS) nerve cells to regenerate lengthy axons and reform synapses with distant neurons results in permanent anatomical and functional disconnection. In contrast to the well documented failure of these interrupted axons to regrow more than a mm or so, it is now known that sustained regenerative elongation of CNS axons is possible in adult mammals if the non-neuronal environment of the damaged axons is changed. One experimental strategy that has been used to change the environment of injured CNS axons consists of grafting a segment of peripheral nerve (for review, see Aguayo, 1985). Such a capacity of central neurons to extend their axons into segments of peripheral nerve was suspected for many years on the basis of light microscopic preparations by Ramón y Cajal (1914) and his students, as well as several subsequent investigators (for review, see Bray et al., 1987). However, without the use of more specific anatomical or electrophysiological tracing techniques, the extent to which the observed growth into the nerve grafts arose from intrinsic CNS neurons remained controversial. Ramón y Cajal (1914) recognized that some of the axons seen in the grafted nerve segments were derived from peripheral nerve fibers, and Clark (1942) considered that all

axons in the experimental grafts arose from such extraneous sources. Thus, in spite of evidence to the contrary, these technical impediments helped to entrench the concept that the regrowth of CNS axons was impossible.

The application of retrogradely transported tracer substances eventually proved that some of the axons that grow into peripheral nerve grafts originate from intrinsic CNS neurons. Richardson et al. (1980) inserted short segments of sciatic nerve into the transected spinal cords of adult rats and used the retrograde transport of horseradish peroxidase (HRP) to show that spinal cord neurons had regrown their axons across the grafted segments of peripheral nerve. Using segments of peripheral nerve up to 3 cm in length, David and Aguayo (1981) applied tracer substances to document that neurons in the spinal cord and medulla oblongata of adult rats could elongate for distances equal to or greater than the longest CNS fiber pathways in these animals. Peripheral nerve "bridges" were subsequently used to document that neurons in other regions of the CNS are also capable of this axonal regrowth into the changed milieu provided by the grafts (Benfey and Aguayo, 1982; Aguayo, 1985; So and Aguayo, 1985), and that neurons with such regenerated axons are able to respond to physiological stimuli (Keirstead et al., 1985, Munz et al., 1985; Gauthier and Rasminsky, 1987).

With these demonstrations that several different classes of CNS neurons retain their developmental potential to regrow lengthy

Neural Regeneration and Transplantation, pages 67–78
© 1989 Alan R. Liss, Inc.

axons, it has become feasible to study the possibility that nerve cells injured in mature experimental animals may also be able to express other developmental capacities necessary for the restoration of damaged neural circuitries. Such considerations require an assessment of the widespread and diverse effects of axotomy. Thus we discuss here certain effects of axotomy and describe the results of nerve grafting experiments designed to modify neuronal responses in the mature CNS of laboratory animals. In this review, we emphasize the responses of neurons to injury and experimental manipulations rather than the nature of the environmental influences that determine these responses. The reader will find current information on investigations aimed at clarifying the role of molecular components of the cellular and noncellular neuronal environment in Chapter 7 (Varon et al.) of this volume.

WIDESPREAD EFFECTS OF AXOTOMY

Injuries or diseases that affect nerve fiber pathways not only interrupt axons and disconnect interrelated neural centers but also cause dynamic and widespread changes in the structure and function of the directly damaged neurons, their associated nerve cells and target tissues, and the cellular and noncellular components of the neuronal environment.

Retrograde Changes in Axotomized Neurons

Interruption of axons leads to perikaryal changes that range from chromatolysis to the death of axotomized neurons, particularly if the lesion is near the cell body (for review, see Lieberman, 1974). The thalamic projection neurons (Barron et al., 1973; Lieberman, 1974) and the cholinergic neurons of the nucleus basalis (Williams et al., 1986) are two of many examples of CNS neurons in which retrograde death has been documented following axotomy. In this review, we emphasize the retrograde effects of optic nerve (ON) lesions on the ganglion cells of the retina (RGCs), a group of CNS neurons in which the effects of axotomy can be more readily quantitated. The loss of retinal neurons caused by ON transection in adult mammals varies from 50% to more than 90%, depending on the techniques used to identify RGCs, the proximity of the lesion to

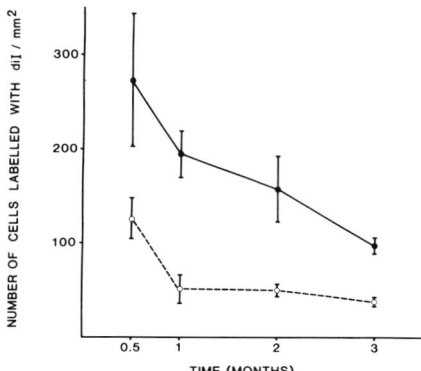

Figure 5–1. Survival of ganglion cells (RGCs) in the retinas of adult rats following optic nerve (ON) transection with and without attachment of peripheral nerve (PN) grafts. RGC survival was estimated by determining the densities of retinal neurons retrogradely labeled with the persistent tracer, diI (Honig and Hume, 1986), at the time of ON transection and PN grafting. In the retinas without PN grafts (open circles), axotomy caused the loss of more than 90% of the diI-labeled RGCs. In the retinas with PN grafts (closed circles), the survival of the axotomized RGCs was enhanced two- to fourfold (Reproduced from Villegas-Perez et al., 1988 by permission of the publisher.)

the eye, and the age and species of the animal. For example, in a study in adult rats, in which retrogradely transported tracers were used to distinguish RGCs from displaced amacrine cells (Villegas-Perez et al., 1988), we found that ON transection near the eye can lead to the loss of more than 90% of the RGCs (Fig. 5–1). However, when RGCs are axotomized 2–3 cm from the eye, the death of RGCs is delayed and less frequent (Misantone et al., 1984). When the ON is transected in newborn mammals, nearly all RGCs die (Muchnick-Miller and Oberdorfer, 1981; Allcutt et al., 1984). Fewer RGCs are lost after optic nerve transection in amphibia (Humphrey and Beazley, 1985; Scalia et al., 1985; Stelzner and Strauss, 1986); in goldfish all of these cells appear to be able to overcome the retrograde effects of axotomy (Murray et al., 1982; Grafstein, 1986).

In the different species of laboratory animals

studied, the exact cause of the axotomy induced retrograde changes, including neuronal death, is unknown. On the basis of experiments in which retrograde transport was blocked (Singer et al., 1982), it was postulated that retrogradely relayed signals from the site of injury might be responsible. The deprivation of peripherally derived influences is another commonly accepted explanation for the retrograde degeneration of axotomized neurons in adult animals. There is abundant evidence that such peripheral influences are important for the survival of neurons during development (for review, see Purves and Lichtman, 1985). In mature animals, the influence of retrogradely transported trophic factors on neuron survival might also explain the phenomenon of enhanced survival of axotomized neurons that have "sustaining collaterals" (Fry and Cowan, 1972). The results of several experimental approaches (reviewed below), which have been used to enhance the survival of axotomized neurons, support the concept that a loss of peripherally derived influences is at least partly involved in the retrograde degeneration of neurons following the interruption of their axons in adult mammals.

Axon interruption also causes extensive rearrangements in the size and shape of the dendrites of the neurons that survive axotomy (Sumner and Watson, 1971; Yawo, 1987). Within the retina, axotomized RGCs show a fivefold reduction in the branching of their dendrites, as well as increases in the diameters of their somata (S. Thanos and A.J. Aguayo, unpublished observations). Axotomy can also lead to transneuronal retrograde changes ranging from the retraction of synapses (for review, see Mendell, 1984) to the degeneration and loss of neurons (Cowan, 1970). However, in sections of axotomized retinas examined by light microscopic immunocytochemistry using antibodies to receptor, horizontal, bipolar, and several subclasses of amacrine cells, no substantial changes have been observed among these different populations of intrinsic retinal neurons up to 1 1/2 years after optic nerve transection (Carter et al., 1987). These results suggest that little or no transsynaptic retrograde degeneration occurs within the retinas of adult rats, even when most RGCs are lost as a result of axotomy.

Orthograde Effects on Neurons and Other Targets

In addition to degeneration of the synaptic terminals and distal segments of transected axons, axonal interruption causes transsynaptic changes in target cells—effector organs, sensory receptors, or other neurons. For example, reflecting the normal regulatory influences of neurons on target cells, denervation of skeletal muscle, smooth muscle, or exocrine glands leads to the development of extrasynaptic chemoreceptors and the development of the phenomena of denervation sensitivity (for review, see Thesleff, 1987). When peripheral nerves are cut in adult animals, there are rearrangements in the representations of sensory receptive fields in the spinal cord (Devor and Wall, 1978) and the cerebral cortex (Kaas et al., 1983). Within the CNS, the interruption of neural circuitry can also be followed by the replacement of lost synaptic contacts by newly formed terminals from local neurons (for review, see Vaughan and Peters, 1985), leading to increased densities of synaptic contacts of one particular neurotransmitter type, e.g., GABAergic (Houser et al., 1983). Thus experimental attempts to reconstitute the neural circuitries that are interrupted by CNS lesions must take into account these widespread effects of axotomy.

ENHANCEMENT OF THE SURVIVAL OF AXOTOMIZED CNS NEURONS IN ADULT MAMMALS

Attempts to enhance the survival of axotomized neurons in experimental animals can be classified into three broad categories: 1) neurotrophic factors; 2) target coculture or grafting; and 3) peripheral nerve grafts.

Neurotrophic Factors

Several substances, which have now been identified, purified and sequenced, support the survival of neurons both in vitro and in vivo. The best known of these is nerve growth factor (NGF), which has trophic effects on developing sympathetic and sensory neurons (for review, see Purves and Lichtman, 1985). When NGF is injected into peripheral nerves in vivo, it binds to high-affinity receptors (Richardson and Riopelle, 1984) and is transported retrogradely to the neuronal cell bodies (Richardson and Riopelle, 1984; Abrahamson et al., 1987). NGF also enhances the survival of axotomized peripheral sympathetic (Hendry and Campbell, 1976) and sensory neurons (Yip and Johnson, 1984) and prevents the retrograde loss of neurons in the basal forebrain caused by fimbria-fornix lesions (Hefti, 1986; Williams et al., 1986; Kromer, 1987).

FIBROBLAST GROWTH FACTOR

Fibroblast growth factor (FGF) which exists in acidic or basic forms, is a mitogen for glial and endothelial cells as well as many cells of mesodermal origin (reviewed by Thomas and Gimenez-Gallego, 1986). FGF is also present in the CNS (Gospardarowicz et al., 1984) and both enhances survival and promotes neurite outgrowth of central and peripheral neurons in vitro (Morrison et al., 1986; Walicke et al., 1986; Unsicker et al., 1987). Furthermore, it has been reported that single applications of small amounts (40–50 ng) of FGF enhanced the survival of axotomized RGCs in vivo (Seivers et al., 1987); it remains to be determined if this is a direct effect on axotomized neurons or an indirect one mediated through glial or endothelial cells.

BRAIN-DERIVED NEUROTROPHIC FACTOR

Brain-derived neurotrophic factor (BDNF), which enhances the survival of RGCs in vitro (Barde et al., 1982; Johnson et al., 1986), has been purified (Barde et al., 1983) and shown to have homologies with NGF (Y. Barde, personal communication).

OTHER SUBSTANCES

Ciliary neuronotrophic factor (CNTF) is also present in peripheral nerve, brain, and the eye (Williams et al., 1984), but its function in vivo has not been defined. Purpurin is a retinol-binding protein derived from the chick retina; its molecular weight is similar to that of CNTF. Purpurin promotes the in vitro survival of chick retinal cells as well as ciliary ganglion cells (Schubert et al., 1986). It has not been determined if the retinal neurons supported by this substance are receptor cells or ganglion cells. Additional substances (for review, see Manthorpe et al., 1986) are also growth factor candidates but, until they have been purified

in significant amounts, it remains possible that they are not unique trophic entities.

Target Coculture or Grafting

The viability of RGCs in vitro is enhanced by coculturing with their target tissues (e.g., Nurcombe and Bennett, 1981; McCaffery et al., 1982). It is reasonable to speculate that this enhancement may be related to the high concentrations of BDNF that are apparently present in the superior colliculus (Johnson et al., 1986). In vivo, the implantation of fetal CNS target tissues has been reported to protect other axotomized neurons in the CNS of neonatal rodents (Björklund and Stenevi, 1984; Bregman and Reier, 1986; Cunningham et al., 1987).

Peripheral Nerve Grafts

In experiments involving axotomy of RGCs, which can be more readily quantitated than is possible with other groups of CNS neurons, it has been found that peripheral nerve (PN) grafts enhance the survival of RGCs whose axons have been interrupted by lesions within the retina (Turner et al., 1987) or by transecting the ON near the eye (Berry et al., 1986; Villegas-Perez et al., 1986, 1988). Furthermore, the data of Turner et al. (1987) suggest that the placement of a PN graft in a retinal lesion delays the onset of neuronal death by 1 week. In the experiments of Villegas-Perez et al. (1988), in which the long-lasting tracer diI (Honig and Hume, 1986) was used to label RGCs at the time of axotomy and PN graft placement, an ameliorative effect of the grafts on the axotomized RGCs ranged from two-to-fourfold between 2 weeks and 3 months after axotomy (Fig. 5–1). Moreover, qualitative observations of the intraretinal portions of RGC axons indicated that such effects persisted for 6 and 9 months after ON transection (Fig. 5–2).

Possible Mechanisms

There is considerable evidence that segments of peripheral nerve, such as those used as grafts in the experiments cited above, contain trophic substances. Injured or excised segments of peripheral nerve synthesize NGF and other neurotrophic factors (Riopelle et al., 1981; Richardson and Ebendal, 1982; Varon et al., 1983/84; Abrahamson et al., 1986; Heu-

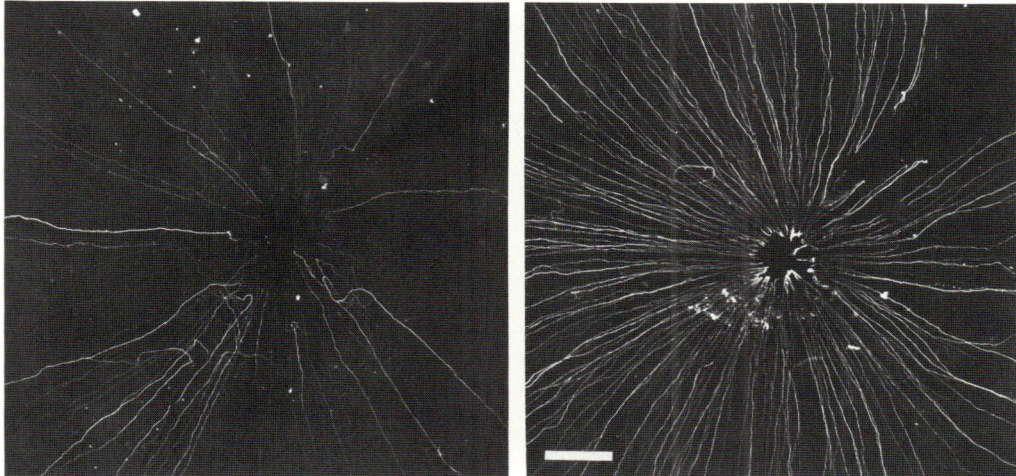

Figure 5–2. The central portions of flat-mounted retinas from adult rats 9 months after ON transection with (right) or without (left) attachment of PN grafts. The intraretinal axons of the RGCs are delineated by their immunoreactivity to RT 97, a monoclonal antibody that reacts with phosphorylated 200-kD neurofilament subunits (Anderton et al., 1982), as visualized with fluorescein isothiocyanate-labeled secondary antibodies. The densities of immunoreactive RGC axons are greater in the retina with a PN graft (right) than in the retina without a graft (left). Fluorescence micrograph, scale bar = 500 μm. (Reproduced from Villegas-Perez et al., 1988, by permission of the publisher.)

mann et al., 1987). Moreover, nerve sheath cells contain mRNA specific for NGF (Shelton and Reichardt, 1984), and there are increases in the content of NGF and its mRNA (Heumann et al., 1987) as well as NGF receptors (Tainuchi et al., 1986) in degenerating peripheral nerve segments such as those used for PN grafts. However, the possible relevance of NGF to the survival and regrowth of RGCs is, at present, unclear. Although developing optic nerves show NGF immunoreactivity (Ayer-Lelievre et al., 1983; Finn et al., 1987), RGCs of adult rodents are apparently not responsive to NGF and do not express NGF receptors. Nevertheless, it remains possible that injured RGCs may have different trophic requirements. Alternatively, growth factors other than NGF may be released by the PN graft and influence the survival and growth of the axotomized RGCs. It is also possible that the extracellular matrix components (Liesi et al., 1984; Carbonetto et al., 1987;Sandrock and Matthew, 1987) of the transplanted PN segments influence the responses of these regenerating axons.

Whatever components of the PN grafts are involved, our observations suggest that their early and late effects on neuronal survival may be related to different trophic modes of action and/or that different populations of RGCs (and presumably other CNS neurons) may have differing requirements for survival following axotomy. The earliest effect may involve substances that diffuse from the graft (Berry et al., 1986; Villegas-Perez et al., 1986, 1988; Turner et al., 1987). Growth factors in the grafted segments of peripheral nerve (Riopelle et al., 1981; Richardson and Ebendal, 1982; Varon et al., 1983/84; Abrahamson et al., 1986; Heumann et al., 1987) could be candidates for this early effect. A later effect of the PN grafts on neuronal survival may be a result of more complex interactions with Schwann cells or other components of the PN grafts into which they have grown their axons. Such a conclusion is suggested by the data of Villegas-Perez et al. (1988), in which the survival of RGCs whose axons had grown into the grafts by 3 months appeared to depend on contact with Schwann cells and other nonneuronal components of

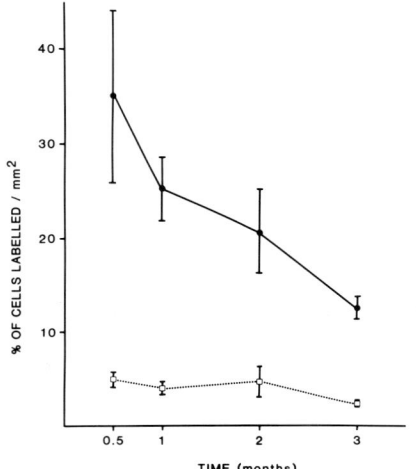

Figure 5–3. Survival and regrowth of RGCs in the retinas of adult rats following ON transection and attachment of PN grafts. Expressed as proportions of the labeling with the respective tracer substances in control retinas, the ratios of surviving RGCs (filled circles) were determined by calculating the densities of neurons labeled with diI applied to the ON stump at the time of axotomy and graft placement, while the proportions of RGCs that had grown to the ends of grafts were determined by calculating the densities of neurons retrogradely labeled with Fast Blue applied to the end of the graft 2 days prior to examination of the retinas. Although the densities of surviving RGCs decreased significantly between 1 and 3 months, the densities of neurons that had regenerated to the end of the graft remained relatively stable, suggesting that contact with components in the PN graft may have contributed to the later survival of these neurons. (Reproduced from Villegas-Perez et al., 1988, by permission of the publisher.)

the PN grafts or substances they secrete (Fig. 5–3).

The long-term survival of axotomized neurons may ultimately depend on the formation of synapses. Such a dependency would not be surprising, since the survival of neurons during development in vertebrates appears to be related to the formation of synaptic connections (for review, see Purves and Lichtman, 1985). However, evidence for such a relationship between connectivity and the survival of axotomized neurons in adult mammals is still indirect. Neurons regenerating into PN grafts from the retina (Keirstead et al., 1985) or the brainstem of adult rats (Gauthier and Rasminsky, 1987) showed apparently normal electrophysiological properties during the first 5 months, but fewer responses were detectable 9–12 months after grafting. Furthermore, fetal CNS neurons transplanted into peripheral nerves of adult rats showed prominent degenerative changes after being in this isolated state for more than 5 months (Doering and Aguayo, 1987). The late declines in the functional and structural integrity of neurons may indicate that either the critical influences provided by the blind-ended PN grafts are not persistently expressed after the regenerating axons have penetrated the grafts, or that their survival is ultimately dependent on the establishment of terminal contacts with target tissues.

Guided Regrowth and Terminal Connectivity of Regenerating CNS Axons

In addition to enhancing neuronal survival, an important element in any attempt to reconstitute neural circuitries interrupted by the injury of fiber pathways in the CNS, PN grafts can also be used experimentally to guide the regenerating axons of CNS neurons to the vicinity of their natural targets. Because the retina contains well characterized populations of neurons whose structure and function are particularly suited for investigations of the regenerative capacities of the CNS, autologous PN grafts, attached to the orbital stump of the optic nerve transected near the eye in adult rats (Fig. 5–4), were used to determine if regenerating RGC axons 1) could be directed along the PN grafts to the vicinity of their natural targets; 2) would penetrate the adjacent CNS tissues when the ends of the grafts were inserted into the superior colliculus; and 3) would reform synapses with neurons in the CNS.

Guidance

Studies in which retrogradely transported tracer substances were applied to the ends of the grafts documented that between 1% and 11% (mean 3.3%) of the original normal population of RGCs regrew axons along the graft for 3–4 cm (Vidal-Sanz et al., 1987), distances that were nearly double those of the normal

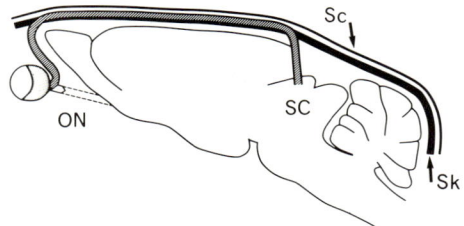

Figure 5–4. Diagram of an adult rat brain in sagittal section showing a PN graft used to replace the transected optic nerve (ON). One end of an autologous peroneal nerve graft was attached to the orbital stump of the ON transected near the eye. The other end of the graft was initially ligated and left between the scalp (Sc) and the skull (Sk). Two to three months later, the distal end of the graft was inserted into the superior colliculus (SC). (Modified from Vidal-Sanz et al., 1987, and reproduced by permission of the publisher.)

Penetration

Although it has been known since the time of Ramón y Cajal (1914) that axons could not regrow for long distances within the CNS of adult mammals, there are documented examples of local axonal growth for several mm after injuries near cell bodies in the retina (Leoz-Ortin and Arcaute, 1914; Goldberg and Frank, 1980; McConnell and Berry, 1982; So et al., 1986) and spinal cord (Risling et al., 1983; Havton and Kellerth, 1987). In keeping with such findings of limited, but unequivocal growth of axons within the adult CNS, our observations, based on the orthograde transport of tracer substances, documented that some RGC axons that had regrown along the PN grafts were able to penetrate the PNS-CNS interface for distances of approximately 1 mm following the insertion of the ends of the grafts into the SC. Thus, on reentering the CNS, either a lack of critical growth-promoting molecules in the environment or the presence of influences that inhibit fiber extension prevented elongation of axons that had grown the entire length of the PN grafts linking the eye and the dorsal midbrain in these animals.

Connectivity

Within the SC, the orthogradely transported RITC or HRP outlined individual fibers that usually formed multiple branched arborizations (Vidal-Sanz et al., 1987; Carter et al., 1988). When the territories of these arborizations were examined by electron microscopy, we observed HRP-labeled axon terminals in the neuropil of the superficial SC within approximately 0.5 mm of the ends of the grafts. Because the PN grafts were the only direct link between the tracer-injected eyes and the SC, these labeled structures are considered to be the terminals of the regenerated RGC axons.

The ultrastructural characteristics of the regenerated and control RGC terminals, identified in the SC by the presence of orthogradely transported HRP, were compared in a series of adult hamsters (Carter et al., 1988). Six to eight weeks after graft insertion, some of the regenerated terminals were larger than normal, but most resembled the HRP-labeled RGC terminals of the control SCs in terms of their densely packed, spherical synaptic vesicles; the presence of large, pale mitochondria; the propor-

retinocollicular projections in adult rats. However, in such experiments it was not possible to relate the extent of this axonal regrowth along the PN grafts to the numbers of surviving RGCs. This was subsequently determined by using a persistent fluorescent tracer, applied at the time of grafting, to estimate the densities of surviving RGCs; in such experiments, it was found that as many as 20% of the surviving RGCs had grown to the ends of the PN grafts, where they contacted and became retrogradely labeled by a second fluorescent tracer (Villegas-Perez et al., 1988).

When orthogradely transported tracers (HRP, rhodamine isothiocyanate-RITC, or tritiated aminoacids) were used to identify regenerated axons, labeled axon profiles were found along the lengths of the PN grafts and in the superior colliculus (SC) (Trecarten et al., 1986; Vidal-Sanz et al., 1987). Within the PN grafts, the labeled ends of the regenerating RGC axons resembled the growth cones seen in the optic nerves of immature birds (Thanos and Bonhoeffer, 1983) or mammals (Williams et al., 1986), and appeared to have grown preferentially between the basal laminae and plasma membranes of the Schwann cells that populate the grafts.

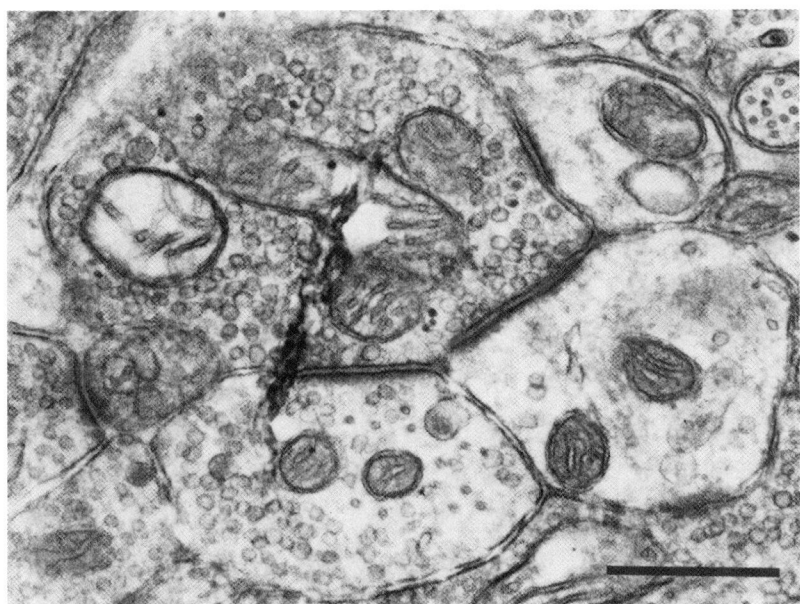

Figure 5–5.   The regenerated terminal of an RGC axon that has regrown along a peripheral nerve graft into the superficial superior colliculus of an adult hamster. The retinal origin of this axon terminal is indicated by the presence of crystalline reaction product formed by horseradish peroxidase (HRP) that had been orthogradely transported from the eye to which the superior colliculus was connected by the graft. (As sometimes occurs with the technique used to visualize the HRP reaction product, the crystalline reaction product has penetrated the plasma membrane of the terminal. For method, see Vidal-Sanz et al., 1987.) This terminal forms three asymmetric synaptic contacts (Gray type I) with dendritic processes, some of which contain synaptic vesicles. The fourth synapse, on the left, does not directly involve the labeled terminal. Electron micrograph, scale bar = 0.5 μm.

tions that showed well-differentiated synaptic specializations in single sections; the tendency to form synaptic complexes; the predominance of synaptic specializations of asymmetric type (Gray type I); and the proportions of contacts with dendritic profiles that either did or did not contain vesicles (Fig. 5–5). Thus most of the regenerating RGC axons that reentered the SC of these adult hamsters underwent pre- and postsynaptic differentiations that resemble those of normal retinofugal synapses in the SC (Lund, 1969). Such re-formed retino-collicular synapses appear to be persistent (Bray et al., 1988) and are able to cause transynaptic activation of SC neurons in response to light (S. Keirstead, M. Rasminsky. Y. Fukada, D.A. Carter, A.J. Aguayo, and M. Vidal-Sanz, unpublished observations). We do not know if they are retinotopically arranged.

Integration

The replacement or substitution of certain populations of lost or abnormal CNS neurons in experimental animals by the transplantation of immature cells into neonatal or even mature hosts can lead to an amelioration of some functional deficits (for review, see Björklund et al., 1987). Such experiments have also provided important insights into the ability of the injured adult CNS to receive inputs from and to respond to the transplanted cells. For example, when grafts of fetal neurons are introduced into developing or denervated sites in the neostriatum (Björklund et al., 1987; Bolam et al., 1987), hippocampus (Clarke et al., 1986), or cerebellum (Sotelo and Alvarado-Mallart, 1987), the extension of immature axons was generally curtailed within the adult host CNS.

However, if the grafted and target neurons were placed in close apposition to each other, the transplanted cells made anatomical and functional contacts with the mature nerve cells of the recipient animals. Such results suggest that it may eventually be possible to show that the axons of RGCs and other CNS neurons, which have regenerated to distant targets along PN grafts, can also be integrated both anatomically and functionally into the interrupted circuitry of the mature CNS.

CONCLUSIONS

We have reviewed briefly the results of an experimental approach to the reestablishment of synaptic contacts between widely separated neurons that have been disconnected by interruption of their fiber tracts in the CNS of adult rodents. This was accomplished by grafting segments of peripheral nerve between the source and target groups of neurons. Such a change in the nonneuronal environment enhanced the survival of the axotomized source neurons, promoted the regrowth of their axons, and guided these axons to the vicinity of target neurons, where relatively normal-appearing synaptic contacts have been observed in rats and hamsters. In other words, by changing the milieu of their severed axons, these neurons in the adult CNS were able to effect some of the steps necessary to act as sources of target reinnervation such as that achieved by the grafting of fetal neurons. Furthermore, since synaptic contacts can be established after an extensive growth of axons, it is reasonable to suggest that such connections might also occur spontaneously between neurons that are closer to each other.

Because most fibers that enter the graft regrow its entire length and most axons that penetrate the SC appear to form synapses, these results suggest that the expression of certain characteristic features of axonal regrowth and terminal differentiation by regenerating CNS neurons may be mandated by conditions in their environment. Thus, components of the two different environments—PNS and CNS—may trigger distinct intrinsic neuronal processes that influence the extension and synaptogenesis of central axons in a manner similar to that observed in regenerating peripheral nerves in which motor, sensory, or autonomic

axons regrow extensively until they reach muscle, skin, or other targets, where they form synapses or other differentiated terminals. The identification of the intrinsic neuronal mechanisms that regulate these responses and the definition of their extrinsic molecular determinants should lead to important advances in this field of biomedical research.

One of the ultimate goals of both the neuronal transplant and the nerve graft experiments is the reconstitution of interrupted neural circuitries. However, it would be premature to equate the morphological demonstration of regenerated synapses in the superior colliculi of rats and hamsters with the reformation of neural circuits until it can be established that such new connections are appropriately integrated into the complex system of excitatory and inhibitory influences that make up such a point-to-point pathway. Indeed, if such regrowth were to lead to the formation of inappropriate connections, it is possible that unwanted functions could result. Thus speculations as to the possible implications of these findings for the treatment of neurological illnesses in humans are not justified at present.

ACKNOWLEDGMENTS

The authors thank Drs. M. Vidal-Sanz, M.-P. Villegas-Perez, D. Carter, and S. Thanos for their collaboration and M. David, S. Harrington, S. Shinn, J. Trecarten, and W. Wilcox for technical assistance. Research grants were provided by The Medical Research Council, the Multiple Sclerosis Society of Canada, the Spinal Cord Research Foundation, and the Daniel Heumann Fund.

REFERENCES

Abrahamson IK, Wilson PA, Rush RA (1986): Production and transport of endogenous trophic activities in a peripheral nerve following target removal. Dev Brain Res 27:117–126.

Abrahamson IK, Bridges D, Rush RA (1987): Transport of endogenous nerve growth factor in the proximal stump of sectioned nerves. J Neurocytol 16:417–422.

Aguayo AJ (1985): Axonal regeneration from injured neurons in the adult mammalian central nervous system. In Cotman CW (ed): 'Synaptic Plasticity.'' New York: Guilford Press, pp 457–484.

Allcutt D, Berry M, Sievers J (1984): A quantitative comparison of the reactions of retinal ganglion cells to optic nerve crush in neonatal and adult mice. Dev Brain Res 16:219–230.

Anderton BH, Downes MJ, Green PJ, Tomlinson BE, Ulrich J, Wood JN, Kahn J (1982): Monoclonal antibodies show that neurofibrillary tangles and neurofilaments share antigenic determinants. Nature 298:84–86.

Ayer-Lelievre LA, Ebendal T, Olson S, Seiger A (1983): Localization of nerve growth factor like immunoreactivity in rat nervous tissue. Med Biol 61:293–304.

Barde YA, Edgar D, Thoenen H (1982): Purification of a new neurotrophic factor from mammalian brain. EMBO J 1:549–553.

Barde YA, Edgar D, Thoenen H (1983): New neurotrophic factors. Annu Rev Physiol 45:601–612.

Barron KD, Means ED, Larsen E (1973): Ultrastructure of retrograde degeneration in thalamus of rat. I. Neuronal somata and dendrites. J Neuropathol Exp Neurol 32:218–244.

Benfey M, Aguayo AJ (1982): Extensive elongation of axons from rat brain into peripheral nerve grafts. Nature 296:150–152.

Berry M, Rees L, Sievers J (1986): Unequivocal regeneration of rat optic nerve axons into sciatic nerve isografts. In Das GD, Wallace RB (eds): "Neural transplantation and regeneration." New York: Springer-Verlag, pp 63–79.

Björklund A, Stenevi U (1984): Intracerebral neural implants: Neural replacement and reconstruction of damaged circuitries. Annu Rev Neurosci 7:279–308.

Björklund A, Lindvall O, Isacson O, Brundin P, Wictorin K, Strecker RE, Clarke DJ, Dunnett SB (1987): Mechanisms of action of intracerebral transplants: Studies on nigral and striatal grafts to the lesioned striatum. Trends Neurosci 10:509–516.

Bolam JP, Freund TF, Björklund A, Dunnett SB, Smith AD (1987): Synaptic input and local output of dopaminergic neurons in grafts that functionally reinnervate the host neostriatum. Exp Brain Res 68:131–146.

Bray GM, Vidal-Sanz M, Aguayo AJ (1987): Regeneration of axons from the central nervous system of adult rats. Prog Brain Res 71:373–379.

Bray GM, Vidal-Sanz M, Aguayo AJ (1988): Regenerated retino-collicular synapses eighteen months after substitution of the optic nerve by a peripheral nerve graft in adult rats. Soc Neurosci Abstr 14: (in press).

Bregman BS, Reier P (1986): Neural tissue transplants rescue axotomized rubrospinal cells from retrograde death. J Comp Neurol 244:86–95.

Carbonetto S, Evans D, Cochard P (1987): Nerve fiber growth in culture on tissue substrata from central and peripheral nervous system. J Neurosci 7:610–620.

Carter D, Vidal-Sanz M, Aguayo AJ (1987): Long term preservation of intrinsic retinal neurons after axotomy induced death of retinal ganglion cells. Neurosci Abst 13:1390.

Carter D, Bray GM, Aguayo AJ (1988): Normal ultrastructural characteristics of regenerated retino-collicular synapses in adult hamsters. Neurosci Lett Suppl 32:575.

Clark, WE Legros (1942): The problem of neuronal regeneration in the central nervous system. I. The influence of spinal ganglia and nerve fragments grafted in the brain. J Anat 77:20–48.

Clarke DJ, Gage FH, Nilsson OG, Björklund A (1986): Grafted septal neurons form cholinergic synaptic connections in the dentate gyrus of behaviorally impaired aged rats. J Comp Neurol 252:483–492.

Cowan WM (1970): Anterograde and retrograde transneuronal degeneration in the central and peripheral nervous systems. In Nauta WJH, Ebbeson SOE (eds): "Contemporary Research Methods in Neuroanatomy." Berlin: Springer-Verlag, pp 217–251.

Cunningham TJ, Sutilla CB, Haun F (1987): Trophic effects of transplants following damage to the cerebral cortex. Ann NY Acad Sci 495:153–167.

David S, Aguayo AJ (1981): Axonal elongation into PNS "bridges" after CNS injury in adult rats. Science 214:931–933.

Devor M, Wall PD (1978): Reorganization of spinal cord sensory map after peripheral nerve injury. Nature 275:75–76.

Doering L, Aguayo AJ (1987): Hirano bodies and other cytoskeletal abnormalities develop in fetal rat CNS grafts isolated for long periods in peripheral nerve. Brain Res 401:178–184.

Finn PJ, Ferguson IA, Wilson PA, Vahaviolos J, Rush RA (1987): Immunocytochemical evidence for the distribution of nerve growth factor in the embryonic mouse. J Neurocytol 16: 639–647.

Fry FJ, Cowan WM (1972): A study of retrograde cell degeneration in the lateral mamillary nucleus of the cat, with special reference to the role of axonal branching in the preservation of the cell. J Comp Neurol 144:1–24.

Gauthier P, Rasminsky M (1987): Activity of medullary respiratory neurons regenerating axons into peripheral nerve grafts in the adult rat. Brain Res 438:225–236.

Goldberg S, Frank B (1980): Will central nervous systems in the adult mammal regenerate after bypassing a lesion? A study in the mouse and chick visual systems. Exp Neurol 70: 675–689.

Gospodarowicz D, Cheng J, Lui GM, Baird A, Bohlen P (1984): Isolation of brain fibroblast growth factor by heparin-sepharose affinity chromatography: Identity with pituitary fibroblast growth factor. Proc Natl Acad Sci USA 81:6963–6967.

Grafstein B (1986): Regeneration in ganglion cells. In Adler R, Farber D (eds): "The Retina." Orlando: Academic Press, pp 275–335.

Havton L, Kellerth JO (1987): Regeneration by supernumerary axons with synaptic terminals in spinal motoneurons of cats. Nature 325:711–714.

Hefti F (1986): Nerve growth factor promotes survival of septal cholinergic neurons after fimbrial transections. J Neurosci 6:2155–2162.

Hendry IA, Campbell J (1976): Morphometric analysis of rat superior cervical ganglion after axotomy and nerve growth factor treatment. J Neurocytol 5:351–360.

Heumann R, Kersching S, Bandtlow C, Thoenen H (1987): Changes of nerve growth factor synthesis in nonneuronal cells in response to sciatic nerve transection. J Cell Biol 104:1623–1631.

Honig MG, Hume RI (1986): Fluorescent carbocyanine dyes allow living neurons of identified origin to be studied in long-term cultures. J Cell Biol 103:171–187.

Houser CR, Lee M, Vaughn JE (1983): Immunocytochemical localization of glutamic acid decarboxylase in normal and deafferented superior colliculus: Evidence for reorganization of gamma-aminobutyric acid synapses. J Neurosci 3:2030–2042.

Humphrey MF, Beazley LD (1985): Retinal ganglion cell death during optic nerve regeneration in the frog *Hyla moorei*. J Comp Neurol 236:382–402.

Johnson JE, Barde YA, Schwab M, Thoenen H (1986): Brain-derived neurotrophic factor supports the survival of cultured rat retinal ganglion cells. J Neurosci 6:3031–3038.

Kaas JH, Merzenich MM, Killackey HP (1983): The reorganization of somatosensory cortex following peripheral nerve damage in adult and developing animals. Ann Rev Neurosci 6:325–356.

Keirstead SA, Vidal-Sanz M, Rasminsky M, Aguayo AJ, Levesque M, So KF (1985): Responses to light of retinal neurons regenerating axons into peripheral nerve grafts in the rat. Brain Res 359:402–406.

Kromer LF (1987): Nerve growth factor treatment after brain injury prevents neuronal death. Science 235:214–216.

Leoz Ortin G, Arcuate LR (1914): Procesos regenerativos del nervio óptico y retina con ocasión de injertos nerviosos. Trab Lab Invest Biol 11:239–254.

Lieberman AR (1974): Some factors affecting retrograde neuronal responses to axonal lesions. In Bellairs G, Gray EG (eds): "Essays of the Nervous System." Oxford: Clarendon pp 71–105.

Liesi P, Dahl D, Vaheri A (1984): Neurons cultured from developing rat brain attach and spread preferentially on laminin. J Neurosci Res 11:241–251.

Lund RD (1969): Synaptic patterns of the superficial layers of the superior colliculus of the rat. J Comp Neurol 135:179–208.

Manthorpe M, Rudge JS, Varon S (1986): Astroglial cell contributions to neuronal survival and neuritic growth. In Fedoroff S, Vernadakis A (eds): "Astrocytes," vol 2. Orlando: Academic Press, pp 315–376.

McCaffery CA, Bennet MR, Dreher B (1982): The survival of neonatal rat ganglion cells *in vitro* is enhanced in the presence of appropriate parts of the brain. Exp Brain Res 48:377–386.

McConnell P, Berry M (1982): Regeneration of axons in the mouse retina after injury. Bibl Anat 23:26–37.

Mendell LM (1984): Modifiability of spinal synapses. Physiol Rev 64:260–324.

Misantone LJ, Gershenbaum M, Murray M (1984): Viability of retinal ganglion cells after optic nerve crush in adult rats. J Neurocytol 13:449–465.

Morrison RS, Sharma A, deVellis J, Bradshaw RA (1986): Basic fibroblast growth factor supports the survival of cerebral cortical neurons in primary cultures. Proc Natl Acad Sci USA 83:7537–7541.

Muchnick-Miller N, Oberdorfer M (1981): Neuronal and neuroglial responses following retinal lesions in the neonatal rats. J Comp Neurol 202:493–504.

Munz M, Rasminsky M, Aguayo AJ, Vidal-Sanz M, Devor M (1985): Functional activity of rat brainstem neurons regenerating axons along peripheral nerve grafts. Brain Res 340:115–125.

Murray M, Sharma S, Edwards MA (1982): Target regulation of synaptic number in the compressed retinotectal projection of the goldfish. J Comp Neurol 209:374–385.

Nurcombe V, Bennett MR (1981): Embryonic chick retinal ganglion cells identified *in vitro*. Their survival is dependent on a factor from the optic tectum. Exp Brain Res 44:249–258.

Purves D, Lichtman JW (1985): "Principles of Neural Development." Sunderland, MA: Sinauer Associates, pp 155–178.

Ramón y Cajal S (1914): "Estudios Sobre la Degeneración y Regeneración del Sistema Nervioso T. II." Madrid: Imprenta de Hijos de Nicolás Moya. pp 203–218.

Richardson PM, Ebendal T (1982): Nerve growth activities in the rat peripheral nerve. Brain Res 246:47–64,

Richardson PM, Riopelle RJ (1984): Uptake of nerve growth factor in rat peripheral and spinal nerves of primary sensory neurons. J Neurosci 4:1683–1689.

Richardson PM, McGuinness U, Aguayo AJ (1980): Axons from CNS neurons regenerate into PNS grafts. Nature 284:265–265.

Riopelle RJ, Boegman RJ, Cameron DA (1981): Peripheral nerve contains heterogeneous growth factors that support sensory neurons *in vitro*. Neurosci Lett 25:311–316.

Risling M, Cullheim S, Hildebrand C (1983): Reinnervation of the ventral root L7 from ventral horn neurons following intramedullary axotomy in adult rats. Brain Res 280:15–23.

Sandrock AW, Matthew WD (1987): An *in vitro* neurite promoting antigen functions in axonal regeneration *in vitro*. Science 237:1605–1608.

Scalia F, Arango V, Singman EL (1985): Loss and displacement of ganglion cells after optic nerve regeneration in adult *Rana pipiens*. Brain Res 344:267–280.

Schubert D, LaCorbiere M, Esch F (1986): A chick neural retina adhesion and survival molecule is a retinal-binding protein. J Cell Biol 102:2295–2301.

Shelton DL, Reichardt LF (1984): Expression of the nerve growth factor gene correlates with density of sympathetic innervation in effector organs. Proc Natl Acad Sci USA 81:7951–7955.

Sievers J, Hausmann B, Unsicker K, Berry M (1987): Fibroblast growth factors promote the survival of adult rat retinal ganglion cells after transection of the optic nerve. Neurosci Lett 76:157–162.

Singer PA, Mehler S, Fernandez HL (1982): Blockade of retrograde axonal transport delays the onset of metabolic and morphologic changes induced by axotomy. J Neurosci 2:1299–1306.

So KR, Aguayo AJ (1985): Lengthy regrowth of cut axons from ganglion cells after peripheral nerve transplantation into the retina of adult rats. Brain Res 328:349–354.

So KF, Xiao YM, Diao YC (1986): Effects on the growth of damaged ganglion cell axons after peripheral nerve transplantation in adult hamsters. Brain Res 377:168–172.

Sotelo C, Alvarado-Mallart RM (1987): Reconstruction of the defective cerebellar circuitry in adult Purkinje cell degeneration mutant mice by Purkinje cell replacement through transplantation of solid embryonic implants. Neurosci 20:1–22.

Stelzner DJ, Strauss JA (1986): A quantitative analysis of frog optic nerve regeneration: Is retrograde ganglion cell death or collateral axonal loss related to selective innervation? J Comp Neurol 245:83–106.

Sumner BEH, Watson WE (1971): Retraction and expansion of the dendritic tree of motor neurons of adult rats induced in vivo. Nature 233:273–275.

Tainuchi M, Clark HB, Johnson EM (1986): Induction of nerve growth factor receptor in Schwann cells after axotomy. Proc Natl Acad Sci USA 83:4094–4098.

Thanos S, Bonhoeffer F (1983): Investigations on the development and topographic order of retinotectal axons: Anterograde and retrograde staining of axons and perikarya with rhodamine in vivo. J Comp Neurol 219:420–430.

Thesleff S (1987): Denervation sensitivity. In Adelman G (ed): "Encyclopedia of Neuroscience." Boston: Birkhauser, pp. 322–323.

Thomas KA, Gimenez-Gallego G (1986): Fibroblast growth factors: Broad spectrum mitogens with potent angiogenic activity. TINS 11:81–84.

Trecarten MJ, Villegas-Perez MP, Vidal-Sanz M, Thanos S, Aguayo AJ (1986): Growth of axons along peripheral nerve system grafts inserted into the retina of adult rats. Soc Neurosci Abstr 12:701.

Turner JE, Blair JR, Chappel ET (1987): Peripheral nerve implant effects on survival of retinal ganglion layer cells after axotomy initiated by a penetrating lesion. Brain Res 419:46–54.

Unsicker K, Reichert-Preibsch H, Schmidt R, Pettmann B, Labourdette G, Sensenbrenner M (1987): Atroglial and fibroblast growth factors have neurotrophic functions of cultured peripheral and central nervous system neurons. Proc Natl Acad Sci USA 84:5459–5463.

Varon S, Manthorpe M, Williams LR (1983–84): Neuro-notrophic and neurite promoting factors and their clinical potential. Dev Neurosci 6:73–100.

Vaughan DW, Peters A (1985): Proliferation of thalamic afferents in cerebral cortex altered by callosal deafferentation. J Neurocytol 14:705–716.

Vidal-Sanz M, Bray GM, Villegas-Perez MP, Thanos S, Aguayo AJ (1987): Axonal regeneration and synapse formation in the superior colliculus by retinal ganglion cells in the adult rat. J Neurosci 7:2894–2907.

Villegas-Perez MP, Vidal-Sanz M, Aguayo AJ (1986): Effects of axotomy and PN grafting on adult rat retinal ganglion cells. Soc Neurosci Abstr 12:700.

Villegas-Perez MP, Vidal-Sanz M, Bray GM, Aguayo AJ (1988): Influences of peripheral nerve grafts on the survival and regrowth of axotomized retinal ganglion cells in adult rats. J Neurosci 8:265–280.

Walicke P, Cowan WM, Keno N, Baird A, Guillemin R (1986): Fibroblast growth factor promotes survival of dissociated hippocampal neurons and enhances neurite extension. Proc Natl Acad Sci USA 83:3012–3016.

Williams LR, Varon S, Peterson GM, Wictorin K, Fisher W, Björklund A, Gage FH (1986): Continuous infusion of nerve growth factor prevents basal forebrain neuronal death after fimbria fornix transection. Proc Natl Acad Sci USA 83:9231–9235.

Williams RW, Bastiani MJ, Lia M, Chalupa LM (1986): Growth cones, dying axons, and developmental fluctuations in the fiber population of the cat's optic nerve. J Comp Neurol 246:32–69.

Yawo H (1987): Changes in the dendritic geometry of mouse superior cervical ganglion cells following postganglionic axotomy. J Neurosci 7:3703–3711.

Yip HK, Johnson EM (1984): Developing dorsal root ganglion neurons require trophic support from their central processes: Evidence for a role of retrogradely transported nerve growth factor from the central nervous system to the periphery. Proc Natl Acad Sci USA 81:6245–6249.

6

Neuronal Responses to Axotomy: Consequences and Possibilities for Rescue From Permanent Atrophy or Cell Death

KEVIN D. BARRON, MD

Research Service, Veterans Administration Medical Center and Department of Neurology, Albany Medical College, Albany, New York 12208

Although this chapter will focus primarily on somal responses to axotomy, completeness requires some mention of dendritic changes and alterations in the axonic segment proximal to the site of an injury. The axon, the subject of axotomy, is the efferent process of the neuron. This definition poses difficulties in the case of the primary sensory neuron, whose distally directed process is termed an axon, although it conducts impulses toward the parent soma (Bodian, 1962). Nevertheless, the definition is generally applicable. Indeed, interruption of the peripherally directed process of the primary sensory neuron provokes the axon reaction (see below).

The severance of an axon invariably results in prograde Wallerian degeneration manifested by rapid and total disintegration of the axonic segment separated from the cell body and by concomitant dissolution of associated myelin sheaths. Myelin dissolution may proceed more slowly than axonal disintegration. In the peripheral nervous system (PNS), the stump of the amputated axon that remains attached to the parent cell undertakes regenerative sprouting (Ramón y Cajal, 1928), with formation of an average of four to eight new processes (regenerative sprouts). Generally, one sprout survives, extends as a new axonic segment distal to the locus of injury, and is

completed to a site of termination. The terminus may or may not be the normal end station of the regenerated fiber, but some degree of functional return often follows this anatomic reconstitution of the severed part, especially if the ends of an interrupted peripheral nerve remain apposed and the growing fibers are not largely misdirected.

In contrast to the situation in the injured PNS, axons of the mammalian central nervous system (CNS) most often show none or only abortive attempts at axonic reconstitution (Barron, 1983a,b). As a result, fiber pathways interrupted by trauma or by other processes, e.g., ischemic infarction, whether in the brain or spinal cord, remain devoid of axons distal to the lesion, and more or less permanent loss of function is the unhappy result.

Unlike the mammalian CNS, which lacks an innate, spontaneous capacity for axonic repair, the CNS of lower vertebrates, such as goldfish and certain amphibia (Grafstein, 1986; Stelzner et al., 1986), shows a remarkable capacity for regeneration of axons. The retinotectal projection of goldfish is restored anatomically and functionally within 5 or 6 weeks after crushing or sectioning of the optic nerve or tract (Grafstein, 1986), and the spinal cord of this animal is also capable of rapid repair and functional return after complete transection (Bernstein and Geldred, 1973). Even in mammals, some central pathways, especially the hypothalamohypophyseal projection, are ca-

Neural Regeneration and Transplantation, pages 79–99
© 1989 Alan R. Liss, Inc.

pable of spontaneous regeneration with restoration of function (Barron, 1983a,b), but such regeneration is very much the exception.

Neurogenesis of mammalian central and peripheral neurons apparently occurs postnatally, even into adulthood (Bayer et al., 1982; Devor and Govran-Lippman, 1985), and is well documented for lower vertebrates (Grafstein, 1986). However, proliferation of new neurons and the appropriate insertion of their processes into the existing circuitry has not been shown to be a source of repair of the mammalian CNS. Furthermore, although tissue transplants from fetal CNS have the potential to replace central neuronal aggregates or their products after destruction by trauma, toxins, or disease (Freed et al., 1985), sociopolitical and technical considerations militate against the early use of this aspect of transplant methodology in man (see Chapters 13–15, this volume). In large measure, hopes for attainment of functional and structural regeneration in mammalian CNS depend upon successful stimulation of the regrowth of interrupted central axons and their reconnection with appropriate target tissues. To this end, as will be brought out below, some forms of tissue transplantation technique have yielded important results, probably because the transplants serve as sources of neurotrophins that are carried to injured nerve cells from the lesion site by retrograde axoplasmic transport.

Historically, the search for the cause of regeneration failure in mammalian CNS has had two major foci of concentration: 1) the soma of the axotomized neuron and its surround; and 2) the macro- and microenvironment at the lesion site. We have hypothesized (Barron et al., 1966; Barron, 1983a,b) that the key to regeneration failure lies in the nature of the axotomy response, which in central or intrinsic neurons is characterized innately by a failure to mount the biosynthetic effort essential to the spinning out of a new axonic segment as replacement for the degenerated, separated part. By definition, the somata and processes of central neurons are confined to the CNS (Barron, 1983a,b). Axotomy of these neurons is often associated with declines in RNA and protein synthesis and with a cellular atrophy that may culminate in cell death (Barron, 1983a,b; Barron et al., 1986) (Fig. 6–1). In contrast, peripheral or ex-

trinsic neurons, whose processes lie in whole or in part outside the CNS (e.g., craniospinal motoneurons, neurons of posterior root and autonomic ganglia), typically react to axotomy by cellular hypertrophy and heightened metabolism of RNA and protein and increased glucose utilization (Rodichok et al., 1984). Since it is an inviolable axiom of neurobiology that the axon is dependent on the soma of origin for both growth and maintenance, the failure of an axotomized nerve cell to mobilize its synthetic machinery to the task of axonic reconstitution must lead to failure of axonal regeneration. The axon itself has little autochthonous capacity for protein synthesis. An emphasis on an innately regressive somal response to axotomy in explanation of CNS regeneration failure need not ignore the importance of the environment at the site of axonic injury, cited above as a second major focus of CNS regeneration research. There is abundant evidence that events at the site must impact upon the soma (Barron, 1983a,b), as work with transplants of PNS segments to optic nerve stumps clearly shows (Berry et al., 1986; Vidal-Sanz et al., 1987). The mandate of this review, however, precludes detailed consideration of events at the site of interruption of central fiber pathways and peripheral nerves. Here, discussion will center on the nature of the axon reaction in central and peripheral neurons, with particular emphasis on the former class of nerve cell. However, modification of the axon reaction of the mammalian intrinsic neuron in an anabolic direction (Barron et al., 1967; Barron and Dentinger, 1979) by pharmacologic and other interventions, including tissue transplants made at the injury site, has opened exciting and long-awaited possibilities for CNS regeneration in mammals; this avenue of approach will be discussed in the section on neuronal rescue.

THE AXON REACTION (AXOTOMY RESPONSE)

Initiation of the Response

The signal (Cragg, 1970) that induces axon reaction is unknown, but it appears to have similar properties in both central and peripheral neurons (Torvik and Heding, 1969). Whether the axonal reaction is brought about by lack of some factor ordinarily delivered

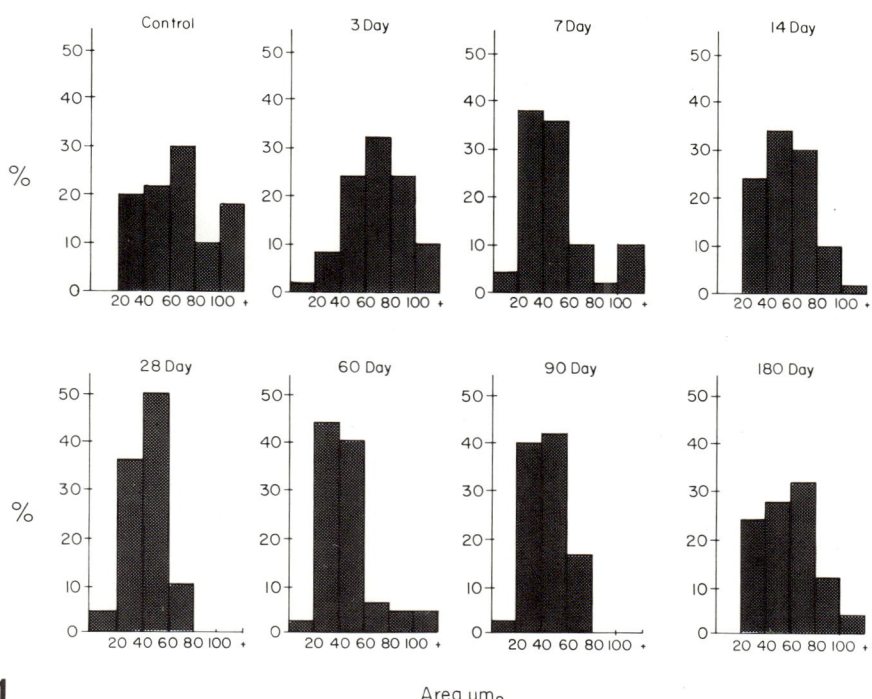

1

Distribution By Somal Area Of Retinal Ganglion Cells
After Intra-Orbital Optic Nerve Crush

Area um₂

Figure 6–1.   Histograms of somal areas of rat retinal ganglion cells ipsilateral to intraorbital crush of one optic nerve performed 3 days to 6 months before sacrifice, two animals per survival period. Note shift to the left, especially 28–90 days postoperatively. At 6 months, neuronal density in the ganglion cell layer is reduced to 32% of normal.

continuously from a peripheral target or whether it is connected to delivery of an abnormal substance or extraordinary quantities and/or proportions of normal metabolites, it would seem likely that the "message" is conveyed to the axotomized cell by retrograde axoplasmic transport (Kristensson, 1981). At the soma, the signal induces changes in DNA-directed RNA synthesis that can be blocked by actinomycin D when this antimetabolite is injected into the brain within 9, but not 15, hours after axotomy (Torvik and Heding, 1969).

Light Microscopic Cytology

Central chromatolysis is an important feature of the axotomy response, developing to the fullest 3–14 days after injury of either central or peripheral neurons. It is marked by a clearing of Nissl granules from the cytocentrum and by a concentration of those that remain under the plasma membrane, while the nucleus moves to an eccentric position opposite the axon hillock (Fig. 6–2). The displaced nucleus is often indented and apposed by a deeply basophilic rim of Nissl substance (the nuclear "cap"). Peripheral dispersion (retispersion) of the Golgi apparatus and increases in size and number of lysosomes and neurofibrils may occur. In regenerating nerve cells, the axotomized soma may be enlarged, its profile may appear rounded, and the nucleus and nucleolus may be hypertrophied, with prominent vacuolation of the latter. In contrast, the retrogressive axotomy response of mammalian intrinsic neurons is, almost without exception, a monotonously atrophic process and is char-

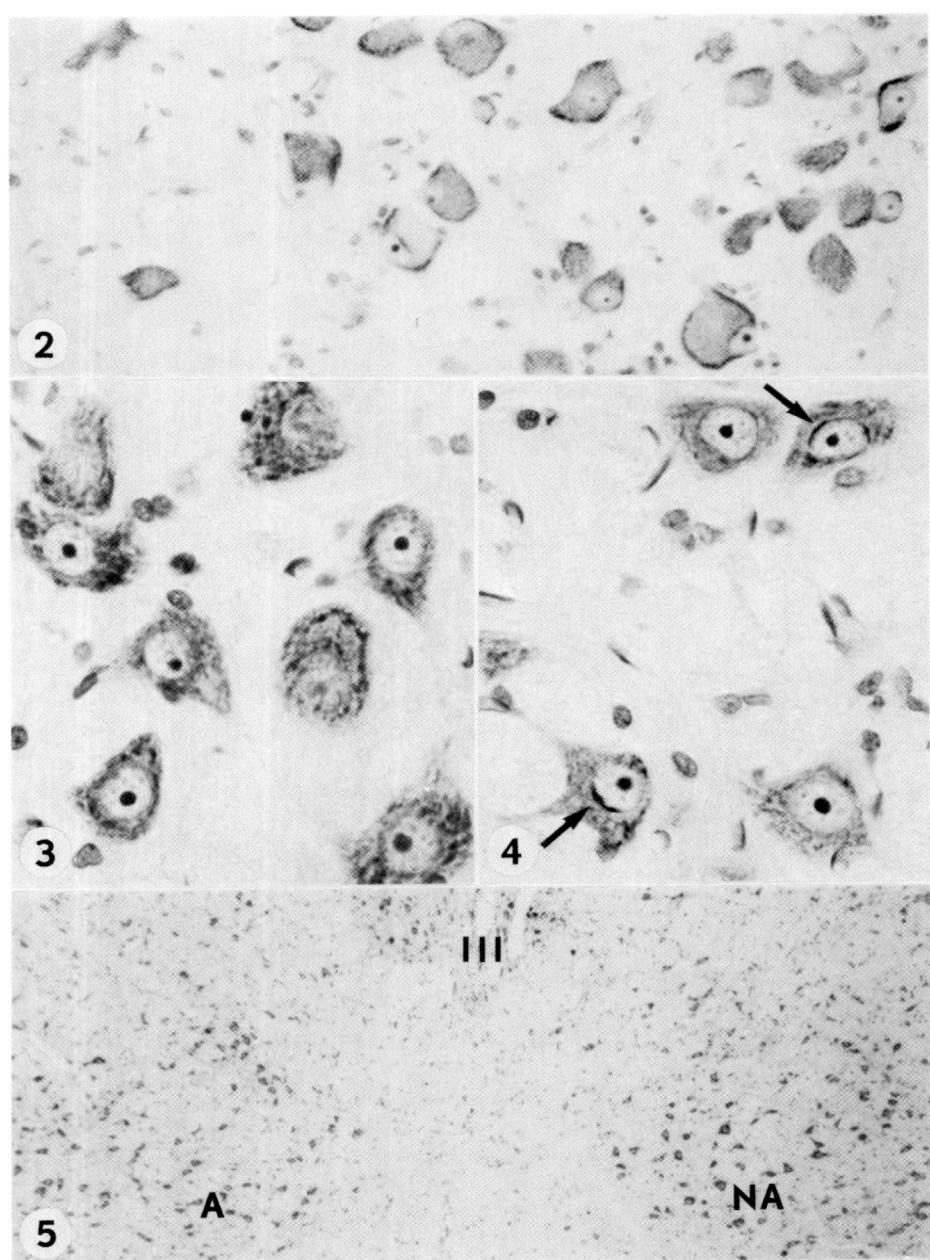

Figure 6–2. Three days after cervical rubrospinal tractotomy, axotomized rubral neurons show nuclear eccentricity and peripheral displacement of Nissl substance characteristic of central chromatolysis. Azure B stain, × 180.

Figures 6–3, 6–4. Illustrations of magnocellular neurons of the nonaxotomized (Fig. 6–3) and axotomized (Fig. 6–4) red nucleus 14 days after one-sided rubrospinal tractotomy. Note prominent nuclear caps (Fig. 6–4), as in cells marked by arrows, and partial reversal of the chromatolytic reaction. Azure B stain, × 560.

Figure 6–5. At a level near the rostral pole of the rat oculomotor nucleus (III), pallor and atrophy of neurons of the axotomized (A) red nucleus is evident under the scanning lens, 60 days after unilateral cervical rubrospinal tractotomy. Cresyl violet stain, × 18. NA, nonaxotomized nucleus.

acterized by measurable and progressive cyto-plasmic, nuclear, and nucleolar shrinkage within 1–2 weeks of axonic interruption. The cytologic changes of axon reaction are highly variable among species and specific neuronal aggregates (Barron et al., 1977, 1982; Barron, 1982). In some nerve cells, disintegration of Nissl granules (chromatolysis sensu strictu) oc-curs diffusely or begins at the periphery of the perikaryon. None of the chromatolytic reac-tions is specific for axotomy and, indeed, light microscopically evident cytologic alterations may be absent in axotomized neurons (Payne et al., 1984). Chromatolysis probably denotes no more than a nonspecific injury response (Graf-stein, 1983). The chromatolyzed neuron gener-ally reverts toward a normal appearance within 2 weeks to 2 months (Figs. 6–3, 6–4), but the process is incomplete in central nerve cells (Fig. 6–5) or is markedly, even indefinitely, delayed in peripheral neurons that are pre-vented from regenerating by experimental ma-nipulations, e.g., by ligature of the central ends of sectioned peripheral nerves.

Electron Microscopic Cytology

The greater resolving power of the electron microscope permits more detailed insights into the structural accompaniments of the axon re-action. The ultrastructural counterpart of the Nissl granule consists of ordered arrays of cisternae of the rough endoplasmic reticulum (RER), which are bounded by ribosome-studded membranes and associated with in-tervening cytoplasmic ribosomal granules arranged in clusters (free cytoplasmic polyribo-somes). Early in the course of the axon reaction, cisterns of RER characteristically become shorter, lose their orderly parallel arrange-ments, and disperse through the cytoplasm. An intracisternal, electron-dense product may ap-pear. Quantitative assay of total cisternal mem-brane per chromatolyzed cell may or may not show depletion of this element (Dentinger et al., 1979). Concentrations of RER may be seen un-der the plasma membrane and adjacent to the nucleus (predictable from light microscopic ob-servations). Axotomized central neurons of mammals do differ from their peripheral coun-terparts in that dispersal and disaggregation of cytoplasmic polyribosomes into single units and degranulation of cisternal membranes in-

variably seem to accompany the chromatolytic reaction. Ribosomal disaggregation is often as-sociated with reduction in the amount of RER (Figs. 6–6, 6–7) and with vacuolation and ve-siculation of its component cisternae (Barron, 1983a; Barron et al., 1986). In contrast, axoto-mized intrinsic neurons of lower vertebrates that regenerate their axons, such as retinal gan-glion cells of the goldfish, retain tightly clus-tered polyribosomal configurations. Qualita-tive alterations of the RER in axotomized mammalian central neurons may revert toward normal (Barron and Dentinger, 1979; Barron, 1983a,b) but quantitative assay ultimately shows a sustained and serious depletion of cisternae (Barron et al., 1986). The changes in the RER of central mammalian neurons that undergo a retrograde atrophy after axotomy may well relate to the suppression of protein synthesis that marks the axon reaction in this circumstance (Barron, 1983a,b).

Jones and Lavelle (1986) have examined de-veloping and mature hamster facial neurons with reference to nucleolar and nuclear alter-ations induced by axotomy. In this cell type, the axotomy response is a regenerative one. In mature facial neurons, the nucleolus contains a dense, central aggregate of ribonucleoprotein (RNP) granules, the intranucleolar body (INB). It is surrounded by interwoven strands of RNP granules that constitute the nucleoloneme and enclose "vacuolar" (although nonmembrane-delimited) areas. A crescent-shaped mass of heterochromatin particles, the nucleolus-associated chromatin, covers a part of the nu-cleolar circumference. Two days after axot-omy, and prior to full development of chromatolytic alterations in the cytoplasm on the fourth postoperative day, nucleolar swell-ing, enlargement of vacuolar areas, and disper-sion of the INB were evident. Clusters of inter-chromatin granules, characteristic of normal adult nuclei, were largely dispersed 4 days af-ter axotomy, and nuclei were enlarged. As a result the nucleoplasm had a homogeneous, finely granular appearance. These changes re-sulted in a nuclear and nucleolar morphology resembling that of actively growing immature neurons and were interpreted as morphologic expressions of an increased, genomically driven, ribosomal RNA synthesis that under-lies the heightened protein production neces-

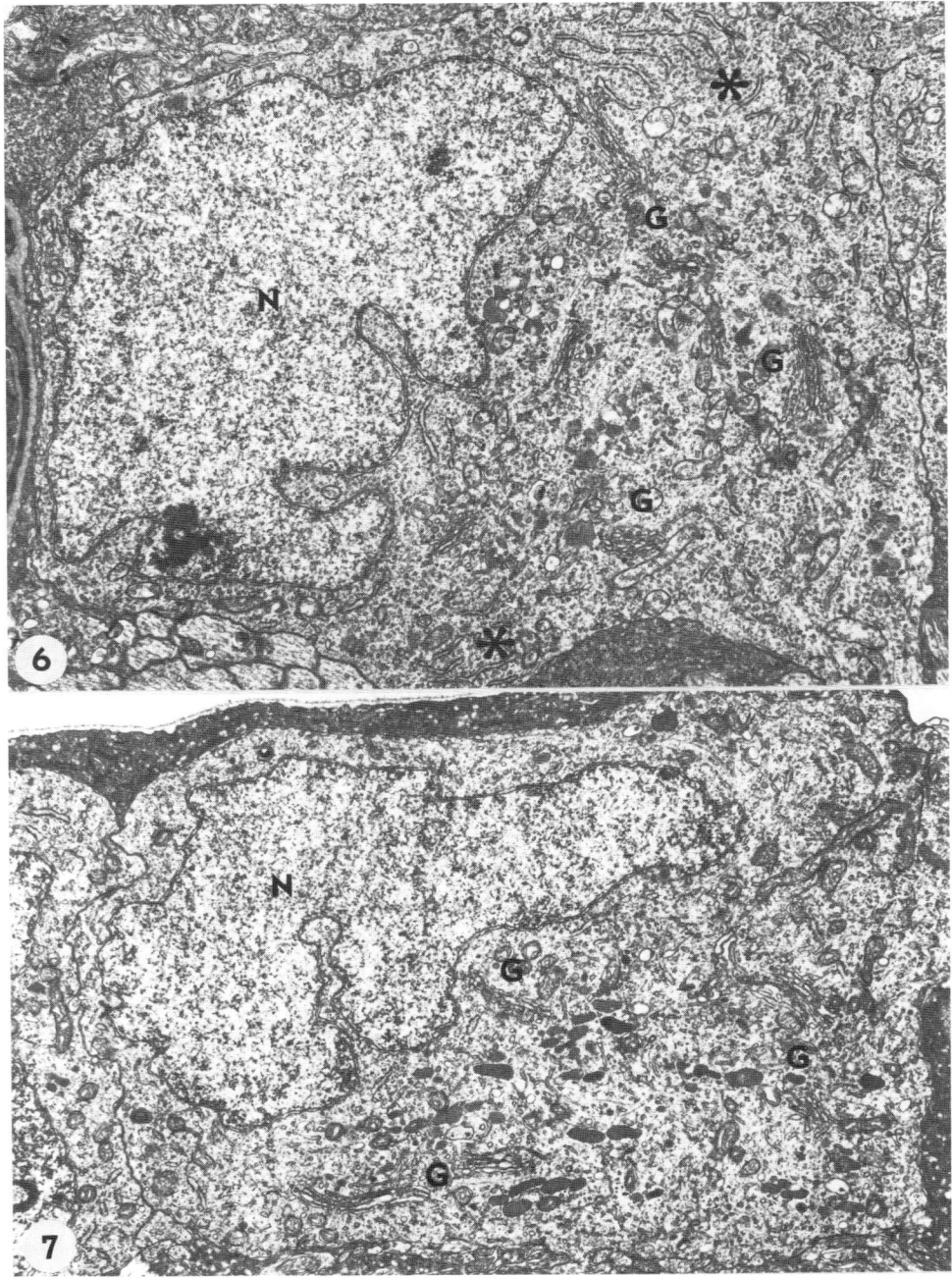

Figures 6–6, 6–7.   Illustration of control (Fig. 6–6) and axotomized (Fig. 6–7) rat retinal ganglion cells. The axotomy was performed by unilateral intraorbital optic nerve crush 3 days prior to fixation. Electron microscopically, arrays of rough endoplasmic reticulum are present in the nonaxotomized neuron (asterisks in Fig. 6–6) but are absent in the axotomized cell (Fig. 6–7). Nuclei (N), Golgi apparatus (G), and other organelles show no essential change. ×9250 and ×10,400.

sary for cellular repair. Although nucleolar vacuoloids may appear in axotomized mammalian intrinsic neurons (Barron et al., 1977), the nuclear changes in the main differ sharply from those described above for hamster facial neurons in that neuronal nuclei typically accumulate focal, densely packed aggregations of chromatin granules, while nucleoli come to contain homogeneous, electron-dense bodies and both nuclei and nucleoli are atrophied (Barron et al., 1967, 1986).

Dramatic increases in neurofilament content, which may reflect failure of (or reduction in) "export" to the axon of these cytoskeletal proteins, and development of conspicuous nuclear furrowing occur in extrinsic and intrinsic neurons under some circumstances, and may portend cell death (Barron et al., 1975). The Golgi apparatus, apart from unpredictable changes in disposition, is relatively resistant to change, even in cells severely depleted of RER (Barron et al., 1986). Golgi elements, however, are rarely incorporated into autophagic bodies (Barron et al., 1975). When retispersion of the Golgi organelle occurs, its constituent cisternae and vesicles appear normal in electron micrographs (Barron and Dentinger, 1979). Mitochondrial, lysosomal, and microtubular alterations show no consistent pattern, but enlargement of the mitochondria is frequent.

Cytochemical Observations on Axotomized Neurons

NUCLEIC ACIDS

The binding of radiolabeled actinomycin D to nuclear DNA is increased through the first 11 days of the axonal response of peripherally projecting motor and sensory neurons (Barron, 1983b; Wells, 1984). This finding suggests a change in the conformation of the deoxyribonucleoprotein of the axotomized cells to an uncoiled, metabolically active state. Axotomized neurons of the cerebral cortex (Wells and Hall, 1985) and thalamus (Means et al., 1972) show similar DNA alterations when assessed by actinomycin D-binding and Feulgen cytophotometry. However, the increase in DNA labeling by tritiated actinomycin D (Wells and Hall, 1985) is short-lived in cortical neurons, where it does not persist beyond the fifth day after axotomy. Perhaps mammalian intrinsic neurons respond to axotomy by attempts at changes in genomic

expression, which could lead to adaptive alterations in types and amounts of RNA transcribed and proteins synthesized, but the regenerative attempt is a precarious one that cannot be maintained. We do not know whether transplants of neural tissues and other experimental manipulations that "rescue" axotomized intrinsic neurons would alter the experimental results recorded above, nor is it known whether the brief period of increased actinomycin D-binding induced by axotomy represents a critical postaxotomy interval during which restorative measures would need to be instituted.

Its crucial role in cellular synthesis of protein has led to many studies of RNA metabolism in axotomized neurons. In general, regenerating cells, whether extrinsic neurons of mammals or retinal ganglion cells of fish and amphibia, exhibit increased content of ribosomal RNA and increased incorporation of radiolabeled RNA precursors at some point in the retrograde response, although the increases may be slight (e.g., 10–15% above control values) and, rarely, delayed until terminal contacts are reestablished (Barron et al., 1982, 1985, 1986; Barron, 1983a,b). Cytoplasmic RNA is invariably increased, but nucleolar RNA content is occasionally unaffected (Barron et al., 1982). Even when 70% of an axotomized population of extrinsic neurons die, as in the dorsal motor vagal nucleus of rat, striking accumulations of cytoplasmic RNA occur early in the axotomy response (Aldskogius et al., 1980). The extrinsic neuron of the adult mammal seems programmed to respond to axotomy with a basically anabolic reaction that is independent of the eventual fate of the neuron and its success or failure in reestablishing connections. In contrast, mammalian intrinsic neurons show progressive declines in cytoplasmic and nucleolar RNA content after axotomy (Barron et al., 1977, 1985; Barron, 1983a,b), while concomitantly there is reduced incorporation of the tritiated RNA precursor, uridine (Barron et al., 1985).

Recent studies of the axotomized rat nodose ganglion have centered attention on RNAs of small molecular weight (Austin and Langford, 1980). Two classes of small nuclear (sn) RNAs, associated with the nucleolus, show increased turnover rates during axon reaction in this system. They appear to relate to the regulation of DNA-directed, RNA-mediated protein synthesis and to be involved in increased production of ribosomal (r) RNAs. Changes also occur in transfer and messenger (m) RNAs. These may well relate to altered rates of synthesis of cellular substituents, including tubulin, actin, and neurofilament proteins, which are crucial to the formation of a new axonic process, while synthesis of proteins characteristic of the growing, immature CNS (see below for growth-associated polypeptides, or GAPs) is expressed anew (Willard and Skene, 1982). These changes in the classes and rates of turnover of the RNAs formed in the axotomized neuron may be large in the absence of considerable, even appreciable, alterations in the cellular content of RNA. It follows that profound alterations in the amounts and types of proteins synthesized could occur in cells that show little change in total RNA content. Nevertheless, in point of fact, increased incorporation of RNA precursors into (r)RNA and increases in the cellular content of (r)RNA are biologic hallmarks of axon reaction in many neurons that are capable of axon regeneration (Barron, 1983a,b), while the converse holds for nonregenerating nerve cells (Barron et al., 1985).

PROTEINS

Radiolabeled amino acid precursors of protein synthesis are taken up at increased rates by axotomized extrinsic neurons. This process is associated with an overall increase in synthesis of proteins by the soma (Aldskogius et al., 1984; Smith et al., 1984). Although dorsal motor vagal neurons ultimately die or atrophy after axotomy, they too show increased uptake of [^{3}H] leucine, injected 15 and 60 min before sacrifice, during days 7–14 postoperative (unilateral vagotomy) (Aldskogius et al., 1984). This process is independent of restitution of contact with terminal end stations (Aldskogius et al., 1984). In contrast to their peripheral counterparts, mammalian intrinsic neurons, e.g., those of the red nucleus, hippocampus, and retina (Barron et al., 1976; Barron, 1983b; Tsang et al., 1985) show sharply reduced levels of protein precursor incorporation after axotomy, once more emphasizing the metabolic differences in the axon reactions of mammalian extrinsic and intrinsic nerve cells. However, the axotomized retinal ganglion cells of the goldfish, a regenerating population of intrinsic neurons of a lower vertebrate, incorporate amino acids into protein at elevated rates during axon reaction (Murray and Grafstein, 1969).

Perhaps more important to the regeneration of the axon than overall rates or amounts of protein synthesis are qualitative changes in the types of proteins synthesized by the axotomized soma. Because the neuron is normally engaged in an active program of axoplasmic renewal, growth of a new axon may not require gross readjustments of protein metabolism (Perry and Wilson, 1981), and quantitative changes, both increases and decreases in types of protein manufactured, may result in a sum total of protein synthesis that shows little departure from the normal condition. Some proteins, especially enzyme and receptor proteins associated with neurotransmitter metabolism (Barron, 1983a,b), are reduced in chromatolyzed neurons, both those that regenerate and those that go on to atrophy and/or death, but the particulars of this phenomenon may differ between central and peripheral neurons. Thus axotomized neurons of the pontine nuclei are markedly less susceptible to loss of muscarinic receptors after axotomy than are those of the hypoglossal nucleus (Rotter et al., 1979). Presumably synthesis of neurotransmitter-related proteins is neglected by an injured cell whose metabolic machinery is redirected to the production of proteins necessary for regrowth of a severed axon.

Although they are present in small amounts in adult CNS, expression of the GAPs (Willard and Skene, 1982), of which GAP43 has been most intensively studied (Meiri et al., 1986), is greatly increased by neurons that are regenerating their axons or extending them during development. GAP43 moves in the fast phase of axonal transport, is present in neurites and, especially, in growth cones, and is readily identified in regenerating peripheral and optic (fish and amphibia) nerves and in neonatal optic nerve of the rat (Meiri et al., 1986; Reh et al., 1987). It declines precipitously as the animal matures and is not reexpressed when optic axons and corticospinal axons (Reh et al., 1987) are interrupted. The failure to express GAPs may relate causally to regeneration failure and may result from the absence of an inducer molecule in injured mammalian CNS. A nonneuronal 37 kD protein (Muller et al., 1985), which is synthesized by both CNS and PNS at increased rates after injury, but which does not accumulate extracellularly in CNS tissue (and therefore may not be available for axonal uptake), is a candidate for such an inducer molecule; it proves to be apolipoprotein E (apo E), a constituent of normal serum. Apo E is present in astrocytes of uninjured rat CNS but rapidly disappears from astroglia after CNS lesions (Stoll and Muller, 1986). That protein metabolism may be fundamentally different in PNS and CNS after axotomy is further supported by the failure of posttranslational modification of axoplasmic proteins in crushed mammalian optic nerve (Shyne-Athwal et al., 1986) and the absence of a decline in the S1 protein of fast transport in mammalian corticospinal axons after axotomy. In contrast, fast transport of the S1 protein is markedly diminished during regeneration of the optic nerve (Reh et al., 1987) of submammalian vertebrates.

Changes in the synthesis of enzyme proteins and alterations in levels of enzyme activities might be expected to occur in association with the wrenching rearrangements of cellular structure and metabolism that follow axotomy. In general, changes in an enzyme activity have been found to correlate well with corresponding alterations in the amounts of that enzyme protein present in the tissue when such estimations have been done by immunochemical assay, for example. In any case, although an enormous number of qualitative and quantitative studies of enzymatic activities in axotomized neurons has been recorded (Barron, 1983a,b), few comparative investigations of regenerating and nonregenerating axotomized cells have been done (Barron, 1983a,b). Cole has used histochemical methods for oxidative enzymes to compare the axon reaction of feline intrinsic neurons (nuclei gracilis and cuneatus, nucleus ruber) with that of extrinsic nerve cells (facial and hypoglossal motoneurons). He and others have shown that an increase in NADPH (TPNH) tetrazolium reductase (diaphorase) staining occurs in chromatolyzed cranial motoneurons (Cole, 1968; Meyer and Cole, 1970; Barron, 1983a,b). In-

deed, raised NADPH diaphorase activity marks the axotomy response of dorsal vagal motor neurons (Gonzalez et al., 1987), despite the largely necrobiotic nature of the reaction in this peripherally projecting neuronal population. In contrast, NADPH diaphorase activity declines in neurons of axotomized medullary sensory nuclei and nucleus ruber, although at the latter locus a temporary increase in enzymatic staining is said to occur during the first 6 days after axotomy, only to be followed by a decrease 16–60 days into the response (Cole, 1968). Oxidative enzymes associated with the hexose monophosphate shunt (HMP), namely glucose-6-phosphate dehydrogenase and 6-phosphogluconate dehydrogenase, are also increased in axotomized extrinsic neurons, both by qualitative assessment and by quantitative assay (Barron, 1983a,b; Kreutzberg, 1986). The formation of ribose, necessary to ribonucleoprotein synthesis, occurs through the activity of the HMP enzymes, and increases in their activities appear to be invariable for regenerating neurons, including those of the axotomized mammalian locus coeruleus (Kaufman et al., 1976), one of the rare intrinsic neuronal populations that is spontaneously capable of regenerative axonal sprouting (Barron, 1983a,b).

Although enzymes of the Krebs cycle and glycolytic pathway are not affected in consistent fashion by axotomy (Barron, 1983a,b), the $[^{14}C]$2-deoxyglucose technique of Sokoloff and colleagues has documented striking increases of glucose utilization in rat facial and hypoglossal nuclei after neurotomy (Barron, 1983a,b). This increase persists longer (60 vs. 30 days) when the transected hypoglossal nerve is prevented from regenerating by ligation (Singer and Mehler, 1986). In striking contrast, the red nucleus, axotomized by cervical and thoracic rubrospinal tractotomies, shows no change in glucose utilization by quantitative assay 1–100 days after operation (Rodichok et al., 1984). Although the relative contributions of neurons, neuroglia, and vasculature to glucose incorporation by a neuronal aggregate and its surround is not determinable by the Sokoloff method, the data do indicate a striking difference between centrally and peripherally projecting nuclei in their respective metabolic responses to axotomy and may further support the contention that central neurons often fail to react anabolically to severance of their axons.

By slide histochemical techniques, Barron et al. (1966) studied hydrolytic enzymes in feline lateral geniculate body after corticectomy and compared the results with those observed in prior studies of axotomized extrinsic neurons of this species. A major finding was the loss of acid beta-glycerophosphatase from geniculate neurons after corticectomy. In contrast, axotomized feline motor neurons showed enhancement of this activity (Barron, 1983a,b). Acid phosphatase may play a role in the generation of phosphate radicals for the synthesis of nucleotides, including adenosine triphosphate and polynucleotides (RNA), phospholipids, and neurofilament proteins (see below). Changes in enzymes related to polyamine metabolism will be mentioned under the subject of neuronal rescue.

Immunohistochemical stains have shown accumulations of neurofilament (NF) protein in perikarya of mammalian motor and sensory neurons and retinal ganglion cells (Drager and Hofbauer, 1984; Rosenfeld et al., 1987; Schlaepfer, 1987) after axotomy. The accumulated protein is of a kind enriched in phosphorylated sites and would belong to the 145kD and 200kD, rather than to the 68 kD, molecular species of the NF protein triplet. NF proteins recognized by antibodies to their phosphorylated epitopes are normally present largely or wholly in axons. After axonic interruption, the richly phosphorylated NF proteins appear in an abnormal location, namely the perikarya, where their presence may be due to a failure of axoplasmic transport. The abnormal staining may persist longer after reversible than after irreversible nerve injuries (Rosenfeld et al., 1987). Three and six days after section of, respectively, the optic nerve and tract (Drager and Hofbauer, 1984), an antibody (RT97) to phosphorylated epitopes of the 200kD neurofilament subunit selectively stains a class of large retinal ganglion cells of the mouse in "Golgi-like" fashion. In normal mice, these neurons are unstained. They project to the lateral geniculate body. The abnormal staining pattern persists for several weeks after optic nerve lesions but wanes by 60 days (Drager and Hofbauer, 1984). Neurofilaments are essential to maintenance of the structure and function of

neurons, and results of their study by immunohistochemical methods seem particularly germane to this review.

Immunohistochemical preparations for enzymes, e.g., neuron-specific enolase and choline acetyltransferase, show reductions of these proteins after, respectively, axotomy of motor neurons (Kirino et al., 1983) and the intrinsic nerve cells of the nucleus basalis (Cuello et al., 1986). In the latter experiments, the immunohistochemical method was used to monitor the response of axotomized neurons of the nucleus basalis (corticectomy) to ganglioside treatment. Increasing use of immunohistochemical techniques in the study of axon reaction and its modification by pharmacologic agents may be expected. Radioautographic, ligand-binding methods for display of receptor sites for neurotransmitters and neurotrophins also are likely to find wide application.

MISCELLANEOUS SUBSTITUENTS

The literature on changes in carbohydrates and lipids during the axon reaction is scant and is referred to elsewhere (Barron, 1983b).

General Biological Factors Bearing on the Axotomy Response

The importance of distinguishing between the axonal reactions of extrinsic and intrinsic neurons of mammals, when consequences of the axotomy response are concerned, has been alluded to repeatedly above. In view of suggestions that the 37kD (Muller et al., 1985) or other proteins may induce peripheral neurons to undertake protein syntheses that are growth-oriented, one may speculate on whether the injured CNS of mammals fails to produce such a molecule or in some way denies an inducer protein access to axotomized central neurons. The ability of some feline spinal motor neurons to regenerate axons through a lesion within the ventral funiculus (Risling et al., 1983), extending them through an astrocytic scar and into a denervated ventral root in the process, may speak to an innate biologic difference between these extrinsic neurons and intrinsic nerve cells of the same species or, alternatively, may relate to the immediate proximity of a denervated ventral root that could be a source from which powerful growth-promoting substances diffuse.

There are many examples of the profound effect of species on the nature of the axonal response (Barron, 1983a,b) of both peripheral and central neurons. Thus the distinctive regenerative capacities of retinal ganglion cells of submammalian vertebrates, such as the goldfish and the frog (Grafstein, 1986; Stelzner et al., 1986), stand apart from the generally feeble regenerative attempts (Barron et al., 1985, 1986) mounted by axotomized mammalian retinal ganglion cells in the absence of experimental manipulations such as those recently reported by Villegas-Perez et al. (1988). Within mammals, profound species differences in the axotomy response of the retinal ganglion cell also occur. Thus interruption of optic axons leads to a slowly progressive loss of ganglion cells in the feline retina (Hollander et al., 1985), contrasting to the rapid atrophy and neuronal loss observed in rabbits and primates, including man (Quigley et al., 1977; Barron et al., 1986).

Both the location and the functional differentiation of a neuron may impact upon its response to axotomy. Within a neuronal population of like function, the cat's retinal ganglion cell layer, cell death after axotomy is greatest and earliest in the medium-sized beta cells, the small (gamma) and large (alpha) cells being less affected (Hollander et al., 1984). Within the visual system of the frog (*Rana pipiens*), tectal neurons fail to show a regenerative response to axotomy, in sharp contrast to the retinal ganglion cells of this species (Lyon and Stelzner, 1987). The motoneurons of different brainstem nuclei differ sharply in their susceptibility to axotomy-induced cell death (Aldskogius et al., 1980; Durica and Jacob, 1980). The ability of hypothalamic neurons, including those of primates, to reestablish a functioning hypothalamohypophyseal pathway after its physical interruption (Antunes et al., 1980; Barron, 1983b) seems to be unique among intrinsic neurons of mammals, especially since it occurs without pharmacologic or other extraneous interventions.

It has long been a neurobiologic maxim, following from the work of Gudden more than a century ago (reviewed in Bleier, 1969), that axotomy induces a particularly rapid and severe nerve cell atrophy, which is characteristically succeeded by necrosis, when immature central or peripheral neurons of neonatal animals are the subjects of experimental injury. While the "Gudden effect" certainly holds for some systems, and can be so sweeping as to preclude regeneration of an interrupted pathway, striking exceptions occur (Bryz-Gornia and Stelzner, 1986; Villablanca et al., 1986). One exception is of particular interest because of the physiological importance of the corticospinal tract. Kalil and Reh (1982) reported regeneration of corticospinal axons after pyramidotomy in neonatal hamsters. Regenerated axons pursued an aberrant course but contributed to functional return. The possibility that section of a tract in neonates will not interrupt all the axons destined to run there is always a consideration, since axons do not go through a tract en masse and simultaneously. Late arrivals may escape axotomy and may grow around and beyond a lesion and be mistaken for regenerative sprouts. This may have happened in the experiments of Kalil and Reh (Tolbert and Der, 1987).

Other factors that may modify the axotomy response include the severity and permanence of the axonic injury, the proximity of the axonic interruption to the parent soma, the concomitant production of deafferentation by lesions producing axotomy (e.g., corticectomy), and the sparing or involvement of collaterals, the latter possibly functioning as a factor when lesions placed close to the cell body result in neuronal necrobiosis or delayed or incomplete regeneration. The nature of an experimental or naturally occurring injury, e.g., avulsion vs. simple crush, determines the severity of the impact on the cell body. The greater the amount of axoplasm removed by a lesion, the more deleterious is the effect on the integrity of the parent soma. Lesions made close to the cell body will remove more axoplasm than those made more distally and are more likely to remove collaterals from contact with the soma. The considerations enumerated above doubtless account for many of the variables associated with the axotomy response (Barron, 1983a,b), but they cannot always explain the essentially unpredictable consequences of the axon reaction.

That unilateral lesions affect nonaxotomized neurons of the uninjured side may be mentioned here and must always be considered when assessment of the axotomy response is made by comparison of injured cells with their companions of the nontraumatized side (Barron et al., 1985). Considerable changes may occur in the noninjured neurons.

Changes in the Processes of the Axotomized Neuron

The degenerative response of mammalian central neurons to axotomy is associated early with electron-dense and electron-lucent abnormal dendrites. Contained mitochondria may enlarge and exhibit bizarre cristal patterns while postsynaptic membrane specializations are lost and glycogen is accumulated. Similar changes occur pari passu in the axotomized somata and may also be encountered during prograde transneuronal degeneration (Barron, 1975). In some situations, dendrites may exhibit neurofilamentous hyperplasia (Barron, 1975). Whether these react with antibodies to phosphorylated neurofilaments, as deafferented, hypertrophied dendrites of Purkinje cells and neurons of inferior olive do (Shiurba et al., 1987), is not known. During axon reaction of the rat hypoglossal motoneuron, retraction and expansion of the dendritic tree can be measured morphometrically while the cell undergoes the initial response to, followed by recovery from, axotomy (Sumner and Watson, 1971). Kreutzberg et al. (1975) have described secretion of acetylcholinesterase by axotomized motoneuron dendrites and suggest that dendritic secretion of proteins may enable the injured cell to regulate blood flow and otherwise manipulate the perineuronal environment. A unique phenomenon occurs in feline motoneurons axotomized by intramedullary cord lesions. Axon-like processes develop from dendrites. These may be myelinated and may enter the adjacent PNS compartment (Linda et al., 1985).

The axon proximal to the site of axonic severance also undergoes alteration. Retrograde degeneration of the axons of axotomized central neurons is of particular importance. Kalil and Schneider (1975) described a progressive dying back of corticospinal axons of the adult hamster following section of the pyramidal tract at a medullary level. The process is preceded by a notable atrophy of axotomized pyramidal cell bodies of the motor cortex, proceeds slowly rostrad from the lesion site, and is to be sharply distinguished from retrograde Wallerian degeneration, in which the cell body dies and axonal disintegration proceeds rapidly in a temporospatial sequence away from the degenerated soma. Pallini et al. (1988) have measured the rate of retrograde degeneration of rat corticospinal axons following spinal cord transection and report rates of 28.8–88.4 μm per day at different postoperative intervals. A similar phenomenon may occur in man (Bronson et al., 1978), but Fishman (1987) has reported that the retraction of corticospinal axons from a spinal cord injury site does not progress in humans beyond the high cervical level, even many years after the cord lesion. Barron and Dentinger (1978) have encountered occasional degenerating axonal profiles at a cortical level in cat following cervical corticospinal tractotomy. In any case, after axotomy, the atrophied central neuron, if it survives, may not be capable of sustaining an axon of normal length and caliber. This fact is of significance when a delay ensues between production of a lesion and the subsequent injection nearby of a retrogradely transported tracer in order to label the somata of origin of the previously severed axons (Barron, 1984).

Regenerating neurons respond to axotomy by a temporary reduction in caliber of the axonic stump central to the lesion coincident with a reduction in the amount of NF proteins transported distally by the axotomized soma (Rosenfeld et al., 1987).

The Surround of the Axotomized Neuron

Following axotomy of rodent and lagomorph craniospinal neurons, striking glial responses ensue. Processes of proliferated microglia ensheath and appear to "strip" axosomatic and axodendritic boutons from the surfaces of the axotomized cells (Blinzinger and Kreutzberg, 1968). This phenomenon may also be seen around axotomized central neurons (Barron, 1982) and has excited much interest among neurophysiologists. It is not an invariable accompaniment of the axotomy response, however. The reactive microglia have plasma membranes rich in glycoconjugates, demonstrable by lectin histochemistry, and derive from cells normally resident in the CNS (Streit and Kreutzberg, 1987). By baring neuronal plasma membrane to the neuropil, bouton "stripping" may allow greater metabolic interchange, needed by the regenerating neuron, with neuroglia and intercellular space, or the deafferentation induced by the process may permit the injured nerve cell to shift metabolic effort toward axonic reconstitution and away from synaptic transmission (Barron, 1982). Bouton separation is reversible when the affected neurons achieve renewed contact with the periphery.

Astrocytes, and to a lesser extent oligodendroglia, participate in the axotomy response (Barron, 1982) and are reported to incorporate radiolabeled precursors of RNA and protein. The great majority of the astrocytes in the normal facial nucleus of rat are protoplasmic in type, and their filaments are negative immunohistochemically for glial fibrillary acidic protein (GFAP), even at the ultrastructural level. Under the stimulus of axotomy, they hypertrophy, become highly GFAP-positive, and are transformed into fibrous astrocytes (Graeber and Kreutzberg, 1986). The physiologic significance of this astroglial response is not known, but the response probably is neuron-supportive in character and is excited by the axotomized nerve cells.

We have recently studied astroglial, oligodendroglial, and microglial responses in axotomized rat hypoglossal and rubral neurons by quantitative histological and cytochemical, including immunohistochemical, methods. In the red nucleus, after cervical rubrospinal tractotomy, we did not find the hypertrophy and hyperplasia of neuroglia and the histochemical changes in these elements that occur in craniospinal motor nuclei after neurotomy. If this negative observation holds for other axotomized intrinsic neuronal populations that undergo a slowly progressive atrophy, it may indicate that the injured intrinsic neuron fails to signal (Graeber and Kreutzberg, 1986) a supportive physiologic response by neighboring neuroglia. The lack of participation of glial cells in the axotomy response may then play a role in the failure of CNS regeneration. Of course, astrocytes and microglia show pathologic responses to necrosis of axotomized central neurons, the former by scarring (gliosis) and the latter by phagocytosis (microglia).

Vascular alterations have also been described adjacent to axotomized peripheral neurons, including increases in capillary alkaline phosphatase activity (Barron, 1982). Capillary alterations may relate to an augmentation in transvascular transport of metabolites required by actively metabolizing, regenerating neurons. Alterations in the neuropil of the feline anterior horn are readily detectable by enzyme histochemistry after brachial plexotomy (Barron and Doolin, 1969), but their significance and cytological locus are unknown.

Retrograde Transneuronal Degeneration

Transneuronal or transsynaptic degeneration (TND) or atrophy (Cowan, 1970) is generally thought of as progressing from one neuronal aggregate to another of a functionally related chain by following the usual direction of impulse propagation (prograde TND). It may be due in some measure to stimulus deprivation. Recently Saji and Reis (1987) proposed a novel interpretation for the cause of prograde TND in substantia nigra, namely disinhibition and excessive excitation of nigral neurons following destruction of the GABA-ergic, inhibitory, strionigral input. Prograde TND is readily demonstrable in the visual system, especially in the lateral geniculate body, after lesions of the retina, optic nerve, or optic tract. Although prograde TND may well have crucial significance for possible restoration of function after interruption of some CNS fiber tracts, it is not directly related to the subject of this review. In contrast, retrograde TND occurs upstream, as it were, to the ordinary direction of passage of nerve stimuli. It involves secondarily, i.e., indirectly, neurons projecting on those that have undergone retrograde degeneration following interruption of their axons in a fiber tract or terminal field. Thus removal of the visual cortex will induce atrophy of the ganglion cell layer of the retina, especially in younger animals, and may selectively affect X cells (Tong et al., 1982). The neuronal relay intervening between the affected retinal population and the visual cortex, namely the lateral geniculate body, rapidly undergoes a degenerative axotomy response (retrograde neuronal degeneration) after extirpations of the visual cortex. Retrograde TND also occurs in neurons of the inner nuclear layer (INL) of the human and feline retina following lesions of the optic nerve and chiasm (van Buren, 1963; Gills and Wadsworth, 1967; Hollander et al., 1984). Retrograde TND is an indirect consequence of a degenerative axotomy response and has great relevance for CNS regeneration. Thus, in the visual system, little might be gained if a measure of optic nerve regeneration by surviving axotomized retinal ganglion cells were achieved in the presence of substantial cell loss or degenerative atrophy of the INL or permanent changes in the circuitry of the inner plexiform layer. The INL makes connections to ganglion cell elements that are requisite to retinal function. Retrograde TND also occurs in the limbic system of several species (Bleier, 1969; Cowan, 1970) and in the human corticopontine projection (Smith, 1975). It is most evident in the immature CNS (Bleier, 1969) and may involve more than two neurons in a chain. It is by no means a universal phenomenon and its occurrence is partly species-dependent. We may presume that it results from a lack of trophic material conveyed by retrograde axoplasmic transport from one neuron, or elements of its surround, to another. Nerve growth factor (NGF) is an example of such a trophin, as will be discussed below. The length of time that the second neuron in a chain, back from the injury site, is vulnerable to irreversible retrograde TND, when that process occurs, is unknown.

Theoretically, the primary retrograde neuronal degeneration, which leads ultimately to retrograde TND, could occur following death of target nerve cells, but in the absence of direct damage to axon terminals impinging on the necrosed target. Such a process could underlie system degenerations in human pathology. It is difficult, however, to visualize a necrotizing process that would destroy the neurons of a nucleus without impacting upon the integrity of axon terminals within the degenerating field (Bleier, 1969).

RESCUE OF THE AXOTOMIZED NEURON

The proportion of neurons within a system that would need to be rescued in order to restore and maintain function has only begun to be explored (Barron et al., 1986). In any case, there are two approaches to neuronal rescue, an objective that primarily concerns the central or intrinsic mammalian neuron. One approach involves the application of soluble trophic agents in such a way that they can reach and act on damaged nerve cells. A second approach involves the insertion of tissue implants at the lesion site. Both approaches appear to accomplish a common goal, namely the provision to the axotomized neuron of trophic factors essential to cellular survival and neuritic elongation. Implants may also provide a physical substratum that aids axonal elongation.

Neurotrophins and Growth-Promoting Agents/Factors

These are "nourishing" substances (Varon et al., 1983; Chapter 7, this volume) that interact with nerve cells in a way that supports their survival, differentiation, and neurite extension. Survival promotion and neurite stimulation have in general been conjoined properties of neurotrophic agents. Because these agents have diverse tissue origins and biological effects outside the CNS and PNS, they might more appropriately be termed growth-promoting or biosynthetic agents or factors.

NERVE GROWTH FACTOR

NGF is a hydrosoluble polypeptide of known amino acid sequence (Hefti and Weiner, 1986); it is target-derived and moved by retrograde axoplasmic transport to the cell bodies of its peripheral neuronal dependents, sympathetic and primary sensory neurons (Hendry and Campbell, 1976; Levi-Montalcini, 1987). It prevents nerve cell death in rat superior cervical ganglion during development and after axotomy (Hendry and Cambell, 1976) and protects adult sensory neurons from axotomy-induced atrophy and necrosis (Otto et al., 1987; Rich et al., 1987).

In recent years, there has been clear demonstration that NGF is a neurotrophic factor for cholinergic neurons of the forebrain (Hefti and Weiner, 1986). The mRNA encoding for NGF and the NGF receptor protein are present in multiple sites in rodent, monkey, and human CNS, including the hippocampus, which receives major cholinergic inputs from the medial septal nucleus and the diagonal band of Broca (Raivich and Kreutzberg, 1987; Riopelle et al., 1987). Of dramatic importance is the demonstration by a number of laboratories that

NGF infusion intraventricularly prevents cell death in cholinergic septal neurons after lesions, partly or completely interrupting their projections to the dorsal hippocampus (Hefti and Weiner, 1986; Williams et al., 1986; Kromer, 1987). NGF also rescues noncholinergic neurons of the nuclei, originating the septohippocampal cholinergic input, but this effect may be an indirect one (Williams et al., 1986; Kromer, 1987). The "window of time" after axotomy during which NGF injection remains effective and the degree to which neuronal survival is accompanied by regenerative axonal sprouting is under active investigation in several laboratories. The effectiveness of NGF in the "rescue" of axotomized neurons of the basal forebrain for the first time holds out a realistic and specific prospect for successful pharmacologic treatment of CNS injury. The distribution of NGF and NGF receptor in brain is relatively wide and is neither limited to cholinergic neurons nor present in all cholinergic systems (Hefti and Weiner, 1986; Raivich and Kreutzberg, 1987). This fact, as well as the enhanced axonal outgrowth produced in crushed optic nerve of goldfish by intravitreal injection of NGF (Grafstein, 1986), suggests that it may have a role in the prevention of cell death after axotomy of CNS neurons other than those of the basal forebrain.

BRAIN-DERIVED NEUROTROPHIC FACTOR (BDNF)

Barde et al. (1982) have derived a neuronotrophic factor from pig brain. BDNF is a basic protein of molecular weight 12,300. It supports the survival of and neurite outgrowth by chick sensory neurons (Barde et al., 1982; Kalcheim et al., 1987) in vitro and in vivo, the latter observations made in embryos. The presence of laminin is a necessary condition for the BDNF effect. A fraction of brain extract derived from an intermediate stage of BDNF purification stimulates neurite outgrowth and supports neuronal maturation and survival in fetal retinal explants and dissociated fetal rat retinal cultures (Turner, 1985).

POLYAMINES

Certain polyamines, putrescine, spermidine, and spermine, are present in high concentrations in developing and regenerating tissues, where rapid growth and cell replication are occurring. Ornithine decarboyxlase (ODC) catalyzes the conversion of ornithine to putrescine in the metabolic step thought to be rate-limiting for synthesis of spermine and spermidine. ODC activity is demonstrable immunohistochemically in neurons of rat brain during the first 14 days of postnatal development (Dorn et al., 1987). A short-lived burst of increased ODC activity marks facial motoneurons after axotomy (Tetzlaff and Kreutzberg, 1985). Enzyme activity is greatest 8–24 hours after the injury and reverts toward normal after the third postoperative day. Polyamines can be involved in the regulation of DNA and RNA synthesis and could conceivably initiate the "regeneration program" (Tetzlaff and Kreutzberg, 1985). After sciatic nerve crush in frog, inhibition of ODC activity by injection of the specific ODC inhibitor, alpha-difluoromethyl ornithine (DFMO), results in prevention of regeneration of sensory axons (Kanje et al., 1986). Gilad and Gilad (1983) reported that intraperitoneal injections of inhibitors of ODC and S-adenosylmethionine decarboxylase activites, both important to polyamine biosynthesis, prevented the chromatolytic response and increased nerve cell death in adult rat superior cervical ganglion after section of the postganglionic nerve. On the other hand, injection of spermine intraperitoneally in rats speeds the rate of recovery of motor function in the sciatic and in peripheral sympathetic nerves (Dornay et al., 1986). Whether the administration of polyamines will encourage CNS regeneration is unanswered and awaits a systematic inquiry.

GANGLIOSIDES

Gangliosides, especially in the GM1 molecular form, have been reported to rescue dopamine neurons of the substantia nigra after partial lesions of the nigrostriatal pathway (Agnati et al., 1983) and cholinergic nerve cells of the nucleus basalis after corticectomy (Cuello et al., 1986). In our laboratory we studied the impact of GM1 on the axotomy response of rubral nerve cells of rat (Barron, 1988). The degree of nerve cell atrophy was not significantly affected by GM1 treatment, and regeneration of the severed rubrospinal axons did not occur.

UNCHARACTERIZED NEUROTROPHINS EFFECTIVE IN VIVO

Growth-associated triggering factors (GATFs) (Hadani et al., 1984; Lavie et al., 1987) are obtained from media conditioned by regenerating goldfish optic nerve or by growing optic nerves of neonatal rabbits. When applied to injured optic nerve of adult rabbits, for instance by wrap-around silastic tubes coated with conditioned medium, GATFs induce regeneration-associated biochemical changes in adjacent retina, including increased protein synthesis, and promote extension of optic neurites in vitro and, temporarily, in vivo (Lavie et al., 1987). The nature of the soluble substance or substances termed GATFs is unknown.

In experiments of great potential significance, performed on rat brain, Cunningham et al. (1987) concentrated a soluble protein from culture medium conditioned by explants of embryonic occipital cortex and implanted it in cavitary lesions produced by extirpation of the posterior neocortex in neonates. The conditioned medium accomplished a threefold increase in survival of neurons of the dorsal nucleus of the lateral geniculate body (dLGB), compared with control rats treated only with unconditioned medium. The trophin preliminarily characterized by Cunningham et al. (1987) is target-derived. If its action is specific for the dLGB and if others of the many nuclei within the brain have similarly idiosyncratic needs, the pharmacologic treatment of neuronal degeneration induced by axotomy will be complex indeed!

MISCELLANEOUS NEUROTROPHINS AND IN VITRO STUDIES

Some blood-borne proteins have been shown to support neuronal survival in vitro or to encourage axonal elongation (Kaufman and Barrett, 1983; Oorschot and Jones, 1986; Walicke et al., 1986). The supportive action of catalase (Walicke et al., 1986), an erythrocyte constituent, is related to the peroxidatic capacity of the enzyme. This reduces neuronal damage caused by toxic peroxides produced in culture media. The catalase effect is not due to a direct interaction with neuronal constituents and is not neurotrophic in the strict sense. Other neuronotrophic factors that have been studied in tissue culture have derived from cortical wounds, cerebrospinal fluid after head trauma, and conditioned medium obtained from cultures of neonatal rat astrocytes (Banker, 1980; Nieto-Sampedro et al., 1983; Walicke et al., 1986).

Fibroblast and astroglial growth factors, closely related if not identical mitogenic proteins, support survival of, and neurite extension by, a variety of peripheral and central neurons in tissue culture (Morrison, 1987; Unsicker et al., 1987). One in vivo study of fibroblast growth factor has appeared (Otto et al., 1987). The basic form of fibroblast growth factor is localizable immunohistochemically to neurons of the developing postnatal rat brain (Pettmann et al., 1986), is synthesized within the brain, and is active in the picomolar range (Morrison, 1987). Another polypeptide, epidermal growth factor (Morrison et al., 1987), supports survival and neuritic outgrowth by neonatal rat telencephalic neurons in tissue culture in a dose-dependent manner and is effective in concentrations as low as 100 pg/ml.

Reports about the effects of ACTH, glucocorticoids, and thyroid hormones on neurons and neuroglia of injured CNS are conflicting. Androgens, however, may accelerate axonal regeneration by peripheral motoneurons (Jones, 1988).

Transplantation of PNS and CNS Tissues to the Injured Mammalian CNS

PNS IMPLANTS

In a series of landmark experiments spanning a decade, Aguayo and colleagues have shown that PNS segments grafted into brain and spinal cord stimulate axonal elongation by damaged intrinsic neurons (Aguayo, 1985; Bray and Aguayo, Chapter 5, this volume). Recently Aguayo and colleagues (Villegas-Perez et al., 1988) have shown that peripheral nerve segments grafted to rat optic nerve sectioned at the disc enhance survival of axotomized retinal ganglion cells by two- to fourfold. In the absence of PNS grafts, 90% of the ganglion cells die within 1 month. Twenty per cent of the neurons surviving after grafting grow lengthy axons into the PNS implant. Unfortunately, only a few of these fibers make synaptic connection within the superior colliculus, where the distal end of the PNS isograft is introduced. It is probable that the protective and stimulatory effects of the grafting procedure relate to diffusible substances (trophins) derived from the nerve that are available to the axotomized retinal neurons when the grafts are apposed to the globe rather than along the intracranial course of the nerve (Villegas-Perez et al., 1988). Turner et al. (1987) calculated that diffusible factors from PNS segments implanted in the eye exert trophic effects over a distance of 1–2 mm. Berry and colleagues (1986) have also reported neuronal rescue in rat retina after anastomosis of PNS grafts to severed optic nerves. These grafts, in addition to supplying soluble trophins to nerve cell bodies, may also provide axons of intrinsic neurons with one or more substrate-bound factors that promote neurite elongation (Sandrock and Matthew, 1987) and that are absent from mature CNS. GATFs may activate glial cells of adult rabbit optic nerve to synthesize laminin (Zak et al., 1987), which is known to play a role in neurite outgrowth and elongation.

CNS IMPLANTS

A major contribution to this field is the demonstration by Bregman and Reier (1986) that fetal spinal cord tissue grafted into midthoracic spinal cord lesions, made in neonates, prevents the massive retrograde degeneration that ordinarily occurs when rubral neurons are axotomized soon after birth. The rescuing effect persists for at least 1 year and is associated, at least in part, with regrowth of some rubrospinal axons beyond (caudal to) the site of transplantation. The fetal cord transplants appear to rescue neurons of other brain systems projecting to the cord, notably the lateral vestibular nucleus (Bregman and Reier, 1986). The rescue effect is, at the least, relatively target-specific and probably trophin-mediated. It is not duplicated by implantation into the lesioned cord of embryonic hippocampus or neonatal sciatic nerve. In important work of a related character, Cunningham et al. (1987) have found that a beneficial impact is exerted by embryonic, posterior cortical implants on survival of neurons in the axotomized dLGB of neonatal and adult rats. The rescuing effect is due to the action of a diffusible, proteinaceous neurotrophic factor released by explants of posterior cortex into media in which they are cocultured with fetal diencephalon (Cunningham et al., 1987).

ACKNOWLEDGMENTS

Studies from the author's laboratory were supported by the Veterans Administration.

REFERENCES

Agnati LF, Fuxe K, Calza L, Benfenati F, Cavicchioli L, Toffano G, Goldstein M (1983): Gangliosides increase the survival of lesioned nigral dopamine neurons and favour the recovery of dopaminergic synaptic function in striatum of rats by collateral sprouting. Acta Physiol Scand 119:347–363.

Aguayo AJ (1985): Axonal regeneration from injured neurons in the adult mammalian central nervous system. In Cotman CW (ed): "Synaptic Plasticity." New York: The Guilford Press, pp 457–484.

Aldskogius H, Barron KD, Regal R (1980): Axon reaction in dorsal motor vagal and hypoglossal neurons of the adult rat. Light microscopy and RNA-cytochemistry. J Comp Neurol 193:165–177.

Aldskogius H, Barron KD, Regal R (1984): Axonal reaction in hypoglossal and dorsal motor vagal neurons of adult rat: Incorporation of [³H]leucine. Exp Neurol 85:139–151.

Antunes JL, Louis KM, Huang S, Zimmerman E, Carmel PW, Ferin M (1980): Section of the pituitary stalk in the Rhesus monkey: Morphological and endocrine observations. Ann Neurol 8:308–316.

Austin L, Langford CJ (1980): Nerve regeneration: A biochemical view. Trends Neurosci 3:130–132.

Banker GA (1980): Trophic interactions between astroglial cells and hippocampal neurons in culture. Science 209:809–810.

Barde Y-A, Edgar D, Thoenen H (1982): Purification of a new neurotrophic factor from mammalian brain. EMBO J 1:549–553.

Barron KD (1975): Ultrastructural changes in dendrites of central neurons during axon reaction. In Kreutzberg GW (ed): "Physiology and Pathology of Dendrites. Advances in Neurology," vol. 12. New York: Raven Press, pp 381–399.

Barron KD (1982): Axon reaction and its relevance to CNS trauma. In Grossman RG, Gildenberg PL (eds): "Head Injury: Basic and Clinical Aspects." New York: Raven Press, pp 45–55.

Barron KD (1983a): Comparative observations on the cytologic reactions of central and peripheral nerve cells to axotomy. In Kao CC, Bunge RP, Reier PJ (eds): "Spinal Cord Reconstruction." New York: Raven Press, pp 7–40.

Barron KD (1983b): Axon reaction and central nervous system regeneration. In Seil FJ (ed): "Nerve, Organ and Tissue Regeneration: Research Perspectives." New York: Academic Press, pp 3–36.

Barron KD (1984): Retrograde transport of injured neurons. Neurology 34:401–403.

Barron KD (1988): The effect of GM1 ganglioside administration on the axotomy response of rat rubral neurons. In Reier PJ, Bunge RP, Seil FJ (eds): "Current Issues in Neural Regeneration Research." New York: Alan R. Liss, Inc.

Barron KD, Doolin PF (1969): Neuronal responses to axon injury. In Norris FH, Kurland L (eds): "Contemporary Neurology Symposia,"· vol. II. New York: Grune and Stratton, pp 301–318.

Barron KD, Dentinger MP (1978): Abnormal ultrastructural appearances in axons of feline pericruciate cortex after lateral funiculotomy. Acta Neuropathol 44:1–8.

Barron KD, Dentinger MP (1979): Cytologic observations on axotomized feline Betz cells. 1. Qualitative electron microscopic findings. J Neuropathol Exp Neurol 38:128–151.

Barron KD, Oldershaw JB, Bernsohn J (1966): Hydrolase cytochemistry of retrograde neuronal degeneration in feline lateral geniculate body with observations on the identification of multiple forms of neural hydrolases having overlapping substrate affinities. J Neuropathol Exp Neurol 25:443–478.

Barron KD, Doolin PF, Oldershaw JB (1967): Ultrastructural observations on retrograde atrophy of lateral geniculate body. I. Neuronal alterations. J Neuropathol Exp Neurol 26:300–326.

Barron KD, Dentinger MP, Nelson LR, Mincy JE (1975): Ultrastructure of axonal reaction in red nucleus of cat. J Neuropathol Exp Neurol 34:222–248.

Barron KD, Dentinger MP, Nelson LR, Scheibly ME (1976): Incorporation of tritiated leucine by axotomized rubral neurons. Brain Res 116:251–266.

Barron KD, Schreiber SS, Cova JL, Scheibly ME (1977): Quantitative cytochemistry of RNA in axotomized feline rubral neurons. Brain Res 130:469–481.

Barron KD, Cova J, Scheibly ME, Kohberger R (1982): Morphometric measurements and RNA content of axotomized feline cervical motoneurons. J Neurocytol 11:707–720.

Barron KD, McGuinness CM, Misantone LJ, Zanakis MF, Grafstein B, Murray M (1985): RNA content of normal and axotomized retinal ganglion cells of rat and goldfish. J Comp Neurol 236:265–273.

Barron KD, Dentinger MP, Krohel G, Easton SK, Mankes R (1986): Qualitative and quantitative ultrastructural observations on retinal ganglion cell layer of rat after intraorbital optic nerve crush. J Neurocytol 15:345–362.

Bayer SA, Yackel JW, Puri PS (1982): Neurons in the rat dentate gyrus granular layer substantially increase during juvenile and adult life. Science 216:890–892.

Bernstein JJ, Geldred JB (1973): Synaptic reorganization following regeneration of goldfish spinal cord. Exp Neurol 41:402–410.

Berry M, Rees L, Sievers J (1986): Unequivocal regeneration of rat optic nerve axons into sciatic nerve isografts. In Das GD, Wallace RB (eds): "Neural Transplantation and Regeneration." New York: Springer-Verlag, pp 63–79.

Bleier R (1969): Retrograde transsynaptic cellular degeneration in mammillary and ventral tegmental nuclei following limbic decortication in rabbits of various ages. Brain Res 15:365–393.

Blinzinger K, Kreutzberg G (1968): Displacement of synaptic terminals from regenerating motorneurons by microglial cells. Z Zellforsch 85:145–157.

Bodian D (1962): The generalized vertebrate neuron. Science 137:323–326.

Bregman BS, Reier PJ (1986): Neural tissue transplants rescue axotomized rubrospinal cells from retrograde death. J Comp Neurol 244:86–95.

Bronson R, Gilles FH, Hall J, Hedley-Whyte ET (1978): Long term post-traumatic retrograde corticospinal degeneration in man. Hum Pathol 9:602–607.

Bryz-Gornia Jr WF, Stelzner DJ (1986): Ascending tract neurons survive spinal cord transection in the neonatal rat. Exp Neurol 93:195–210.

Cole M (1968): Retrograde degeneration of axon and soma in the nervous system. In Bourne GH (ed): "The Structure and Function of Nervous Tissue. Structure I," vol. I. New York: Academic Press, pp 269–300.

Cowan WM (1970): Anterograde and retrograde transneuronal degeneration in the central and peripheral nervous system. In Nauta WJ, Ebbeson SOE (eds): "Contemporary Research Methods in Neuroanatomy." New York: Springer-Verlag, pp 217–251.

Cragg BG (1970): What is the signal for chromatolysis? Brain Res 23:1–21.

Cuello AC, Stephens PH, Tagari PC, Sofroniew MV, Pearson RCA (1986): Retrograde changes in the nucleus basalis of the rat, caused by cortical damage, are prevented by exogenous ganglioside GM_1. Brain Res 376:373–377.

Cunningham TJ, Haun F, Chantler PD (1987): Diffusible proteins prolong survival of dorsal lateral geniculate neurons following occipital cortex lesions in newborn rats. Dev Brain Res 37:133–141.

Dentinger MP, Barron KD, Kohberger RC, McLean B (1979): Cytologic observations on axotomized feline Betz cells. II. Quantitative ultrastructural findings. J Neuropathol Exp Neurol 38:551–564.

Devor M, Govrin-Lippman R (1985): Neurogenesis in adult rat dorsal root ganglia. Neurosci Lett 61:189–194.

Dorn A, Muller M, Bernstein H-G, Pajunen A, Jarvinen M (1987): Immunohistochemical localization of L-ornithine decarboxylase in developing rat brain. Int J Dev Neurosci 5:145–150.

Dornay M, Gilad VH, Shiler I, Gilad GM (1986): Early polyamine treatment accelerates regeneration of rat sympathetic neurons. Exp Neurol 92:665–674.

Drager UC, Hofbauer A (1984): Antibodies to heavy neurofilament subunit detect a subpopulation of damaged ganglion cells in retina. Nature 309:624–626.

Durica TE, Jacob SK (1980): Comparison of the facial, vagal, and hypoglossal neuronal populations following axotomy in the adult hamster. Anat Rec 196:51A.

Fishman PS (1987): Retrograde changes in the corticospinal tract of posttraumatic paraplegics. Arch Neurol 44:1082–1084.

Freed WJ, de Medinaceli L, Wyatt RJ (1985): Promoting functional plasticity in the damaged nervous system. Science 227:1544–1552.

Gilad GM, Gilad VH (1983): Polyamine biosynthesis is required for survival of sympathetic neurons after axonal injury. Brain Res 273:191–194.

Gills JP, Wadsworth JAC (1967): Retrograde transsynaptic degeneration of the inner nuclear layer of the retina. Invest Ophthalmol 6:437–448.

Gonzalez MF, Sharp FR, Sagar SM (1987): Axotomy increases NADPH-diaphorase staining in rat vagal motor neurons. Brain Res Bull 18:417–427.

Graeber MB, Kreutzberg GW (1986): Astrocytes increase in glial fibrillary acidic protein during retrograde changes of facial motor neurons. J Neurocytol 15: 363–373.

Grafstein B (1983): Chromatolysis reconsidered: A new view of the reaction of the nerve cell body to axon injury. In Seil FJ (ed): "Nerve, Organ and Tissue Regeneration: Research Perspectives." New York: Academic Press, pp 37–50.

Grafstein B (1986): The retina as a regenerating organ. In Adler R, Farber DB (eds): "The Retina: A Model for Cell Biology Studies," Part II. New York: Academic Press, pp 275–335.

Hadani M, Harel A, Solomon A, Belkin M, Lavie V, Schwartz M (1984): Substances originating from the optic nerve of neonatal rabbit induce regeneration-associated response in the injured optic nerve of adult rabbit. Proc Natl Acad Sci USA 81:7965–7969.

Hefti F, Weiner WJ (1986): Nerve growth factor and Alzheimer's disease. Ann Neurol 20:275–281.

Hendry IA, Campbell J (1976): Morphometric analysis of rat superior cervical ganglion after axotomy and nerve growth factor treatment. J Neurocytol 5:351–360.

Hollander H, Bisti S, Maffei L, Hebel R (1984): Electroretinographic responses and retrograde changes of retinal morphology after intracranial optic nerve section. A quantitative analysis in the cat. Exp Brain Res 55: 483–493.

Hollander H, Bisti S, Maffei L (1985): Long term survival of cat retinal ganglion cells after intracranial optic nerve transection. Exp Brain Res 59:633–635.

Jones KJ (1988): Steroid hormones and neurotrophism: Relationship to nerve injury. Metab Brain Dis 3:1–18.

Jones KJ, Lavelle A (1986): Differential effects of axotomy on immature and mature hamster facial neurons: A time course study of initial nucleolar and nuclear changes. J Neurocytol 15:197–206.

Kalcheim C, Barde Y-A, Thoenen H, Le Douarin NM (1987): In vivo effect of brain-derived neurotrophic factor on the survival of developing dorsal root ganglion cells. EMBO J 6:2871–2873.

Kalil K, Schneider GE (1975): Retrograde cortical and axonal changes following lesions of the pyramidal tract. Brain Res 89:15–27.

Kalil K, Reh T (1982): A light and electron microscopic study of regrowing pyramidal tract fibers. J Comp Neurol 211:265–275.

Kanje M, Fransson I, Edstrom A, Lowkvist B (1986): Ornithine decarboxylase activity in dorsal root ganglia of regenerating frog sciatic nerve. Brain Res 381:24–28.

Kauffman FC, Ross RA, Reis DJ (1976): Reversible effects of axotomy on locus coeruleus glucose-6-P dehydrogenase. Trans Am Soc Neurochem 7:86.

Kaufman LM, Barrett JN (1983): Serum factor supporting long-term survival of rat central neurons in culture. Science 220:1394–1396.

Kirino T, Brightman MW, Oertel WH, Schmechel DE, Marangos PJ (1983): Neuron-specific enolase as an index of neuronal regeneration and reinnervation. J Neurosci 3:915–923.

Kreutzberg GW (1986): The motoneuron and its microenvironment responding to axotomy. In Das GD, Wallace RB (eds): "Neural Transplantation and Regeneration." New York: Springer-Verlag, pp 271–276.

Kreutzberg GW, Toth L, Kaiya H (1975): Acetylcholinesterase as a marker for dendritic transport and dendritic secretion. In Kreutzberg GW (ed): "Physiology and Pathology of Dendrites, Advances in Neurology," vol 12. New York: Raven Press, pp 269–281.

Kristensson K (1981): Retrograde signaling of nerve cell body response to trauma. In Gorio A, Millesi H, Mingrino S (eds): "Posttraumatic Nerve Regeneration: Experimental Basis and Clinical Implications." New York: Raven Press, pp 27–34.

Kromer LF (1987): Nerve growth factor treatment after brain injury prevents neuronal death. Science 235:214–216.

Lavie V, Harel A, Doron A, Solomon A, Lobel D, Belkin M, Ben-Basat S, Sharma S, Schwartz M (1987): Morphological response of injured adult rabbit optic nerve to implants containing media conditioned by growing optic nerves. Brain Res 419:166–172.

Levi-Montalcini R (1987): The nerve growth factor 35 years later. Science 237:1154–1162.

Linda H, Risling M, Cullheim S (1985): "Dendraxons" in regenerating motoneurons in the cat: Do dendrites generate new axons after central axotomy? Brain Res 358:329–333.

Lyon ML, Stelzner DJ (1987): Tests of regenerative capacity of tectal efferent axons in the frog, *Rana pipiens*. J Comp Neurol 255:511–525.

Means ED, Barron KD, Copeland A (1972): Retrograde atrophy of rat thalamus. J Neuropathol Exp Neurol 31:168.

Meiri KF, Pfenninger KH, Willard MB (1986): Growth-associated protein, GAP-43, a polypeptide that is induced when neurons extend axons, is a component of growth cones and corresponds to pp46, a major polypeptide of a subcellular fraction enriched in growth cones. Proc Natl Acad Sci USA 83:3537–3541.

Meyer DD, Cole M (1970): Comparison of certain retrograde oxidative reactions after section of axons in central and peripheral nervous systems. Neurology 20: 918–924.

Morrison RS (1987): Fibroblast growth factors: Potential neurotrophic agents in the central nervous system. J Neurosci Res 17:99–101.

Morrison RS, Kornblum HI, Leslie FM, Bradshaw RA (1987): Trophic stimulation of cultured neurons from neonatal rat brain by epidermal growth factor. Science 238:72–75.

Muller HW, Gebicke-Harter PJ, Hange DH, Shooter EM (1985): A specific 37,000-Dalton protein that accumulates in regenerating but not in nonregenerating mammalian nerves. Science 228:499–501.

Murray M, Grafstein B (1969): Changes in the morphology and amino acid incorporation of regenerating goldfish optic neurons. Exp Neurol 23:544–560.

Nieto-Sampedro M, Manthrope M, Barbin G, Varon S,

Cotman CW (1983): Injury-induced neuronotrophic activity in adult rat brain: Correlation with survival of delayed implants in the wound cavity. J Neurosci 3: 2219–2229.

Oorschot DE, Jones DG (1986): Tissue culture analysis of neurite outgrowth in the presence and absence of serum: Possible relevance for central nervous system regeneration. J Neurosci Res 15:341–352.

Otto D, Unsicker K, Grothe C (1987): Pharmacological effects of nerve growth factor and fibroblast growth factor applied to the transectioned sciatic nerve on neuron death in adult rat dorsal root ganglia. Neurosci Lett 83:156–160.

Pallini R, Fernandez E, Sbriccoli A (1988): Retrograde degeneration of corticospinal axons following transection of the spinal cord in rats. A quantitative study with anterogradely transported horseradish peroxidase. J Neurosurg 68:124–128.

Payne BR, Pearson HE, Berman N (1984): Deafferentation and axotomy of neurons in cat striate cortex: Time course of changes in binocularity following corpus callosum transection. Brain Res 307:201–215.

Perry GW, Wilson DL (1981): Protein synthesis and axonal transport during nerve regeneration. J Neurochem 37:1203–1217.

Pettmann B, Labourdette G, Weibel M, Sensenbrenner M (1986): The brain fibroblast growth factor (FGF) is localized in neurons. Neurosci Lett 68:175–180.

Quigley HA, Davis EB, Anderson DR (1977): Descending optic nerve degeneration in primates. Invest Ophthalmol Visual Sci 16:841–849.

Raivich G, Kreutzberg GW (1987): The localization and distribution of high affinity β-nerve growth factor binding sites in the central nervous system of the adult rat. A light microscopic autoradiographic study using [^{125}I]β-nerve growth factor. Neuroscience 20:23–36.

Ramón y Cajal S (1928): "Degeneration and Regeneration of the Nervous System," vol 1. London: Oxford University Press.

Reh TA, Redshaw JD, Bisby MA (1987): Axons of the pyramidal tract do not increase their transport of growth-associated proteins after axotomy. Mol Brain Res 2:1–6.

Rich KM, Luszczynski JR, Osborne PA, Johnson EM Jr (1987): Nerve growth factor protects adult sensory neurons from cell death and atrophy caused by nerve injury. J Neurocytol 16:261–268.

Riopelle RJ, Richardson PM, Verge VMK (1987): Distribution and characteristics of nerve growth factor binding on cholinergic neurons of rat and monkey forebrain. Neurochem Res 12:923–928.

Risling M, Cullheim S, Hildebrand C (1983): Reinnervation of the ventral root L7 from ventral horn neurons following intramedullary axotomy in adult cats. Brain Res 280:15–23.

Rodichok LD, Barron KD, Popp AJ, Dentinger MP, Scheibly ME (1984): Glucose utilization is unchanged in red nucleus after axotomy. Brain Res 324:253–259.

Rosenfeld J, Dorman ME, Griffin JW, Sternberger LA, Sternberger NH, Price DL (1987): Distribution of neurofilament antigens after axonal injury. J Neuropathol Exp Neurol 46:269–282.

Rotter A, Birdsall NJM, Burgen ASV, Field PM, Smolen A, Raisman G (1979): Muscarinic receptors in the central nervous system of the rat. IV. A comparison of the effects of axotomy and deafferentation on the binding of [^{3}H]propylbenzilylcholine mustard and associated synaptic changes in the hypoglossal and pontine nuclei. Brain Res Rev 1:207–224.

Saji M, Reis DJ (1987): Delayed transneuronal death of substantia nigra neurons prevented by γ-aminobutyric acid agonist. Science 235:66–69.

Sandrock AW Jr, Matthew WD (1987): Identification of a peripheral nerve neurite growth-promoting activity by development and use of an in vitro bioassay. Proc Natl Acad Sci USA 84:6934–6938.

Schlaepfer WW (1987): Neurofilaments: Structure, metabolism and implications in disease. J Neuropathol Exp Neurol 46:117–129.

Shiurba RA, Eng LF, Sternberger NH, Sternberger LA, Urich H (1987): The cytoskeleton of the human cerebellar cortex: An immunohistochemical study of normal and pathological material. Brain Res 407:205–211.

Shyne-Athwal S, Riccio RV, Chakraborty G, Ingoglia NA (1986): Protein modification by amino acid addition is increased in crushed sciatic but not optic nerves. Science 231:603–605.

Singer P, Mehler S (1986): Glucose and leucine uptake in the hypoglossal nucleus after hypoglossal nerve transection with and without prevented regeneration in the Sprague-Dawley rat. Neurosci Lett 67:73–77.

Smith CB, Crane AM, Kadekaro M, Agranoff BW, Sokoloff L (1984): Stimulation of protein synthesis and glucose utilization in the hypoglossal nucleus induced by axotomy. J Neurosci 4:2489–2496.

Smith MC (1975): Histological findings after hemicerebellectomy in man: Anterograde, retrograde and transneuronal degeneration. Brain Res 95:423–442.

Stelzner DJ, Bohn RC, Strauss JA (1986): Regeneration of the frog optic nerve. Comparisons with development. Neurochem Pathol 5:255–288.

Stoll G, Muller HW (1986): Macrophages in the peripheral nervous system and astroglia in the central nervous system of rat commonly express apolipoprotein E during development but differ in their responses to injury. Neurosci Lett 72:233–238.

Streit WJ, Kreutzberg GW (1987): Lectin binding by resting and reactive microglia. J Neurocytol 16:249–260.

Sumner BEH, Watson WE (1971): Retraction and expansion of the dendritic tree of motor neurons of adult rats induced in vivo. Nature 233:273–275.

Tetzlaff W, Kreutzberg GW (1985): Ornithine decarboxylase in motoneurons during regeneration. Exp Neurol 89:679–688.

Tolbert DL, Der T (1987): Redirected growth of pyramidal tract axons following neonatal pyramidotomy in cats. J Comp Neurol 260:299–311.

Tong L, Spear PD, Kalil RE, Callahan EC (1982): Loss of retinal X-cells in cats with neonatal or adult visual cortex damage. Science 217:72–75.

Torvik A, Heding A (1969): Effect of actinomycin D on retrograde nerve cell reaction. Further observations. Acta Neuropathol 14:62–71.

Tsang D, Yew DT, Lam STL (1985): Acute responses of

rat retina after optic nerve ligation: A biochemical and histochemical study. Brain Res 336:289–295.

Turner JE (1985): Promotion of neurite outgrowth and cell survival in dissociated fetal rat retinal cultures by a fraction derived from a brain extract. Dev Brain Res 18:265–274.

Turner JE, Blair JR, Chappel ET (1987): Peripheral nerve implant effects on survival of retinal ganglion layer cells after axotomy initiated by a penetrating lesion. Brain Res 419:46–54.

Unsicker K, Reichert-Preibsch H, Schmidt R, Pettmann B, Labourdette G, Sensenbrenner M (1987): Astroglial and fibroblast growth factors have neurotrophic functions for cultured peripheral and central nervous system neurons. Proc Natl Acad Sci USA 84:5459–5463.

Van Buren JM (1963): Trans-synaptic retrograde degeneration in the visual system of primates. J Neurol Neurosurg Psychiatry 26:402–409.

Varon S, Manthrope M, Williams LR (1983): Neuronotrophic and neurite-promoting factors and their clinical potentials. Dev Neurosci 6:73–100.

Vidal-Sanz M, Bray GM, Villegas-Perez MP, Thanos S, Aguayo AJ (1987): Axonal regeneration and synapse formation in the superior colliculus by retinal ganglion cells in the adult rat. J Neurosci 7:2894–2909.

Villablanca JR, Burgess JW, Benedetti F (1986): There is less thalamic degeneration in neonatal-lesioned than in adult-lesioned cats after cerebral hemispherectomy. Brain Res 368:211–225.

Villegas-Perez MP, Vidal-Sanz M, Bray GM, Aguayo AJ (1988): Influences of peripheral nerve grafts on the survival and regrowth of axotomized retinal ganglion cells in adult rats. J Neurosci 8:265–280.

Walicke P, Varon S, Manthrope M (1986): Purification of a human red blood cell protein supporting the survival of cultured CNS neurons, and its identification as catalase. J Neurosci 6:1114–1121.

Wells MR (1984): Alterations of [³H]actinomycin D binding to axotomized dorsal root ganglion cell nuclei: An autoradiographic method to detect changes in chromatin structure and RNA synthesis. Exp Neurol 86:303–312.

Wells MR, Hall MF (1985): Neuronal chromatin changes in layer V pyramidal cells of somatomotor cortex after pyramidal tract lesions as demonstrated by [³H]actinomycin D binding. Exp Neurol 87:393–402.

Willard M, Skene JHP (1982): Molecular events in axonal regeneration. In Nicholls JG (ed): "Repair and Regeneration of the Nervous System." New York: Springer-Verlag, pp 71–89.

Williams LR, Varon S, Peterson GM, Wictorin K, Fischer W, Björklund A, Gage FH (1986): Continuous infusion of nerve growth factor prevents basal forebrain neuronal death after fimbria fornix transection. Proc Natl Acad Sci USA 83:9231–9235.

Zak NB, Harel A, Bawnik Y, Benbasat S, Vogel Z, Schwartz M (1987): Laminin-immunoreactive sites are induced by growth-associated triggering factors in injured rabbit optic nerve. Brain Res 408:263–266.

7

Neuronal Growth Factors

S. VARON, MD, T. HAGG, MD, AND M. MANTHORPE, PhD

Department of Biology, School of Medicine, University of California at San Diego, La Jolla, California 92093

Clinicians and basic scientists view the nervous system with perspectives that are different but complementary. The goal is a common one: to expand our knowledge and understanding of the functioning nervous system and project that knowledge toward the correction of its pathological dysfunctions. The clinician, with his or her firsthand exposure to the human patient, can best identify the problem and describe detailed observations that may hold clues to the underlying, although still poorly understood, processes. The basic neuroscientist has the task of analyzing normal and pathological behaviors of neural tissue at the cellular and molecular levels, devising in vitro and in vivo animal models amenable to experimental manipulations, and generating concepts and molecular tools that might provide new avenues for clinical interventions. It is up to the clinician, once again, to assess these new avenues, try them out in the clinical context, and generate a new cycle of challenges.

This chapter will illustrate such basic/clinical linkages by reviewing one field of neurobiology that is expanding very rapidly, with increasing promise for clinical consideration—that of special neuroactive proteins ("factors"), which control directly or indirectly the maintenance, growth, repair, and differentiated functional capabilities of selected nerve cell populations. The operation of these factors is subject to physiological and pathological modulations at different levels and by different agents, thereby providing interfaces with a variety of other conditions of neurologic interest.

DIFFERENT CLASSES OF NEUROACTIVE PROTEIN FACTORS
Neuronotrophic Factors (NTFs)

During development, a given population of neurons is generated in excess numbers that will be trimmed down to the future adult numbers by a process called "developmental neuronal death" (Hamburger and Oppenheim, 1982), which takes place at the defined developmental period when the axons of these neurons reach and connect with their innervation (or "target") territory. For example, the cholinergic neurons in the ciliary ganglion undergo a 50% reduction when they interact with the intraocular (choroid, ciliary body, iris) musculature, and the cholinergic motor neurons of the ventral spinal cord drop by as much as 80% when they reach the corresponding skeletal muscles. The magnitude of this neuronal death depends on the size of the innervation territory: early ablation of it increases the neuronal death, and early implantation of additional target tissue reduces it. These observations have led to the concepts that 1) the innervation territory produces and supplies one or more "neuronotrophic" factors, necessary for the survival of innervating neurons; 2) the target-derived NTFs are recognized by specific receptors on the nerve endings, internalized, and brought to the nerve cell body by retrograde axonal transport; and 3) the NTF/receptor binding triggers, via second messages, a sequence of transduction events leading to the activation of survival-promoting cellular and molecular machineries.

The discovery of nerve growth factor (NGF), the first and best known of such NTFs (see below), has prompted the search for other neuronotrophic proteins (Varon and Adler, 1981;

Neural Regeneration and Transplantation, pages 101–121

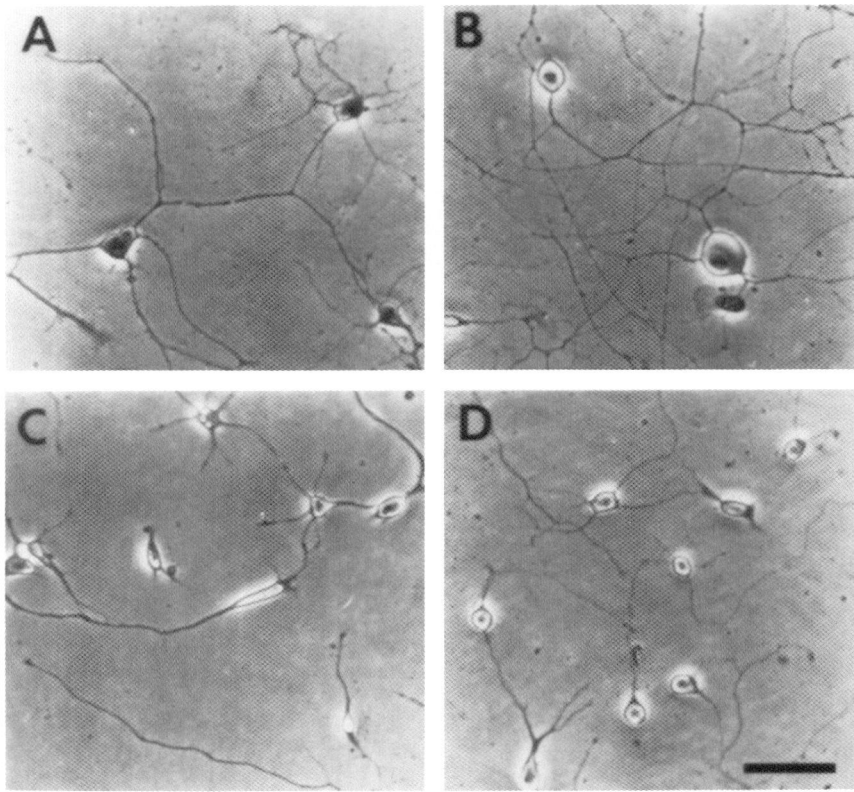

Figure 7–1. Examples of neuronal cultures for bioassays of neuronotrophic (or toxic) factors. Enriched neuronal cell suspensions were obtained from **A:** E12 chick sympathetic ganglia. **B:** Neonatal mouse dorsal root ganglia. **C:** E8 chick forebrain. **D:** E18 rat hippocampus. Scale bar = 100µm.

Varon, 1985), such as a ciliary neuronotrophic factor (CNTF) for ciliary ganglion cells from their intraocular innervation territory (Manthorpe and Varon, 1985; Manthorpe et al., 1988). Crucial to these investigations has been the use of in vitro neuronal cell cultures (Fig. 7–1). The neurons for which an NTF is sought are dissociated from prenatal tissue, purified from most of the accompanying nonneuronal cells, and seeded on an adhesive culture substratum and with an appropriate culture medium that includes the putative NTF source at serial dilutions, thereby allowing the definition of a trophic titer for the original material under test (1 trophic unit (TU) per ml = activity in the culture medium that promotes half-maximal survival). The same neuronal cultures with which one recognizes the presence of a trophic (or a toxic) factor can then be used

to monitor the purification of the active molecule and also to study cellular and molecular mechanisms of its action.

In vitro cultures are also essential to investigate the cells that produce NTFs. An increasingly recognized concept in neurobiology is that of neuron-glia interactions (Hydèn, 1967; Varon and Somjen, 1979), more recently extended to include neuronotrophic and gliotrophic interrelations. Cultures of purified glial cells, from both peripheral (Schwann cells) and central (astroglia) origins, have been shown to be capable of producing and releasing into their medium neuronotrophic agents addressing cultured neurons from peripheral and central neural tissues (Varon and Manthorpe, 1982; Manthorpe et al., 1986). These findings emphasize the fact that nerve cells live and operate in the context of a cellular

TABLE 7.1. CNS Neuronotrophic (NTF) Hypothesis

Postulates
  NTFs regulate CNS (as well as PNS) and adult (as well as developing) neurons
  Adult CNS neurons depend on NTFs for maintenance, function, and repair
Corollaries
  Endogenous NTF deficits could lead to CNS neuronal dysfunction and degeneration
  Exogenous NTF administration may alleviate or prevent CNS damage
  NTF deficits and/or NTF administration may be relevant to human CNS pathologies and regeneration

society, and that neuronal behaviors are largely dictated by their social context. Thus it is likely that changes in neuronal behaviors could be imposed secondarily by primary alterations in their neighboring glial cells, a concept of importance in pathogenic processes as well as in potential therapeutic approaches. A research direction under current investigation is the use of astroglial cell cultures to identify treatments (hormones, mitogens, etc.) that would modulate the glial production or secretion of neuronotrophic agents (Manthorpe et al., 1987).

Most of the work of NTFs has involved neurons that are in relatively early (perinatal) stages of development and that belong to the peripheral nervous system (PNS). Neuronal cultures from perinatal central nervous system (CNS) comprise a much larger variety of neuronal subsets, which makes it difficult to use them as bioassays for subset-specific putative NTFs rather than for NTFs with a wide spectrum of responsive neurons. Nevertheless, it has been attractive to formulate a CNS neuronotrophic hypothesis along the lines given in Table 7.1 (Varon et al., 1984, 1988). The hypothesis is that NTFs play equally important roles for CNS (not only PNS) and for adult (not only developing) neurons, and that adult CNS neurons actually depend on appropriate NTF supplies for their maintenance, function, and repair capabilities. It would follow that CNS dysfunction and degeneration can result from a relative neuronotrophic deficit, whether an increased need beyond the normal availability

of NTF or a decreased availability of endogenous NTF (e.g., deficient production or release by the source cells, reduced retrograde axonal transport capabilities, or an impaired competence of the neuron to recognize and benefit from the available factors). The CNS neuronotrophic hypothesis, if substantiated, would have important clinical implications: 1) endogenous NTF deficits could be the basis for certain degenerative or involutive CNS situations in the human (Varon, 1975a; Appel, 1981; Varon et al., 1982; Hefti, 1983); 2) inadequate supplies of NTF or neurite-promoting factors (see below) may underlie the known failure of CNS axons to regenerate after a traumatic lesion (Varon, 1977); and 3) administration of exogenous NTFs may either compensate for an endogenous deficit or supplement the endogenous supplies to prevent or reduce the corresponding CNS damages.

Nerve Growth Factor

The existence of NTFs might have remained a mere speculation had it not been for the discovery of Nerve Growth Factor (Levi-Montalcini and Hamburger, 1951; Levi-Montalcini, 1987), for which Rita Levi-Montalcini was awarded a Nobel prize in 1986. The NGF purified from an unexpectedly rich source, the submaxillary gland of the adult male mouse, is a basic, 26,000-dalton, dimeric protein. Cloning of the mouse NGF gene has led to the cloning of the human NGF gene and the recognition of a high homology between them, implying the evolutionary conservation of this important factor. NGF receptors, demonstrated in all the NGF-targeted cells, occur in two subsets: a high-affinity subset that presumably mediates the action of NGF, and a lower-affinity but more abundant one whose role remains to be fully understood. The lower-affinity receptors were purified from the rat, their gene was cloned, and monoclonal antibodies were raised against the receptor protein, providing a new battery of tools for the investigation of NGF-related cells (Varon, 1975b; Greene and Shooter, 1980; Varon et al., 1988).

PNS neuronal targets have demonstrated three major roles for NGF:

1. Neuronotrophic action. Administration of exogenous NGF protects embryonic ganglionic

neurons against their developmental death and causes massive hypertrophy of sympathetic ganglionic neurons in the neonatal rodent. Administration of NGF to pregnant animals leads to production of antibodies against their own endogenous NGF and the destruction of both dorsal root and sympathetic ganglia in their fetuses. Direct administration of anti-NGF antibodies to neonatal rodents elicits a dramatic destruction of sympathetic (but not dorsal root) ganglia—an "immunosympathectomy" response. These observations not only prove the physiologic need for endogenous NGF by its target neurons, they also reveal changing NGF requirements with developmental age.

2. Neurite promotion. As the name "nerve Growth" Factor indicates, NGF was first recognized for its stimulation of nerve fiber ("neurite") growth. Neurite elongation could be viewed as a secondary expression of the trophic action of NGF. That is, an NGF-enhanced anabolic activity of the target neuron could be expressed not only with a cell body enlargement (hypertrophy) but also with an extension of processes from a cell, such as a neuron, already programmed and equipped for such a behavior. Later experiments, however, have shown that neurite extension requires direct action by NGF on the growth cones, the elongating machinery at the end of a growing nerve process (Campenot, 1977). Moreover, local sources of NGF can dictate the direction and not only the amplitude of this neuritic growth (Gundersen and Barrett, 1980). Both such actions of NGF, neurite stimulation and neurite guidance, together with its trophic action, remain important contributors to axonal regeneration by its PNS target neurons.

3. Neurotransmitter function. Nerve cells operate by signaling to their postsynaptic partners through the release of specific chemical transmitters (e.g., acetylcholine, catecholamines). The availability of a transmitter, in turn, depends on the activities of the enzymes that produce and degrade it. A third action of NGF is to stimulate the production of transmitter-synthesizing enzymes. Stimulation of transmitter enzymes by NGF applies to adult as well as developing neurons.

Although NGF was viewed for a long time to be only targeted to select PNS neurons, recent studies have demonstrated a role of NGF also for certain central neurons, specifically cholinergic neurons in developing and adult brain. In the basal forebrain, cholinergic neurons of the medial septum and diagonal band nuclei project to the hippocampus and dentate gyrus, largely via a tract called fimbria-fornix, whereas cholinergic neurons of the nucleus basalis magnocellularis project to the cerebral cortex. The basal forebrain cholinergic neurons and their projections are important components of cognitive activities (e.g., Hepler et al., 1985) and display prominent defects in the aged brain (Bartus et al., 1982) and Alzheimer's disease (Coyle et al., 1983); both conditions are accompanied by deficits in memory and learning behaviors. Unlike those of the basal forebrain, cholinergic neurons in the striatum and nucleus accumbens do not project outside these territories. All these cholinergic neurons are responsive to exogenous NGF and may, in fact, depend on endogenous NGF as one (if not the only one) of their neuronotrophic factors. For example: 1) both messenger RNA for NGF and its NGF protein product are present in the hippocampal formation and cerebral cortex, the innervation territories of basal forebrain cholinergic neurons (Korsching et al., 1985, 1986; Shelton and Reichardt, 1986); 2) radiolabeled NGF injected into these innervation territories is retrogradely transported to and selectively accumulated in the corresponding basal forebrain cholinergic cell bodies (Seiler and Schwab, 1984); 3) CNS cholinergic neurons specifically display receptors for NGF (Richardson et al., 1986; Taniuchi et al., 1986; Raivich and Kreutzberg, 1987; Springer et al., 1987b); and 4) NGF stimulates choline acetyltransferase, the acetylcholine-producing enzyme, in developing CNS cholinergic neurons (Hefti et al., 985; Martinez et al., 1985; Mobley et al., 1985).

Neurite-Promoting Factors

In vitro investigations of neural cell cultures have revealed the existence of another family of neuroactive protein factors, devoid of direct neuronotrophic activity and specifically promoting the outgrowth of neuronal processes (Varon and Adler, 1980; Davis et al., 1985). These neurite-promoting factors (NPFs) were first recognized in media conditioned by glial and other cell populations because of their ability to perform after anchorage to polycationic culture substrata (PNPFs). Further observations led to the hypothesis that PNPFs might belong to a larger class of biological molecules present on certain cell surfaces and/or in the extracellular matrix bridging cells of different embryologic derivation. Evaluation of purified extracellular matrix constituents (e.g., collagens, proteoglycans, fibronectin, and laminin) showed the highest neurite-promoting competence in the glycoprotein laminin and the participation of laminin complexed with proteoglycans in the PNPFs derived from conditioned media. The neurite-promoting competence of rat laminin and rat Schwann cell-derived PNPF on PNS neuronal cultures is illustrated in Fig. 7–2. Similar competences are demonstrable for a variety of perinatal neurons, including those derived from several CNS tissues.

The NPF property of laminin is expressed even more dramatically in intact extracellular matrices (Danielsen et al., 1987a; Davis et al., 1987a). One such preparation has been obtained from human amnion membrane matrix (HAMM). After collection of the amnion membrane from otherwise discarded human placentae and removal of its single layer of epithelial cells (Fig. 7–2D), the HAMM consists of a flexible sheet with two distinct layers: a compact basement membrane (or basal lamina) composed of laminin, proteoglycans, and collagen type IV, and a looser stroma, mainly composed of collagen type VI and VII. The HAMM can be made to adhere to a nitrocellulose sheet, leaving either the basement membrane or the stroma surfaces exposed, or it can be folded onto itself to generate a multilayered HAMM material. Neurons seeded on the basement membrane, but not the stroma, surface will display a dramatic neuritic outgrowth, often oriented in parallel bundles (Fig. 7–2E). Neurons seeded on cross sections of multilayered HAMM will grow neurites preferentially along the basement membrane surfaces, traceable immunochemically by their laminin content (Fig. 7–2F). It appears, therefore, that laminin and related extracellular matrix components can not only perform as a potent neurite-pro-

moting surface but can also provide directional guidance to the growing axons.

We have already reviewed the neurite-promoting and neurite-guiding properties of NGF. NGF and other trophic factors such as CNTF have long been assumed to act as humoral agents. Nevertheless, evidence that they can operate after firm anchorage to a surface has been recently provided by a new in vitro technique called cell blot (Carnow et al., 1985; Pettmann et al., 1987). Crude preparations of NGF and CNTF, or the purified factors themselves, are subjected to SDS electrophoresis (which separates protein bands according to molecular mass), and the bands are then transferred electrophoretically to nitrocellulose strips (the so-called Western blots), where they retain their isolated positions. When neurons are cultured on these blots without any NTF in the medium, neuronal survival and, in the case of NGF, neurite outgrowth only occur over the corresponding NTF bands.

Growth Factors

Yet another impact of the early NGF studies has been a branch investigation that led Stanley Cohen to the discovery of epidermal growth factor (EGF), the prototype for a new family of proliferation-stimulating proteins, or growth factors, for which Cohen shared with Levi-Montalcini the 1986 Nobel prize (Cohen, 1987). The field of growth factors has expanded in several directions that are beyond the boundaries of this chapter (for reviews, see Bradshaw and Prentis, 1987; Guroff, 1987). Here we shall merely note a number of features by which growth factors may overlap neuroactive factors.

It has become increasingly clear that molecular control of normal cell growth, i.e., proliferation of developing cell populations or turnover of adult cells, utilizes basically similar mechanisms as does control (or lack of control) of tumoral growth. In the adult nervous system, glial cells retain their ability to proliferate in pathological situations and are the major sources of indigenous neural tumors. Proliferation of both Schwann cells from the PNS and astroglial cells from the CNS (Krikorian et al., 1982; Pettmann et al., 1985; Skaper and Varon, 1987) are stimulated in vitro by several growth factors: EGF itself, fibroblast growth factor

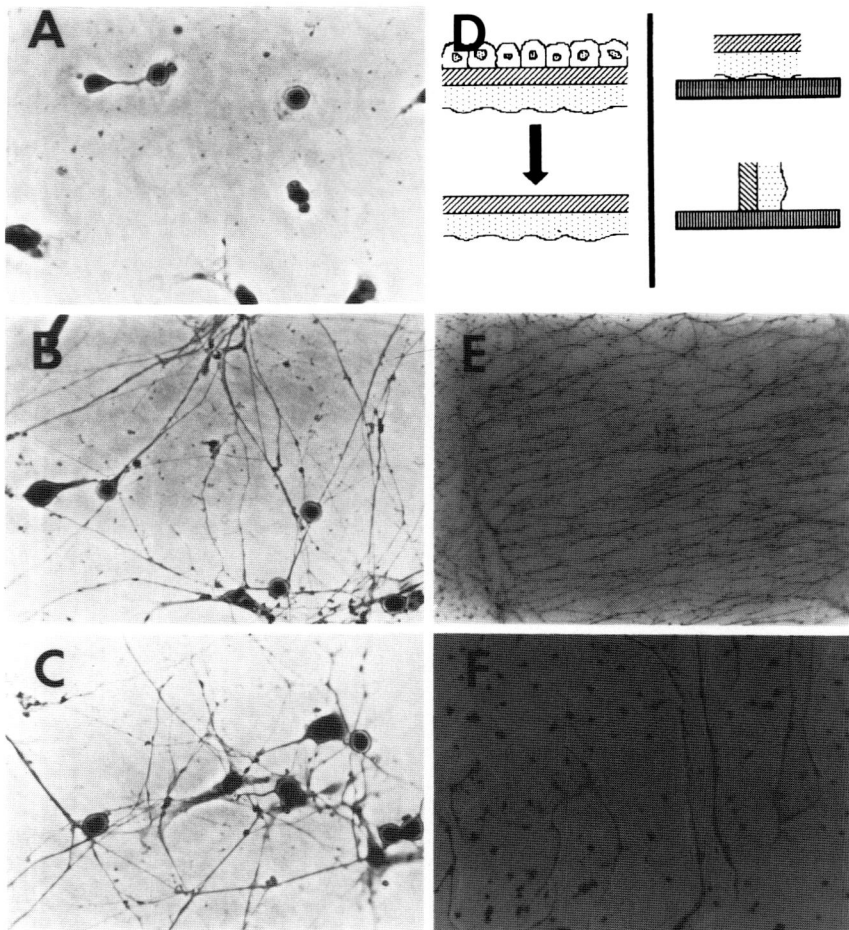

Figure 7–2. In vitro testing of neurite promoting factors (NPFs) and human amnion membrane matrix (HAMM). Polyornithine-coated wells are pretreated with no NPF (**A**), an NPF purified from rat Schwannoma cell-conditioned medium (**B**), or purified rat laminin (**C**). Alternatively, HAMM is prepared and anchored to a nitrocellulose support (**D**) either as a sheet with its basement membrane facing up (**E**) or as a multilayered cross section (**F**), and then placed into culture wells. E8 chick ciliary ganglionic neurons are seeded and cultured for 24 hr on all such substrata in a CNTF-containing medium (to sustain their survival).

(FGF), platelet-derived growth factor (PDGF), and the insulin-like growth factors (IGF-1 and IGF-2, previously known as somatomedins). In addition, FGF is a most potent angiogenic agent, causing proliferation of endothelial cells and their assembly into newly formed blood vessels (Gospodarowicz et al., 1986; Folkman and Klagsbrun, 1987).

While the term "growth factors" reflects the stimulation of cell proliferation (i.e., a growth in cell numbers), many growth factors have also been found to promote the expression of differentiated cell behaviors. Such observations blur the boundary between growth and trophic factors and encourage a speculation that members of both classes may share common molecular mechanisms leading to different growth modalities and/or differentiated behaviors, depending on 1) type or age of the targeted cell; 2) the conditions under which a targeted cell operates; and/or 3) the dynamic convergence of several extrinsic signals. Hypothetically, then, glial cells could respond to a growth factor in different circumstances with either an increased proliferation or an increased output of neuronoactive agents.

Several of the known growth factors occur in the brain and some have, in fact, been isolated and characterized from a neural source (e.g., FGF). Some recent work indicates that neuronal survival and neurite outgrowth in vitro can be supported by FGF (Morrison et al., 1986; Walicke et al., 1986a) or by EGF (Herschman et al., 1983; Morrison et al., 1987). In particular, FGF purified from bovine brain shares with CNTF the ability to support the survival of the cholinergic neurons of embryonic ciliary ganglia (Schubert et al., 1986; Unsicker et al., 1987).

Gangliosides

Gangliosides are a family of sialidated glycosphingolipid components of the plasma membrane of vertebrate cells, especially abundant in the nervous tissue. While they are clearly distinct from any of the protein factors discussed in this section, gangliosides have drawn increasing attention from both basic scientists and clinicians because of their apparent ability to mimic or synergize the effects of neuronotrophic factors in a variety of experimental situations, in vivo as well as in vitro. For updated surveys of ganglioside studies, the reader is referred to the proceedings of recent symposia (Tettamanti et al., 1986; Masland et al., 1987; Ledeen et al., 1988).

AXONAL REGENERATION IN PERIPHERAL NERVE

PNS vs. CNS Regeneration

It has long been held that, in the adult mammal, axonal regeneration cannot occur in the CNS, although it usually does in the PNS. The work of Aguayo and collaborators (Aguayo et al., 1982; Bray and Aguayo, Chapter 5, this volume), however, has repeatedly demonstrated in recent years that the axons of adult CNS neurons do retain the ability to regrow into pieces of peripheral nerve used as bridges between, for example, brain and spinal cord. Besides reopening the question of CNS regeneration, these findings point out that adult

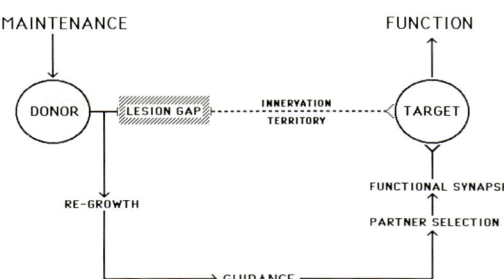

Figure 7–3. The major steps in a neural regeneration process.

peripheral nerve tissue is a regeneration-competent terrain far superior to adult CNS tissue. A crucial task, therefore, is to identify the cellular and molecular features of nerve tissue that confer this axonal regeneration-supportive competence.

Both PNS and CNS regeneration requires a coordinated sequence of neuronal behaviors, depicted in Fig. 7–3. The axotomized neuron ("donor") must be protected against irreversible damage and maintained in a healthy and growth-supportive condition. The healthy neuron must regenerate a growth cone, and elongation of a new axon (and axonal branches) must be stimulated. The regrowing axon must be guided through the lesion gap and into its proper innervation territory. Once there, axonal growth cones must seek and recognize appropriate synaptic partners ("targets") and establish new, functional synapses with them. Lastly, the reinnervated target neurons must resume activity within the appropriate and properly maintained networks, in order to restore the corresponding behavioral functions. The current neurobiological view is that all those steps are controlled by, and thus require, the intervention of the corresponding factors: neuronotrophic factors for the protection and maintenance of the neurons, neurite-promoting factors for axonal regrowth and guidance, possibly glia-modulating factors (e.g., growth factors) to optimize the glial contributions to the process, and recognition- and synapse-promoting factors yet to be adequately identified.

Silicone Chamber Model for Nerve Regeneration

Cellular and molecular bases for the regeneration competence of peripheral nerve could be fruitfully explored with in vivo models for nerve regeneration if the latter were both amenable to a detailed analysis and accessible to experimental manipulations. Lundborg and collaborators in Sweden have sought in vivo model systems in which regenerating nerve fibers would grow, organize, and mature within a preformed space of defined geometry (Lundborg and Hansson, 1979; Lundborg et al., 1981). They developed "mesothelial" chambers produced by the host rat around a subcutaneously implanted solid core. A sciatic nerve was then exposed and resected in the same animal, and its proximal and distal stumps were sutured into the opposite ends of the collected mesothelial tube (after removal of its solid core), leaving interstump gaps ("chambers") of selected lengths. An organized nerve developed across such chambers within 1–3 months, and its axons grew on into the distal nerve segment to reach and connect with the appropriate end organs (muscle, skin, vessels). These pioneering studies have fostered considerable investigations by several other research groups using chamber models with modified wall materials and initial gap contents (e.g., Politis et al., 1982; Uzman and Villegas, 1983; Seckel et al., 1984; Jenq and Coggeshall, 1985; Madison et al., 1985). An early modification of the mesothelial chamber was the adoption of an impermeable silicone tube as the nerve stump entubating material (Lundborg et al., 1982a; for reviews, see Varon and Williams, 1986 and Lundborg et al., 1987). As illustrated in Fig. 7–4, this simpler "silicone chamber" model also allowed the generation of a new nerve structure across the interstump gap (as well as eventual reconnections with the end organs), but provided the additional advantage of considerable insulation from the surrounding tissue and, thus, better control over intracellular environment and events.

A spatial-temporal analysis of the events underlying the formation of a nerve regenerate in the silicone chamber (Williams et al., 1983) has led to the recognition of the sequence illustrated in Fig. 7–5A. Within the first day, the chamber fills with fluid exuded from both nerve stumps. Within 1 week, the two nerve stumps become physically connected by a cell-free matrix composed of coaxially oriented fibrin polymers. Over the next 1–2 weeks, the

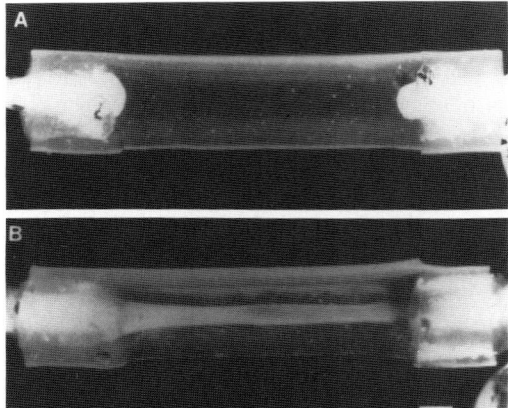

Figure 7–4. Macrophotographs of the silicone chamber model for nerve regeneration. **A:** At implantation time. **B:** One month later. Scale bar = 1 mm.

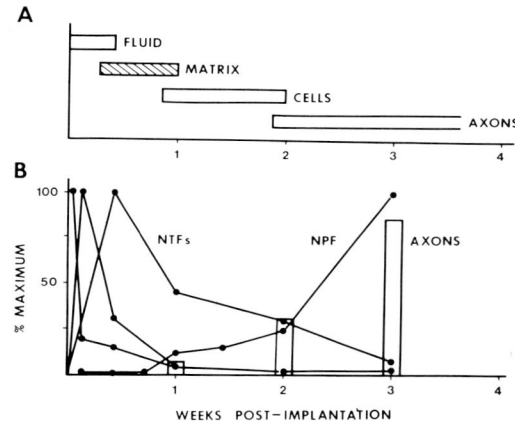

Figure 7–5. Sequential events in the silicone chamber model. **A:** Appearance of nerve stump exudate in the chamber fluid leads to formation of a fibrin matrix and the migration into it of various cell populations, followed by the axonal outgrowth. **B:** The fluid acquires NTFs sequentially for sensory, sympathetic, and spinal cord neurons, in an early phase. NPF activity appears only later and is matched by the axonal advance.

matrix is invaded by several cell populations migrating out of both stumps: some occupy the outer region of the matrix (perineurial-like cells), while others penetrate the matrix core (Schwann cells and vessel-forming endothelial cells). Axons emerge from the proximal stump only after Schwann cell immigration, to form with them typical "regeneration units," and acquire in many cases a progressively thicker myelin sheath. Axons reach the distal nerve stump by the fourth week, and will later elongate all the way to the end organs.

Investigation of the chamber fluid has provided the first evidence that neuronotrophic and neurite-promoting factors may be involved in adult nerve repair (Lundborg et al., 1982b; Longo et al., 1983a,b, 1984a). As shown in Fig. 7–5B, NTFs accumulate in rapid succession for all the neurons (sensory, sympathetic, and motor) that contribute axons to the sciatic nerve. The early peaking of these NTF activities suggests a primary importance for the maintenance and repair processes of the axotomized neurons, rather than the triggering of axonal regrowth that begins much later. In contrast, the laminin-containing neurite-promoting factors are detected much later in temporal coincidence with the Schwann cell invasion (and the appearance of laminin in the regenerate), and their progressive accumulation is closely matched by the axonal advance into the chamber.

The temporal sequence of these events points to a crucial role for the chamber matrix which must coalesce from the chamber fluid. The fibrin matrix and its coaxial organization appear essential for a timely cell immigration, which in turn leads to vascularization of the regenerate, modification of the fibrin matrix to a laminin-containing matrix (laminin is a known product of Schwann cells as well as endothelial cells), and the presentation of a neurite-promoting terrain for the advance of regenerating axons. Experimental modifications of the chamber matrix have already led to significant improvements of both the size and the timetable of the intrachamber nerve regenerate. For example, prefilling the chamber with a plasma-enriched saline has made regeneration possible across chamber gaps 15–20 mm long, more than a previously assumed 10-mm gap limit (Williams et al., 1987a). Investigations of a rat amnion membrane matrix, still in a preliminary stage, have raised the possibility of segregating the regrowing axons along laminin-lined pathways, as illustrated in Fig. 7–6 (Danielsen et al., 1988a).

Another variation of the silicone chamber, in which the chamber is divided into two longitudinal compartments by a nitrocellulose partition, opens up possibilities of investigating the process of fasciculation within the nerve regenerate (Danielsen et al., 1988b). Moreover, the ability of nitrocellulose to anchor protein factors firmly permits the evaluation of their potential influences in the regeneration process, the first example of which, illustrated in Fig. 7–7, has been a dramatic stimulation of blood vessel formation by the angiogenic factor, FGF (Danielsen et al., 1987).

The silicone chamber model has clearly provided valuable information on processes and control mechanisms underlying peripheral nerve regeneration. In clinical practice, nerve regeneration occurs in adult humans with still variable degrees of success, despite the best surgical approaches. The use of autologous nerve grafts and microsurgical apposition techniques often remain inadequate in cases presenting sizable reconstruction challenges. Valuable help is likely to come from a better understanding of the neurobiological basis on which nerve regeneration is founded and a new availability of molecular factors and prosthetic materials to improve the natural regeneration process. Perhaps equally important are the contributions that such experimental advances may generate toward the much more complex problem of CNS regeneration.

REGENERATION IN THE ADULT MAMMALIAN CNS

The CNS neuronotrophic hypothesis proposes that adult CNS neurons continue to need neuronotrophic factors for maintenance and function, as well as for repair activities. Similarly, neurite-promoting factors may become important contributors when axonal regrowth and guidance are required. Figure 7–8 offers an overview of these concepts. If a retrograde supply of the presumptive endogenous NTF from the innervation territory (A) is interrupted, e.g., by axotomy, the trophically deprived neuronal body should suffer damage and possibly death (B). Administration of exogenous NTF should protect the neuron against such damage (C) and perhaps stimulate its ability to regrow axonal processes (sprouting). If a neurite-promoting bridge were to be inserted across

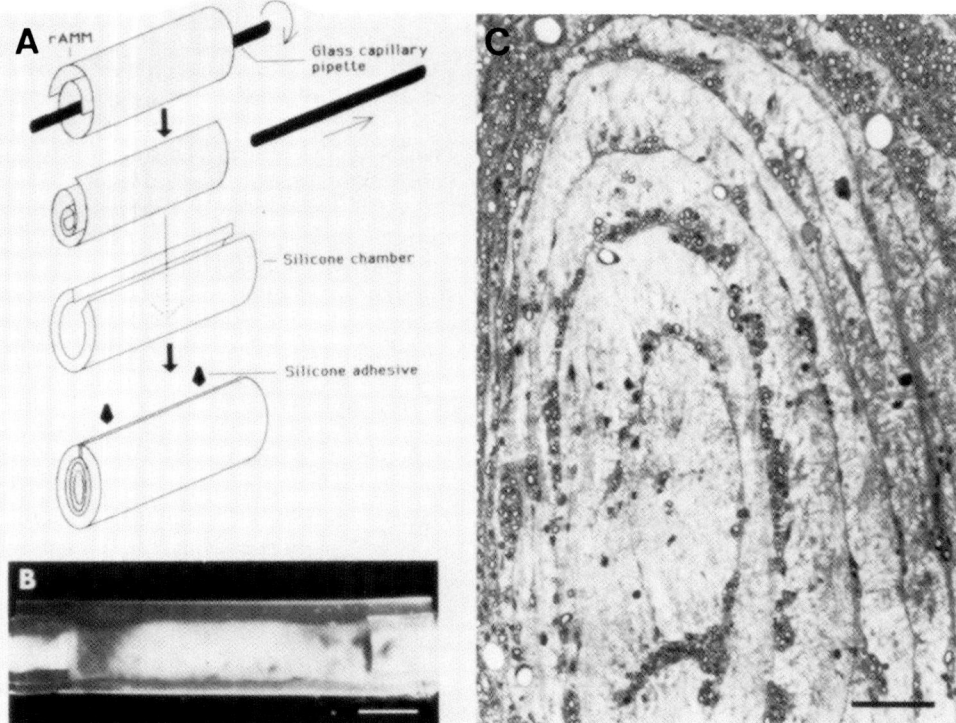

Figure 7–6. Silicone chambers prefilled with rat amnion membrane matrix (RAMM). **A:** The RAMM is rolled into a cylinder and inserted into the chamber. **B:** The chamber receives the two nerve stump inserts and is implanted in situ. **C:** A cross section taken 16 days later from the proximal portion of the chamber shows that profiles of the regenerating axons trace the spiral arrangement of the RAMM. Scale bars = 2 mm (B) and 25 μm (C).

the lesion, the sprouting axons could be coaxed to grow along the bridge, reach the innervation territory on the other side, and invade it (D). It might be possible to discontinue the exogenous NTF administration after the new axons recapture a supply of endogenous NTF in the innervation territory (E).

Inspired by the studies of peripheral nerve chamber fluid, neuronotrophic activities were sought in fluid collected from mechanical wounds in the CNS of young and adult rats (Nieto-Sampedro et al., 1982, 1983; Manthorpe et al., 1983). NTF activity in these CNS wound fluids increased with postlesion time, and the increase was paralleled by increasing survival and neuritic growth capability of cholinergic neurons in fetal septal grafts implanted into the lesion cavity. The lesion-induced appear-

ance of NTFs in the adult CNS and its correlation with fetal CNS neuronal behaviors in vivo provided the first explicit evidence in favor of the CNS neuronotrophic hypothesis.

One limitation of those early studies was that the CNS wound fluid activities were assessed with cultures of peripheral sensory and sympathetic ganglionic neurons and of PNS-projecting spinal cord motor neurons, and not with test cultures of brain-derived nerve cells (which were not available as NTF bioassays at that time). Another study, using embryonic forebrain neurons, did reveal CNS-addressing neuronotrophic activity in the cerebrospinal fluid of head trauma human patients (Longo et al., 1984b). Detailed studies of several CNS and PNS neuronal cultures produced the interesting observation that many, if not all, of these

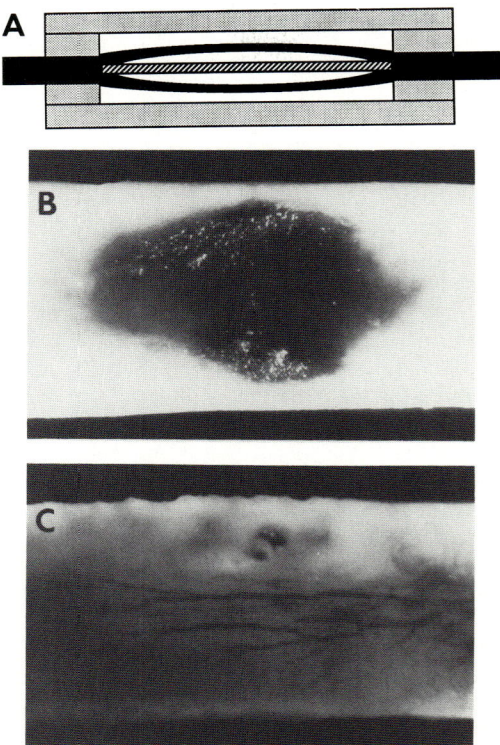

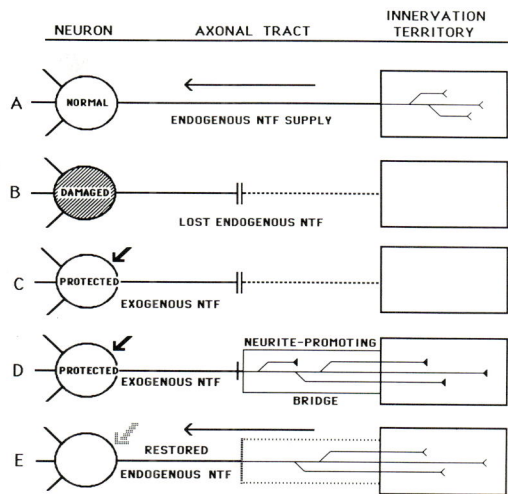

Figure 7–8. Putative roles of neuronotrophic and neurite-promoting factors in adult CNS axonal regeneration. See text for further explanation.

Figure 7–7. Silicone chambers with a longitudinal nitrocellulose partition, presoaked with fibroblast growth factor. **A:** Diagram of the nerve fascicles regenerating in each of the two chamber compartments. **B,C:** Top views of 16-day regenerates in chambers partitioned with untreated (B) or FGF-treated (C) nitrocellulose.

As with the PNS regeneration, more explicit advances toward the recognition and understanding of molecular controls on CNS damage and repair depend on the development of adult CNS in vivo models amenable to detailed analysis and experimental manipulations.

Septohippocampal Model in the Adult Rat

The septohippocampal cholinergic system has proved particularly suitable for further investigations of the CNS neuronotrophic hypothesis, in that 1) the cholinergic neuron subset is identifiable from other neuronal elements; 2) the system has defined anatomical location and projections; and 3) an NTF related to it (NGF) has been identified. Cholinergic neurons and their axons can be specifically distinguished through their content of acetylcholine-related enzymes, choline acetyltransferase (ChAT) by immunocytochemistry and acetylcholinesterase (AChE) by enzyme cytochemistry. As mentioned above, cholinergic neurons of the medial septum and vertical diagonal band nuclei project to the hippocampal formation via the fimbria-fornix tract. A complete fimbria-fornix transection should deprive these neurons of their hippocampal NTF supply and lead to their degeneration, without

cultured neurons were unable to use glucose for their energy needs and would thus survive only if supplied with intermediate metabolites such as pyruvate (Selak et al., 1985). Alternatively, the same neurons could regain the use of glucose if provided with catalase, vitamin E, or other antioxidants (Walicke et al., 1986b), encouraging the interpretation that they were particularly vulnerable to attack by free radicals (Chau et al., 1987; Varon et al., 1987). It is attractive to speculate that peroxidation processes may also be a major mechanism of neuronal damage to the CNS of adult animals and humans in a variety of traumatic, infectious, or toxic neuropathologies as well as in brain aging (Halliwell and Gutteridge, 1985).

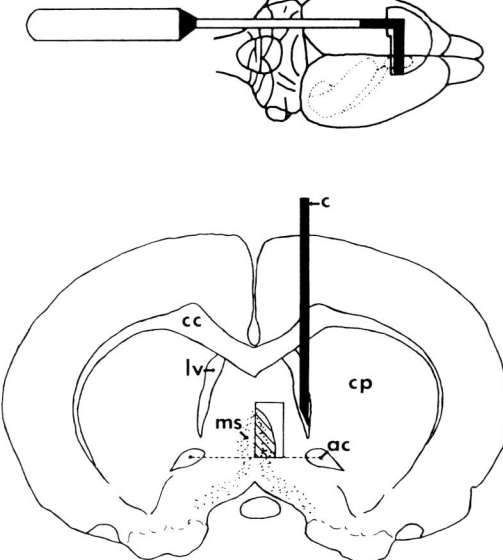

Figure 7–9. Diagrammatic representation of the cannula device for continuous NGF infusion (top), and of the intraventricular location of a unilaterally implanted cannula (bottom). The brain coronal section also shows cc, corpus callosum; lv, lateral ventricle; ms, medial septum; ac, nucleus accumbens; cp, caudate-putamen.

direct damage to the majority of neighboring septal neurons that do not participate in such a projection. The serendipitous discovery that NGF fits the role of an endogenous NTF for septal (and other CNS) cholinergic neurons made it possible to verify whether its exogenous administration would compensate for the postulated loss of endogenous NTF support and provide the postulated protection against axotomy-induced damage (Fig. 7–8A–C).

An additional component for an optimal model would be the means of administering the exogenous NTF (or other relevant agents) with an adequate and quantitative control of the dosage and duration of the treatment. One step in this direction has been the development of a microcannula device connected to an osmotic minipump, whereby exogenous NGF loaded into the pump with an appropriate vehicle can be continuously infused into the lateral ventricle on the same side of the lesion (Williams et al., 1987b). Fig. 7–9 illustrates the infusion device and the position of the intraventricular cannula relative to the medial septum nucleus in a coronal section of the brain.

Neuronal Damage After Axotomy and NGF-Induced Protection

A complete aspirative unilateral transection of the supracallosal stria and fimbria-fornix causes a nearly complete disappearance of the hippocampal cholinergic innervation. It also induces, over a 2-week period after surgery, the disappearance of a majority of the AChE- and ChAT-positive neuronal cell bodies in the medial septum and the vertical limb of the diagonal band on the side of the lesion, without significantly affecting the contralateral side (Gage et al., 1986). Cholinergic neurons in the horizontal limb of the diagonal band and their hippocampal projection are spared by the fimbria-fornix lesion, as the projection follows a separate, more ventral pathway. Continuous administration of exogenous NGF into the ipsilateral ventricle, starting 3 days before and proceeding for 2 weeks after the fimbria-fornix transection, led to nearly complete preservation of AChE-positive neuronal cell bodies in the medial septum and vertical diagonal band, while there was no effect on cholinergic fiber disappearance in the hippocampus (Williams et al., 1986). Similar results have been obtained by other research groups. Hefti and co-workers (Heft et al., 1984; Hefti, 1986) used multiple intraventricular injections of NGF after a partial unilateral fimbrial lesion, and observed NGF protection of both septal cholinergic neurons and hippocampal cholinergic innervation. Kromer (1987) reported that continuous unilateral intraventricular NGF infusion after bilateral fimbria-fornix transection provided extensive protection of cholinergic septal neurons on both sides.

Fig. 7–10 shows the ChAT-immunoreactive neurons of the medial septum in coronal sections taken from an adult rat 14 days after complete unilateral fimbria-fornix lesion. The dramatic disappearance of ChAT-positive cells on the side ipsilateral to the lesion is almost entirely prevented by the continuous NGF treatment. The same percentage loss (relative to the contralateral side), as well as the NGF-induced protection, occurs across most of the medial septum, permitting the economical use of a

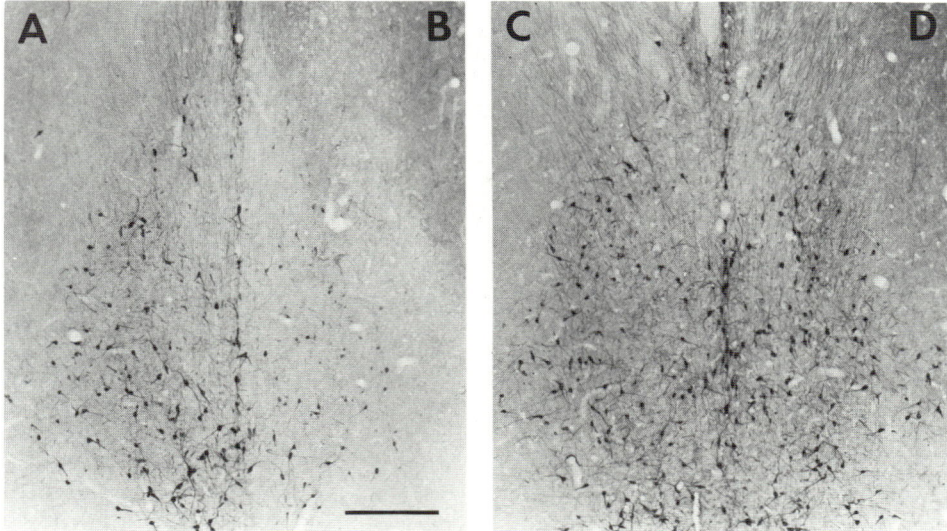

Figure 7–10. Coronal sections, immunostained for choline acetyltransferase (ChAT), taken from adult rats 14 days after unilateral complete fimbria-fornix transection. **A,B:** Untreated animals. Most of the ChAT-positive neurons in the medial septum have disappeared on the lesion side (B). **C,D:** NGF-treated animals. The lesion side (D) displays as many ChAT-positive neurons as its contralateral counterpart. Scale bar = 250 μm.

single representative section to monitor the extent of these events in further studies (Hagg et al., 1987). It is crucial to stress that the apparent loss or persistence of these cholinergic neurons is defined by the number of cells that can be detected through their stainability for either ChAT or AChE. An apparent loss of neurons (including the large ones presumed to be cholinergic) is also seen using traditional neuronal stains (e.g., toluidine blue), which reveal the nucleic acid content of the perinuclear Nissl substance, a classical feature of mature nerve cells. Such observations have encouraged the interpretation that the cholinergic neurons' disappearance reflects an actual cell death.

An alternate possibility, however, could be that the cholinergic neurons lose, upon axotomy, the expression of their cholinergic "markers" rather than, or well before, degenerating and dying. Such a phenomenon has been noted in the PNS, where axotomy leads to structural rearrangements paralleled by a shift from functional to repair-related protein synthesis (Grafstein, 1975). To test this possibility

in the septohippocampal model (Hagg et al., 1987), the 14-day administration of NGF was delayed by 7 days (at which time 50% of the medial septum ChAT-positive neurons have already disappeared) or by 14 and 21 days (at which times the neurons have dropped to a baseline 20% of the starting numbers). Several possible outcomes might be expected, as illustrated in Figure 7–11: 1) NGF delayed by 7 days can no longer interfere with an irreversible process already started (a 50% death already incurred, plus another 30% of neurons already committed to die); 2) the 7-day delayed NGF stops the process but does not reverse it, holding the cell death at its 7-day 50% level; 3) NGF reverses the already occurred 50% disappearance, beside protecting against further losses; or 4) NGF achieves decreasing reversal levels as its administration is increasingly delayed. The actual results are seen in Figure 7–11B. A 14-day NGF treatment starting only at 7 days postlesion fully reversed the already incurred 50% loss of ChAT-positive neurons. Delays of 14 and 21 days still allowed for some reversal but only about halfway back to maxi-

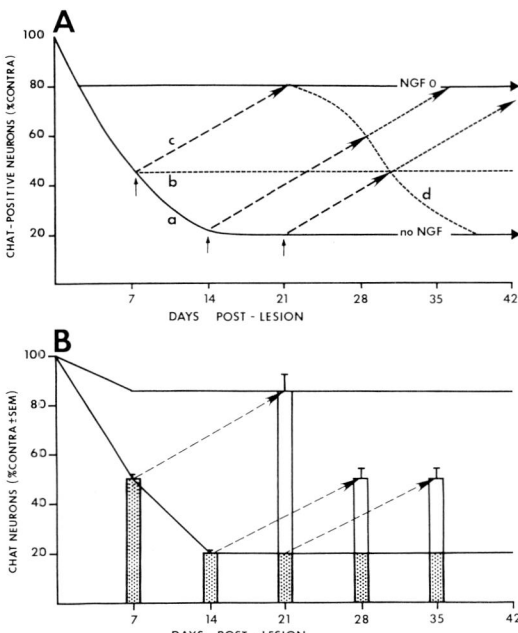

Figure 7–11. Consequences on medial septum ChAT-positive neurons of delaying the NGF treatment after fimbria-fornix transection. **A:** Potential effects. Delaying the onset of a 14-day NGF treatment by 7 days could: a) have no effect; b) prevent future neuronal losses but not those already incurred; c) fully reverse already incurred losses; or d) achieve decreasing reversals with increasing delay times. **B:** Experimental data. A 7-day delay fully reversed the 50% loss already incurred, and 14- or 21-day delays still raised ChAT-positive neuronal numbers well above the 20% residual baseline.

mal numbers. It remains to be determined whether the lesser effectiveness of longer delayed NGF administration could be improved upon by altering the dosages, duration, or other conditions of the NGF treatment itself.

These observations indicate that the disappearance of ChAT-positive neurons in the medial septum after fimbria-fornix transection is primarily due to a loss in their transmitter enzyme content, which may or may not be followed by irreversible cell degeneration. Many clinical situations are characterized by an apparent loss of cholinergic neurons or cholinergic innervation, e.g., during brain aging (Bartus et al., 1982; McGeer et al., 1984; Hepler et al.,

1985) or in Alzheimer's disease (Terry and Davies, 1980; Coyle et al., 1983). Since such losses are recognized by a decrease in cholinergic enzyme activity or immunochemical detectability, they need not document an actual, irreversible degenerative event. Moreover, neuronal and innervation losses in many other CNS systems (whether in experimental models or in human pathology) are similarly evaluated by use of transmitter-related markers (e.g., dopamine in Parkinson's disease) and they, too, might require some careful reevaluation.

The delayed NGF treatments, beside clarifying the viable status of apparently lost cholinergic neurons, also reveal aspects of NGF action that have crucial implications for clinical intervention: 1) there can be a "grace" period between lesion time and onset of treatment (in the present model, at least 7 days) that still allows for successful intervention; and 2) NGF can regulate functional competences of its adult CNS target neurons, beside cell maintenance and repair capabilities, and might be able to do so in chronic as well as acute lesions (see below).

Axonal Regeneration and Neurite-Promoting Bridges

The septohippocampal model also provides opportunities to investigate conditions and tools that might foster adult CNS axonal regeneration and bring the regenerating axons back to their hippocampal innervation territory. Such investigations include (cf. Fig. 7–8D and E): 1) identification of neurite-promoting materials to be implanted into the lesion as successful "bridges"; 2) determination of their effectiveness when combined with the continuous administration of exogenous NTF; and 3) evaluation of the final outcome with regard to the restoration of both an endogenous NTF supply to the regenerating neurons and of a functional competence in the reinnervated territory. Research along these lines is still at an early stage and is almost entirely limited to the first point, the evaluation of various materials as potential bridges. The use of peripheral nerve implants in several model systems is an excellent example of such possibilities (see Bray and Aguayo, Chapter 5, this volume).

In the septohippocampal model, promising

results were obtained a few years ago by use of fetal hippocampal implants (Kromer et al., 1981). Fetal hippocampal tissue represents the "natural" innervation territory for septal cholinergic neurons and could, therefore, provide a competent terrain for the regeneration of their axons. The hippocampal implants did become invaded by a heavy plexus of AChE-positive fibers, and some of them extended beyond the "bridge" to invade the hippocampus of the adult host. No information was provided on possible effects of the fetal hippocampal implant on the cholinergic cell bodies within the septum. In current terms, it is conceivable that fetal hippocampal tissue may also supply "endogenous" neuronotrophic factors to the axotomized septal neurons and thus bring them into participating in the regenerative events without a concurrent, direct administration of exogenous NGF.

In a more recent approach (Davis et al., 1987b; Gage et al., 1988), the septohippocampal model has been used to explore potential "bridge" competences of the human amnion membrane matrix. As illustrated in Figure 7–12A, HAMM material was rolled into a cylinder, and a cylinder segment was implanted into the fimbria-fornix lesion cavity so that the two ends of the HAMM cylinder were closely apposed against the septal and hippocampal tissues, respectively. After 2–4 weeks, AChE-positive fibers could be seen both on the HAMM bridge and within the host hippocampus (Fig. 7–12B). There were no signs of immunological reactions to the presence of the HAMM, and HAMM implants often preserved their emplacement and configuration. Similar results were obtained by use of HAMM laid down on nitrocellulose strips (Fig. 7–2) rather than rolled into a coil. In both studies, no exogenous NGF was infused intraventricularly to support the axotomized septal cholinergic neurons, suggesting that the cholinergic axons growing on the HAMM and in the hippocampal tissue may have derived from other cholinergic cell bodies.

These preliminary results encourage further efforts to optimize both the configuration and the positioning of a HAMM implant. Particular attention should be directed toward maximizing the opportunity for the axons of NGF-supported neurons to enter the bridge and thus

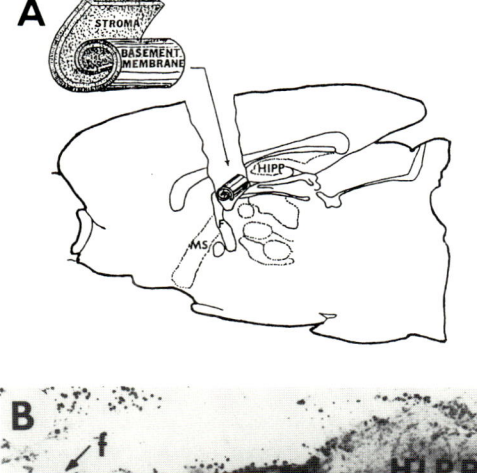

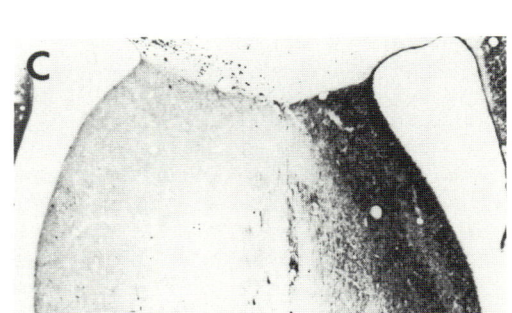

Figure 7–12. Cholinergic axonal regrowth after fimbria-fornix transection in adult rats. **A:** Preparation and insertion of a HAMM bridge into the lesion cavity. **B:** AChE-stained sagittal sections showing cholinergic fibers (f) in both the HAMM bridge and the host hippocampus (HIPP), in rat not treated with NGF. **C:** NGF-infused animals lacking a bridge display substantial cholinergic sprouting within the dorsal lateral septum and only on the side of lesion and NGF-infusing cannula. m, matrix; ms, medial septum.

reach their host innervation territory. It has been observed previously (Williams et al., 1986) that NGF causes conspicuous ipsilateral sprouting of cholinergic fibers in the dorsal lateral region of the septum, as illustrated in Figure 7–12C. While constrained within the septal confines in the absence of a potential outlet, these NGF-promoted cholinergic axons could well take advantage of an appropriately presented HAMM bridge. Success in this model would validate the potential use of HAMM bridges in other discrete lesions (e.g., spinal cord, optic nerve). Unlike the fetal hippocampal tissue, HAMM materials have no region-specific limitations, are available in large quantities (from human placentae normally discarded in hospitals) without any ethical difficulties, and can be manipulated in a number of ways because of their mechanical resilience.

CHRONIC DEGENERATION IN MAMMALIAN CNS

Many degenerative diseases of the human CNS involve defined subpopulations of CNS neurons. For example, amyotrophic lateral sclerosis affects lower and upper CNS motor neurons, Parkinson's disease affects the dopaminergic neurons of the substantia nigra, and Alzheimer's disease involves a prominent deficit in CNS cholinergic systems. It has been pointed out (Appel, 1981; Varon et al., 1982; Hefti, 1983) that such neuronal target specificities would fit well with the concept of underlying deficits in the corresponding neuronotrophic factors. Cognitive deficiencies associated with the aging of the brain also correlate with cholinergic deficits and may thus reflect some insufficiency in neuronotrophic support (Varon, 1977). As described above, NGF has proved to be an effective exogenous agent for acutely injured septal cholinergic neurons, and its ability to restore enzymes regulating the transmitter competence of these neurons makes it likely that NGF might also provide help for chronically impaired cholinergic systems.

In a recent study, Fischer and coworkers (1987) utilized the intraventricular cannula device for continuous NGF infusion to probe the possibility that NGF treatment might improve cognitive behaviors impaired in aged rats. Two-year-old rats were tested on a Morris water maze task for their ability to identify and remember the location of a submerged platform in a swimming tank. A series of daily pre-

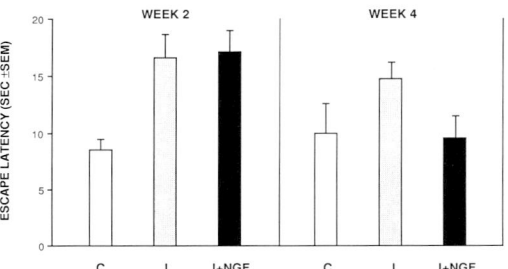

Figure 7–13.   Aged rat performance in a cognitive water maze task. Unimpaired control rats (C) rapidly learn to reach and climb on a submerged platform in a swimming tank within some 10 s (escape latency time), whereas impaired rats (I) have more difficulty even in achieving longer escape latency times. Continuous unilateral infusion of NGF in impaired rats (I + NGF) fails to improve this behavior for 2 weeks, but fully restores an unimpaired performance by 4 weeks of treatment.

trials distinguished a rat subset that rapidly achieved a short escape latency (i.e., the time needed to seek and climb the platform in a given trial) from the rest of the aged population, which settled on escape latency times three- to fourfold longer, thus defining a learning and/or retention impairment. All the impaired rats were implanted unilaterally with the cannula device, half of them to receive NGF and half to receive vehicle only. The three sets of animals (unimpaired controls, impaired rats without NGF, and impaired rats with continuous NGF infusion) were retested for several days on the water maze task 2 and 4 weeks later.

Figure 7–13 summarizes the behavioral results. After 2 weeks the impaired rats, while slightly improved relatively to the pretrial tests, continued to exhibit two- to threefold worse performances than controls, and they did so regardless of the presence or absence of NGF in the infusate. By 4 weeks, however, the behavior of the NGF-treated subset had become undistinguishable from that of the unimpaired rats, in marked contrast to the impaired rats receiving no NGF. Other data suggested that the NGF-induced improvement involved memory retention rather than learning (or motor) performances. Histologic examinations at the end of the 4-week period revealed smaller

AChE-stained neuronal cell bodies in all the basal forebrain nuclei (medial septum, vertical diagonal band, nucleus basalis) as well as in the striatum, on both sides of the impaired vs. nonimpaired rats—a cellular hypotrophy presumably underlying the age-related behavioral impairment. In the NGF-treated rats, however, there were some modest but significant increases (relatively to those receiving no NGF) of cholinergic cell body sizes (but not numbers) in the nucleus basalis ipsilateral to the infusion side.

Several interesting points emerge from such a study and encourage some provocative speculations. First, age-related "atrophy" of cholinergic CNS neurons is not necessarily indicative of permanent cell loss—a conclusion similar to that already discussed for acutely damaged neurons. Second, NGF does have the ability to affect beneficially chronically impaired CNS neurons in an animal model in which no experimental lesions are imposed. Third, the NGF benefits extend to cholinergic-mediated behaviors and not only to the cholinergic cells themselves. The NGF effect is not likely to be a result of protection of cholinergic neurons against further degeneration (since the cell numbers appeared unaffected), or to merely reflect stimulation of cholinergic enzyme production (which would be expected to occur more rapidly than the several weeks required for behavioral improvement). One can only speculate, at present, on relationships between neuronal cell size and cognitive behavior and a possible additional involvement of NGF-induced changes in axonal sprouting and/or synaptic competences in the cholinergic innervation territories. Most important, from a clinical perspective, is the strong support these findings give to the speculation that NGF treatments may prove beneficial to human patients with Alzheimer's disease, as well as to those with age-related functional brain deficits.

SUMMARY AND PROJECTIONS

We have endeavored in this chapter to offer a dynamic view of how the progressive unfolding of basic neurobiological research can reach into the realm of clinical neurology. The concept of neuronotrophic factors inspired by the developmental neuronal death phenomenon acquired a reality with the discovery of NGF NGF studies have fostered research on additional NTFs and opened up new avenues of research on neurite- and growth-promoting protein factors. A CNS neuronotrophic hypothesis has been articulated to include NTF involvements not only in regeneration after acute injury but also in the basis and/or modulation of chronic degenerative or involutive processes. Animal models have been developed to validate the involvement of such protein factors in both PNS and CNS injury and repair. In addition, evidence has been obtained with at least one NTF, the Nerve Growth Factor, and one CNS system, the cholinergic one, that in vivo administration of an exogenous factor can lead to remarkable cellular and behavioral improvements.

We are entering an exciting era, with a vast number of challenging tasks still ahead. Among them are 1) the acquisition of further details on the septohippocampal model and its NGF treatments—delivery control, doses, duration, and the permanence of the effects; 2) the extension of similar studies to other factors and agents, as well as their combinations—new NTFs, hormones, antioxidants, and gangliosides, among others; 3) a corresponding extension to other modes of injury of the CNS cholinergic system—other mechanical lesions and ischemic and toxic lesions; and 4) similar demonstrations of possible benefits from NGF or other treatments on different, noncholinergic CNS models. With regard to CNS regeneration, an equally long and challenging list includes: 1) refinement of HAMM and other bridges to obtain efficient prosthetic materials for promotion and guidance of regenerating axons; 2) validation of such materials as bridges for other discrete CNS lesions, particularly those of the spinal cord and optic nerve; and, eventually, 3) evaluation of an effective reinnervation of the denervated territory at morphologic, electrophysiologic, and behavioral levels.

How close are we to clinical applications of current and future advances? In the area of neural regeneration, the road ahead is still a long one, although some benefits from the entubation models and the neurite-promoting bridges may materialize in the not-too-distant future. In the view of these writers, however, treatment of Alzheimer's patients with NGF is a highly credible and accessible possibility. Here the participation of the clinician is essential for rapid progress. Even moderate success in a few clinical trials, restricted to extreme cases, would give an overwhelming impetus to the energetic pursuit of some questions that are crucial for more extended pharmaceutical applications: the large-scale production of human NGF by bioengineering techniques, its long-term testing in primates, and more practical modes of administration. In this last context, exploration of two exciting possibilities has begun: the intracerebral implantation of NGF-producing living cells (Springer et al., 1987a), and the pharmacological stimulation of local glial cells to resume or increase their NGF production (Manthorpe et al., 1987).

ACKNOWLEDGMENTS

Much of the work reviewed here has been supported by grants from the National Science Foundation (BNS-81-8847 and BNS-86-17034) and the National Institute for Neurological and Communicative Diseases and Stroke (NS-16349 and NS-25011).

REFERENCES

Aguayo A, Davis S, Richardson P, Bray G (1982): Axonal elongation in peripheral and central nervous system transplants. Adv Cell Neurobiol 3:215–234.

Appel SH (1981): A unifying hypothesis for the cause of amyotrophic lateral sclerosis, parkinsonism, and Alzheimer disease. Ann Neurol 10:499–505.

Bartus RT, Dean RL, Beer B, Lippa AS (1982): The cholinergic hypothesis of geriatric memory dysfunction. Science 217:408–417.

Bradshaw RA, Prentis S (eds) (1987): "Oncogenes and Growth Factors." New York: Elsevier.

Campenot R (1977): Local control of neurite development by nerve growth factor. Proc Natl Acad Sci USA 74:4516–4519.

Carnow TB, Manthorpe M, Davis GE, Varon S (1985): Localized survival of ciliary ganglionic neurons identifies neuronotrophic factor bands on nitrocellulose blots. J Neurosci 5:1965–1971.

Chau RMW, Skaper SD, Varon S (1988): Peroxidative block of glucose utilization and survival in CNS neuronal cultures. Neurochem Res, 13:611–616.

Cohen S (1987): Epidermal growth factor. In Vitro Cell Dev Biol 23:239–246.

Coyle JT, Price DL, DeLong MR (1983): Alzheimer's disease: A disorder of cortical cholinergic innervation. Science 219:1184–1190.

Danielsen N, Muller H, Pettmann B, Williams LR, Manthorpe M, Engvall E, Davis GE, Varon S (1988a): Rat amnion membrane matrix as a substratum for regenerating axons from peripheral and central neurons: Effects in a silicone chamber model. Dev Brain Res 39:39–50.

Danielsen N, Vahlsing HL, Manthorpe M, Varon S (1988b): A two-compartment modification of the silicone chamber model for nerve regeneration. Exp Neurol, in press.

Danielsen N, Vahlsing HL, Pettmann B, Manthorpe M, Varon S (1987): Immobilized fibroblast growth factor affects peripheral nerve regeneration in a silicone chamber model. Soc Neurosci Abstr 13:1207.

Davis GE, Varon S, Engvall E, Manthorpe M (1985): Substratum-binding neurite-promoting factors: Relationships to laminin. Trends Neurosci 8:528–532.

Davis GE, Engvall E, Varon S, Manthorpe M (1987a): Human amnion membrane as a substratum for cultured peripheral and central nervous system neurons. Dev Brain Res 33:1–10.

Davis GE, Blaker SN, Engvall E, Varon S, Manthorpe M, Gage FH (1987b): Human amnion membrane serves as a substratum for growing axons in vitro and in vivo. Science 236:1106–1109.

Fischer W, Wictorin K, Björklund A, Williams LR, Varon S, Gage FH (1987): Amelioration of cholinergic neuron atrophy and spatial memory impairment in aged rats by nerve growth factor. Nature 329:65–68.

Folkman J, Klagsbrun M (1987): Angiogenic factors. Science 235:442–447.

Gage FH, Wictorin K, Fischer W, Williams LR, Varon S, Björklund A (1986): Retrograde cell changes in medial septum and diagonal band following fimbria-fornix transection: Quantitative temporal analysis. Neuroscience 19:241–255.

Gage FH, Blaker SN, Davis GE, Engvall E, Varon S, Manthorpe M (1988): Human amnion membrane matrix as a substratum for axonal regeneration in the central nervous system. Exp Brain Res, in press.

Gospodarowicz D, Neufeld G, Schweigerer L (1986): Fibroblast growth factor. Mol Cell Endocrinol 46:187–204.

Grafstein B (1975): The nerve cell body response to axotomy. Exp Neurol 48:32–51.

Greene LA, Shooter EM (1980): The nerve growth factor: Biochemistry, synthesis, and mechanism of action. Annu Rev Neurosci 3:353–402.

Gundersen RW, Barrett JN (1980): Characterization of the turning response of dorsal root neurites toward nerve growth factor. J Cell Biol 87:546–554.

Guroff G (ed) (1987): "Oncogenes, Genes and Growth Factors." New York: John Wiley & Sons.

Hagg T, Vahlsing HL, Manthorpe M, Varon S (1987): Delayed intraventricular NGF infusion reverses axotomy-induced loss of medial septum ChAT-positive neurons. Soc Neurosci Abstr 13:922.

Halliwell B, Gutteridge JMC (1985): Oxygen radicals and the nervous system. Trends Neurosci 8:22–26.

Hamburger V, Oppenheim RN (1982): Naturally occurring neuronal death in vertebrates. Neurosci Comment 1:39–55.

Hefti F (1983): Alzheimer's disease caused by a lack of nerve growth factor? Ann Neurol 13:109–110.

Hefti F (1986): Nerve growth factor promotes survival of septal cholinergic neurons after fimbrial transections. J Neurosci 6:2155–2162.

Hefti F, Dravid A, Hartikka J (1984): Chronic intraventricular injections of nerve growth factor elevate hippocampal choline acetyltransferase activity in adult rats with partial septo-hippocampal lesions. Brain Res 293:305–311.

Hefti F, Hartikka JJ, Eckenstein F, Gnahn H, Heumann R, Schwab M (1985): Nerve growth factor increases choline acetyltransferase but not survival or fiber outgrowth of cultured fetal septal cholinergic neurons. Neuroscience 14:55–68.

Hepler DJ, Wenk GL, Cribbs BL, Olton DS, Coyle JT (1985): Memory impairments following basal forebrain lesions. Brain Res 346:8–14.

Herschman HR, Goodman R, Chandler C, Simpson D, Cawley D, Cole R, DeVellis J (1983): Is Epidermal growth factor a modulator of nervous system function? In Haber B, Regino Perez-Polo J, Hashim GA, Giuffrida Stella AM (eds): "Nervous System Regeneration." Alan R. Liss for the March of Dimes Birth Defect Foundation. BD: OAS 19(4):79–94.

Hydèn H (1967): RNA in brain cells. In Quarton GC, Melnechuk T, Schmitt FO (eds): "Neuroscience Study Program." New York: University Press, pp 248–266.

Jenq C-B, Coggeshall RE (1985): Numbers of regenerating axons in parent and tributary peripheral nerves in the rat. Brain Res 326:27–40.

Korsching S, Auburger G, Heumann R, Scott J, Thoenen H (1985): Levels of nerve growth factor and its mRNA in the central nervous system of the rat correlate with cholinergic innervation. EMBO J 4:1389–1393.

Korsching S, Heumann R, Thoenen H, Hefti F (1986): Cholinergic denervation of the rat hippocampus by fimbrial transection leads to a transient accumulation of nerve growth factor (NGF) without change in mRNA NGF content. Neurosci Lett 66:175–180.

Krikorian D, Manthorpe M, Varon S (1982): Purified mouse Schwann cells: Mitogenic effects of fetal calf serum and fibroblast growth factor. Dev Neurosci 5:77–91.

Kromer LF (1987): Nerve growth factor treatment after brain injury prevents neuronal death. Science 235:214–216.

Kromer LF, Björklund A, Stenevi U (1981): Regeneration of the septohippocampal pathways in adult rats is promoted by utilizing embryonic hippocampal implants as bridges. Brain Res 210:173–200.

Ledeen R (ed) (1988): "New Trends in Ganglioside Research: Neurochemical and Neuroregenerative Aspects. Fidia Research Series. Padova, Italy: Liviana Press, in press.

Levi-Montalcini R (1987): The Nerve growth factor thirty-five years later. Science 237:1154–1162.

Levi-Montalcini R, Hamburger V (1951): Selective growth stimulating effects of mouse sarcoma on sensory and sympathetic nervous systems of the chick embryo. J Exp Zool 116:321–362.

Longo FM, Manthorpe M, Skaper SD, Lundborg G, Varon S (1983a): Neuronotrophic activities accumulate in vivo within silicone nerve regeneration chambers. Brain Res 261:109–117.

Longo FM, Skaper SD, Manthorpe M, Williams LR, Lundborg G, Varon S (1983b): Temporal changes in neuronotrophic activities accumulating in vivo within nerve regeneration chambers. Exp Neurol 81:756–769.

Longo FM, Hayman EG, Davis GE, Ruoslahti E, Engvall E, Manthorpe M, Varon S (1984a): Neurite promoting factors and extracellular matrix components accumulating in vivo within nerve regeneration chambers. Brain Res 309:105–117.

Longo FM, Selak I, Zovickian J, Manthorpe M, Varon S, U H-S (1984b): Neuronotrophic activities in cerebrospinal fluid of head trauma patients. Exp Neurol 84:207–218.

Lundborg G, Hansson HA (1979): Regeneration of peripheral nerve through a preformed space. Preliminary observations on the reorganization of regenerating nerve fibers and perineurium. Brain Res 179:573–576.

Lundborg G, Dahlin LB, Danielsen N, Hansson HA, Larsson K (1981): Reorganization and orientation of regenerating nerve fibers, perineurium and epineurium in preformed mesothelial tubes—an experimental study on the sciatic nerve of rats. J Neurosci Res 6:265–281.

Lundborg G, Dahlin LB, Danielsen N, Gelberman RH, Longo FM, Powell HC, Varon S (1982a): Nerve regeneration in silicone chambers: Influence of gap length and presence of distal stump components. Exp Neurol 76:361–375.

Lundborg G, Longo FM, Varon S (1982b): Nerve regeneration model and trophic factors in vivo. Brain Res 232:157–161.

Lundborg G, Rydevik B, Manthorpe M, Varon S, Lewis JL (1988): Peripheral nerves: The physiology of injury and repair. In Wood S, Buckwelter JA (eds): "Injury and Repair of the Musculoskeletal Soft Tissues." Am Acad Orthop Surg, pp. 297–352.

Madison R, DaSilva CF, Dikkes P (1985): Modification of the microenvironment allows axonal regeneration across a 20 mm nerve gap using entubation repair. Soc Neurosci Abstr 11:1253.

Manthorpe M, Varon S (1985): Regulation of neuronal survival and neuritic growth in the avian ciliary ganglion. In Guroff G (ed): "Growth and Maturation Factors, vol 3. New York: John Wiley & Sons, pp 77–117.

Manthorpe M, Nieto-Sampedro M, Skaper SD, Lewis ER, Barbin G, Longo FM, Cotman CW, Varon S (1983): Neuronotrophic activity in brain wounds of the developing rat. Correlation with implant survival in the wound cavity. Brain Res 267:47–56.

Manthorpe M, Rudge J, Varon S (1986): Astroglial cell contributions to neuronal survival and neuritic growth. In Fedoroff S, Vernadakis A (eds): "Astrocytes, vol 2. New York: Academic Press, pp 315–376.

Manthorpe M, Pettmann B, Varon S (1988): Modulation of astroglial cell output of neuronotrophic and neurite promoting factors. In Norenberg M, Schousboe A (eds): "Biochemical Pathology of Astrocytes." New York: Alan R. Liss, Inc., pp. 41–57.

Manthorpe M, Ray J, Pettmann B, Varon S (1988): Studies on the ciliary neuronotrophic factor. In Rush RA (ed): "Nerve Growth Factors. Methods in the Neurosciences (IBRO Handbook Series)." New York: John Wiley & Sons, in press.

Martinez HJ, Dreyfus CF, Jonakait GM, Black IB (1985): Nerve growth factor promotes cholinergic development in brain striatal cultures. Proc Natl Acad Sci USA 82:7777–7781.

Masland R, Portera-Sanchez A, Toffano G (eds) (1987): "Neuroplasticity: A New Therapeutic Tool in CNS Pathology." Fidia Research Series. Padova, Italy: Liviana Press, in press.

McGeer PL, McGeer EG, Suzuki J, Dolman CE, Nagai T (1984): Aging, Alzheimer's disease and the cholinergic system of the basal forebrain. Neurology 34:741–745.

Mobley WC, Rutkowski JL, Tennekoon GI, Buchanan K, Johnston MV (1985): Nerve growth factor increases choline acetyltransferase activity in the striatum of neonatal rats. Science 229:284–287.

Morrison RS, Sharma A, DeVellis J, Bradshaw RA (1986): Basic fibroblast growth factor supports the survival of cerebral cortical neurons in primary culture. Proc Natl Acad Sci USA 83:7537–7541.

Morrison RS, Kornblum HI, Leslie FM, Bradshaw RA (1987): Trophic stimulation of cultured neurons from neonatal rat brain by epidermal growth factor. Science 238:72–75.

Nieto-Sampedro M, Lewis ER, Cotman CW, Manthorpe M, Skaper SD, Barbin G, Longo FM, Varon S (1982): Brain injury causes a time-dependent increase in neuronotrophic activity at the lesion site. Science 217:860–861.

Nieto-Sampedro M, Manthorpe M, Barbin G, Varon S, Cotman CW (1983): Injury-induced neuronotrophic activity in adult rat brain. Correlation with survival of delayed implants in a wound cavity. J Neurosci 3:2219–2229.

Pettmann B, Weibel M, Sensenbrenner M, Labourdette G (1985): Purification of two astroglial growth factors from bovine brain. FEBS Lett 189:102–108.

Pettmann B, Varon S, Manthorpe M (1987): Visualization of nerve growth factor biological activities by a cell-blot technique using ganglionic neurons as probes. Soc Neurosci Abstr 13:1608.

Politis MJ, Ederle K, Spencer PS (1982): Tropism in nerve regeneration in vivo. Attraction of regenerating axons by diffusible factors derived from cells in distal nerve stumps of transected peripheral nerves. Brain Res 235:1–12.

Raivich G, Kreutzberg GW (1987): The localization and distribution of high affinity β-nerve growth factor binding sites in the central nervous system of the adult rat. A light microscopic autoradiographic study using [^{125}I]-β-nerve growth factor. Neuroscience 20:23–36.

Richardson PM, Verge Issa VMK, Riopelle RJ (1986): Distribution of neuronal receptors for nerve growth factor in the rat. J Neurosci 6:2312–2321.

Schubert D, LaCorbierre M, Esch F (1986): A chick neural adhesion and survival molecule is a retinol binding protein. J Cell Biol 102:2295–2301.

Seckel BR, Chiu TH, Nyilas E, Sidman RL (1984): Nerve regeneration through synthetic biodegradable nerve guides: Regulation by the target organ. Plast Reconstr Surg 74:173–181.

Seiler M, Schwab ME (1984): Specific retrograde transport of nerve growth factor (NGF) from neocortex to nucleus basalis in the rat. Brain Res 300:33–39.

Selak I, Skaper SD, Varon S (1985): Pyruvate participation in the low molecular weight trophic activity for CNS neurons in glia-conditioned media. J Neurosci 5:23–28.

Shelton DL, Reichardt LF (1986): Studies on the expression of β nerve growth factor (NGF) gene in the central nervous system: Level and regional distribution of NGF mRNA suggest that NGF functions as a trophic factor for several distinct populations of neurons. Proc Natl Acad Sci USA 83:2714–2718.

Skaper SD, Varon S (1987): Ionic responses and growth stimulation in rat astroglial cells: Differential mechanisms of gangliosides and serum. J Cell Physiol 130:453–459.

Springer JE, Collier TJ, Notler MFD, Sladek JR, Loy R (1987a): Transplants of NGF-rich tissue facilitate survival and regeneration of axotomized cholinergic neurons in the medial septum and diagonal band. Soc Neurosci Abstr 13:185.

Springer JE, Koh S, Tayrien MW, Loy R (1987b): Basal forebrain magnocellular neurons stain for nerve growth factor receptor: Correlation with cholinergic cell bodies and effects of axotomy. J Neurosci Res 17:111–118.

Taniuchi M, Schweizer JB, Johnson EM (1986): Nerve growth factor receptor molecules in rat brain. Proc Natl Acad Sci USA 83:1950–1954.

Terry RD, Davies P (1980): Dementia of the Alzheimer type. Annu Rev Neurosci 3:77–95.

Tettamanti G, Ledeen R, Sandhoff K, Nagai Y, Toffano G (eds) (1986): "Neuronal Plasticity and Gangliosides," vol 6. Fidia Research Series. Padova, Italy: Liviana Press.

Unsicker K, Reichert-Preibsch H, Schmidt R, Pettmann B, Labourdette G, Sensenbrenner M (1987): Astroglial and fibroblast growth factors have neurotrophic functions for cultured peripheral and central nervous system neurons. Proc Natl Acad Sci USA 84:5459–5463.

Uzman BG, Villegas GM (1983): Mouse sciatic nerve regeneration through semipermeable tubes: A quantitative model. J Neurosci 9:325–338.

Varon S (1975a): In vitro approaches to the study of neural tissue aging. In Maletta G (ed): "Survey of the Aging Nervous System." DHEW Pub (NIH) 74-296, pp 59–76.

Varon S (1975b): Nerve growth factor and its mode of action. Exp Neurol 48:75–92.

Varon S (1977): Neural growth and regeneration: A cellular perspective. Exp Neurol 54:1–6.

Varon S (1985): Factors promoting the growth of the nervous system. In "Discussions in Neuroscience," vol 2. Geneva: FESN (Foundation for the Study of the Nervous System), no 3, pp 1–62.

Varon S, Adler R (1980): Nerve growth factors and control of nerve growth. Curr Top Dev Biol 16:207–252.

Varon S, Adler R (1981): Trophic and specifying factors directed to neuronal cells. Adv Cell Neurobiol 2:115–163.

Varon S, Manthorpe M (1982): Schwann cells: An in vitro perspective. Adv Cell Neurobiol 3:35–95.

Varon S, Somjen G (1979): Neuron-glia interactions. Neurosci Res Prog Bull 17:1–239.

Varon S, Williams LR (1986): Peripheral nerve regeneration in a silicone model chamber: Cellular and molecular aspects. Periph Nerve Repair Regen 1:9–25.

Varon S, Manthorpe M, Longo FM (1982): Growth factors and motor neurons. In Rowland LR (ed): "Human Motor Neuron Diseases. Advances in Neurology," vol 36. New York: Raven Press, pp 453–472.

Varon S, Manthorpe M, Williams LR (1984): Neuronotrophic and neurite promoting factors and their clinical potentials. Dev Neurosci 6:73–100.

Varon S, Skaper SD, Manthorpe M (1987): Trophic and toxic mechanisms in neuronal survival. In Vernadakis A, Privat A, Lauder JM, Timiras PS, Giacobini E (eds): "Model Systems of Development and Aging of the Nervous System." Boston: M. Nijhoff Publ. Co., pp 277–295.

Varon S, Manthorpe M, Davis GE, Williams LR, Skaper SD (1988): Growth factors. In Waxman SG (ed): "Functional Recovery in Neurological Disease. Advances in Neurology," vol 47. New York: Raven Press, pp 493–521.

Walicke P, Cowan WM, Ueno N, Baird A, Guillemin R (1986a): Fibroblast growth factor promotes survival of dissociated hippocampal neurons and enhances neurite extension. Proc Natl Acad Sci USA 83:3012–3016.

Walicke P, Varon S, Manthorpe M (1986b): Purification of a human red blood cell protein supporting the survival of cultured CNS neurons, and its identification as catalase. J Neurosci 6:1114–1121.

Williams LR, Longo FM, Powell HC, Lundborg G, Varon S (1983): Spatial-temporal progress of peripheral nerve regeneration within a silicone chamber: Parameters for bioassay. J Comp Neurol 218:460–470.

Williams LR, Varon S, Peterson G, Wictorin K, Fischer W, Björklund A, Gage FH (1986): Continuous infusion of nerve growth factor prevents basal forebrain neuronal death after fimbria-fornix transection. Proc Natl Acad Sci USA 83:9231–9235.

Williams LR, Danielsen N, Muller H, Varon S (1987a): Exogenous matrix precursors promote functional regeneration across a 15 mm gap within a silicone chamber in the rat. J Comp Neurol, 264:284–290.

Williams LR, Vahlsing HL, Lindamood T, Varon S, Gage FH, Manthorpe M (1987b): A small gauge cannula device for continuous infusion of exogenous agents into the brain. Exp Neurol 95:743–754.

8

Axonal Sprouting in Response to Injury

FREDRICK J. SEIL, MD

Office of Regeneration Research Programs, Veterans Administration Medical Center and Department of Neurology, Oregon Health Sciences University, Portland, Oregon 97201

Axonal sprouting refers to the growth of processes from an axon or an axon terminal. There are basically two types of axonal sprouting, terminal and collateral (Cotman et al., 1981). Terminal sprouting includes the outgrowth of processes from a cut or otherwise damaged proximal axonal stump (regenerative sprouting; Fig. 8–1A) or the extension of a pre-existing intact axon terminal (Fig. 8–1B). Collateral sprouting is the growth of collateral processes from an intact axon (Fig. 8–1C). If the collateral sprout originates from a node of Ranvier, it is referred to as a nodal sprout.

Axonal sprouting occurs normally during neural development and in mature animals where there is an apparent normal turnover of neural connections, such as at neuromuscular junctions (Barker and Ip, 1965). Axonal sprouting also occurs as a consequence of damage to a nerve or in response to denervation or inactivation of an axonal target. The focus of this chapter will be on axonal sprouting as a response to injury and on the contribution of sprouting to the restoration or change of neural structural and/or functional organization.

As axonal sprouting is common to both peripheral (PNS) and central (CNS) nervous systems, experimental studies in both systems will be reviewed. Initiating events for terminal and collateral sprouting will be considered, as well as the concept of an hierarchical order for synapse formation by sprouted axons. Examples of sprouting at several different CNS levels will be given, since organizational changes resulting from axonal sprouting may vary in different CNS regions. Finally, the question of

whether or not axonal sprouting is beneficial to the injured organism will be addressed.

AXONAL SPROUTING IN THE PERIPHERAL NERVOUS SYSTEM
Terminal Sprouting

Terminal sprouting of the regenerative variety occurs vigorously in the PNS. When successful, such sprouting results in the rematching of the original axon with its target, thereby establishing conditions for restoration of normal function. Regenerative sprouting is often associated with direct injury to a peripheral nerve, such as cut, crush, or tear.

The rate at which sprouting is initiated varies with the type of nerve injury, with the nature of the injury, and with the species (Grafstein and McQuarrie, 1978). In rat sciatic nerve, for example, the delay after injury until initial outgrowth was noted as 1.3 days for adrenergic axons, 1.6 days for sensory axons, and 2.2 days for motor axons. Greater delays were observed after nerve sectioning than after crush. Initiation of sprouting after crush in rat sciatic nerve sensory axons (1.6 days) was considerably faster than in rabbit sciatic nerve sensory axons (5.2 days). According to Grafstein and McQuarrie (1978), there may be some sprouting by 4–6 hr after axotomy in mammalian nerves, but such early sprouts may degenerate or involute, and definitive sprouting for most axons does not occur until after 24 hr.

The rate of growth after initiation of axonal sprouting is subject to similar variation (Grafstein and McQuarrie, 1978). Rates of 0.15 mm/day were reported in mouse sciatic nerve after excision, compared with 4.3 mm/day in rat sciatic sensory nerve after crush. Axonal outgrowth rate can be accelerated after lesion-

Neural Regeneration and Transplantation, pages 123–135
© 1988 Alan R. Liss, Inc.

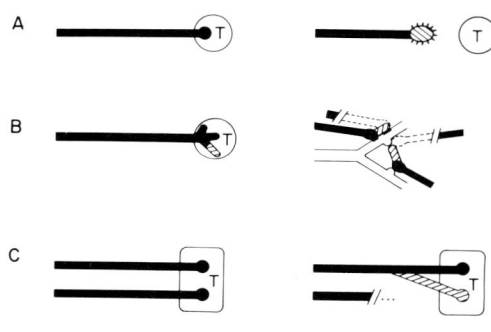

Figure 8–1. Varieties of axonal sprouting. **A:** Shown on the left is a schematic representation of an intact nerve innervating a target (T). After nerve section, as shown on the right, there is an outgrowth (hatched) from the proximal axonal stump toward the denervated target (regenerative sprouting). **B:** The extension (hatched) of an intact axon terminal to innervate an increased portion of its target is illustrated on the left. This form of terminal extension is often seen in the peripheral nervous system, especially at neuromuscular junctions. Forms of terminal extension more frequently seen in the central nervous system are shown on the right, where terminal extension (hatched) results in an increase of synaptic area or in innervation of a denervated dendritic spine. **C:** On the left, two adjacent nerve fibers innervate a target. After lesioning of one of the axons, as shown on the right, a collateral sprout (hatched) emanates from the undamaged axon and innervates the territory previously occupied by the lesioned axon.

ing if the axons have been injured within 2 weeks before the neural lesion (McQuarrie and Grafstein, 1973; McQuarrie et al., 1977; McQuarrie, 1985, Chapter 3, this volume). The initial injury is referred to as a "conditioning" lesion.

Terminal sprouting may be induced by a mechanical injury to a nerve (reviewed in Grafstein and McQuarrie, 1978; Cotman et al., 1981), by denervation or disuse of the target tissue (Guth, 1956; Snider and Harris, 1979), by blocking of axonal transport (Aguilar et al., 1973), by the degeneration products of nerve injury (Hoffmann, 1950; Brown et al. 1978),

and by trophic factors (Levi-Montalcini and Hamburger, 1951; Diamond et al., 1976). A mechanical injury such as a cut or crush may produce partial or complete denervation, interruption of axonal transport, and the production of nerve degeneration products, thus representing a complex situation in which several sprout inducing stimuli may be at play.

Motor nerve terminal sprouting can be induced with botulinum toxin, which blocks the release of acetylcholine from the terminals (Watson, 1966; Snider and Harris, 1979), and with tetrodotoxin, which blocks action potentials but does not interfere with axonal transport (Brown and Ironton, 1977). The sprouting induced by drug-mediated target disuse is exclusively a terminal sprouting, in contrast to denervation or blockade of axoplasmic flow with colchicine (Aguilar et al., 1973; Guth et al., 1980), in which both terminal and collateral sprouting occur.

Hoffmann (1950) and later Brown et al. (1978) provoked terminal sprouting of motoneurons on intact muscle with extracts of degenerating nerve. Other investigators (Vrbová, 1967; Jones and Vrbová, 1974) showed that nerve degeneration products induced extrajunctional neurotransmitter hypersensitivity in innervated muscle, and that extrajunctional acetylcholine receptors were associated with motor nerve terminal sprouting (Pestronk and Drachman, 1978). These studies suggest that nerve degeneration products induce the formation of extrajunctional receptors, which then stimulate terminal sprouting. What factor(s) in degenerating nerve might initiate such a reaction is not clear.

The best characterized trophic factor, nerve growth factor (NGF), is a potent stimulus for the outgrowth of sympathetic ganglia axons and of sensory axons during certain stages of development (Levi-Montalcini and Hamburger, 1951; Levi-Montalcini, 1987). It is conceivable that denervated targets might produce similar trophic factors that induce axonal sprouting. As a variant of this notion, Diamond et al. (1976) postulated that target tissue continuously produces a sprout-promoting factor, which is normally held in check by a neuronally secreted sprout-inhibiting factor that is axonally transported. The inhibitory factor production is halted by denervation or interference with axonal transport, and sprouting is no longer prevented. This is an interesting but unproven hypothesis.

Collateral Sprouting

Collateral sprouting, which is also well represented in the PNS, can be induced by denervation (partial or complete) and by block of axonal transport (Edds, 1953; Cooper et al., 1977; Guth et al., 1980). The signal for collateral sprouting by intact axons may arise from damaged axons or may be mediated by trophic factors, as postulated above. Another possibility is stimulation of sprouting by glia (Cotman et al., 1981). Speidel (1935) reported axon collateral sprouting in the presence of dividing glia in tadpoles. Glial-conditioned medium has been shown to promote axonal elongation in vitro (Rudge et al., 1985; Manthorpe et al., 1986). Both Schwann cells and astrocytes may produce NGF, as well as other trophic factors (Lindsay, 1979; Varon and Somjen, 1979; Heuman et al., 1987). It is conceivable that glia have a role in inducing collateral sprouting by intact axons.

Collateral sprouts may innervate target territory vacated by damaged primary axons. For example, lizards losing tails as a defensive or escape mechanism regenerate new tails, but not new sensory ganglia (Pannese, 1963). The newly grown tails are, instead, cutaneously innervated by collateral sprouts from the most caudal remaining ganglia. One of the concomitants of the increase of target territory is hypertrophy of the sensory ganglia neuron somata. This kind of territorial expansion of innervation represents a permanent change, as there is no source for regenerated primary axons.

When primary sensory nerve axons are damaged, but their parent cell bodies survive, undamaged fibers may undergo collateral sprouting and reinnervate the denervated region well before regenerative growth from the primary axons is complete. When the regenerated primary fibers arrive at the target zone, they displace the sprouted axon collaterals, and the original axon-target relationship is restored (Zander and Weddell, 1951; Devor et al., 1979; Jackson and Diamond, 1981). Thus the primary axons originally programmed for a specific target have priority for that target site in a later

competitive situation. The sprouted sensory axon collaterals may provide a temporary innervation to a denervated zone, but they give way to regenerated primary axons. Similarly, if a muscle is denervated, reinnervation may occur early by collateral sprouts from undamaged axons, followed by the later appearance of regenerating primary motor axons (van Harreveld, 1945; Guth, 1956). After arrival of the regenerated primary axons, the endplates formed by the collateral sprouts are displaced by the primary terminals (Brown and Ironton, 1978; Thompson, 1978).

The displacement of sprouted collateral terminals by primary axons is not always complete. If preganglionic afferents in autonomic ganglia are interrupted, remaining intact fibers sprout and reestablish the normal quantity of synapses on partially deafferented cells (Guth and Bernstein, 1961; Njå and Purves, 1978; Roper and Ko, 1978). The interrupted primary axons may regenerate and displace some, but not all, of the sprouted collateral terminals. In the case of frog cardiac ganglia, there is a resultant hyperinnervation of the ganglia neurons (Roper and Ko, 1978). The implications of these studies are that in some cases reinnervation by collateral sprouts may at least partially interfere with the reestablishment of normal functional reinnervation. Thus sprouting may have some detrimental as well as beneficial consequences.

Sprouting of Peripheral Axons in Response to Central Denervation

Sympathetic noradrenergic nerve fibers originating from the superior cervical ganglia are normally present on the surface of the brain, where they innervate pial blood vessels. Injuries of the hippocampus (Loy and Moore, 1977), specifically of cholinergic septohippocampal fibers originating from the medial septal nucleus (Stenevi and Björklund, 1978), instigate a collateral sprouting and ingrowth of sympathetic fibers into the hippocampal formation, remote from the lesion site (Fig. 8–2). The peripheral noradrenergic sprouts appear to replace lesioned central cholinergic axons (Crutcher et al., 1981). Similar sympathetic ingrowth into CNS areas is found after lesions of the septohabenular pathway, leading to ingrowth of the habenula (Crutcher and Davis,

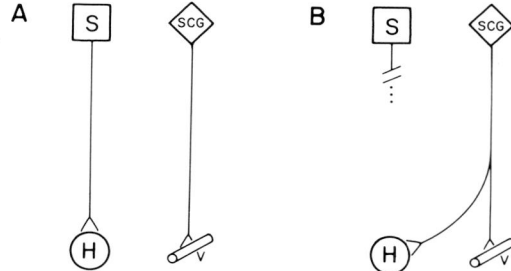

Figure 8–2. Ingrowth of sprouted peripheral noradrenergic fibers into the central nervous system. **A:** Cholinergic fibers from the septal nucleus (S) project to the hippocampus (H). Sympathetic noradrenergic fibers from the superior cervical ganglion (SCG) innervate pial blood vessels (V) over the surface of the brain. **B:** In response to a lesion of the septohippocampal pathway, sympathetic fibers undergo collateral sprouting and grow into the hippocampal formation where they appear to replace the lesioned central cholinergic fibers.

1980), and of the nucleus basalis to cortex pathway, also cholinergic, leading to ingrowth into the cerebral cortex (Crutcher, 1981). In the case of the hippocampus, evidence has been presented to suggest that the sprouting is directed by a hippocampus-derived factor (Davis, 1983). The target trophic factor is not produced by degenerating septal fibers, but may originate from the mossy fiber axons of dentate granule cells.

These studies indicate that peripheral noradrenergic fibers may sprout in response to central denervation and grow into the CNS, where they appear to replace lesioned central cholinergic fibers. The sympathetic sprouting appears to be regulated by a trophic factor. The functional consequences of such sympathetic ingrowth are uncertain.

AXONAL SPROUTING IN THE CENTRAL NERVOUS SYSTEM

While collateral sprouting and extension of preexisting terminals are frequently seen in the CNS (Cotman et al., 1981), regenerative sprouting, although it may be initiated, is usually not successful in the adult mammalian CNS. This may, at least in part, be due to a less favorable environment for axonal growth in the CNS,

compared with the PNS. This notion is supported by the studies of Aguayo and coworkers (Richardson et al., 1980; David and Aguayo, 1981; Aguayo, 1985; Bray and Aguayo, Chapter 5, this volume), who have shown remarkable growth of CNS axons placed in a peripheral nerve environment. Central axons may grow well beyond their normal lengths in a peripheral nerve bridge, but growth stops 1–2 mm after reentry into the CNS. The cessation of axonal growth is consistent with the concept that substrate conditions within the adult CNS inhibit or fail to promote axonal growth. Also contributing significantly to the lack of a central regenerative sprouting response is the generally regressive reaction and reduced survival of adult mammalian CNS neurons after axotomy (Barron, 1983, Chapter 6, this volume).

Exceptions to the general rule about the lack of regenerative axonal growth in the CNS are the monoaminergic neurons, which are capable of regenerative and collateral sprouting in response to denervation of their targets (Björklund et al., 1973; Björklund and Lindvall, 1979). Monoaminergic axons may regenerate over long distances in the CNS to reconstruct their normal innervation patterns. Monoaminergic fibers include adrenergic, noradrenergic, dopaminergic, and serotonergic axons.

Because of the complex and varied organization of the CNS, different modes of organizational change are seen as a consequence of injury-induced axonal sprouting in different CNS regions. It would therefore be of benefit to use a "systems" approach in the CNS, and look at examples of sprouting at several CNS levels. An in vitro model of CNS sprouting will also be examined as an illustration of some principles of organizational change associated with induction and regression of axonal sprouting.

Spared Dorsal Root Preparation

Sprouting in the adult mammalian CNS was first described by Liu and Chambers (1958) in a classical study in which all lumbar and sacral dorsal roots but one (L6) were sectioned unilaterally in cats. They demonstrated an increased intraspinal projection of the spared root compared with the same dorsal root on the unlesioned side. The increase in density of projections was found in all of the spinal cord segments to which the spared root normally projected, including dorsal horn, zona intermedia, and Clarke's nucleus, and in the nucleus gracilis. The increased projection was considered a result of collateral sprouting of the axons of the spared root. McCouch et al. (1958) found a correlation between increased dorsal root projections, as determined morphologically, and an increased electrophysiological response to stimulation of the spared root that was associated with ipsilateral hyperactivity of spinal reflexes. In the totally hind limb deafferented preparation, Goldberger and Murray (1974) correlated the time course of collateral sprouting with the recovery of reflexes. They considered that hyperactivity of reflexes mediated by descending spinal pathways, which sprout only with total deafferentation and not when a single root is spared, was of functional benefit for behavioral recovery. These studies demonstrated that axonal sprouting occurred in the CNS, and that, in the preparations described, it may contribute to functional improvement.

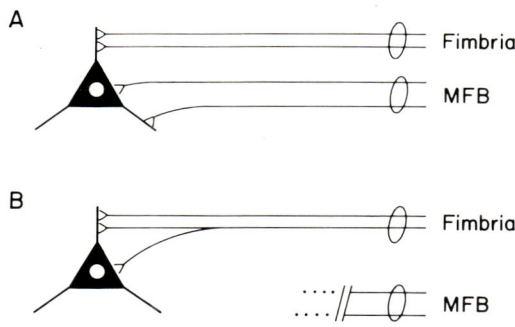

Figure 8–3. Collateral sprouting in the septal nucleus. **A:** Lateral septal nucleus neurons receive an afferent input from the hippocampus via the fimbria, which terminates exclusively on dendrites. A second projection, via the medial forebrain bundle (MFB), originates in the ventral tegmental area and lateral hypothalamus and terminates on both dendrites and somata of lateral septal nucleus neurons. **B:** After lesioning the medial forebrain bundle, fimbrial axons undergo collateral sprouting and project to the somata as well as the dendrites of lateral septal nucleus neurons.

Septal Nucleus

The first morphological demonstration of CNS axonal sprouting was in the partially deafferented adult rat septal nucleus (Raisman, 1969; Raisman and Field, 1973). With ultrastructural studies, Raisman and his coworkers showed that surviving axons increased their projection to maintain a constant number of synapses in the septal nucleus.

Neurons in the principal portion of the lateral septal nucleus receive afferents from the hippocampus via the fimbria and another afferent projection from the ventral tegmental area and lateral hypothalamus through the medial forebrain bundle (MFB). The fimbrial axons synapse exclusively on dendrites (97% on spines and the remainder on dendritic shafts), while a substantial number of the MFB axons terminate on cell bodies (Fig. 8–3A). The MFB was lesioned, and several weeks were allowed to elapse until all degenerating synapses had been removed. Then the fimbria was lesioned. Ultrastructural examination 2 days after the second lesion revealed a considerable number of degenerating axosomatic as well as axodendritic synapses. The axosomatic

synapses had been formed by fimbrial axons that had sprouted to extend their territory after the first (MFB) lesion (Fig. 8–3B). Thus the somatic synapses normally made by MFB axons had been replaced by somatic synapses formed by collaterally sprouted fimbrial axons.

Further extensions of these studies (Field et al., 1980; Raisman, 1985) focused on the dorsolateral quadrant of the lateral septal nucleus, which receives 43% of its afferents from the ipsilateral fimbria, 24% from the contralateral fimbria, and 33% from nonfimbrial axons. If one fimbria was cut, its distribution was completely taken over by sprouted axons from the other fimbria. If bilateral fimbrial lesions were made, then the nonfimbrial axons sprouted and reinnervated the sites normally occupied by fimbrial axon terminals. These studies demonstrated an hierarchical order for replacement of synapses, with like (homotypical) synapses from other fimbrial axons having precedence over unlike (heterotypical) synapses from nonfimbrial axons. Thus an effect of nonfimbrial axon sprouting was not evident unless there were no surviving fimbrial axons to respond to the denervation.

Red Nucleus

The red nucleus also represents a region in which inputs from two different sources converge. Red nucleus neurons receive somatic afferents from the contralateral cerebellar interpositus nucleus, while afferents from ipsilateral sensorimotor cortex synapse on distal portions of dendrites (Nakamura and Mizuno, 1971). The large neurons of the red nucleus are subject to intracellular electrophysiological recording. Tsukahara and colleagues recorded excitatory postsynaptic potentials (EPSPs) from large red nucleus neurons of adult cats while stimulating either sensorimotor cortex or interpositus nucleus (Tsukahara et al., 1974, 1975). Stimulation of the interpositus nucleus produced fast-rising EPSPs, consistent with axosomatic synapses, while cortical stimulation produced slow-rising EPSPs, consistent with axon terminals being located on distal dendrites away from the recording electrode. By 10 or more days after lesion of the interpositus nucleus, the rise time of EPSPs induced by sensorimotor cortex stimulation decreased. These findings were interpreted as indicative of sprouting of cortical axons to increase their projection to sites closer to or on the red nucleus neuronal somata. This interpretation of the electrophysiological data was supported by morphological studies (Nakamura et al., 1974; Murakami et al., 1982; Tsukahara, 1985).

These elegant studies not only demonstrated CNS axonal sprouting and synapse replacement in response to deafferentation, but also indicated that the newly formed synapses, although heterotypical, were functional. Thus a cellular basis for possible recovery of some degree of function after injury was established.

Hippocampus

The dentate gyrus of the hippocampal formation is a well-characterized structure that is amenable to studies of the effects of deafferentation (Lynch et al., 1972, 1976; Cotman et al., 1973; Steward et al., 1974; Matthews et al., 1976a, b; Cotman and Nadler, 1978; Scheff, Chapter 9, this volume). A single row of granule cells project their dendrites into the molecular layer of the dentate gyrus. Here they receive a dense input from the ipsilateral entorhinal cortex and from ipsilateral (associational fibers) and contralateral (commissural

fibers) pyramidal neurons of area CA4 of the hippocampus, as well as sparse projections from the contralateral entorhinal cortex and the septal nuclei (Fig. 8–4A). The entorhinal cortex fibers project to the outer three-quarters of the molecular layer, while the CA4 fibers project to the inner quarter (Cotman, 1983). Septal fibers project largely to the outer portion of the molecular layer and are very sparse in the CA4 zone. A denser layer of septal fibers is found below the CA4 region (not shown in Fig. 8–4).

Unilateral destruction of the entorhinal cortex in the adult rat resulted in loss of approximately 60% of the synapses on the granule cells of the ipsilateral dentate gyrus. The deafferentation triggered sprouting of contralateral entorhinal cortex fibers, septal fibers, and both associational and commissural CA4 fibers. The CA4 fibers extended their projection by sprouting partially into the entorhinal fiber zone and occupied the inner 35% of the molecular layer (Fig. 8–4B). Septal and contralateral entorhinal cortex fibers proliferated only in the denervated area and withdrew from the expanded territory of the CA4 projection (Fig. 8–4B). Thus a degree of laminar reorganization was associated with the lesion-induced sprouting and synapse replacement.

The new synapses formed by sprouted contralateral entorhinal cortex fibers were homotypical, as they originated from the same type of cells as the original fibers. The synapses formed by sprouted septal and CA4 associational and commissural fibers were heterotypical. Both homotypical and heterotypical synapses appeared to be electrophysiologically functional (Steward et al., 1973; West et al., 1975).

Not all fibers found in the dentate gyrus sprouted in response to an entorhinal lesion (Cotman et al., 1981). There was no apparent increase of the sparse GABA-ergic terminals that end on granule cell somata, and the density of noradrenergic locus coeruleus fibers in the granule cell dendritic zone did not increase.

These studies indicated that some fairly complex reorganization and rearrangement of previously existing connections could occur after lesion-induced sprouting. No new pathways were formed, however, in the lesioned adult animal. All of the afferents that reinner-

A

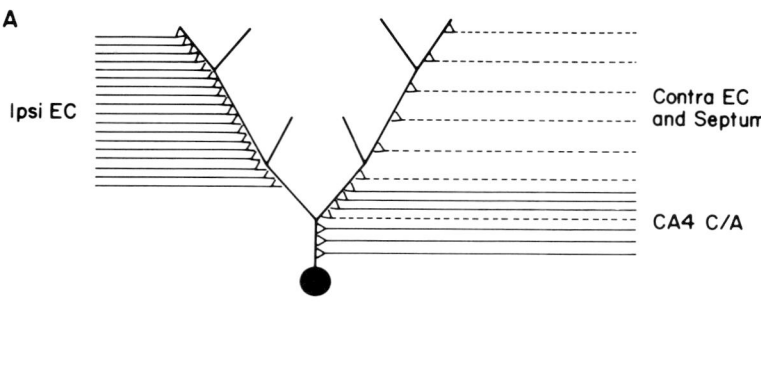

B

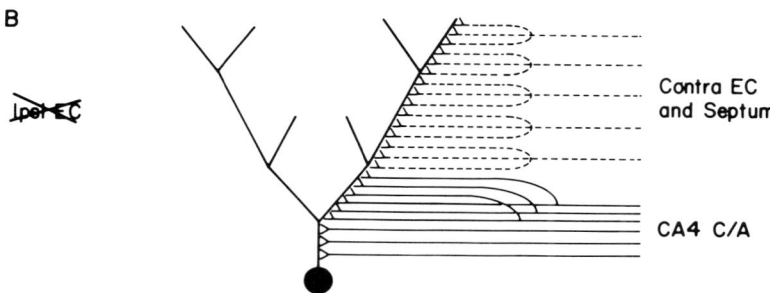

Figure 8–4.   Collateral sprouting and laminar reorganization in the adult hippocampus. **A:** Granule cell dendrites in the dentate gyrus of the hippocampal formation receive a dense input from the ipsilateral entorhinal cortex (Ipsi EC, solid lines) and from both ipsilateral (associational) and contralateral (commissural) hippocampal area CA4 pyramidal cell axons (CA4 C/A, solid lines). In addition, there is a sparse input from the contralateral entorhinal cortex and septal nuclei (Contra EC and Septum, dashed lines). Entorhinal cortex fibers project to the outer 75% of the granule cell dendritic tree, while CA4 fibers project to the inner 25%. **B:** After destruction of the ipsilateral entorhinal cortex, CA4 fibers, septal fibers, and fibers from the contralateral entorhinal cortex all undergo collateral sprouting to replace the lost synapses. The CA4 fibers extend their projection to the inner 35% of the dendritic tree by sprouting partially into the entorhinal fiber zone, while entorhinal cortex and septal fibers sprout only in the denervated area, and retreat from the expanded CA4 territory.

vated the denervated dentate gyrus molecular layer had overlapping projections with the destroyed afferents. This is consistent with a general principle of CNS collateral sprouting observed in mature animals, that an afferent fiber will reinnervate a denervated zone only if its field overlaps that of a damaged afferent (Cotman, 1983).

An In Vitro Model of CNS Axonal Sprouting

Tissue cultures of CNS can be easily manipulated in a variety of ways, and thus are useful for studies of neural plasticity. A culture model that we have worked with is the cerebellar explant exposed to cytosine arabinoside to destroy one of the cortical neuronal groups, the granule cells (Seil et al., 1983a). This model has its limitations in that it is a developing rather than a mature system, and thus may have a greater reorganizational capacity than adult tissue. Nevertheless, this culture system illustrates some of the same principles of neural response to injury that have been observed in studies of adult mammalian CNS in vivo.

There are five major groups of neurons in the cerebellar cortex, including Purkinje, Golgi, basket, stellate, and granule cells (Eccles et al., 1967). The granule cells are excitatory and project their axons (the parallel fibers) to the dendrites of all other cortical neurons. The other four neuronal groups are inhibitory. The only cells that project axons out of the cerebellar cortex are the Purkinje cells. The Purkinje cell axons give off recurrent collateral branches within the cortex that project to all other cortical neurons (including other Purkinje cells) except for the granule cells. The basket and stellate cells project to Purkinje cell somata and proximal dendrites and to distal Purkinje cell dendrites, respectively. The complexly branched Golgi cell axons synapse with granule cell dendrites. Excitatory extracerebellar afferents include climbing fibers, which originate from the inferior olive and project to Purkinje cell dendrites, and mossy fibers, which represent all the remaining extracerebellar input and project to the granule cell dendrites. The same cortical neuronal groups, with the same interneuronal relationships, are present in explant cultures of mouse cerebellum (Seil, 1979) (Fig. 8–5A, normal culture). The major difference from the cerebellum in vivo is the absence or vast reduction of extracerebellar afferents.

Granule cells are dividing neuroblasts at the time that cerebellar cultures are explanted from newborn mice. Exposure of the explants to cytosine arabinoside (Ara C), an inhibitor of DNA synthesis, for the first 5 days in vitro destroyed the granule cells, and thus affected a major denervation of the remaining cortical neurons (Seil et al., 1980). In response to the absence of parallel fibers, there was a tremendous sprouting of Purkinje cell recurrent axon collaterals, which projected to the somata and dendritic spines of other Purkinje cells (Blank et al., 1982) (Fig. 8–5B, granuloprival culture).

The presence of recurrent axon collateral terminals on Purkinje cell dendritic spines in Ara C-treated cultures suggested that inhibitory terminals now occupied sites that were normally contacted by excitatory parallel fibers. Indeed, extracellular electrophysiological studies indicated that the sprouted recurrent axon collateral terminals were functional and were inhibitory, as antidromic stimulation of Purkinje cell axons produced a profound inhibition of spontaneous cortical discharges, an atypical response due to the collateral inhibition. This kind of reorganization is different from what occurs in vivo with cerebellar granule cell destruction. In ferrets treated with panleukopenia virus to eliminate granule cells, mossy (primarily) and climbing fibers synapsed with Purkinje cell dendritic spines, and appreciable sprouting of Purkinje cell recurrent axon collaterals did not occur (Llinas et al., 1973) (Fig. 8–5C, granuloprival animal). Although these were heterotypical synapses, nevertheless the sites usually occupied by excitatory parallel fibers were taken over by excitatory extracerebellar afferents. Such animals were, however, severely ataxic. In the extreme case of the cerebellar culture system, which is devoid of extracerebellar afferents, inhibitory fibers sprouted in the absence of any available excitatory afferents and synapsed with the denervated Purkinje cell dendritic spines. Comparing the in vivo and in vitro studies, an hierarchical order of priorities for Purkinje cell dendritic spine synapses is apparent, with excitatory terminals having preference over inhibitory terminals as replacements for missing excitatory axons, even though the excitatory neurotransmitters may be different. However, inhibitory terminals may serve as substitutes when no excitatory axons are available.

Once the Ara C-treated cerebellar cultures had become reorganized, could the reorganization be reversed by the reintroduction of granule cells? To address this question, we exposed cerebellar explants to kainic acid, an analog of glutamic acid, to destroy all cerebellar cortical neurons except granule cells, which are highly resistant to kainate neurotoxicity (Seil et al., 1979). Such cultures were superimposed upon 9- or 16-day-old Ara C-treated cerebellar cultures. Granule cells and glia migrated from the kainate-treated explants to the Ara C-exposed cultures and triggered a series of changes that produced a return toward a normal structural and functional organization (Blank and Seil, 1983; Seil et al., 1983b) (Fig. 8–5D, transplanted culture). Significant among these changes were the appearance of parallel fiber-Purkinje cell dendritic spine synapses, the disappearance of most recurrent collateral-Purkinje cell dendritic spine synapses, and a

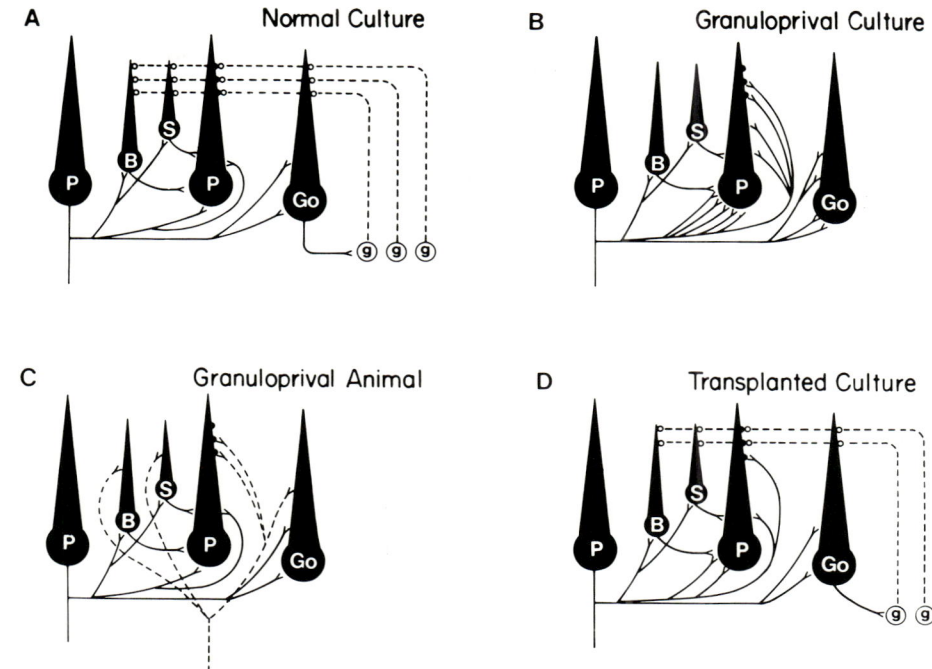

Figure 8–5. Axonal sprouting and withdrawal in cerebellar cultures. **A:** Normal cerebellar culture with Purkinje (P), basket (B), stellate (S), Golgi (Go), and granule (g) cells. Purkinje cells project recurrent axon collaterals to all other cortical neurons except granule cells, including the somata and dendritic shafts of other Purkinje cells. Granule cells project to the dendritic spines of Purkinje cells and to all other cortical neurons except granule cells. Excitatory axons are shown as dashed lines, and inhibitory axons are solid. Extracerebellar afferents (mossy and climbing fibers) are absent or severely reduced. **B:** After destruction of the granule cells by exposure to cytosine arabinoside (granuloprival culture), inhibitory Purkinje cell recurrent axon collaterals in cerebellar cultures undergo remarkable sprouting, and project densely to other Purkinje cells, including the dendritic spines normally occupied by excitatory granule cell axons. **C:** A similar destruction of cerebellar granule cells in vivo (granuloprival animal) evokes a sprouting of excitatory extracerebellar afferents (MF) that project to sites normally occupied by granule cell axons. A sprouting of Purkinje cell recurrent collateral axons does not occur in this situation. **D:** If granule cells are introduced into a reorganized granuloprival culture (transplanted culture), granule cell axons synapse with Purkinje cell dendritic spines, most of the recurrent collateral-dendritic spine synapses disappear, and there is a reduction of the sprouted Purkinje cell recurrent collateral axons, as the collaterally sprouted axons retreat upon the appearance of primary axons. (Modified from Seil et al., 1983a, and reproduced by permission of the publisher.)

reduction of the excess sprouted Purkinje cell recurrent axon collaterals to an almost normal density. That the presence of granule cells was necessary for this reduction was shown by an experiment in which fragments of optic nerve, a source of glia without granule cells, were superimposed upon Ara C-treated explants, with a resultant failure of elimination of sprouted

recurrent axon collaterals (Meshul and Seil, 1988). Antidromic stimulation of Purkinje cell axons in Ara C-exposed cultures with superimposed kainic acid-treated explants no longer produced inhibition of spontaneous cortical discharges (Seil et al., 1983b).

These studies demonstrated that in the CNS, as in the PNS, sprouted axon collaterals may retreat upon the reappearance of primary axons. The synapses that had been formed by the sprouted collaterals became disconnected, even though they were functional, and the appropriate synapses were formed. Again, this shows the priority of the originally programmed axons for their synaptic sites, and the plasticity of the nervous system in its ability to form substitute connections in response to injury, and then to form its normal synapses when the appropriate elements become available.

AXONAL SPROUTING AS A REPAIR MECHANISM

Other examples of axonal sprouting could have been cited as well, such as sprouting after spinal cord injury (Bernstein and Bernstein, 1971) or after cerebral neocortex lesions (Kristt, 1987). It is evident from all of the illustrations of axonal sprouting in both the CNS and PNS that such sprouting is a common, although not invariable, response to injury. Is axonal sprouting beneficial to the injured organism?

In the case of regenerative sprouting, if the original nerve-target relationship is accurately restored and functional recovery is attained, there is little doubt that this is of benefit. That accurate or complete restoration does not always occur is well known to clinicians who have seen aberrant function following recovery from peripheral nerve injuries.

Collateral sprouting presents more of a problem. In some instances of collateral sprouting in the PNS, such as in the cutaneous innervation by sensory nerve collaterals of the regrown lizard tail after amputation, the collateral sprouting would appear to be advantageous. Collateral sprouts might also provide interim innervation to a target until the regenerative sprouting of primary axons is complete, and then give way to the primary axons to allow reformation of the normal nerve-target pattern. This process has been shown to occur with some peripheral sensory and motor axons and, as indicated by the tissue culture studies, could at least theoretically occur in the CNS as well. In other instances, such as with autonomic ganglia, the displacement of collaterally sprouted fibers by regenerating primary axons may not be complete, as the sprouted axons

may interfere with the reestablishment of normal connections.

In the CNS, where, except for monoaminergic neurons, regenerative sprouting is minimal, the picture is even less clear. Interference with regenerative sprouting by collateral sprouting has been postulated to occur in the CNS, as local growth after lesioning may be achieved at the expense of regenerative growth in the mammalian spinal cord (Bernstein et al., 1978). In the case of the formation of synapses by collaterally sprouted central fibers, as occurs in the partially denervated septal nucleus, it has not been established whether such synapses improve or augment the functional deficit induced by the original lesion (Raisman, 1985). The hierarchical order for synapse replacement seen in septal nucleus, hippocampus, and cerebellum, with like axons having preference over similar axons and similar axons having preference over dissimilar axons, as well as the occurrence of collateral sprouting only in axons whose projection fields overlap those of the damaged axons, suggests that the nervous system is programmed to attempt to preserve or restore function by collateral sprouting. There is some evidence indicating that heterotypical synapses formed as a result of collateral sprouting in the red nucleus may result in partial recovery of normal movement (Tsukahara, 1985). However, the collateral sprouting of mossy and climbing fibers in animals without cerebellar granule cells did not prevent ataxia. In the more extreme case of the cerebellar culture devoid of parallel fibers and extracellular afferents, the formation of heterotypical synapses with terminals of opposite function to the original suggests a potentially maladaptive consequence of collateral sprouting, if this can be taken as a model of what could occur in vivo.

It is conceivable that the results of collateral sprouting and either homotypical or heterotypical synapse formation in the CNS vary from area to area and from projection to projection as to whether function is improved, unaffected, or made worse. Much more needs to be learned about the consequences of collateral axonal sprouting in various parts of the CNS in order to know if and when and where such sprouting should be encouraged or discouraged. That sprouting can, at least to some extent, be manipulated is indicated by a retarding effect of systemic administration of adrenal corticosteroids on axonal sprouting in the hippocampal dentate gyrus (Scheff et al., 1980), and an enhancing effect of electrical stimulation in partially denervated superior cervical ganglion (Maehlen and Njå, 1979). Other strategies for the manipulation of axonal sprouting are under investigation.

More critical for the CNS, however, is to learn how to promote regenerative sprouting. This is the condition most suitable for the reestablishment of normal function. Studies of central axonal growth in peripheral nerve bridges are very encouraging in this regard. Speculations as to why central axons grow well in a PNS environment include the presence of trophic or substrate factors that are no longer supplied by the mature CNS, or presence in the CNS of inhibitory factors that prevent growth. The definition of such factors represents one of the many tasks that lie ahead on the road to understanding the mechanisms of neural regeneration, and to the successful application of our acquired knowledge to the achievement of functional recovery in neurally injured man.

ACKNOWLEDGMENTS

Studies from the author's laboratory were supported by the Veterans Administration and NIH Grant NS 17493.

REFERENCES

Aguayo AJ (1985): Axonal regeneration from injured neurons in the adult mammalian central nervous system. In Cotman CW (ed): "Synaptic Plasticity." New York: Guilford Press, pp 457–484.

Aguilar CE, Bisby MA, Cooper E, Diamond J (1973): Evidence that axoplasmic transport of trophic factors is involved in the regulation of peripheral nerve fields in salamanders. J Physiol (Lond) 234:449–464.

Barker D, Ip MC (1965): The probable existence of motor end-plate replacement. J Physiol (Lond) 176:11P–12P.

Barron KD (1983): Axon reaction and central nervous system regeneration. In Seil FJ (ed): "Nerve, Organ, and Tissue Regeneration: Research Perspectives." New York: Academic Press, pp 3–36.

Bernstein JJ, Bernstein ME (1971): Axonal regeneration and formation of synapses proximal to the site of the lesion following hemisection of the rat spinal cord. Exp Neurol 30:336–351.

Bernstein JJ, Wells MR, Bernstein ME (1978): Spinal cord regeneration: Synaptic renewal and neurochemistry. In Cotman CW (ed): "Neuronal Plasticity." New York: Raven Press, pp 49–71.

Björklund A, Lindvall O (1979): Reformation of normal terminal innervation patterns by central noradrenergic neurons after 5,7-dihydroxytryptamine-induced axotomy. Brain Res 171:275–293.

Björklund A, Novin A, Stenevi U (1973): Regeneration of central serotonin neurons after axonal degeneration induced by 5,6-dihydroxytryptamine. Brain Res 50: 214–220.

Blank NK, Seil FJ (1983): Reorganization in granuloprival cerebellar cultures after transplantation of granule cells and glia. II. Ultrastructural studies. J Comp Neurol 214:267–278.

Blank NK, Seil FJ, Herndon RM (1982): An ultrastructural study of cortical remodeling in cytosine arabinoside induced granuloprival cerebellum in tissue culture. Neuroscience 7:1509–1531.

Brown MC, Ironton R (1977): Motor neuron sprouting induced by prolonged tetrodotoxin block of nerve action potentials. Nature (Lond) 265:459–461.

Brown MC, Ironton R (1978): Sprouting and regression of neuromuscular synapses in partially denervated mammalian muscles. J Physiol (Lond) 278:325–348.

Brown MC, Holland RL, Ironton R (1978): Degenerative nerve products affect innervated muscle fibers. Nature (Lond) 275:652–654.

Cooper E, Diamond J, Turner C (1977): The effects of nerve section and of colchicine treatment on the density of mechanosensory nerve endings in salamander skin. J Physiol (Lond) 264:725–749.

Cotman CW (1983): Reactive synaptogenesis. In Seil FJ (ed): "Nerve, Organ, and Tissue Regeneration: Research Perspectives." New York: Academic Press, pp 269–282.

Cotman CW, Nadler JV (1978): Reactive synaptogenesis in the hippocampus. In Cotman CW (ed): "Neuronal Plasticity." New York: Raven Press, pp 227–271.

Cotman CW, Matthews DA, Taylor D, Lynch G (1973): Synaptic rearrangement in the dentate gyrus: Histochemical evidence of adjustments after lesions in immature and adult rats. Proc Natl Acad Sci USA 70:3473–3477.

Cotman CW, Nieto-Sampedro M, Harris EW (1981): Synapse replacement in the nervous system of adult vertebrates. Physiol Rev 61:684–784.

Crutcher K (1981): Cholinergic denervation of rat neocortex results in sympathetic innervation. Exp Neurol 74:324–329.

Crutcher K, Davis JN (1980): Noradrenergic sprouting in response to cholinergic denervation: The sympathohabenular connection. Exp Neurol 70:187–191.

Crutcher K, Brothers L, Davis JN (1981): Sympathetic noradrenergic sprouting in response to central cholinergic denervation: A histochemical study of neuronal sprouting in the rat hippocampal formation. Brain Res 210:115–128.

David S, Aguayo A (1981): Axonal elongation into PNS "bridges" after CNS injury in adult rats. Science 214: 931–933.

Davis J (1983): Target regulation of neuronal sprouting. In Seil FJ (ed): "Nerve, Organ, and Tissue Regeneration: Research Perspectives." New York: Academic Press, pp 157–169.

Devor M, Schonfeld D, Seltzer Z, Wall PD (1979): Two

modes of cutaneous reinnervation following peripheral nerve injury. J Comp Neurol 185:211–220.

Diamond J, Cooper E, Turner C, McIntyre L (1976): Trophic regulation of nerve sprouting. Science 193:371–377.

Eccles JC, Ito M, Szentágothai J (1967): "The Cerebellum as a Neuronal Machine." New York: Springer-Verlag, pp 4–31.

Edds MV Jr (1953): Collateral nerve regeneration. Q Rev Biol 206:260–276.

Field PM, Coldham DE, Raisman G (1980): Synapse formation in the adult rat brain: Preferential reinnervation of denervated fimbrial sites by axons of the contralateral fimbria. Brain Res 189:103–113.

Goldberger ME, Murray M (1974): Restitution of function and collateral sprouting in the cat spinal cord: The deafferented animal. J Comp Neurol 158:37–54.

Grafstein B, McQuarrie I (1978): Role of nerve cell body in axonal regeneration. In Cotman CW (ed): "Neuronal Plasticity." New York: Raven Press, pp 155–195.

Guth L (1956): Regeneration in the mammalian peripheral nervous system. Physiol Rev 36:461–478.

Guth L, Bernstein JJ (1961): Selectivity in the reestablishment of synapses in the superior cervical ganglion of the cat. Exp Neurol 4:59–69.

Guth L, Smith S, Donati EJ, Albuquerque, EX (1980): Induction of intramuscular collateral nerve sprouting by neurally applied colchicine. Exp Neurol 67:513–525.

Heumann R, Korshing S, Bantlow C, Thoenen H (1987): Changes of nerve growth factor synthesis in nonneuronal cells in response to sciatic nerve transection. J Cell Biol 104:1623–1631.

Hoffmann HL (1950): Local reinnervation in the partially denervated muscle: A histo-physiological study. Aust J Exp Biol Med Sci 28:838–397.

Jackson PC, Diamond J (1981): Regenerating axons reclaim sensory targets from collateral nerve sprouts. Science 214:926–928.

Jones R, Vrbová G (1974): Two factors responsible for the development of denervation hypersensitivity. J Physiol (Lond) 236:517–538.

Kristt DA (1987): Morphological responses to local CNS trauma: Sprouting and synaptogenesis within membranes implanted into mature cerebral cortex of the rat. J Neuropathol Exp Neurol 46:668–681.

Levi-Montalcini R (1987): The nerve growth factor 35 years later. Science 237:1154–1162.

Levi-Montalcini R, Hamburger V (1951): Selective growth stimulating effects of mouse sarcoma on sensory and sympathetic nerve of the chick embryo. J Exp Zool 116:321–362.

Lindsay RM (1979): Adult rat brain astrocytes support survival of both NGF-dependent and NGF-insensitive neurons. Nature (Lond) 282:80–82.

Liu C-N, Chambers WW (1958): Intraspinal sprouting of dorsal root axons. Arch Neurol Psychiatry 79:46–61.

Llinás R, Hillman DE, Precht W (1973): Neuronal circuit reorganization in mammalian agranular cerebellar cortex. J Neurobiol 4:69–94.

Loy R, Moore RY (1977): Anomolous innervation of the hippocampal formation by peripheral sympathetic axons following mechanical injury. Exp Neurol 57:645–650.

Lynch GS, Matthews DA, Mosko S, Parks T, Cotman CW (1972): Induced acetylcholine-rich layer in rat dentate gyrus following entorhinal lesions. Brain Res 42:311–318.

Lynch G, Gall C, Rose G, Cotman, CW (1976): Changes in the distribution of the dentate gyrus associational system following unilateral or bilateral entorhinal lesion in the adult rat. Brain Res 110:57–71.

Maehlen J, Njå A (1979): Sprouting after partial denervation in the superior cervical ganglion: Effect of preganglionic nerve stimulation. Acta Physiol Scand 105: 18A–19A.

Manthorpe M, Rudge JS, Varon S (1986): Astroglial cell contributions to neuronal survival and neurite growth. In Fedoroff S, Vernadakis A (eds): "Astroctyes," vol 2. Orlando: Academic Press, pp 315–376.

Matthews DA, Cotman CW, Lynch G (1976a): An electron microscopic study of lesion-induced synaptogenesis in the dentate gyrus of the adult rat. I. Magnitude and time course of degeneration. Brain Res 115:1–21.

Matthews DA, Cotman CW, Lynch G (1976b): An electron microscopic study of lesion-induced synaptogenesis in the dentate gyrus of the adult rat. II. Reappearance of morphologically normal contacts. Brain Res 115:23–41.

McCouch GP, Austin GM, Liu C-N, Liu CY (1958): Sprouting as a cause of spasticity. J Neurophysiol 21: 205–216.

McQuarrie IG (1985): Effect of a conditioning lesion on axonal sprout formation at nodes of Ranvier. J Comp Neurol 231:239–249.

McQuarrie IG, Grafstein B (1973): Axon outgrowth enhanced by a previous nerve injury. Arch Neurol 29:53–55.

McQuarrie IG, Grafstein B, Gershon MD (1977): Axonal regeneration in the rat sciatic nerve: Effect of a conditioning lesion and of dbcAMP. Brain Res 132:443–453.

Meshul CK, Seil FJ (1988): Transplanted astrocytes reduce synaptic density in the neuropil of cerebellar cultures. Brain Res, 441:23–32.

Murakami F, Katsumaru H, Saito K, Tsukahara N (1982): A quantitative study of synaptic reorganization in red nucleus neurons after lesion of the nucleus interpositus in the cat: An electron microscopic study involving intracellular injection of horseradish peroxidase. Brain Res 242:41–53.

Nakamura Y, Mizuno N (1971): An electron microscopic study of the interpositorubral connections in the cat and rabbit. Brain Res 35:283–286.

Nakamura Y, Mizuno N, Konishi A, Sato M (1974): Synaptic reorganization of the red nucleus after chronic deafferentation from cerebellorubral fibers: An electron microscopic study in the cat. Brain Res 82:298–301.

Njå A, Purves D (1978): Specificity of initial synaptic contacts made on guinea pig superior cervical ganglion during regeneration of the cervical sympathetic trunk. J Physiol (Lond) 281:45–62.

Pannese E (1963): Investigations on the ultrastructural

changes of the spinal ganglion neurons in the course of axon regeneration and cell hypertrophy. Z Zellforsch Mikrosk Anat 61:561–586.

Pestronk A, Drachman DB (1978): Motor nerve sprouting and acetylcholine receptors. Science 199:1223–1225.

Raisman G (1969): Neuronal plasticity in the septal nuclei of the adult rat. Brain Res 14:25–48.

Raisman G (1985): Synapse formation in the septal nuclei of adult rats. In Cotman CW (ed): "Synaptic Plasticity." New York: Guilford Press, pp 13–38.

Raisman G, Field PM (1973): A quantitative investigation of the development of collateral reinnervation after partial deafferentation of the septal nuclei. Brain Res 71:1–16.

Richardson PM, McGuinness UM, Aguayo AJ (1980): Axons from CNS neurons regenerate into PNS grafts. Nature (Lond) 284:264–265.

Roper S, Ko C-P (1978): Synaptic remodeling in the partially denervated parasympathetic ganglion in the heart of the frog. In Cotman CW (ed): "Neuronal Plasticity." New York: Raven Press, pp 1–25.

Rudge JS, Manthorpe M, Varon S (1985): The output of neuronotrophic and neurite-promoting agents from rat brain astroglial cells: A microculture method for screening potential regulatory molecules. Dev Brain Res 19:161–172.

Scheff SW, Benardo LS, Cotman, CW (1980): Hydrocortisone administration retards axon sprouting in rat dentate gyrus. Exp Neurol 68:195–201.

Seil FJ (1979): Cerebellum in tissue culture. In Schneider DM (ed): "Reviews of Neuroscience," vol 4. New York: Raven Press, pp 105–177.

Seil FJ, Leiman AL, Blank NK (1979): Toxic effects of kainic acid on mouse cerebellum in tissue culture. Brain Res 161:253–265.

Seil FJ,. Leiman AL, Woodward WR (1980): Cytosine arabinoside effects on developing cerebellum in tissue culture. Brain Res 186:393–408.

Seil FJ, Blank NK, Leiman AL (1983a): Circuit reorganization in granuloprival and transplanted cerebellar cultures. In Seil FJ (ed): "Nerve, Organ and Tissue Regeneration: Research Perspectives." New York: Academic Press, pp 283–300.

Seil FJ, Leiman AL, Blank NK (1983b): Reorganization in granuloprival cerebellar cultures after transplantation of granule cells and glia. I. Light microscopic and electrophysiological studies. J Comp Neurol 258–266.

Snider WD, Harris GL (1979): A physiological correlate of disuse-induced sprouting at the neuromuscular junction. Nature (Lond) 281:69–71.

Speidel CC (1935): Studies on living nerves. III. Phenomena of nerve irritation and recovery, degeneration and repair. J Comp Neurol 61:1–80.

Stenevi U, Björklund A (1978): Growth of vascular sympathetic axons into the hippocampus after lesions of the septohippocampal pathway: A pitfall in brain lesion studies. Neurosci Lett 78:219–224.

Steward O, Cotman CW, Lynch GS (1973): Reestablishment of electrophysiologically functional entorhinal cortical input to the dentate gyrus deafferented by ipsilateral entorhinal lesions: Innervation by contralateral entorhinal cortex. Exp Brain Res 18:396–414.

Steward O, Cotman CW, Lynch GS (1974): Growth of a new fiber projection in the brain of adult rats: Reinnervation of the dentate gyrus by the contralateral entorhinal cortex following ipsilateral entorhinal lesions. Exp Brain Res 20:45–66.

Thompson W (1978): Reinnervation of partially denervated rat soleus muscle. Acta Physiol Scand 103:81–91.

Tsukahara N (1985): Synaptic plasticity in the red nucleus and its possible behavioral correlates. In Cotman CW (ed): "Synaptic Plasticity." New York: Guilford Press, pp 201–229.

Tsukahara N, Hultborn H, Murakami F (1974): Sprouting of cortico-rubral synapses in red nucleus neurones after destruction of the nucleus interpositus of the cerebellum. Experientia 30:57–58.

Tsukahara N, Hultborn H, Murakami F, Fujito Y (1975): Electrophysiological study of formation of new synapses and collateral sprouting in red nucleus neurons after partial denervation. J Neurophysiol 38:1359–1372.

van Harreveld A (1945): Reinnervation of denervated muscle fibers by adjacent functioning motor units. Am J Physiol 144:477–493.

Varon S, Somjen G (1979): Neuron-glia interactions. Neurosci Res Prog Bull 17:1–239.

Vrbová G (1967): Induction of an extrajunctional chemosensitive area in intact innervated muscle fibres. J Physiol (Lond) 191:20P–21P.

Watson WE (1966): Quantitative observations upon acetylcholine hydrolase activity of nerve cells after axotomy. J Neurochem 13:1549–1550.

West JR, Deadwyler SA, Cotman CW, Lynch G (1975): Time dependent changes in commissural field potentials in the dentate gyrus following lesions of the entorhinal cortex in adult rats. Brain Res 97:215–233.

Zander E, Weddell G (1951): Reaction of corneal nerve fibers to cornea injury. Br J Ophthalmol 35:61–87.

9

Synaptic Reorganization After Injury: The Hippocampus as a Model System

STEPHEN W. SCHEFF, PhD

Department of Anatomy and Neurobiology, Sanders-Brown Research Center on Aging, University of Kentucky College of Medicine, Lexington, Kentucky 40536

Since man first encountered head trauma resulting in a neurological deficit and the subsequent recovery from that deficit, there have been numerous theories and speculations on the mechanisms underlying the "recovery of function." As mankind learned more about the brain and became acutely aware that a certain amount of localization of function is inherent in the brain, an even greater problem arose. It stands to reason that the most effective mechanism for the recovery of a lost neurological function would be the subsequent regrowth of either the neurons that were lost or the regeneration of the pathway that had been destroyed. Numerous investigators failed in their attempts to demonstrate regeneration of tissue in the mammalian central nervous system (CNS). Many early theorists believed that the brain was "hard-wired" (circuitry once formed during development was not amenable to rearrangement during aging) and incapable of reorganization (Finger and Stein, 1982).

One of the earliest theories, *diaschisis*, is attributed to Constantin von Monakow, a Swiss neurologist and neuroanatomist who lived from 1853 to 1930. von Monakow believed that following any acute head trauma, the nervous system undergoes a certain amount of inactivity of normal function, and that over time the injured areas are reactivated, resulting in some recovery. This is not to say that there will not be some permanent loss of function. While the neural shock model can account for some re-

covery, it cannot explain all the present experimental data. Another of the early theories, *vicariation*, is attributed to Herman Munk (1839–1912). This theory holds that following a specific neural trauma, remaining tissue might possibly "take over" the function of the tissue that was lost. One of the strong supporters of this concept was Karl Lashley, who believed in a limited equal potentiality of the brain. Still other theorists relied upon the fact that a certain amount of recovery following neural trauma was not in fact a "true" recovery of the lost function but rather the use of behavioral substitution, by which the organism attains the proper goal through a different mechanism.

A German scientist named Exner published a paper in 1885 describing the apparently anomalous growth of peripheral nerves as a consequence of transection of the nerve supplying the circothyroid muscle. Several other prominent neuroanatomists (e.g., Ramón y Cajal, 1928) supported Exner's findings by demonstrating that sensory axons could develop collaterals even in the absence of specific trauma. Ramón y Cajal, however, held a pessimistic view of any regenerative capacity in the mammalian CNS and its possible role in recovery following injury. One of the pivotal points in our current understanding of CNS plasticity was the elegant study by Geoffrey Raisman in 1969. Raisman used the electron microscope to document collateral sprouting and the replacement of lost synaptic contacts following partial denervation in the septal nuclei of young adult rats. It was previously known that the septal nuclei received different afferent fibers. Following transection of one of

Neural Regeneration and Transplantation, pages 137–156

these major afferent pathways, the fimbria, the hippocampal projection to the septum degenerates and leaves the lateral septal nuclei partially denervated. Afferent fibers from the hypothalamus, which travel via the medial forebrain bundle, grow collaterals, and new terminals make contacts on the dendritic sites evacuated by the degenerating hippocampal projection. In this way the circuitry of the septal area has been reorganized as a result of the lesion. This study demonstrated that the mammalian CNS is not "hard-wired" but amenable to manipulation, thus lending support to the notion that "axon sprouting" and "lesion-induced synaptogenesis" might be utilized as a mechanism for recovery of function.

As a result of the initial experiments by Raisman, numerous studies were carried out exploring the universality of the "sprouting" phenomenon and the extent of the repair process (Cotman et al., 1981). One of the most carefully examined mammalian brain structures is the hippocampal formation, which is noted for its role in learning and memory and which appears to maintain a high degree of anatomical plasticity even in adult animals. Because of the many afferents projecting to the hippocampal formation and their discrete terminal fields within the structure, this area has provided the researcher with a unique advantage in analyzing the response of a brain structure to injury. In order to fully appreciate the magnitude of the "self-repair" process, it is important to understand the normal anatomy of this structure. The information derived from the experiments described below has provided a framework for analyzing synapse replacement in other areas of the mammalian CNS.

NORMAL HIPPOCAMPAL ANATOMY

The hippocampal formation consists of two discrete areas, each governed by a specific neuronal type (Fig. 9–1). The largest portion of the hippocampus is composed of pyramidal neurons, which can be considered "projection" cells because they transmit information away from the hippocampus to such structures as the septal nuclei. The neurons form a "U" shape and have long dendritic trees that radiate out in an area called stratum radiatum. Ramón y Cajal (1893) was one of the first anatomists to describe the normal cytoarchitecture

of this structure. The second major division of the hippocampal formation is formed by granule cells. These neurons also form a "U" shape that appears to interlock the configuration formed by the pyramidal neurons. The granule cells are considered "local circuit" cells because they project information only to other parts of the hippocampus. The region of the hippocampus containing the granule cells is called the dentate gyrus, while that containing most of the pyramidal cells is often called the hippocampus proper or by one of its subregions (CA1–CA4). Many early experiments that examined the anatomical plasticity of the hippocampal formation concentrated on the dentate gyrus because of its relatively simple anatomical structure and because it maintains the same anatomical cytoarchitecture throughout its septal-temporal extent.

The granule cells of the dentate gyrus form a continuous row of densely packed neurons, which have apical dendrites arborizing in a zone called the molecular layer. These dendritic trees receive numerous afferent inputs that appear to be well segregated. The most prominent afferent system projecting to the granule cell dendrites arises from the entorhinal cortex ipsilateral to the hippocampus. Neurons in the entorhinal cortex send axons, which project via the perforant path, to the outer two-thirds of the dendritic tree and make en passant synapses. The terminal field of this excitatory input can be mapped by destroying the entorhinal cortex and then examining sections of the hippocampus prepared with a stain for degeneration, such as the Fink-Heimer silver stain (Fig. 9–2). One quickly realizes that a unique feature of this afferent pathway lies in the fact that the terminals are confined to an extremely precise area of the dendritic tree—the outer two-thirds. The inner one-third of the molecular layer contains no degenerative debris following the entorhinal cortex lesion, because it contains terminals arising from other afferent fiber systems.

The commissural fibers, which arise from CA4 pyramidal neurons in the hilar region of the dentate gyrus, project to the granule cells on the opposite side of the brain. The terminals of these afferents are confined to the inner one-third of the molecular layer just below the terminal area of the entorhinal afferents. This

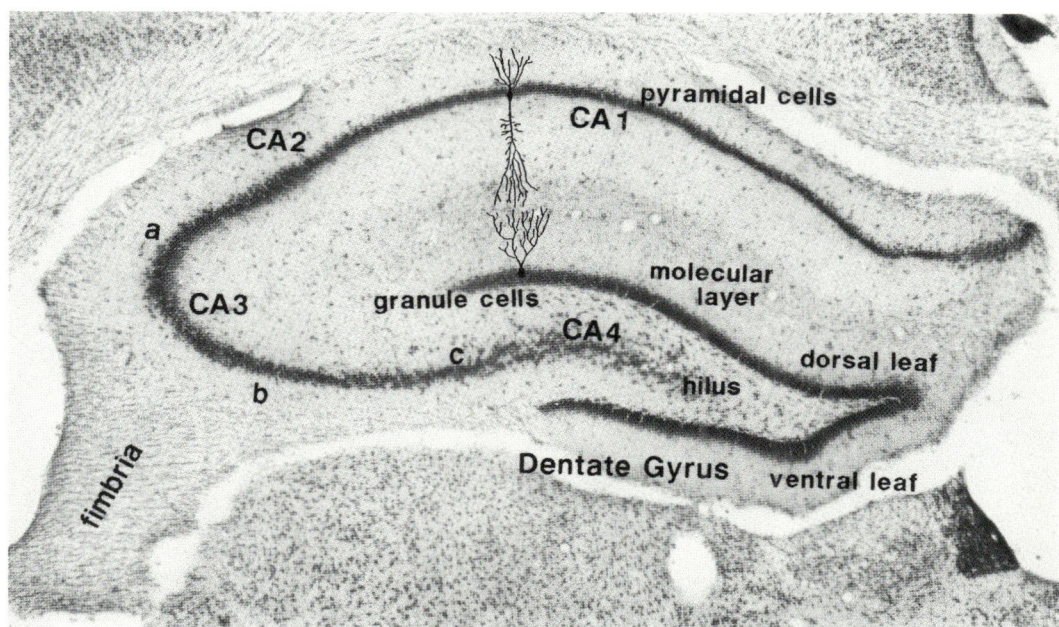

Figure 9–1. Cresyl violet-stained coronal section from the midseptal-temporal axis of the rodent hippocampal formation. Two distinct areas can be defined: the hippocampus proper, composed of pyramidal neurons, and the dentate gyrus, composed of granule cell neurons. The dentate gyrus has been the most common area used to study plasticity following partial denervation in the hippocampal formation. The hippocampal fissure is the boundary separating the dentate gyrus dorsal leaf from the CA1 field of the hippocampus proper. Both hippocampal areas receive afferent fibers via the fimbria.

particular fiber system forms a line of communication between the two hippocampi. The associational fibers use the same terminal field as the commissural afferents. These fibers arise for the ipsilateral CA4 pyramidal neurons of the hilar region. There is some evidence that the cells that give rise to the commissural afferents also give rise to the associational afferents. In this way the same information transmitted to the opposite hippocampus is also projected to the granule cells on the same side. The commissural and associational fibers account for most of the terminals within the inner one-third of the dentate gyrus molecular layer (Fig. 9–2). Like the entorhinal cortex afferents, the commissural and associational inputs provide a strong excitatory influence on the granule cells.

Another prominent afferent fiber system arises from the medial septal nucleus, nucleus of the diagonal band, and intermediolateral regions of the septal area. These fibers are commonly referred to as the cholinergic septohippocampal fibers because acetylcholinesterase (AChE) histochemistry serves as a convenient method to map their projection. This staining method has delineated a band of fibers terminating immediately above the granule cell layer and in the hilar region of the dentate gyrus. A more diffuse and subsequently lighter staining pattern is observed throughout the molecular layer, suggesting a sparser distribution of terminals. Like the entorhinal and commissural-associational afferents, the septohippocampal influence on the granule cells is excitatory.

The above afferent inputs represent the major projections to the dentate gyrus granule cells. There are, however, a few minor inputs, such as those arising from the midbrain locus coeruleus, midbrain raphe, and various interneurons. The most notable of the interneurons

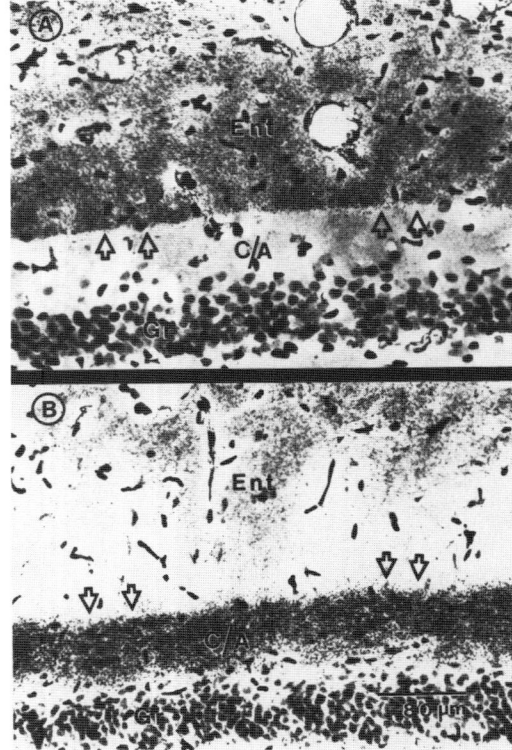

Figure 9–2. The dorsal leaf of the dentate gyrus prepared with the Fink-Heimer silver stain for degeneration. **A:** The entorhinal (Ent) cortex was unilaterally ablated 2 days prior to killing the animal. The small degenerating particulate is contained within the outer two-thirds of the molecular layer. The area immediately above the granule cells (Gr) is devoid of this particulate. **B:** Obtained from a rat 2 days after removal of the commissural and associational (C/A) afferents. The open arrows in both micrographs indicate the extent of the degenerative debris. In B, the degeneration is limited to the inner one-third of the neuropil.

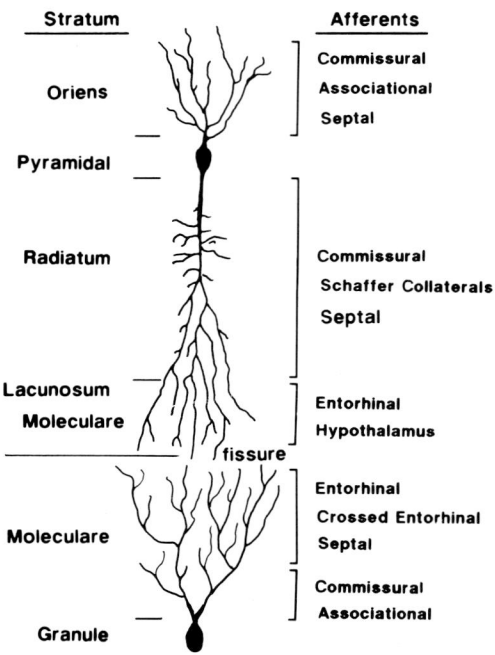

Figure 9–3. One prominent feature of the hippocampal formation is the strictly ordered lamination of the afferents on the dendritic trees of both pyramidal and granule cells. This schematic diagram of the cells portrayed in Figure 9–1 lists the major afferents found in the various strata.

is the basket cell, which is located in the granule cell layer and synapses on the soma and dendritic shaft of the granule cell. One final afferent input is worth mentioning, since it appears to play a significant role in the final remodeling of the dentate gyrus following partial denervation. The contralateral entorhinal cortex sends an extremely sparse projection to the outer two-thirds of the molecular layer within

the same terminal field as the ipsilateral entorhinal projection (Goldowitz et al., 1975). This projection accounts for only about 2% of the normal synaptic contacts in the normal animal. In summary, then, the hippocampal dentate gyrus is a precisely laminated structure that can be selectively denervated (Fig. 9–3).

Normal Ultrastructure of the Dentate Gyrus

A low-power view of the neuropil in the dentate gyrus reveals a neuron-free area containing numerous segments of tangentially cut granule cell dendrites, cross sections of small unmyelinated axons, a relatively small number of myelinated axons, and the profiles of relatively few astrocytes and microglia (Fig. 9–4A). Occasionally one will encounter the cross section of a blood vessel arising from transverse arteries that are branches of the longitudinal hippocampal artery. The penetrating vessels form a capillary plexus in the molecular layer (Coyle, 1978). The astrocytes are usually in close association with these blood vessels. The other prominent feature of the neuropil is the density of synaptic contacts within this structure of the brain. Numerous studies have determined that the density of synaptic contacts is fairly uniform throughout the dentate gyrus molecular layer and along its septal-temporal axis.

The most frequently observed type of synaptic contact in the molecular layer is the asymmetric or Gray type I synapse, which is composed of a relatively straight presynaptic element containing numerous small round vesicles and is in contact with the end of a postsynaptic element, usually a dendritic spine (Fig. 9–4B). These contacts account for approximately 90% of the synaptic population in the outer two-thirds of the molecular layer. It appears that most of the synaptic contacts are *en passant*, rather than terminal (Blackstad, 1958, 1963; Laatsch and Cowan, 1966). Many of the presynaptic elements contain one or two mitochondria, and occasionally microtubules are present. A second type of asymmetric contact can be observed and belongs to the category of complex synapses. These contacts are sometimes referred to as "U"- and "W"-type synapses (Fig. 9–4C, D). Complex synapses appear to make contact with dendritic shafts or main branches of dendrites. They do not appear to be specific to any particular afferent input to the dentate gyrus nor peculiar to any particular region of the granule cell dendrite. Such complex synaptic contacts account for about 10% of the normal synaptic density. Symmetric or Gray type II synapses are extremely uncommon in the molecular layer and probably account for less than 1% of the total number of synapses. When the symmetric type of synapse is observed, most often it is making contact with main dendritic branches. These contacts do not appear to have a preference for any particular portion of the neuropil. The normal density of synapses in the molecular layer of the dentate gyrus is approximately 35 contacts per 100 μm^2, a density that includes the most common type of asymmetric synapses, complex asymmetric synapses, and symmetric synapses regardless of whether they contact dendritic spines or branches.

DEGENERATION FOLLOWING LESIONS

Regardless of whether the outer two-thirds of the molecular layer is denervated as a result of an ipsilateral entorhinal cortex ablation (Matthews et al., 1976a,b; Hoff et al., 1982b; Steward and Vinsant, 1983) or whether the inner one-third of the molecular layer is partially denervated as a result of a commissural and/or associational afferent lesion (McWilliams and Lynch, 1978; Nadler et al., 1980), the degenerative response appears to proceed along the same time course. Most investigators who have detailed the ultrastructural changes in the dentate gyrus during the self-repair process have initiated the analyses at 2 days posttrauma. However, within 24 hours after the trauma a considerable amount of degenerating fibers and synapses can be observed. The density of this degenerative debris increases markedly by 2 days and appears to reach its peak between 2 and 4 days. By 4 days postlesion, the density of degenerating terminals begins to decline. Over time the total number of degenerating synapses is reduced until at very long postlesion intervals only a residual amount of degenerative debris remains (Fig. 9–5).

Many of the synaptic boutons in the outer molecular layer appear to increase in electron density immediately following an entorhinal cortex lesion. The axoplasm becomes very dark, and organelles often appear distorted (Fig. 9–6). Two different classes of degeneration appear in the denervated neuropil, one dark and electron-dense and the other light and electron lucent (Fifkova, 1975). The electron-dense type of profile appears to be significantly smaller or shrunken, compared with the normal synaptic contacts. The intracellular morphology is often difficult to ascertain because of the dark staining. It is not uncommon, however, to observe some vesicles and mitochondria in the darkly stained cytoplasm. Occasionally one can observe what appear to be detached degenerating terminals in the neuropil. Whether or not this detachment is the result of a retraction of the postsynaptic site, such as the reabsorption of a dendritic spine, is unknown at present. In the late stages of the degeneration reaction, the dying boutons appear as extremely electron-dense irregularly shaped masses, in which vesicles or mitochon-

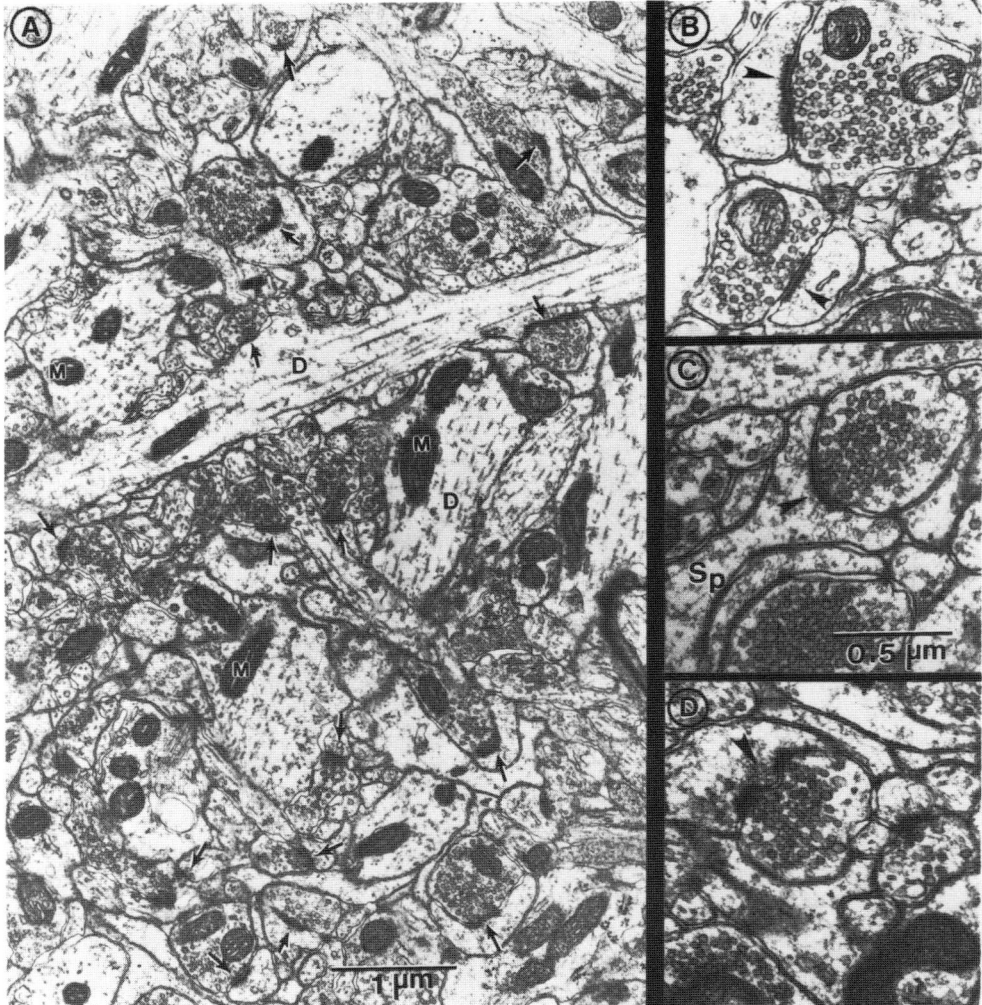

Figure 9–4.   Electron micrographs showing synaptic profiles typically observed in the dorsal leaf molecular layer of the rodent dentate gyrus. **A:** Low-power view of the field typically observed. Long and short segments of dendrites (D) can be seen making contacts with presynaptic endings (arrows). The area is studded with mitochondria (M). **B:** The most common type of synaptic contact observed. These "noncomplex" synapses are formed by the close apposition of a presynaptic element containing three or more synaptic vesicles, presumably containing neurotransmitter, and a postsynaptic specialization. Over 98% of the synapses in the molecular layer of the dentate gyrus are asymmetric and have a prominent postsynaptic density (arrowhead). **C:** One of the two types of complex synapses observed in this neuropil, the "U" type (arrowhead). It is not uncommon to find synapses on dendritic spines (Sp). **D:** Another type of complex synapse observed in this neuropil, the "W" type (arrowhead).

dria are not recogniziable. This transformation presents some problems in determining the density of the degenerating synapses, since the most common definition for a synapse in the dentate gyrus is the presence of synaptic vesicles and presynaptic membrane in association

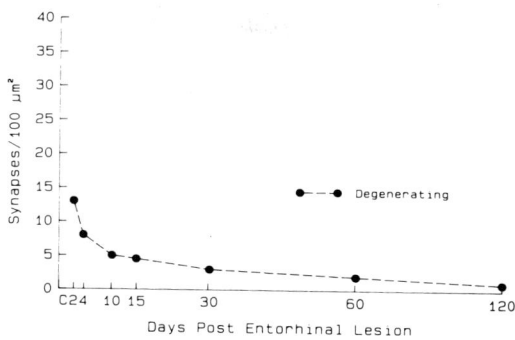

Figure 9–5. Time course of appearance and removal of degenerating synaptic contacts in the dorsal leaf of the rodent dentate gyrus (outer two-thirds of molecular layer) after an ipsilateral entorhinal cortex lesion. Although the removal of degenerating contacts is rapid, there appear to be a few degenerating terminals even at long posttrauma survival.

with a postsynaptic specialization, usually one with a postsynaptic density.

The pale, electron-lucent form of degeneration is primarily observed at early posttrauma time points and is most often described as swollen axonal endings containing a watery cytoplasm with few recognizable organelles. Following a unilateral removal of the ipsilateral entorhinal cortex, the electron-lucent type of degeneration accounts for approximately 25% of the density at the very early stages. After approximately 10 days posttrauma, the electron-lucent degeneration is completely removed, while the electron-dense form is still very noticeable. Whether or not the electron-dense type is a transformation of the electron-lucent type is unknown at present.

The removal of the degenerating boutons proceeds at an extremely rapid rate and is primarily the work of glia. It is not uncommon to observe hypertrophied astrocytes that contain degenerative debris in their cytoplasm. In fact, there is a highly significant increase in the size of the astroglial processes and a highly significant increase in the total number of these cells. It is reasonable to assume that astrocytes phagocytose or engulf the degenerative debris. There are some who believe that the astroyctes are responsible for the final

removal of degenerative contacts from the postsynaptic site (Raisman and Field, 1973). In an excellent study, Rose et al. (1976) detailed the hypertrophy and apparent migratory action of these cells in the dentate gyrus in response to the cortical ablation. It is unknown at present whether or not the astrocytes form the principal guidance mechanism that leads to the formation of new synaptic contacts. Recent experimental results have indicated that the astrocytes release a trophic substance into the denervated neuropil that aids in the survival of the neurons in that region and possibly plays a role in process outgrowth and terminal proliferation (Nieto-Sampedro and Cotman, 1985). It is probably safe to say that the astroglia create a more favorable milieu for the self-repair process. Future experiments will more accurately define their role in this repair process. The possible role played by the microglia has also been investigated, and these cells appear to play an important role in the repair process (Gall et al., 1979).

The residual degeneration observed in the neuropil at extremely long postlesion survival times is quite different morphologically from that observed early in the self-repair process. "Old" degenerating terminals have a simple round shape, unlike the irregular shape of "newly formed" degeneration, and the older dying terminals do not appear as electron-dense. Furthermore, no internal structures can be recognized in the older degeneration.

The fact that degenerative debris is removed immediately signals that a repair process is initiated quickly after the damage and indicates that this particular system is certainly not placed in a state of "shock." One might consider the first phase of the self-repair process as a "clean-up" of the neuropil, preparatory for the "reconstructive" phase. In a recent experiment, in which glucocorticoids were employed as an agent to disrupt the self-repair process, it was shown that some of the replacement of lost synaptic contacts occurs even though extensive amounts of degenerative debris are still present (Scheff et al., 1986). While the removal of degenerative debris may aid in the self-repair, it does not appear to be essential or to be the rate-limiting factor.

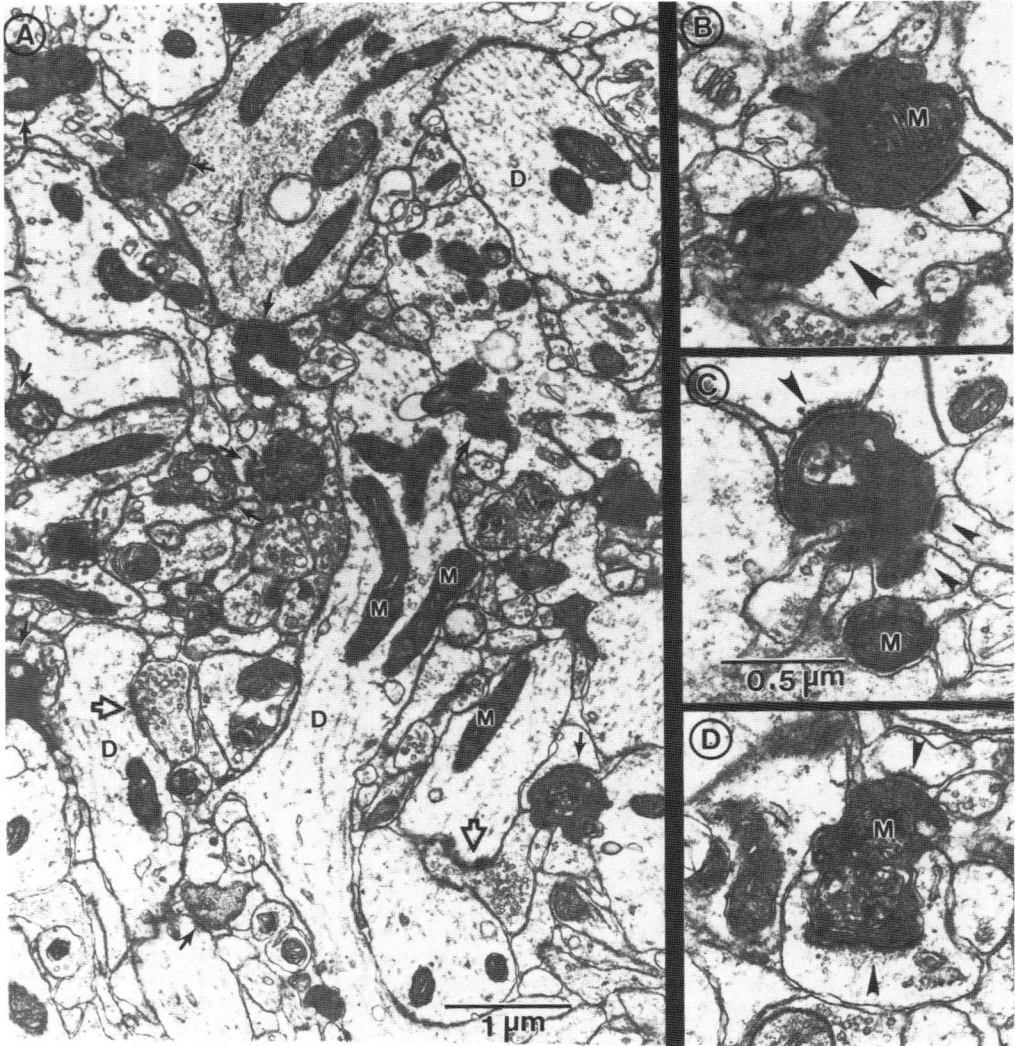

Figure 9–6. Electron micrographs showing degenerating terminals observed in the dorsal leaf molecular layer of the rodent dentate gyrus within 4 days following ipsilateral removal of the entorhinal cortex. **A:** Low-power view of the neuropil showing the extensiveness of the lesion. The closed arrows indicate some of the degenerating contacts observed on dendritic shafts and spines. A small number of nondegenerating synaptic contacts can also be observed (open arrows). The mitochondria (M) often take on irregular shapes. D, dendrites. **B:** Typical degenerating contact consisting of a postsynaptic specialization with a prominent postsynaptic density (arrowheads) in opposition to a deteriorating presynaptic element. Mitochondria (M) can often be observed at early post-trauma survival times. **C:** A degenerating multiple synaptic contact, one presynaptic element making contact with several postsynaptic specializations (arrowheads). **D:** A complex synapse degenerating. These micrographs indicate that the entorhinal afferents are capable of many different types of synaptic configurations.

SYNAPSE REPLACEMENT

The actual replacement of lost synaptic contacts occurs very quickly following the neurological trauma. The simplest method for determining whether or not injury-induced synaptogenesis (replacement of synapses) has occurred is to count the number of intact synapses per area of neuropil immediately before, immediately after, and at some later survival time after the damage. A number of ultrastructural studies have monitored synapse replacement in denervated zones of the hippocampus (e.g., Matthews et al., 1976a,b; Cotman et al., 1977; Lee et al., 1977; McWilliams and Lynch, 1978, 1979; Goldowitz et al., 1979; Nadler et al., 1980; Hoff et al., 1981, 1982a,b; Steward, 1986; Steward and Vinsant, 1983; Anderson et al., 1986a; Scheff et al., 1986). Following an ablation of the entorhinal cortex, there is a dramatic reduction in the numerical density of nondegenerating synaptic contacts in the outer two-thirds of the dentate gyrus molecular layer. By 2 days after the damage, only about 10–15% of the normal synaptic density is present. If the prelesion density is 35 synapses/100 μm2, then at 2 days after the ablation one would only observe three to five intact synaptic contacts in the same area of the neuropil. This means that approximately 85–90% of the normal synaptic input to the outer two thirds of the granule cell dendrites is derived from the ipsilateral entorhinal cortex. By 4 days after the damage, the number of intact synaptic contacts begins to increase, again lending support to the notion that the system responds very quickly to the damage and is not in a temporary state of dysfunction. This synapse replacement continues for many months (Fig. 9–7).

There appear to be two distinct phases to the initial process of synapse replacement: 1) growth and formation of the presynaptic element; and 2) the actual formation or contact of the presynaptic element with the postsynaptic site. The growth of the presynaptic element (sometimes called terminal proliferation) has been monitored in a few ultrastructural studies (McWilliams and Lynch, 1978; Steward and Vinsant, 1983). All of the terminals in the neuropil at different survival periods after deafferentation were counted. Terminals included not

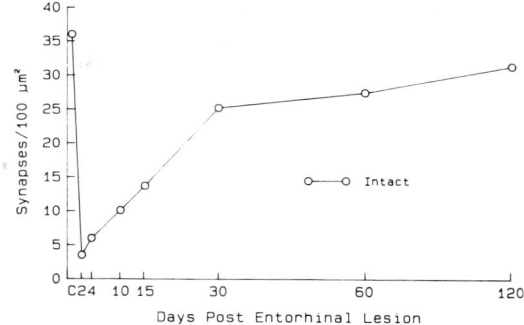

Figure 9–7. The time course of loss and reappearance of nondegenerating (intact) synaptic contacts in the dorsal leaf of the rodent dentate gyrus (outer two-thirds of molecular layer) after ipsilateral removal of the entorhinal cortex. Almost immediately following the trauma, the area initiates a self-repair process that rapidly replaces a portion of the synaptic density. However, even at very long posttrauma survival periods, the snyaptic density does not attain control levels.

only synaptic contacts, in which a presynaptic element with vesicles contacted a postsynaptic site, but also presynaptic elements with vesicles that did not appear to make contact with a postsynaptic site. Then only those terminals that appeared to be synapses were counted. There appear to be twice as many terminals as synapses during the early and more rapid stages of the replacement process. In the later stages of restoration, the number of terminals nearly equals the number of synaptic contacts, indicating that eventually all terminals make contact with postsynaptic elements. This increase in terminals, compared with synapses alone, indicates that the replacement process is not merely the expansion of residual contacts and the formation of multiple synapses, but the actual growth of new terminals. One would expect terminal proliferation prior to synapse formation.

There is a highly significant proliferation of nondegenerating synaptic contacts within the first 2 weeks following the denervation. By 30 days after the initial lesion, the neuropil has begun to assume normal appearance. Most of the degeneration has been removed, and almost 50% of the synaptic density has been restored. To provide an objective evaluation of the reinnervation response, we have employed a "reinnervation index," or RI50, to define the time required after a lesion for the replacement of 50% of the synapses found in the control animals. The RI50 serves as a basis to compare the ability of different experimental groups to initiate and maintain an early reinnervation response. We have determined that following a unilateral entorhinal lesion, the RI50 in the dorsal leaf of the dentate gyrus is approximately 35 days (Hoff et al., 1982a; Scheff et al., 1986). The process continues for a long time, leading to a considerably greater reinnervation. However, several studies have shown that even at a long postlesion survival interval, the synaptic density never reaches control levels (Hoff et al., 1982a (86%); Steward and Vinsant, 1983 (70%); Scheff et al., 1986 (80%)). In an early study, Matthews et al. (1976b) reported hyperinnervation of the middle portion of the dentate gyrus molecular layer following an entorhinal cortex ablation. Normally there appears to be little variability in the density of synapses in various hippocampal areas between animals. Following the initiation of the reinnervation process, the return of lost synaptic contacts proceeds rapidly initially, but levels off in the later stages and rarely exceeds the normal synaptic density. This increase above the normal synaptic density is most unusual but has been reported by other investigators (Goldowitz and Cotman, 1980). A denervation of the inner one-third of the molecular layer following a commissural lesion appears to result in an almost complete reinnervation (97.9%) (McWilliams and Lynch, 1979). The reason for the difference in the extent of the reinnervation between the inner and outer regions of the granule cell dendrite may lie in the fact that a commissural lesion only removes 36% of the terminals, while an entorhinal cortex ablation is responsible for approximately 90%. On the other hand, the difference may be related to a specific portion of the dendritic tree or the afferent fibers that respond to the damage.

Two studies lend support to the notion that the percentage of denervation is not the limiting factor, nor is the location on the dendritic tree. Goldowitz et al. (1979) and Anderson et al. (1986a) utilized the CA1 pyramidal cells as an experimental model to study lesion-induced synaptogenesis in the hippocampus. The CA1 pyramidal cells receive both commissural and associational afferents (Schaffer collaterals) upon the inner three-quarters of the dendritic tree (Fig. 9–3). Unlike the dentate gyrus commissurotomy, which removes only 36% of the terminals in the inner portion of the granule cell dendritic tree, in the two aforementioned studies both the commissural and associational afferents were removed, with resultant elimination of approximately 75% of the synaptic contacts. In both studies complete reinnervation was attained within 60 days after the trauma.

COMPLEX AND NONCOMPLEX SYNAPSES

In the normal neuropil two distinct groups of nondegenerating synaptic contacts have been described. It is of some interest to determine if the proportions of these contacts are maintained in the "repaired" neuropil. Even though the exact function of the complex synapses is unknown at present, it stands to reason that a more complete restoration of the neuropil would dictate that the same type and proportion of synaptic contact be formed. Possible changes in the distribution of these synaptic configurations have been monitored at various postlesion intervals (Matthews et al., 1976b; Hoff et al., 1982a). As stated earlier, the most common synaptic configuration in the dentate gyrus under normal conditions is the simple straight asymmetric contact or noncomplex synapse. These contacts also account for the majority of the contacts in the reinnervated neuropil. Approximately 85% of the synaptic density at long postrauma survival times is composed of noncomplex synapses, which is only a slight reduction from the normal density. The remaining nondegenerating contacts are complex asymmetric synapses (Fig. 9–8A). There appeared to be no change in the number of symmetric or Gray type II contacts. The result, then, is a slight redistribution in the proportion of complex and noncomplex synaptic contacts as a result of the trauma. One is more likely to find complex synapses in the reinnervated neuropil at long postlesion survival times, compared with the normal state. Whether or not the change in the distribution is a function of the postsynaptic element or the result of a specific afferent that reinnervates the neuropil is unknown at present.

MULTIPLE SYNAPTIC CONTACTS

The density of multiple synaptic contacts as a function of time after injury has been monitored in several studies. Multiple synaptic contacts are defined as a single presynaptic element making contact with two or more postsynaptic elements (Fig. 9–8B). Following a lesion of the entorhinal cortex, there appears to be a substantial increase in the density of multiple contacts (Matthews et al., 1976b; Steward and Vinsant, 1983). A time-dependent evaluation of the formation of synapses indicates that multiple synaptic contacts do not contribute to the early phase of the reinnervation but most likely to the later stages. The increase in this form of contact possibly indicates an expansion of pre-existing terminals at late stages of the restoration process, while axon sprouting and new terminal formation would most likely occur during the early stages. One possible reason for the increase in appearance of multiple synaptic contacts late in the restoration process may lie in the fact that they are more resistant to degeneration immediately following the injury. They may also be more resistant to removal by glial cells as opposed to the simple straight contact. Trophic influences from several different postsynaptic elements may help retard the degradation process.

SHRINKAGE

In any study involving the loss and reacquisition of some particular element, it is important to consider what gross morphological effect the initial damage has upon the area itself. For instance, an increase in the density of synapses per unit area might be the result of a collapse of the neuropil (i.e., shrinkage of the tissue) as a result of the denervation, and not the actual formation of any new synapses.

The simplest way to determine whether or not a manipulation results in a significant change in the neuropil is either to measure the various structures in the area or to measure the entire area itself before and sometime after the manipulation. For instance, in the hippocampus, because of its definitive boundaries, it is possible to measure the height of the molecular layer in control material and in subjects following a lesion. Most investigations aimed at determining changes in the hippocampal dentate gyrus following different surgical manipulations have employed light microscopic measurements of the distance between the granule cell layer and the obliterated hippocampal fissure. With tissue that is embedded in plastic for ultrastructural analysis, semithin sections (1–2 μm) can be used for such determinations. The entire molecular layer of the dentate gyrus collapses by about 15–20% following a unilateral removal of the entorhinal cortex. Lesions that denervate only the inner one-third of the granule cell dendritic tree (that area occupied by commissural and associational afferents) do not appear to affect the height (McWilliams and Lynch, 1979; Nadler et al., 1980).

To deal with a change in the neuropil, several reasonable assumptions must be made. First, we must assume that the shrinkage most probably results in a collapse of the neuropil as a result of a loss of neural structures, and has no affect on the size of residual structures. Those remaining structures continue to occupy the same prelesion space, so that the remaining dendrites and synaptic terminals are not affected by the collapse. Second, considering the fact that the inner one-third of the molecular layer does not change, even as a result of massive denervation in that terminal field, it is reasonable to assume that the shrinkage is contained within the outer or denervated zone following a lesion of the entorhinal cortex. Finally, it is important to assume that the measurement of the neuropil height is a valid measure for assessing the percentage of shrinkage.

If the molecular layer of the denate gyrus, which is approximately 240 μm in height, shrinks by 20% (48 μm), and if this shrinkage is restricted to the outer two-thirds (160 μm) of the molecular layer, then the actual reduction in the denervated zone is 30%. Can all of the changes in the denervated zone be accounted for by a 30% decrease in the denervated zone? That answer is definitely no. In fact there appears to be an 85% denervation following the lesion, resulting in a synaptic density of about 5 synapses per 100 μm^2. A 30% reduction in

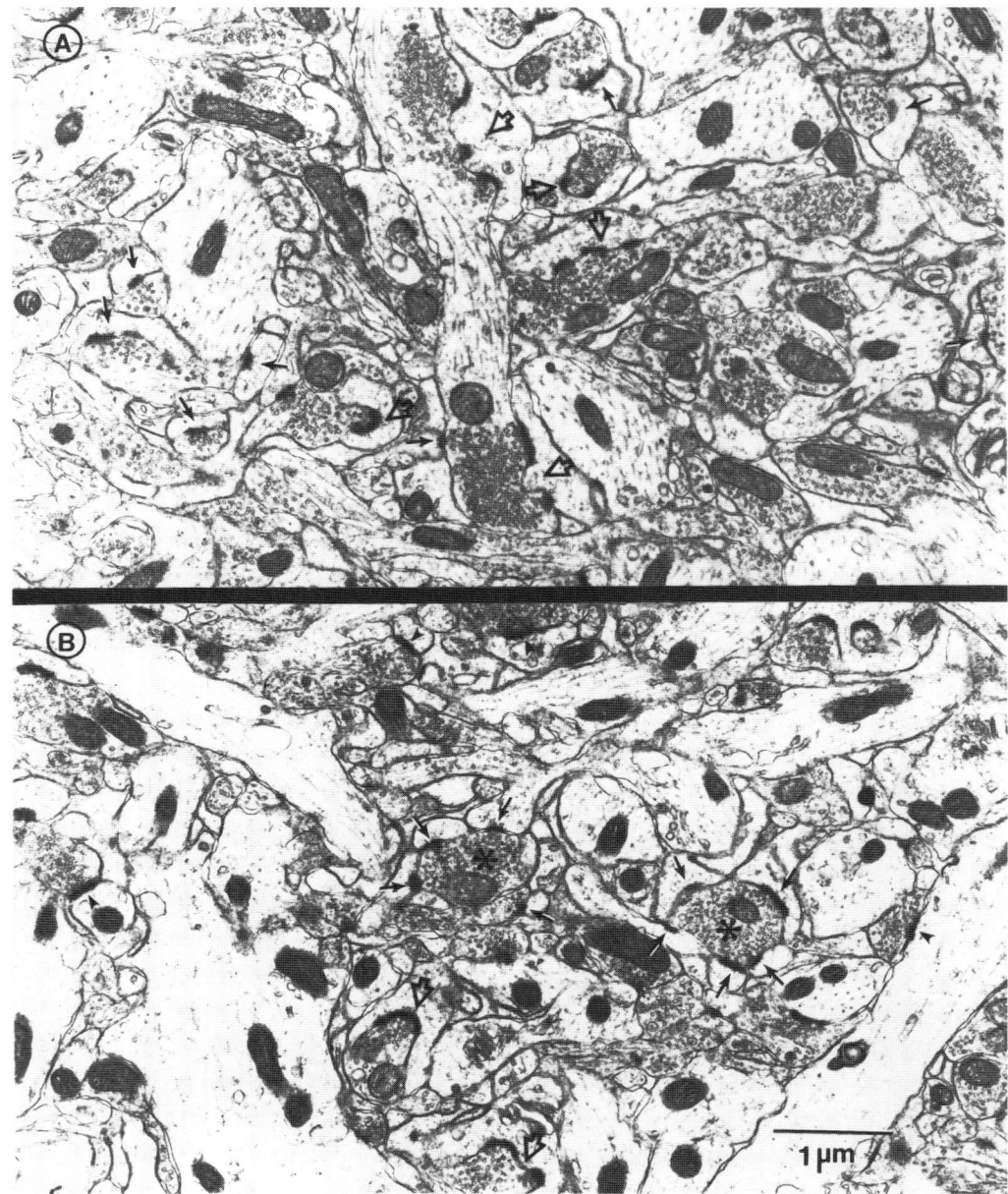

Figure 9–8.   Electron micrographs showing the outer molecular layer of the dentate gyrus 120 days after an ipsilateral entorhinal cortex lesion. The reinnervated neuropil appears very similar to that taken from control animals. **A:** One of the prominent features following the restoration process is the increase in complex synapses (open arrows), along with noncomplex synaptic contacts (closed arrows). **B:** There appears to be an increase in the density of multiple synaptic contacts (*). Typically the multiple contacts consist of a presynaptic element making contact with several simple noncomplex postsynaptic specializations displaying prominent postsynaptic densities (closed arrows).

the neuropil would only increase the density to 14 synapses per 100 μm^2.

Lynch et al. (1975) determined that the shrinkage of the molecular layer does not occur until about 5 days after the entorhinal lesion and progresses in a linear fashion until about day 15 postlesion. Based upon an 80% reinnervation rate of normal synaptic contacts and a 30% decline in the neuropil, the actual lesion-induced synaptogenesis would result in only a 56% replacement of total lost synaptic contacts. This fact does not, however, negate the principal idea that following massive denervation of the neuropil, a significant amount of synaptogenesis occurs.

It is important at this time to draw attention to an interesting aspect of the self-repair process. Regardless of whether or not there is a collapse of the neuropil, the synaptic density in the denervated area appears to approach normal. The most convincing evidence for lesion-induced synaptogenesis and the regulation of synaptic density is derived from those studies that show significant denervation and subsequent reinnervation without shrinkage (McWilliams and Lynch, 1979; Nadler et al., 1980; Anderson et al., 1986a). In these studies, the percentage of innervation was between 85% and 100% of control with no hyperinnervation. A careful look at the neuropil certainly reveals the fact that the area is capable of supporting a greater density of synapses. Perhaps the target neuron signals the inhibition of synapse formation.

TOTAL SYNAPSE COUNT

In every quantitative study evaluating the loss and return of synaptic contacts, one quickly realizes that the number of degenerating contacts summed with the number of nondegenerating contacts does not equal the normal synaptic density. If the number of degenerating synapses were as great as the number of intact synapses lost, a simple relationship would exist, and a mechanism of synapse replacement that is intuitively simple would follow. Unfortunately, that is not the case. Two possibilities might account for the discrepancy in determining the total synaptic count. First, it appears that the degenerating synapses are removed quickly. In a recent study, glucocorticoids, which appear to stabilize cell mem-

branes, were employed to slow the rate of degeneration in the hippocampus following an entorhinal cortex lesion (Scheff et al., 1986). The net effect was a highly significant increase in the density of degenerating synapses at early postlesion survival times, compared with subjects not receiving the steroid. In animals with the steroid, the membranes were not quickly broken down or removed quickly by the glial cells. As was mentioned earlier, the glial cells, which play an important role in the "clean-up" process, are activated almost immediately after the trauma. In the steroid-treated animals, the total number of intact and degenerating synapses more closely approximated the preinjury synaptic density, even at early postlesion survival times. Glucocorticoids by themselves do not appear to disrupt the normal synaptic density.

The second point to consider when assessing the total number of synaptic contacts relates to the morphological changes that can occur during the process of degeneration. Many synaptic contacts may be degenerating, but they no longer appear as synaptic contacts. The usual criteria for identifying a synaptic contact is a presynaptic element with vesicles in association with a postsynaptic element. As the dying contacts become more electron-dense, it is sometimes difficult to identify any of the organelles in the axoplasm. Degenerating synapses might be misinterpreted as debris rather than as actual contacts. It is also known that during the process of degeneration, the dying presynaptic element is often dissociated from the postsynaptic element, once again rejecting the criterion for a synapse. One final possibility to consider in this regard is the fact that the postsynaptic element may retract from the presynaptic terminal before it becomes electron-dense. The target cell may somehow "sense" that certain synaptic contacts are no longer functional and begin to "shed" these synapses. The degenerating synapses then may appear as free terminal endings.

SIZE OF SYNAPSES

Change in synaptic size has only recently been carefully investigated (Hillman and Chen, 1985). Increase in size of new or residual synaptic contacts may be a mechanism to help stabilize transmitter release and receptor activation. It may be a mechanism to increase synaptic efficiency. In one of the early studies in which the loss and reacquisition of synaptic contacts in the denervated hippocampal dentate gyrus were monitored, Matthews et al. (1976b) reported an increase in synaptic profile length. After a long survival time, there appears to be a 16% increase in synaptic diameter. If one considers the simple synaptic contact as a disk, then there is significant increase in total synaptic area in the reinnervated neuropil. Significant change in the length of the synaptic contacts in the denervated neuropil has not been observed in other studies, possibly as a result of many different factors. It is unclear, for instance, whether or not the increase observed by Matthews et al. was limited to simple synaptic contacts and exactly what percentage of the total identified synaptic population was measured. Since it is known that the density of complex synapses does increase as a function of some lesions, one would expect the size of the contact area to increase proportionately. The increase was also observed at extremely long posttrauma survival times, and in many of the other studies in which remodeling has been examined, the same temporal sequence was not employed. Increases in the size of contacts have been observed in other areas of the central nervous system after different manipulations (Hillman and Chen, 1985).

NONDENERVATED AREAS

It appears that not only does the area directly denervated as a result of the damage respond with synaptic remodeling, but also nondenervated areas of the neuropil and areas not directly denervated respond as well (Matthews et al., 1976b; Hoff et al., 1981). As a result of an entorhinal cortex lesion, there is a decrease in the density of synapses in the inner one-third of the dentate gyrus molecular area, that zone normally occupied by commissural and associational afferents. The response appears to be both ipsilateral and contralateral. The ipsilateral inner one-third of the molecular zone shows a sharp decrease in the density of normal synapses, followed by a return to normal levels. At 4 days after the entorhinal lesion, there is a 20% reduction of nondegenerating contacts in the inner one-third. By 10 days af-

ter the trauma, this neuropil has recovered to control levels. Small synapses with noncomplex synaptic junctions appear to participate in this change. At long postlesion survival times, there appears to be a slight increase in density, compared with normal densities.

The contralateral inner one-third of the molecular layer also responds and undergoes a similar decrease in synaptic density, followed by a return in the number of synapses. The time course for this transient change on the contralateral side is much longer than on the ipsilateral side. Little degeneration appears to be associated with the fluctuations in the synaptic densities. However, a number of vacant postsynaptic specializations are present. These changes suggest that an actual remodeling or "turnover" of existing synapases can occur in addition to the lesion-induced direct denervation synaptogenesis.

The mechanism responsible for this "shedding" and reacquisition of contacts in nondenervated zones is largely speculative at present. In the case of entorhinal cortex damage, the turnover might be linked to the subsequent reactive outgrowth of commissural and associational fibers, which play a role in the restoration of the denervated area. On the other hand, the denervated granule cells may somehow temporarily alter the accumulation of trophic material that is used to maintain shaft contacts. As the cells reestablish their equilibrium, the synapses are replaced.

SOURCE OF NEW CONTACTS

While careful evaluation of the loss and replacement of synaptic contacts can provide a direct measurement of the extent of the repair process, it provides little information on the specific afferents that are responsible for the new contacts. Many studies have carefully detailed at least some of these afferents and their time course of growth.

Septohippocampal Pathway

The first afferent pathway known to respond to a lesion of the entorhinal cortex was the cholinergic septohippocampal pathway (Lynch et al., 1972). These fibers, which normally occupy the outer two-thirds of the granule cell dendritic tree, appear to reorganize their afferent input and restrict it to the outer one-third

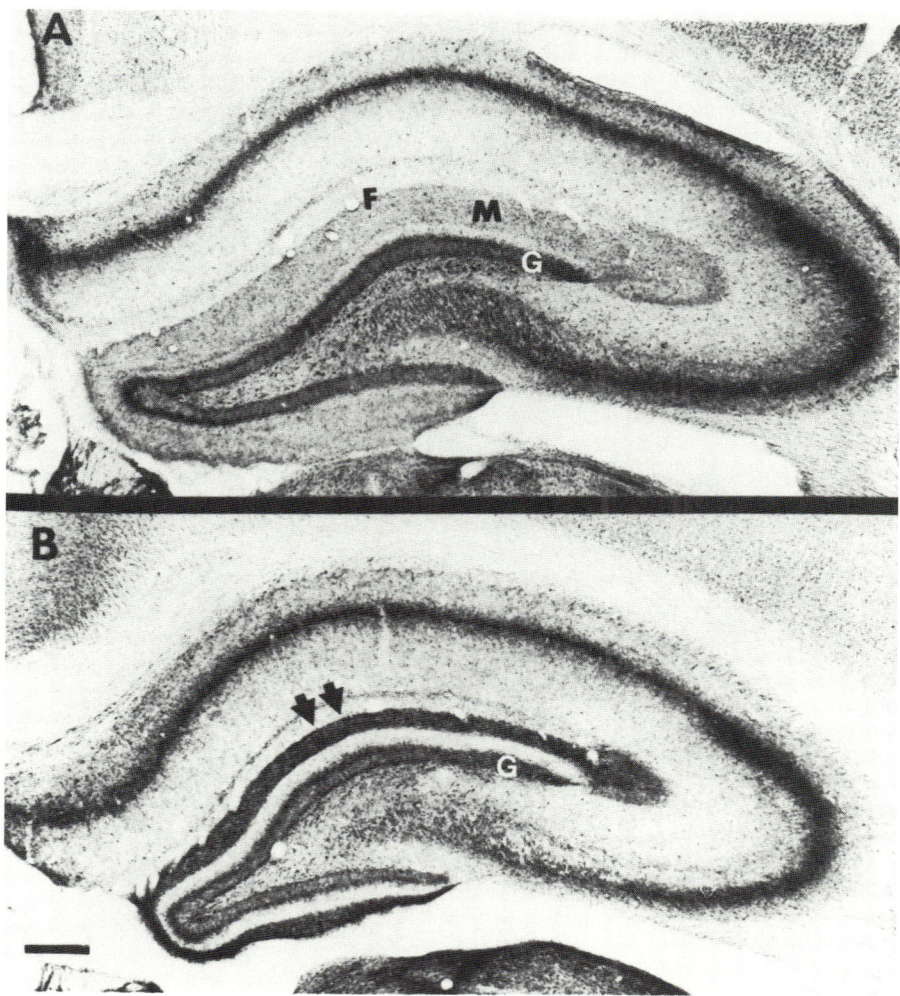

Figure 9–9.   Coronal sections of the rodent hippocampal formation stained for the enzyme acetyl-cholinesterase (AChE), a marker used to monitor the septohippocampal projections. **A:** Normal staining pattern. Note the even distribution of staining in the molecular layer (M) of the dentate gyrus immediately below the hippocampal fissure (F). A small band devoid of staining can be observed above the granule cells (G) and indicates the zone occupied by the commissural and associational afferents. **B:** Staining pattern 15 days after an ipsilateral entorhinal cortex lesion. An intense band of staining (arrows) forms in the outer portion of the molecular layer just below the fissure. The clear zone immediately above the granule cells (G) is more prominent and wider, indicative of the out-growth of commissural and associational fibers in response to the lesion. Scale bar = 300 μm.

of the molecular layer (Fig. 9–9). The most common procedure to monitor changes in this pathway is to monitor the distribution of AChE staining. Between 4 and 6 days after an ento-rhinal lesion, there is a significant intensifica-tion of AChE stain in the outer one-third of the

molecular layer, which further increases with greater posttrauma survival times (Nadler, 1977a,b). Two lines of evidence place the ori-gin of these afferents in the septal area. First, most of the AChE in the hippocampus has been localized to axons and terminals of the

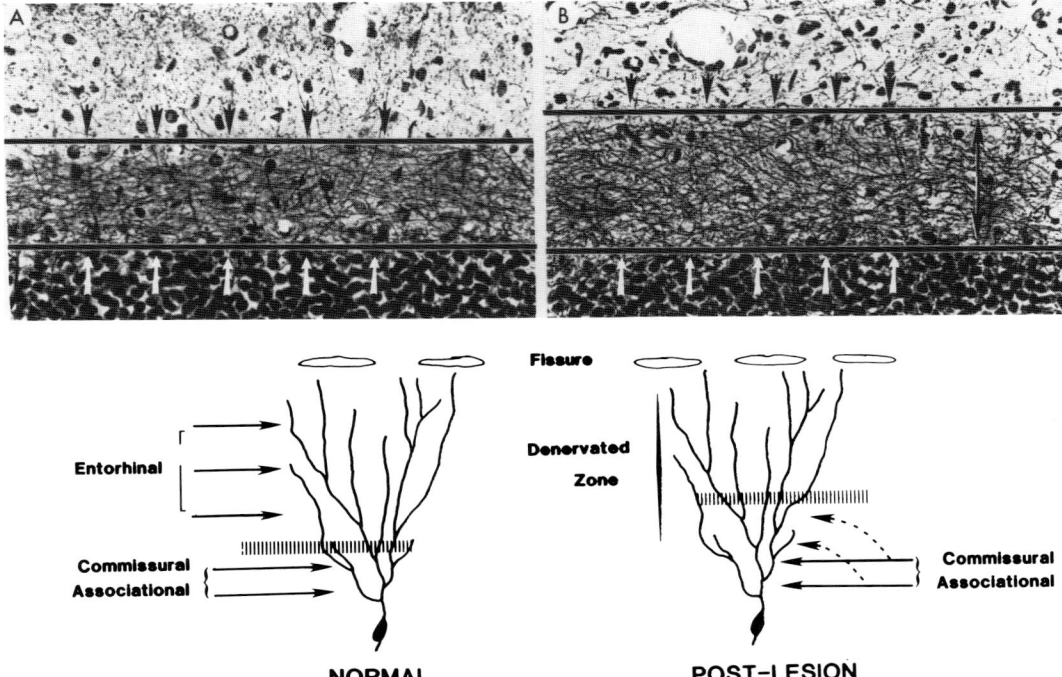

Figure 9–10.   Upper panel: Afferent fibers in the molecular layer of the dentate gyrus demonstrated by the Holmes silver method after an ipsilateral entorhinal lesion. **A:** The ipsilateral entorhinal projection was removed 2 days prior to processing of the tissue and represents the normal width of the commissural-associational projection to the inner one-third of the molecular layer. **B:** The same area of the dentate gyrus molecular layer shown from an animal allowed to survive 15 days after the cortical ablation. Lines, demarcated by arrows, indicate the boundaries used for determination of changes in the width of this fiber plexus. **Lower panel:** Schematic diagram of the response of the commissural and associational fibers following an entorhinal lesion. The fibers, which normally occupy the inner portion of the granule cell dendritic tree, grow axon collaterals, which actually invade the territory previously occupied by the entorhinal afferents. Subsequently the axon sprouting results in the establishment of new synaptic contacts in the denervated zone.

septal area (Shute and Lewis, 1966; Cotman et al., 1973) and second, a secondary lesion of the medial septal nucleus eliminates the appearance of the intense band of staining (Lynch et al., 1972). It is important to note, however, that the histochemical method of evaluating the sprouting of septohippocampal afferents is not a direct measurement of the extent of the projection. While the increase in staining as a result of the lesion could be explained by increases in the number of septohippocampl fibers and terminals, it could also be the result of an increase in the normal population of these terminals. However, the correlation between the time course of terminal proliferation

in the denervated zone and the increase in AChE staining is very striking.

Commissural and Associational Afferents

These afferent fibers, which normally occupy the inner one-third of the granule cell dendritic tree, expand their terminal field in response to an entorhinal lesion (Fig. 9–10). This type of growth is easily monitored by employing normal fiber stains such as the Holmes or Bodian. Because of the entorhinal lesion, the only axons that stain in the inner molecular layer are the commissural and associational fibers. Changes in the width of these fibers can be used to quantitate the outgrowth. In young adult animals this fiber outgrowth begins rapidly following the lesion, and significant growth can be observed within 5 or 6 days (Lynch et al., 1976, 1977; Scheff et al., 1978, 1980). The expansion of this fiber plexus is initially rapid but appears to be virtually complete by 45 days after the injury (unpublished observation). The outgrowth of the commissural and associational afferents closely follows the initial replacement of lost synaptic contacts. Electrophysiological studies have provided considerable evidence that this expanded system is functional as early as 9 days after the trauma (West et al., 1975). It is interesting that the septohippocampal fibers do not appear to overlap with the newly expanded commissural and associational fibers; these systems rigidly adhere to the normal laminar profile. The expanded fiber plexus always appears to be as dense as that found in normal animals, suggesting that new fibers are formed from parent fibers in the old commissural-associational zone.

Contralateral Entorhinal Cortex Afferents

Afferents from the contralateral entorhinal cortex normally send a sparse projection to the outer two-thirds of the dentate gyrus molecular layer. The time course and extent of changes in this pathway have been carefully studied using a variety of neuroanatomical and electrophysiological methods. By employing autoradiographic tract tracing methods, it has been determined that this crossed entorhinal cortex projection increases in density between 6 and 8 days postlesion (Steward and Loesche, 1977). The proliferation of this pathway continues for several months. Considering that the crossed afferents are collaterals of the ipsilateral pathway from the entorhinal cortex to the dentate gyrus (Steward and Vinsant, 1978a,b), the pathway appears to be very important. Electrophysiological experiments have determined that it is functional as early as 6 days after the trauma and closely follows terminal proliferation in the denervated zone, as measured with the electron microscope (Steward et al., 1974). These new cortical synapses appear to account for only a small portion of the new contacts formed in response to the lesion (Cotman et al., 1977).

Other Afferents

Interneurons found in the dentate gyrus (Anderson et al., 1986b) appear to respond to the trauma also. GABA-ergic interneurons increase their enzyme levels and the amount of GABA released (Nadler et al., 1974, 1977a). Not all afferents appear to sprout in response to the denervation. In the case of the entorhinal cortex lesion, which denervates the outer two-thirds of the granule cell dendritic tree, the locus coeruleus afferents and terminals do not proliferate, even though they normally project to the area denervated. A commissural lesion, which partially denervates the inner one-third of the granule cell dendrite, triggers synapse replacement by its ipsilateral homologue, the associational fibers. This commissural lesion, however, fails to elicit any quantitative response from the entorhinal cortex afferents. Combined commissural and Schaffer collateral removal, while resulting in massive denervation of the proximal three-quarters of the CA1 pyramidal cell dendrite, fails to entice changes in septal afferents to the denervated area or translaminar growth of entorhinal fibers found in the lacunosum-moleculare region (Fig. 9–3). Nevertheless, the synaptic density in the CA1 area of the hippocampal formation is restored following such a lesion (Goldowitz et al., 1979; Nadler et al., 1980).

CONCLUSIONS

Although the hippocampal formation has been used extensively as a model system to study the self-repair process in the central nervous system, certain principles can be derived from these studies that can be generalized to other areas of the brain. First, following partial denervation, resulting in the loss of as much as 85–90% of the total synaptic input, the area is almost completely restored. This restoration is not specific to a particular type of denervation.

Second, the self-repair process is initiated quickly, beginning with the immediate removal of degenerative debris and the replacement of lost synaptic contacts. This self-repair process continues for several months, eventually leading to almost complete restoration. The self-repair is composed of two different processes that operate at the same time and follow a similar time course (Fig. 9–11). There

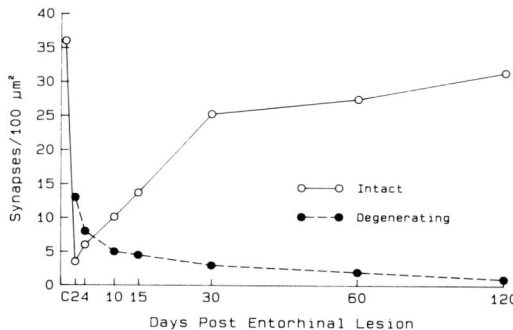

Figure 9–11. Time course of the changes in synaptic density, both intact and degenerating, in the dorsal leaf of the rodent dentate gyrus (outer two-thirds of molecular layer) after ipsilateral removal of the entorhinal cortex. Note the delay in formation of new synaptic contacts and the inverse relationship between the removal of degenerating synapses and the formation of new ones.

is a high correlation between the removal of degenerating synaptic contacts and the replacement of lost synaptic contacts. It appears that the rate of removal of degenerating synapses is proportional to the rate of new synapse construction. While this high correlation would suggest a rate-limiting effect of one upon the other, such an effect does not necessarily appear to be the case (Scheff et al., 1986).

Third, the general appearance of the newly formed synaptic contacts is remarkably similar to those normally present, suggesting that the reinnervation is a property of afferents normally residing within the denervated area itself or within the general vicinity of the neuropil. In the hippocampus, the new synaptic contacts are asymmetric, Gray type I, with round vesicles clustered near the typical synaptic junction. The neuropil has a remarkably similar appearance after long posttrauma survival. The synapses are found on dendritic shafts and spines similar to those lost. There does not appear to be any increase in symmetric or axoaxonic contacts.

Fourth, the density of synaptic contacts in the restored neuropil is almost identical to that prior to the damage. Even though rare cases of hyperinnervation have been noted, the most common finding is a return to normal synaptic

density regardless of whether or not shrinkage is a factor. This finding indicates that the mechanisms that regulate the density, including trophic agents and growth retardants, are fully operational. In the normal state, the neuropil is quiescent, and the partial denervation induces the area to manifest its growth capacity.

Fifth, since no new pathways appear to be created, the reinnervation must occur as a result of translaminar growth or a redistribution of residual terminals within the damaged area. There appears to be some hierarchy, which lies within the residual afferents, in the capacity of afferents to grow in response to a specific lesion. Clearly the reinnervation is selective, since certain afferents do not respond even though the denervation is within their synaptic territory. For example, neither septohippocampal nor entorhinal afferents appear to respond to a commissural and or associational afferent lesion.

Sheer amount of degeneration does not seem to be the principal factor in determining which afferents are responsible for the reinnervation, yet the system appears capable of recovering pretrauma synaptic densities. Which afferent fibers are destroyed may be one of the more important factors in determining the final circuitry. The best possible outcome following partial denervation would be complete reinnervation by the original afferents that were destroyed, "true regeneration." However, in the case of entorhinal cortex removal, that does not appear to be the case. The next best outcome would be repopulation by homologous afferents. Again, employing the outcome after a unilateral entorhinal cortex lesion, proliferation of the crossed entorhinal projection would be appropriate. While the expansion of this normally sparse pathway does occur, it probably is not responsible for the major portion of the reinnervation. The denervated target, the granule cells, appears to receive new synapses from sources not homologous to that lost. Both septal afferents and commissural and associational afferents participate in the restoration, and these afferents have little relation to the circuitry that was destroyed.

One can only speculate as to the functional consequences of this reorganization of the laminar profile within the dentate gyrus. While there has been some attempt at assessing the functional outcome (Steward, 1982), it has been largely correlative in nature. Perhaps the exact origin of the synaptic contacts is not nearly as important as the type (single vs. multiple; excitatory vs. inhibitory; simple vs. complex).

Both light and electron microscopic studies of partial denervation of the hippocampal formation underscore the remarkable capacity of the central nervous system to compensate for the loss of specific afferent input. The system does not appear to enter a state of "shock" immediately following the damage, but instead activates other areas to "take over," so to speak, for the lost connections. Certainly a reorganization occurs. The end result of this reorganization must be a form of "behavioral substitution," since the system must respond in a different manner to a particular stimulus. The significance, then, of the capacity of the central nervous system to reorganize is beyond the morphological changes that can be observed with the light or electron microscope. These studies suggest that synaptic connections are capable of an immense amount of "turnover," which probably occurs on an everyday basis without massive denervation (Cotman et al., 1981). The simple fact that we can adapt to a variety of behavioral situations ensures our survival in an ever-changing environment. Our ability to accept new ideas, to remember those ideas, and to act upon them at some later time is testimony to the plasticity of the nervous system.

ACKNOWLEDGMENTS

Special thanks to my students and collaborators, Drs. Kevin Anderson, Joanne Morse, Steve Hoff, Larry Benardo, and Steve DeKosky. Thanks to Doug Price for technical help in the electron microscopic studies and Le Ann Johnston for help in the light microscopy. The author gratefully acknowledges the support provided by National Institute of Health Research Grants NS 16981 and NS 21541.

REFERENCES

Anderson KJ, Scheff SW, DeKosky ST (1986a): Reactive synaptogenesis in hippocampal area CA1 of aged and young adult rats. J Comp Neurol 252:374–384.

Anderson KJ, Maley BE, Scheff SW (1986b): Immunocytochemical localization of GABA in the rat hippocampal formation. Neurosci Lett 69:7–12.

Blackstad TW (1958): On the termination of some afferents to the hippocampus and the fascia dentata. An experimental study in the rat. Acta Anat 35:202–214.

Blackstad TW (1963): Ultrastructural studies on the hippocampal region. Prog Brain Res 3:122–148.

Cotman CW, Matthews DA, Taylor D, Lynch G (1973): Synaptic rearrangement in the dentate gyrus: Histochemical evidence of adjustments after lesions in immature and adult rats. Proc Natl Acad Sci USA 70:3473–3477.

Cotman C, Gentry C, Steward O (1977): Synaptic replacement in the dentate gyrus after unilateral entorhinal lesion: Electron microscopic analysis of the extent of replacement of synapses by the remaining entorhinal cortex. J Neurocytol 6:455–464.

Cotman CW, Nieto-Sampedro M, Harris EW (1981): Synapse replacement in the nervous system of adult vertebrates. Physiol Rev 61:684–784.

Coyle P (1978): Spatial features of the rat hippocampal vascular system. Exp Neurol 58:549–561.

Exner S (1885): Notiz zu der Frage von der Faservertheilung mehrerer Nerven in einem Muskel. Pfluegers Arch 36:572–576.

Fifkova E (1975): Two types of terminal degeneration in the molecular layer of the dentate fascia following lesion of the entorhinal cortex. Brain Res 96:169–175.

Finger S, Stein DG (1982): "Brain Damage and Recovery: Research and Clinical Perspectives." New York: Academic Press, pp 1–352.

Gall C, Rose G, Lynch G (1979): Proliferative and migratory activity of glial cells in the partially deafferented hippocampus. J Comp Neurol 183:539–550.

Goldowitz D, Cotman CW (1980): Do neurotrophic interactions control synapse formation in the adult rat brain? Brain Res 181:325–344.

Goldowitz D, White W, Steward O, Cotman C, Lynch G (1975): Anatomical evidence for a projection from the entorhinal cortex to the contralateral dentate gyrus of the rat. Exp Neurol 47:433–441.

Goldowitz D, Scheff SW, Cotman CW (1979): The specificity of reactive synaptogenesis: A comparative study in the adult rat hippocampal formation. Brain Res 170:427–441.

Hillman DE, Chen S (1985): Plasticity in the size of presynaptic and postsynaptic membrane specializations. In Cotman CW (ed): "Synaptic Plasticity." New York: Guilford Press, pp 39–76.

Hoff SF, Scheff SW, Kwan AY, Cotman CW (1981): A new type of lesion-induced synaptogenesis: I. Turnover in non-denervated zones of the dentate gyrus in young adult rats. Brain Res 222:1–13.

Hoff SF, Scheff SW, Benardo LS, Cotman CW (1982a): Lesion-induced synaptogenesis in the dentate gyrus of aged rats: I. Loss and reaquisition of normal synaptic density. J Comp Neurol 205:246–252.

Hoff SF, Scheff SW, Benardo LS, Cotman CW (1982b): Lesion-induced synaptogenesis in the dentate gyrus of aged rats: II. Demonstration of an impaired degeneration clearing response. J Comp Neurol 205:253–259.

Laatsch RH, Cowan WM (1966): Electron microscopic studies of the dentate gyrus of the rat. I. Normal structure. J Comp Neurol 128:359–396.

Lee KS, Stanford EJ, Cotman CW, Lynch GS (1977): Ultrastructural evidence for bouton proliferation in the partially deafferented dentate gyrus of the adult rat. Exp Brain Res 29:475–485.

Lynch GS, Matthews DA, Mosko S, Parks T, Cotman CW (1972): Induced acetylcholinesterase-rich layer in the rat dentate gyrus following entorhinal lesions. Brain Res 42:311–318.

Lynch GS, Rose G, Gall C, Cotman CW (1975): The response of the dentate gyrus to partial deafferentation. In Santini M (ed): "Golgi Centennial Symposium: Perspectives in Neurobiology." New York: Raven Press, pp 305–317.

Lynch GS, Gall C, Rose G, Cotman CW (1976): Changes in the distribution of the dentate gyrus associational system following unilateral or bilateral entorhinal lesions in the adult rat. Brain Res 110:57–71.

Lynch GS, Gall C, Cotman C (1977): Temporal parameters of axon "sprouting" in the brain of the adult rat. Exp Neurol 54:179–183.

Matthews DA, Cotman CW, Lynch G (1976a): An electron microscopic study of lesion-induced synaptogenesis in the dentate gyrus of the adult rat: I. Magnitude and time course of degeneration. Brain Res 115:1–21.

Matthews DA, Cotman CW, Lynch G (1976b): An electron microscopic study of lesion-induced synaptogenesis in the dentate gyrus of the adult rat: II. Reappearance of morphologically normal contacts. Brain Res 115:23–41.

McWilliams JR, Lynch G (1978): Terminal proliferation and synaptogenesis following partial deafferentation: The reinnervation of the inner molecular layer of the dentate gyrus following removal of its commissural afferents. J Comp Neurol 180:581–616.

McWilliams JR, Lynch G (1979): Terminal proliferation in the partially deafferented dentate gyrus: Time courses for the appearance and removal of degeneration and the replacement of lost terminals. J Comp Neurol 187:191–198.

Nadler JV, Cotman CW, Lynch GS (1974): Biochemical plasticity of short-axon interneurons: Increased glutamate decarboxylase activity in the denervated area of rat dentate gyrus following entorhinal lesion. Exp Neurol 45:403–412.

Nadler JV, White WF, Vaca KW, Cotman CW (1977a): Calcium-dependent γ-aminobutyrate release by interneurons of rat hippocampal region: Lesion-induced plasticity. Brain Res 131:241–258.

Nadler JV, Cotman CW, Lynch GS (1977b): Histochemical evidence of altered development of cholinergic fibers in the rat dentate gyrus following lesion. I. Time course after complete unilateral entorhinal lesion at various ages. J Comp Neurol 171:561–588.

Nadler JV, Perry BW, Gentry C, Cotman CW (1980): Loss and reacquisition of hippocampal synapses after selective destruction of CA3-CA4 afferents with kainic acid. Brain Res 191:387–403.

Nieto-Sampedro M, Cotman CW (1985): Growth factor induction and temporal order in central nervous system repair. In Cotman CW (ed): "Synaptic Plasticity." New York: Guilford Press, pp 407–455.

Raisman G (1969): Neuronal plasticity in the septal nuclei of the adult rat. Brain Res 14:25–48.

Raisman G, Field PM (1973): A quantitative investigation of the development of collateral reinnervation after partial deafferentation of the septal nuclei. Brain Res 50:241–264.

Ramón y Cajal S (1893): "Über die feinere Struktur des Ammonshornes," translated by von Kölliker A. Z Wissen Zool 56:613–663.

Ramón y Cajal S (1928): "Degeneration and Regeneration of the Nervous System." London: Oxford University.

Rose G, Lynch G, Cotman CW (1976): Hypertrophy and redistribution of astrocytes in the deafferented dentate gyrus. Brain Res Bull 1:87–92.

Scheff SW, Benardo LS, Cotman CW (1978): Effect of serial lesions on sprouting in the dentate gyrus: Onset and decline of the catalytic effect. Brain Res 150:45–53.

Scheff SW, Benardo LS, Cotman CW (1980): Decline in reactive fiber growth in the dentate gyrus of aged rats compared to young adult rats following entorhinal cortex removal. Brain Res 199:21–38.

Scheff SW, Hoff SF, Anderson KJ (1986): Altered regulation of lesion-induced synaptogenesis by adrenalectomy and elevated corticosterone in young adult rats. Exp Neurol 96:1–15.

Shute CCD, Lewis PR (1966): Electron microscopy of cholinergic terminals and acetylcholinesterase-containing neurones in the hippocampal formation of the rat. Z Zellforsch 69:334–343.

Steward O (1982): Assessing the functional significance of lesion-induced neuronal plasticity. Int Rev Neurobiol 23:197–254.

Steward O (1986): Lesion-induced synapse growth in the hippocampus: In search of cellular and molecular mechanisms. In Isaacson RL, Pribram KH (eds): "The Hippocampus," vol 3. New York: Plenum Press, pp 65–111.

Steward O, Cotman CW, Lynch GS (1974): Growth of a new fiber projection in the brain of adult rats: Reinnervation of the dentate gyrus by the contralateral entorhinal cortex following ipsilateral entorhinal lesions. Exp Brain Res 20:45–66.

Steward O, Loesche J (1977): Quantitative autoradiographic analysis of the time course of proliferation of contralateral entorhinal efferents in the dentate gyrus denervated by ipsilateral entorhinal lesions. Brain Res 125:11–21.

Steward O, Vinsant SV (1978a): Identification of the cells of origin of a central pathway which sprouts following lesions in mature rats. Brain Res 147:223–243.

Steward O, Vinsant SV (1978b): Collateral projections of cells in the surviving entorhinal area which reinnervate the dentate gyrus of the rat following unilateral entorhinal lesions. Brain Res 149:216–222.

Steward O, Vinsant SL (1983): The process of reinnervation in the dentate gyrus of the adult rat: A quantitative electron microscopic analysis of terminal proliferation and reactive synaptogenesis. J Comp Neurol 214:370–386.

West JR, Deadwyler SA, Cotman CW, Lynch GS (1975): Time-dependent changes in commissural field potentials in the dentate gyrus following lesions of the entorhinal cortex in adult rats. Brain Res 97:215–233.

10

Recovery Mechanisms in Spinal Cord Injury: Implications for Regenerative Therapy

WISE YOUNG, MD, PhD

Department of Neurosurgery, New York University Medical Center, New York, New York 10016

Spinal cord injury disconnects the brain from the body by damaging the major conduit through which sensory and motor signals pass. The condition has long been believed to be irreversible (Breasted, 1930). Early descriptions of the abortive attempts by injured spinal axons to regrow (Ramón y Cajal, 1928) convinced several generations of neuroscientists that the major obstacle to functional recovery in spinal cord injury is the inability of the central nervous system (CNS) to regenerate. Three decades of research on the subject have shown that not only can injured central neurons sprout neurites that can synapse on other neurons but that these neurites can grow long distances in peripheral nerves, only to stop when they reach central nervous tissues (David and Aguayo, 1981; Bray and Aguayo, Chapter 5, this volume). These findings suggest that the failure of spinal axonal regeneration stems not from an intrinsic inability of central neurons to grow and reconnect but rather from the presence or absence of factors in the CNS that block or stimulate neuronal growth. This notion stimulated an intense search for factors that control neural growth in central nervous tissues (Varon et al., Chapter 7, this volume).

Many neuroscientists believe that regeneration is the only hope for recovery from spinal cord injury. A growing body of evidence, however, suggests that regeneration is neither sufficient nor required for recovery. In this article, I will review evidence showing that substantial functional recovery occurs even in severe spinal cord injuries, that astonishingly few axons are needed to support the recovery, that axonal dysfunction contributes to the functional deficits of spinal cord injury, and that the spinal cord possesses remarkable capabilities for independent segmental function. I shall argue that animals have evolved effective alternative mechanisms for recovery from spinal cord injury and that regeneration may have been selected against in evolution because it is too slow to contribute to survival. The implications of these findings for regenerative therapy of spinal cord injury will be discussed.

TRANSECTIONS VS. CONTUSIONS

Many investigators use physically transected spinal cords for studying spinal cord regeneration. Complete severance of the spinal cord has been stipulated as a prerequisite for rigorous demonstrations of regeneration in the spinal cord (Guth et al., 1980b). A sharp knife drawn across an exposed rat spinal cord will often leave a small ventral portion of the cord intact, allowing rats to recover from such injuries (Guth et al., 1980a). Failure to cut the spinal cord completely has, therefore, been used to dismiss studies claiming treatment effects (Matinian and Andreasian, 1976). Transected spinal cords, however, are rarely encountered in human spinal cord injury. In the vast majority of clinical spinal injuries, the cord is not only physically intact but usually free of continuing compression by bony fragments. At

Neural Regeneration and Transplantation, pages 157–169
© 1989 Alan R. Liss, Inc.

surgery, the injury site often cannot be identified visually from the dural surface.

Protection of the spinal cord against penetrating trauma must have received very high priority in evolution. This is evident from the elaborate vertebral bony armor present in all animals with spinal cords. The spinal cord is protected in other effective but more subtle ways. For example, the cord is situated in a pressurized fluid environment, contained by a tough dural sack. The dural tube redistributes compressive forces, causing the maximum shear to the innermost part of the spinal cord, similar to the way compressing a toothpaste tube will squeeze paste from the center of the tube. Spinal tissues close to the dural surface are relatively protected from stretching and shear forces. Note that the ventral spinal cord is unusually reinforced by a penetrating sulcus. The sulcus will not only deflect compressive forces but will reduce axonal stretching of axons situated close to it. The spinal tracts most important for functional recovery are situated close to the dural surface. Nowhere else is the CNS organized in this manner, with the most critical structures situated closest to the dural surface.

The effectiveness of these protective mechanisms is strongly supported by clinical statistics. The annual incidence of spinal cord injuries causing lasting neurological deficits and requiring hospitalizations is probably less than 10,000 per year in the United States (Anderson and McLaurin, 1980; Bracken et al., 1981; Ergas, 1985). This is a tiny fraction of the millions of vehicular, sports, and work-related accidents that involve possible trauma to the spinal cord. Because of the vertebral armor and the dural tube, almost all spinal cord injuries observed clinically result from blunt, nonpenetrating contusions of the cord with a varying degree of continued compression. The only exceptions are direct knife and gunshot wounds of the spinal cord. Contused spinal cords almost invariably manifest with hemorrhagic lesions centered in gray matter. This pathological pattern occurs in spinal cords injured by a variety of causes. Preservation of a thin rim of white matter close to the dural surface is commonly observed in clinical pathological examinations of injured human spinal cords (Kakulas and Bedbrook, 1976; Kakulas, 1985a,b).

Transected spinal cords therefore fail to model human spinal cord injury in several essential respects. First, due to the natural tension present in spinal cords, the two ends of a cut cord will separate. Such a gap is rarely, if ever, present in human spinal cord injury. Growing axons may not regenerate well in severed spinal cords for the same reasons axons do not regenerate in cut and poorly opposed peripheral nerves. Second, in order to cut the spinal cord, the dura has to be opened, allowing invasion by external cells. These cells may critically alter the environment of the injury site. The consistent failure to demonstrate spontaneous spinal regeneration in the past may have been an artifact of the transection model. As more investigators have begun to look for regeneration in partially lesioned spinal cords, the number of reports of axonal regeneration in the spinal cord has increased (Borgens et al., 1986a,b). Finally, in the vast majority of injured human spinal cords, some axons survive the injury. In transected spinal cords, the interactions between regenerating and surviving axons cannot be studied.

FUNCTIONAL RECOVERY IN SPINAL CORD INJURY

A poor prognosis for severe spinal cord injury is widely accepted among both lay people and professionals who care for the spinal-injured. Although the prospects for survival by spinal-injured patients have improved significantly in the past 3 decades, many clinicians still hold deeply pessimistic views concerning the possibility of functional recovery in spinal cord injury. This pessimism in turn has led to the popular perception that regeneration is the only route to functional recovery in spinal cord injury. A closer examination of the clinical data, however, suggests that this pessimistic view is extreme and may not be applicable to most spinal-injured patients.

In a recent multicenter trial examining the treatment of acute spinal cord injury with methylprednisolone (MP), detailed neurological data were collected on more than 300 patients from nine spinal cord injury centers in the United States. Called the National Acute Spinal Cord Injury Study (NASCIS) (Bracken et al., 1984), the study compared 100-mg and 1,000-mg doses of MP treatments given within

Scores (range 14 to 84)

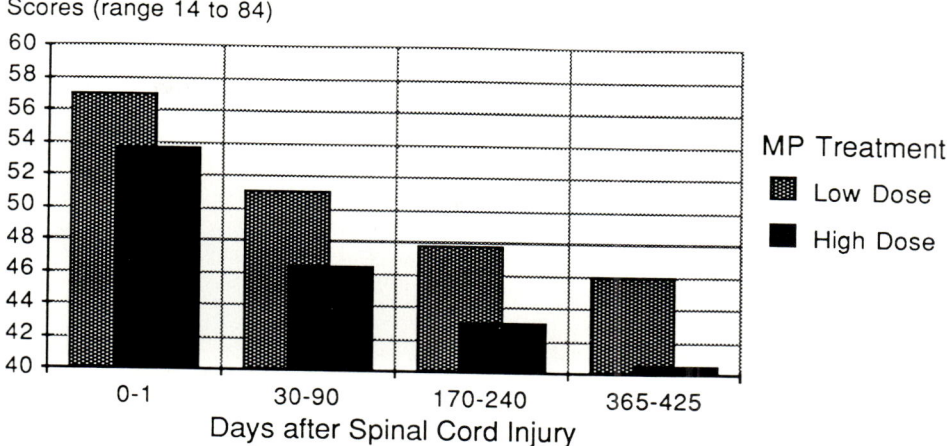

Figure 10–1.   Mean motor deficit scores in patients treated with methylprednisolone (MP) at either 100 mg per day (low dose) or 1,000 mg per day (high dose) for 10 days after spinal cord injury. The mean scores represent summed motor deficits in 14 major muscle groups scored on a scale of 1 to 6 (representing normal to paralysis), where 84 is complete loss of motor function in all major muscle groups tested, and 14 represents no loss. The mean scores were obtained from 130–150 patients per treatment group. The patients include thoracic and cervical spinal cord injuries with motor losses ranging from plegic to paretic.

24 hr after injury and daily for 10 days. The patients were followed for up to a year after their injuries (Bracken et al., 1985). Although the differences between the groups with high- and low-dose treatments did not turn out to be statistically significant, the extent of recovery that occurs in spinal cord injury provides some interesting insights into the potential for recovery in patients with such injury.

Neurological recovery is common in spinal-injured patients. Approximately one-half of spinal-injured patients (51%) studied at these tertiary care centers had complete paralysis and sensory loss below the lesion level at the time of admission, within 48 hr of injury. Patients with paralysis and partial sensory losses accounted for 21% of the population, while 28% had partial motor and sensory deficits. Figure 10–1 shows the mean motor deficit scores in these patients; 84 represents complete loss of motor function in all muscle groups examined, and 14 indicates no loss. Note the definite recovery of motor function from admission to 1 year after injury in both groups ($P < 0.001$). Likewise, there was a significant improvement in sensory responses to

both pinprick and touch (Figs. 10–2, 10–3) in all groups. Thus, even in severe spinal cord injury, some recovery is the rule rather than the exception.

The available clinical data probably underestimate the extent of neurological recovery from spinal cord injury. The population of patients studied in tertiary care centers, such as the NYU-Bellevue Spinal Cord Injury Center and other institutions associated with the NASCIS trial, is skewed toward more severe injuries. Many patients who have suffered mild spinal cord injuries and who subsequently recover are not referred to our centers and are not represented in the data collected in the NASCIS trial. It is likely that a more general population of spinal-injured patients will have fewer severe injuries and a higher incidence of spontaneous recovery. Despite this omission, many of the patients studied in the NASCIS trial, in all categories of injury ranging from complete to partial motor and sensory loss, showed significant recovery. Recovery from spinal cord injury is therefore likely to be much more commonplace than popularly believed.

Scores (range 29 to 87)

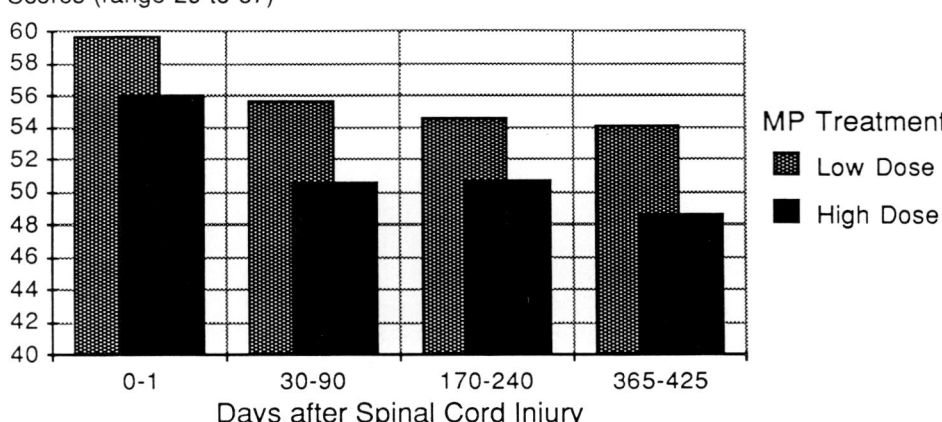

Days after Spinal Cord Injury

Figure 10–2. Mean pinprick sensory deficit scores in patients treated with methylprednisolone (MP) at either 100 mg per day (low dose) or 1,000 mg per day (high dose) for 10 days after spinal cord injury. The mean scores represent summed pinprick scores in 29 dermatomes scored on a scale of 1 to 3 (representing normal, abnormal, and absent sensation), where 87 indicates absent pinprick sensations in all dermatomes tested, and 29 represents no loss. The mean scores were obtained from 130–150 patients per treatment group. The patients include thoracic and cervical spinal cord injuries, with sensory losses ranging from sensory loss in all dermatomes to partial loss.

Scores (range 29 to 87)

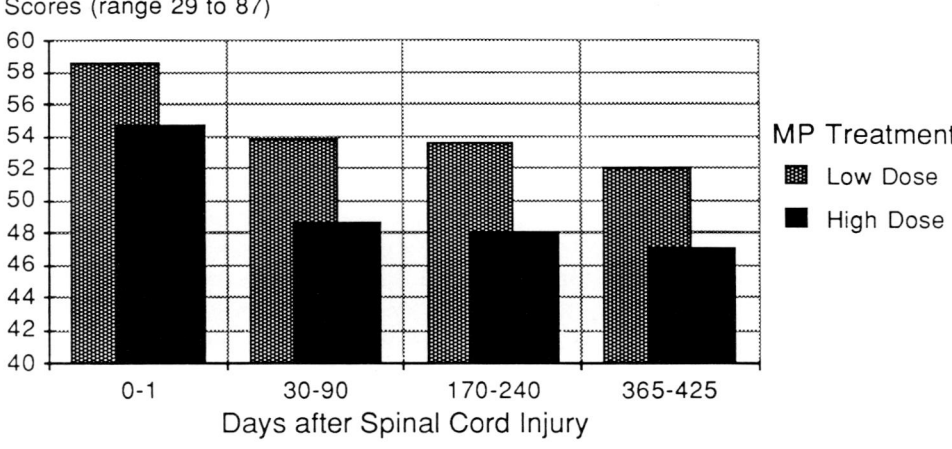

Days after Spinal Cord Injury

Figure 10–3. Mean touch sensory deficit scores in patients treated with methylprednisolone (MP) at either 100 mg per day (low dose) or 1,000 mg per day (high dose) for 10 days after spinal cord injury. The mean scores represent summed touch scores in 29 dermatomes scored on a scale of 1 to 3 (representing normal, abnormal, and no sensation), where 87 indicates absent pinprick sensations in all dermatomes tested, and 29 represents no loss. The mean scores were obtained from 130–150 patients per treatment group. The patients include thoracic and cervical spinal cord injuries, with sensory losses ranging from sensory loss in all dermatomes to partial loss.

Complete vs. Incomplete Spinal Cord Injury

A cherished clinical dogma stipulates that patients with "complete" lesions do not re-cover, while those with "incomplete" lesions tend to recover. Figure 10–4 shows the changes in neurological deficits in the patients shown in Figures 10–1—10–3 segregated into

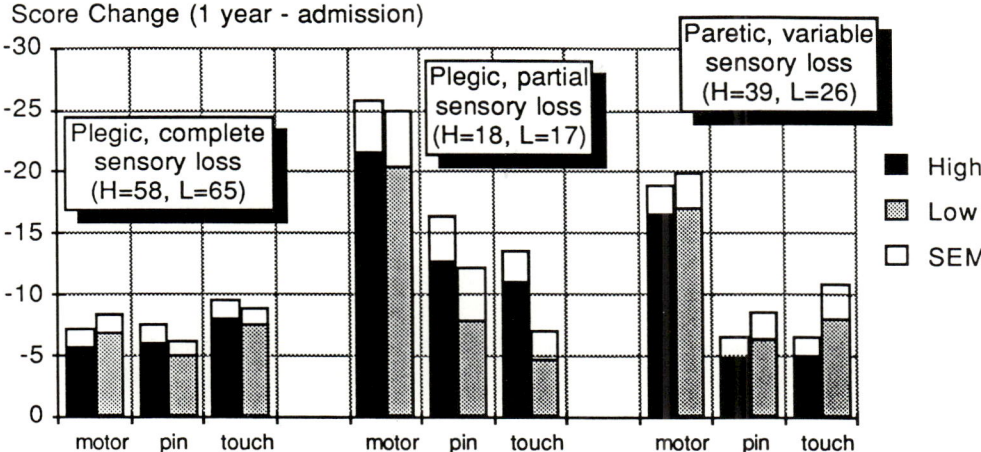

Figure 10–4. Recovery at 1 year after spinal injury. Mean motor, pin, and touch deficit scores in patients treated with methylprednisolone at either 100 mg per day (low) or 1,000 mg per day (high) for 10 days after spinal cord injury. The patients are segregated into three groups: those who were paralyzed and had no sensation below the lesion level (Plegic, complete sensory loss), those who were paralyzed and had some sensory preservation below the lesion level (Plegic, partial sensory loss), and those with incomplete motor and sensory loss below the lesion level (Paretic, variable sensory loss). The number of patients from each treated groups (H and L) within each category is indicated. Standard errors of the means (SEM) are indicated by the white columns above the means.

three categories of injury severity, based on their motor and sensory losses on admission. The score differences were obtained by subtracting scores at 1 year from admission. The more negative scores indicate greater improvement over the 1-year period. A striking feature of the 1-year followup neurological scores is that the changes are statistically significant ($P < 0.01$) across the board in all categories and for all modalities tested. In plegic patients with complete sensory loss, as expected, improvement was slight, limited to -5 to -10 points for all categories, but it was nonetheless statistically significant. Paretic patients with variable sensory loss showed improvement, but less so than plegic patients with partial sensory loss, who had the greatest improvements, particularly in the motor scores.

Averaged neurological scores have the unfortunate tendency to hide the exceptional cases. In the past 8 years, of about 113 patients studied at the NYU-Bellevue Spinal Cord Injury Center with no motor or sensory function below the lesion level for 24 hr, we have observed remarkable recoveries in three patients with cervical spinal injuries. All three recov-

ered sufficiently to stand unaided, with return of definite somatosensory-evoked potentials from their lower limbs, compared with absent responses on admission. Several other investigators (Michaelis, 1969–1970; Ducker et al., 1983; Dimitrijevic et al., 1984; Stauffer, 1984; Meinicke, 1985; Ducker and Walleck, 1986; Cioni et al., 1987; Dimitrijevic, 1988; Young and Ransohoff, 1988) have reported similar percentages of patients recovering from severe spinal cord injuries who had no motor or sensory function below the injury level during the first 24 hr after injury. Clearly, although the dogma of "complete" and "incomplete" injuries is usually predictive of recovery, there are exceptions that are unexplained.

The recovery of spinal-injured patients with severe spinal cord injuries (sufficient to abolish all motor function but leaving slight residual sensory function on admission to the hospital) presents an interesting paradox. A majority of such patients recovered substantial motor function. These patients recovered an average of > 20 motor points, equivalent to return of at least four major muscle groups to normality or more than four muscle groups to partial function. About 20% of plegic patients with some sensory preservation seen at the NYU-Bellevue Spinal Cord Injury Center recovered sufficient motor function to return to functional ambulation and could not, at 4–6 years after injury, be readily distinguished from normal by the untrained eye. Why should the presence of slight sensory function be such a good prognostic sign? These patients were just as paralyzed as the patients with so-called "complete" injuries.

Why do some patients recover function after spinal cord injury? Is it because they are regenerating lost pathways, repairing damaged pathways, or making better use of residual pathways? These questions cannot be answered satisfactorily in humans because injured spinal cords of patients who recover are seldom examined. Morphological analyses of spinal-injured patients who die accidentally have been carried out. Unfortunately, quantitative axons counts or assessments of their origins and distribution cannot be easily done on necropsy material. Also, in many cases, the neurological examinations may not have been completely reliable. Most of what we know about recovery therefore has to be extrapolated from laboratory spinal cord injury models.

Morphological Correlates of Functional Recovery

Laboratory studies suggest that remarkably few axons can support substantial functional recovery. Several investigators have reported that animals with severe spinal cord lesions can recover locomotory capabilities. For example, Windle et al. (1958) found that cats with as much as 90% sections of their spinal cords recovered walking. Eidelberg et al. (1977, 1980, 1981a, 1986) have found that selective preservation of ventral spinal tracts will allow locomotory recovery in cats and ferrets. In fact, a human case has been reported (Windle, 1980) in which a > 90% loss of the spinal cord pathways was observed at surgery, and the patient experienced sufficient motor and sensory recovery to function for more than 30 years. The severity of the spinal injury was confirmed on autopsy. Unfortunately, the patient deteriorated in the later years of her life.

Very small differences in axonal numbers may segregate recovering and nonrecovering

spinal-injured animals. Blight (1983a) systematically counted the number of axons present in the spinal cord in cats that recover and those that do not. Normal cats have ~ 500,000–700,000 axons countable on the light microscopic level in the thoracic spinal cord. After a 20-gm weight dropped 20 cm onto the cord, typically less than 50,000 axons survive. Cats that recover locomotion on an average have more axons than those that do not recover, but this difference is often very small. Some cats recover locomotory capability with less than 50,000 axons present across the lesion site, although 25,000 axons appear to be the lower limit. In at least two published studies in which we (Young et al., 1981, 1988) found marked differences in locomotory recovery of animals after high-dose naloxone and methylprednisolone, we could not detect a major difference in the histological appearance of the lesion site.

A minimum threshold of axons required for recovery may explain the gap in recovery that has been empirically observed between patients who have even the slightest motor or sensory preservation and those who show no function below the lesion level. The former group of patients are often called "incomplete" spinal cord injury, as opposed to those with "complete" spinal cord injuries, who seldom recover. Physical injuries to the spinal cord are unlikely to produce all-or-none losses of axons. The difference between so-called incomplete and complete injury groups may therefore have a biological basis, related to a threshold in number or distribution of axons required to support function. This difference may be so slight that nonquantitative assessments of the injury site cannot detect the difference. Thus quantitative morphometric analyses of spinal cords are essential.

The number and kinds of axons required to support neurological recovery in humans are not known. Dimitrijevic and coworkers (Dimitrijevic et al., 1983, 1984; Cioni et al., 1987; Dimitrijevic, 1988) have reported that as many as 70% of patients with neurological diagnoses of "complete" spinal cord injury have neurophysiological evidence of axonal conduction across the lesion site, a condition that Dimitrijevic (1987) termed "discomplete." Examining the effects of elicited descending activity on segmental reflexes induced by tonic vibratory stimuli or phasic reflexes, they showed that patients can augment or inhibit induced motor activity even when they show no evidence of voluntary motor activity. The presence of such "subclinical" function in these cases suggests that even very severely injured patients often have surviving or perhaps even spontaneously regenerated axons. If most animal species (including subhuman primates (Eidelberg et al., 1977, 1981b)) can recover locomotion with 10% of the spinal cord, humans with normally 10–20 million axons (Blinkov and Glezer, 1968) may likewise recover locomotory function with 500,000 axons. Depending on the number of axons that survive the initial injury, the addition of a small number of axons may have a relatively large effect on functional recovery.

PHYSIOLOGICAL DEFICITS IN SPINAL CORD INJURY

Many investigators tacitly assume that the number of axons crossing the lesion site is the only determinant of functional recovery. Injury to the spinal cord, however, damages not only axons but oligodendroglia and astrocytes at the lesion site (Gledhill et al., 1973). As a result, axons that survive the injury often become demyelinated (Blight, 1983b, 1985). Remyelination may occur through migration or extension of oligodendroglial cells from surrounding cord, but, if the lesion spans too great a distance, remyelination is often incomplete (Waxman, 1982). Thus, even if sufficient axons survive the injury, they may be unable to transmit action potentials to support function.

Demyelination may contribute to the neurological deficits in spinal cord injury. Blight (1983a,b) recorded from axons in the spinal cords of animals that were recovering and that did not recover. Although the axon counts generally correlated with function, there was a significant overlap of axon counts between the two groups. Some animals that remained paralyzed had more axons than those that were recovering. Recordings from axons in these paralyzed animals revealed significantly fewer axons conducting at body temperatures, compared with animals that recovered. At 25°C, more axons conducted across the lesion site. Such temperature sensitivity is typical of de-

myelinated axons (Waxman, 1978). Lowering temperature increases duration of action potentials, increasing the currents generated by action potentials that overcome the leakiness and increased capacitance characteristic of demyelinated axons.

Morphometric analyses of the myelinated axons in animals with spinal cord injury confirmed that a majority of axons crossing the lesion site are demyelinated. Demyelination begins within 24 hr after a contusion of the spinal cord and peaks several days later (Blight and deCrescito, 1987). The mean myelin index, i.e., the ratio of the diameter of the axon plus its myelin to the axonal diameter, falls from a normal value of 1.8 to about 1.2 by 3 days and gradually rises over time to 1.4. The spread of the index indicates a diverse population of axons with demyelination. Note that these indices were obtained in a much smaller number of axons that continue to cross the lesion site after injury. This finding suggests that the number of functioning axons required to support locomotory recovery in cats is very low, indeed.

Regenerating axons should be highly susceptible to the same environmental constraints that limit the function of surviving axons at the lesion site. For example, regenerating axons are naked neurites that require myelination to conduct rapidly. If the conditions at the lesion site are such that the surviving axons do not become remyelinated, it is likely that the regenerating axons will also not be myelinated. Myelination of axons, whether surviving or regenerated, is therefore likely to be an important determinant of functional recovery. Other environmental factors may play a role. For example, the ionic environment of the lesion site may influence conduction of modulated bursts of action potentials.

Improved Axonal Conduction: A Mechanism of Recovery

Several observations indicate that physiological axonal dysfunctions play a major role in neurological deficits in spinal cord injury. In the initial subacute period, days or even weeks after injury, physiological conduction blocks can account for much of the deficits in mildly injured spinal cords. For example, although most cats will recover virtually completely from a mild spinal contusion with a 10-gm weight dropped 20 cm, they nevertheless always suffer a period of functional loss for days. The conduction loss during this period partly results from blood flow (Young, 1985a, 1987) and ionic (Young and Flamm, 1982; Young et al., 1982a,b; Young and Koreh, 1986) changes that occur at the lesion site. Somatosensory-evoked potentials in recovering spinal-injured patients also show a tendency to be initially diminished in amplitude, followed by recovery beginning with the appearance of long latency responses that gradually return to normal over a period of weeks (Young, 1981, 1985b; Young et al., 1982c).

Axonal conduction can be improved in chronically injured spinal cords by pharmacological means. Blight and Gruner (1987) and Gruner et al. (1987) recently investigated the effects of 4-aminopyridine (4-AP) on spinal-injured cats. This drug selectively blocks fast voltage-sensitive K^+ channels in neurons (Sherratt et al., 1980; Bostock et al., 1981) and has been used to treat multiple sclerosis clinically (Jones et al., 1986; Stefoski et al., 1987). Systemic administration of 2 mg/kg of 4-AP remarkably improves descending activation of muscles in spinal-injured animals, as measured by free fall responses (FFRs). FFRs are stereotyped muscle responses in hindlimb muscles during a vestibular stimulation induced by dropping an animal into sudden free fall (Gruner et al., 1984). The response is carried in bulbospinal pathways. Two groups of chronically spinal-injured animals were tested at 3–7 months after injury: a severely injured group with an average of 40,000 ± 15,000 (~ 5%) axons crossing the lesion site and a more moderately injured group with an average of 103,000 ± 36,000 (~ 12%) axons at the lesion site.

The general reactivity of the animals was increased by 4-AP, inducing spontaneous micturation in some. Prior to 4-AP administration, all the animals had very small and delayed, or no, FFRs. Intravenous administration of 2 mg/kg of 4-AP dramatically restored amplitudes and latencies of FFR responses in virtually all the animals tested ($P = 0.006$). In a majority of the animals, there was no detectable response in the vastus lateralis before 4-AP. A robust response of virtually normal latency appeared in this muscle in almost all of the treated animals. The effect wore off by 5 hr after injection. Thus 4-AP not only enhanced a conducted bulbospinal response in spinal-injured cats with a time course expected from the K^+ channel blocking effect of 4-AP, but it induced responses in muscles in which there were none prior to injury and restored existing responses to nearly normal latencies.

The mechanisms of the 4-AP effects on injured spinal cords cannot be attributed entirely to improvement of conduction in demyelinated axons. Blight (1987) examined the effect of 4-AP on axonal conduction in isolated cat spinal cords with chronic spinal cord injury. He found that 4-AP improved the latency and amplitude of conducted action potentials in some of the axons but not sufficiently to explain the dramatic increases in the free fall responses. It may be acting on the spinal cord distal to the lesion site. Clinical implications of the 4-AP effects are limited, since systemically administered 4-AP raises blood pressure, is epileptogenic, and produces only transient improvements of function. However, these results suggest that there are other routes of improving function in chronically injured spinal cords besides regeneration. Furthermore, since regenerated axons are demyelinated, such treatments improve the conduction in regenerated as well as surviving axons.

Segmental Mechanisms of Behavioral Recovery

Loss and recovery of function is not a straightforward outcome of injury sustained by well-studied spinal tracts. The systematic studies of Lundberg (1979) illustrate this clearly in a model of forelimb motor recovery. Cats, when offered a morsel of food placed in a small cylinder, will engage in a stereotyped visually guided feeding behavior. They dip their paws into the cylinder, hook the morsel with a claw, and bring the food to their mouths in a smooth movement. Unilateral lesions in the upper cervical spinal cord, interrupting individually or in combination the corticospinal, rubrospinal, or reticulospinal inputs, revealed an interesting phenomenon. The feeding behavior recovered quickly (within days) from either corticospinal or rubrospinal lesions, done individually or sequentially. However, if the reticulospinal pathways were cut, either at the same time (i.e., a hemisection), before, or soon after the corticospinal or rubrospinal lesions, recovery was prolonged (over months) and incomplete. Considered alone, these experiments suggest that the bulbospinal tracts can substitute for the corticospinal or rubrospinal tracts. However, when bulbospinal pathways were cut 7–10 days after the corticospinal and/or rubrospinal lesions, recovery was rapid. Thus the bulbospinal tracts may not be substituting but rather enhancing recovery by being present for a certain period of time. After this period, the recovered function no longer requires the ipsilateral bulbospinal tract.

Recovery of motor behavior depends on integrity of local spinal circuits. For example, forelimb food-taking and target-reaching ability of cats after rubrospinal or corticospinal lesions depends on propriospinal neurons situated at C3-C4 (Alstermark et al., 1984a,b,c, 1986a,b). After lesions of the rubrospinal or corticospinal sections, interrupting pathways between the forelimb and the ipsilateral C3-C4 propriospinal neurons has profound disruptive effects on the recovered behavior. For example, cutting the ipsilateral dorsal column at C5 or C6 will result in marked hypermetria and protraction, whereas cutting the ipsilateral dorsal column at C2 or C3, rostral to the C3-C4 propriospinal neurons, has little effect on recovery (Alstermark et al., 1986c). Thus this finding is an example of behavioral recovery that requires local spinal circuits and appears to be relatively independent of more rostral pathways.

Kato and coworkers (Kato et al., 1984; Kato, 1987) reported similarly paradoxical findings with experiments examining the effects of single and double spinal cord hemisections on locomotory recovery. Hemisected cats recovered locomotory capabilities within a week after low thoracic or high cervical spinal cord hemisections, although more sophisticated behavior, such as walking on a grid, tended to show greater and more prolonged deficits (Murray and Goldberg, 1974). When Kato did double hemisections, e.g., a left thoracic hemisection and a right cervical hemisection, the animals took much longer to recover. However, if he waited a week or more after the first hemisection before carrying out the second hemisec-

tion, the animals recovered rapidly. Analyses of the locomotory and postural responses in the recovered double-hemisected cats indicated that forelimb and hindlimb movements fall out of phase.

These experiments suggest an ability of spinal-injured animals to recover motor function despite major lesions of the spinal cord. In the double-hemisection model, for example, descending spinal axons innervating the lumbrosacral spinal cord should be virtually eliminated. Yet animals with double hemisections will recover locomotion if the lesions are separated by time. Thus isolated spinal cord appears capable of sophisticated automatic function that can mimic functional recovery. The temporary presence of some residual pathway, particularly the bulbospinal tracts, can enhance at least the rate, if not the ultimate extent, of recovery. If these influences can be identified, it may be possible to supply them to the spinal cord exogenously either in the form of electrical stimulation, drugs, or biological factors.

WHY NOT SPINAL REGENERATION?

Given the importance of the spinal cord for survival, it is surprising that most animals have not evolved the ability to regenerate spinal axons. This inability has been blamed on barriers to regenerating axons in the injured spinal cord. Without question, regenerating spinal axons face a daunting obstacle course. At the lesion site, the axons must cross barriers of glial scars, circumvent fluid-filled cysts, survive the attacks of invading macrophages, and weather the intemperate environments resulting from degenerating cells at the lesion site. Once past the lesion site, the axons must somehow resist the siren calls of other neurons en route to their destination. Nevertheless, effective regeneration has been reported in other parts of the CNS and in the spinal cord of a few animals.

The most formidable barrier to regeneration in the spinal cord, however, is seldom considered. Due to axonal dieback and the length of the spinal cord, injured axons have to grow great distances to reconnect with their original sites. In human spinal cord injuries, for example, these distances may exceed 1,000 mm. At the rate of 1 mm per day, regenerating spinal axons may require 2–3 years to complete their journey. By the time regenerating axons complete their odyssey, their original synaptic sites may have degenerated or become occupied by proliferating axons from more closely located cellular systems. Target muscles and neurons may have atrophied by that time. Successful regeneration thus requires not only that directed axonal growth be sustained for years, but that changes in the remaining nervous system be prevented during this time.

The time factor may be one reason why regeneration has not evolved as a mechanism of recovery in mammals. A spinal-injured animal cannot wait months or years for regeneration to take place. It must recover rapidly enough to find food and escape from predators. Without alternative recovery mechanisms, spinal-injured animals would not survive long enough for spinal cord regeneration to evolve, to exert its beneficial effects, and then to be passed on to offspring. A similar explanation has been offered to explain why lizards can regenerate their tails (which are not crucial to their survival) but not their legs, while salamanders can regenerate their legs but not their tails (which are important for swimming). Distance and time should not pose as serious a problem for small animals. For example, in goldfish, frogs, lampreys or young animals, in which the regeneration path may be 1 cm or less, regeneration may be a feasible mechanism of recovery. Regeneration studies carried out in small animals may not be generalizable to larger mammals.

Regeneration may also interfere with existing recovery strategies. Given the distance and the other obstacles in the path of regenerating axons, the probability of regenerating axons making inappropriate connections is high. The two most critical determinants of functional recovery are balanced excitatory and inhibitory influences and appropriate feedback interactions between neural structures. Some of the most debilitating consequences of spinal cord injury may stem not from disconnections but from imbalance of the remaining pathways. For example, although the Sherringtonian interpretation that spasticity is a product of disinhibition has held sway for more than half a century, several clinical observations argue strongly against this interpretation. Abnor-

mal motor activities are most pronounced in patients with partial preservation of their spinal pathways. Spasticity responds to changes in supraspinal activity (Dimitrijevic and Sherwood, 1980). Likewise, pathological pain syndromes are most common in patients with partial motor and sensory loss, and seldom pose problems in patients with complete sensory and motor deficits.

CONCLUSIONS

We must achieve a better understanding of recovery mechanisms in injured spinal cords before we can begin restoring function by adding new pathways.

1. Contrary to popular opinion, recovery from spinal cord injury is commonplace. Animal studies indicate that locomotory recovery is possible with as few as 5–10% of the axons passing through the thoracic spinal cord. Injured spinal cords possess remarkably effective recovery mechanisms, based partly on the ability of spinal segmental circuitry to take over functions mediated by long spinal tracts. The interaction between these recovery mechanisms and regenerated axons must be considered carefully prior to interposing regenerative therapy on injured spinal cords.

2. Recent studies suggest that demyelination may play a major role in the neurological deficits in spinal cord injury. This has implications not only for surviving axons but for regenerating axons as well. Regenerating axons are unmyelinated. If surviving axons do not get remyelinated, can we expect regenerated axons to become myelinated? Therefore, regenerated axons may not function well.

3. Spinal axons must grow long distances, as far as a meter in humans, to reach their former synaptic sites. At the rate of 1 mm per day, axons may require years to reconnect. Axonal growth and guidance mechanisms must therefore be sustained for prolonged periods. Recovery will be slow, perhaps so slow that recovery resulting from axonal regeneration may provide little or no selective advantage, and hence accounts for the failure of larger mammals to evolve spinal cord regenerative mechanisms.

ACKNOWLEDGMENTS

This work was supported in part by NIH NINCDS grants NS10164 and NS15078.

REFERENCES

Alstermark B, Lundberg A, Sasaki S (1984a): Integration in descending motor pathways controlling the forelimb in the cat. 10. Inhibitory pathways to forelimb motoneurones via C3-C4 propriospinal neurones. Exp Brain Res 56:279–292.

Alstermark B, Lundberg A, Sasaki S (1984b): Integration in descending motor pathways controlling the forelimb in the cat. 11. Inhibitory pathways from higher motor centres and forelimb afferents to C3-C4 propriospinal neurones. Exp Brain Res 56:293–207.

Alstermark B, Lundberg A, Sasaki S (1984c): Integration in descending motor pathways controlling the forelimb in the cat. 12. Interneurones which may mediate descending feed-forward inhibition from the forelimb to C3-C4 propriospinal neurones. Exp Brain Res 56: 308–322.

Alstermark B, Johannisson T, Lundberg A (1986a): The inhibitory feedback pathway from the forelimb to C3-C4 propriospinal neurons investigated with natural stimulation. Neurosci Res 3:451–456.

Alstermark B, Gorska T, Johannisson T, Lundberg A (1986b): Hypermetria in forelimb target-reaching after interruption of the inhibitory pathway from forelimb afferents to C3-C4 propriospinal neurones. Neurosci Res 3:457–461.

Alstermark B, Gorska T, Johannisson T, Lundberg A (1986c): Effects of dorsal column transection in the upper cervical segments on visually guided forelimb movements. Neurosci Res 3:462–466.

Anderson D, McLaurin R (1980): Report on the National Head and Spinal Cord Injury Survey (NHSCIS). J Neurosurg 53:534.

Blight AR (1983a): Cellular morphology of chronic spinal cord injury in the cat: Analysis of myelinated axons by line sampling. Neuroscience 10:521–543.

Blight AR (1983b): Axonal physiology of chronic spinal cord injury in the cat: Intracellular recording in vitro. Neuroscience 10:1471–1486.

Blight AR (1985): Delayed myelination and macrophage invasion: A candidate for "secondary" cell damage in spinal cord injury. CNS Trauma 2:299–315.

Blight AR (1987): Effect of 4-aminopyridine on action potential conduction in myelinated axons of chronically injured spinal cord. Soc Neurosci Abstr 13:62.

Blight AR, DeCrescito V (1987): Morphometric analysis of experimental spinal cord injury in the cat: The relationship of injury intensity to survival of myelinated axons. Neuroscience 19:321–341.

Blight AR, Gruner JA (1987): Augmentation by 4-aminopyridine of vestibulospinal free fall responses in chronic spinal-injured cats. J Neurol Sci 82:145–159.

Blinkov SM, Glezer II (1968): The Human Brain in Figures and Tables—A Quantitative Handbook. New York: Basic Books, Inc., Plenum Press, pp 53–78.

Borgens RB, Blight AR, Murphy DJ (1986a): Axonal regeneration in spinal cord injury: A perspective and new technique. J Comp Neurol 250:157–167.

Borgens RB, Blight AR, Murphy DJ, Stewart L (1986b): Transected dorsal column axons within the guinea pig spinal cord regenerate in the presence of an applied electrical field. J Comp Neurol 250:168–180.

Bostock HT, Sears TA, Sherratt RM (1981): The effects of 4-aminopyridine and tetraethylammonium ions on normal and demyelinated mammalian nerve fibres. J Physiol (Lond) 313:321–341.

Bracken MD, Freeman DH Jr, Hallebrand K (1981): Incidence of acute traumatic hospitalized SCI in the U.S., 1970–1977. Am J Epidemiol 113:615–622.

Bracken MB, Collins WF, Freeman DF, et al. (1984): Efficacy of methylprednisolone in acute spinal cord injury. JAMA 251:45–52.

Bracken MB, Shepard MJ, Hellenbrand KG, et al. (1985): Methylprednisolone and neurological function 1 year after spinal cord injury. J Neurosurg 63:704–713.

Breasted JH (1930): "The Edwin Smith Surgical Papyrus," vol 2. Chicago: University of Chicago Press.

Cioni B, Dimitrijevic MR, McKay WB, Sherwood AM (1987): Voluntary supraspinal suppression of spinal reflex activity in paralyzed muscles of spinal cord injury patients. Exp Neurol 93:574–583.

David S, Aguayo AJ (1981): Axonal elongation into peripheral nervous system "bridges" after central nervous system injury in adult rats. Science 214:931–933.

Dimitrijevic MR (1987): Neurophysiology in spinal cord injury. Paraplegia 25:205–208.

Dimitrijevic MR (1988): Residual motor functions in spinal cord injury. In Waxman SG (ed): "Advances in Neurology, Volume 47: Functional Recovery in Neurological Disease." New York: Raven Press, pp 139–155.

Dimitrijevic MR, Sherwood AM (1980): Spasticity: Medical and surgical treatment. Neurology 30:19–27.

Dimitrijevic MR, Faganel J, Lehmkuhl D, Sherwood A (1983): Motor control in man after partial or complete spinal cord injury. In Desmedt JE (ed): "Motor Control Mechanisms in Health and Disease." New York: Raven Press, pp 915–926.

Dimitrijevic MR, Dimitrijevic M, Faganel J, Sherwood AM (1984): Suprasegmentally induced motor unit activity in paralyzed muscles of patients with established spinal cord injury. Ann Neurol 16:216–221.

Ducker TB, Walleck CA (1986): Recovery from cord injury. In: "Central Nervous System Trauma Status Report—1985." Bethesda: NIH-NINCDS, pp 369–374.

Ducker TB, Lucas JT, Wallace CA (1983): Recovery from spinal cord injury. Clin Neurosurg 30:495–513.

Eidelberg E, Straehley D, Erspamer R (1977): Relationship between residual hindlimb assisted locomotion and surviving axons after incomplete spinal cord injuries. Exp Neurol 56:312–322.

Eidelberg E, Story JL, Meyer B, Nystel J (1980): Stepping by chronic spinal cats. Exp Brain Res 40:241–246.

Eidelberg E, Story JL, Walden JG, Meyer BL (1981a): Anatomical correlates of return of locomotor function after partial spinal cord lesions in cats. Exp Brain Res 42:81–88.

Eidelberg E, Walden J, Nguyen L (1981b): Locomotor control in macaque monkeys. Brain 104:647–663.

Eidelberg E, Nguyen L, Deza L (1986): Recovery of locomotor function after hemisection of the spinal cord in cats. Brain Res Bull 16:507–515.

Ergas Z (1985): Spinal cord injury in the United States: A statistical update. CNS Trauma 2:19–32.

Gledhill RF, Harrison BM, McDonald WI (1973): Demyelination after acute spinal cord compression. Exp Neurol 38:472–487.

Gruner JA, Young W, DeCrescito V (1984): The vestibulospinal free fall response: A test of descending function in spinal-injured cats. CNS Trauma 1:139–159.

Gruner JA, Blight AR, Petruziello M (1987): Recovery of motor function in chronic experimental spinal cord injury enhanced by 4-aminopyridine. Soc Neurosci Abstr 13:62.

Guth L, Brewer CR, Collins WF, Goldberger ME, Perl ER (1980b): Criteria for evaluating spinal cord regeneration experiments. Exp Neurol 69:1–3.

Guth L, Albuquerque EX, Deshpande SS, Barrett CP, Donati EJ, Warnick JE (1980a): Ineffectiveness of enzyme therapy on regeneration in the transected spinal cord of the rat. J Neurosurg 52:73–86.

Jones RE, Heron JR, Foster DH, Snelgar RS, Mason RJ (1986): Effects of 4-aminopyridine in patients with multiple sclerosis. J Neurol Sci 60:353–362.

Kakulas BA (1985a): Pathology of spinal injuries. CNS Trauma 1:117–129.

Kakulas BA, Bedbrook GM (1976): Pathology of injuries of the vertebral column. In Vinken PJ, Bruyn GW, Braakman R (eds): "Handbook of Clinical Neurology. Injuries of the Spine and Spinal Cord," vol 25, part 1. Amsterdam: Elsevier/North-Holland, pp 27–42.

Kakulas BA (1985b): Pathomorphological evidence for residual spinal cord functions. In Eccles JC, Dimitrijevic MR (eds): "Recent Achievements in Restorative Neurology, Volume 1: Upper Motor Neuron Functions and Dysfunctions." Basel: Karger.

Kato M (1987): Motoneuronal activity of cat lumbar spinal cord following separation from descending or contralateral impulses. CNS Trauma.

Kato M, Murakami S, Yasuda K, Hirayama H (1984): Disruption of fore- and hindlimb coordination during overground locomotion in cats with bilateral serial hemisection of the spinal cord. Neurosci Res 2:27–47.

Lundberg A (1979): Multisensory control of spinal reflex pathways. In Granit R, Pompeiano G (eds): "Reflex Control of Posture and Movement. Progress in Brain Research," vol 50. Asmterdam: Elsevier/North Holland Biomedical Press, pp 11–28.

Matinian LA, Andreasian AS (1976): "Enzyme Therapy in Organic Lesions of the Spinal Cord," translated by E. Tanasescu. Los Angeles: Brain Information Service, UCLA.

Meinicke FW (1985): Some thoughts about neurological recovery in spinal cord injuries: A philosophical review. Paraplegia 23:78–81.

Michaelis LS (1969–1970): International inquiry on neurological terminology and prognosis in paraplegia and tetraplegia. Paraplegia 7:1–5.

Murray M, Goldberg ME (1974): Restitution of function and collateral sprouting in the cat spinal cord: The partially hemisected animal. J Comp Neurol 158:19–36.

Ramón y Cajal S (1928): "Degeneration and Regeneration of the Nervous System," translated by R. M. May. London: Oxford University Press.

Sheratt RM, Bostock H, Sears TA (1980): Effects of 4-aminopyridine on normal and demyelinated mammalian nerve fibers. Nature 283:570–572.

Stauffer ES (1984): Neurological recovery following injuries to the cervical spinal cord and nerve roots. Spine 9:532–534.

Stefoski D, Davis FA, Faut M, Schauf CL (1987): 4-aminopyridine improves clinical signs in multiple sclerosis. Ann Neurol 21:71–77.

Waxman SG (1978): Prerequisites for conduction in demyelinated fibers. Neurology 28:27–33.

Waxman SG (1982): Membranes, myelin, and the pathophysiology of multiple sclerosis. New Engl J Med 306:1529–1533.

Windle WF (1980): Concussion, contusion, and severance of the spinal cord. In Windle WF (ed): "The Spinal Cord and Its Reactions to Traumatic Injury." New York: Marcel Dekker, pp 205—217.

Windle WF, Smart JO, Beers JJ (1958): Residual function after subtotal spinal cord transection in adult cats. Neurology 8:518–521.

Young W (1981): Correlation of somatosensory evoked potentials and neurological findings in clinical spinal cord injury. In Tator CH (ed): "Early Management of Cervical Spinal Injury." New York: Raven Press, pp 153–166.

Young W (1985a): Blood flow, metabolism and neurophysiologic mechanisms of spinal cord injury. In Becker DP, Povlishock JT (eds): "CNS Trauma Status Report 1985." Bethesda: NIH-NINCDS, pp 463–473.

Young W (1985b): Cortical somatosensory evoked potential changes in spinal cord injury. In Schramm J, Jones SJ (eds): "Spinal Cord Monitoring." Berlin-New York: Springer Verlag, pp 127–142.

Young W (1987): The post-injury responses in trauma and ischemia: Secondary injury or protective mechanisms? CNS Trauma 4:27–52.

Young W, Flamm ES (1982): Effect of high dose corticosteroid therapy on blood flow, evoked potentials, and extracellular calcium in experimental spinal injury. J Neurosurg 57:667–673.

Young W, Koreh I (1986): Potassium and calcium changes in injured spinal cords. Brain Res 365:42–53.

Young W, Ransohoff J (1988): Acute spinal cord injury: Experimental therapy, pathophysiological mechanisms, and recovery of function. In Sherk H (ed): "Cervical Spine." Cervical Spine Research Society, in press.

Young W, Flamm ES, Demopoulos HB, DeCrescito V, Tomasula JJ (1981): Effect of naloxone on posttraumatic ischemia in experimental spinal contusion. J Neurosurg 55:209–219.

Young W, Koreh I, Yen V, Lindsay A (1982a): Effects of sympathectomy on extracellular potassium activity and blood flow in experimental spinal cord contusion. Brain Res 253:105–113.

Young W, Yen V, Blight A (1982b): Extracellular calcium activity in experimental spinal cord contusion. Brain Res 253:115–123.

Young W, Cohen A, Merkin H, Fisher B, Berenstein A, Ransohoff J (1982c): Somatosensory evoked potential changes in spinal injury and during intraoperative spinal manipulation. J Am Paraplegia Soc 5:44–48.

Young W, DeCrescito V, Flamm ES, Blight AR, Gruner JA (1988): Pharmacological treatments of acute spinal cord injury: A review of naloxone and methylprednisolone. Clin Neurosurg 34:675–697.

11

Spinal Cord Regeneration: The Laboratory/Clinical Interface

BARTH A. GREEN, MD, AND K. JOHN KLOSE, PhD

Department of Neurological Surgery, University of Miami School of Medicine, and Veterans Administration Medical Center, Miami, Florida 33136

In the following pages, we will present some of the practical and theoretical considerations facing basic scientists and clinicians attempting to extrapolate from basic science data a practical treatment for persons paralyzed from injuries or diseases of the human spinal cord. This chapter will focus on victims of traumatic spinal cord injury (SCI). However, it must be appreciated that successful spinal cord regeneration or functional reconnection would also benefit multitudes of persons suffering from other injuries and diseases of the central nervous system (CNS).

While the incidence of SCI has not changed dramatically over the last 2 decades, (i.e., 10,000–12,000 new injuries per year in the United States), the prevalence (i.e., the number of SCIs living in the overall population) is growing as a result of the advances that have been made in preventing morbidity and mortality (Young and Northrup, 1979; Stover and Fine, 1986). The growing numbers have increased the social consequence of SCI for the community at large and emphasized the need for research that will lead to better methods of producing increased recovery of function. In the 1990s advances may come from a new source (one other than surgical instruments, computerized monitors, stimulators, etc.), namely, human experimentation based on data evolving from the basic science laboratories.

SYSTEMS APPROACH TO SCI CARE

In order to better plan for a smooth laboratory/clinical interface for spinal cord regeneration in paralysis victims, one should first consider the "state of the art" of patient care in 1988. The "systems approach" (Green and Eismont, 1984) to spinal cord injury is generally considered to provide the optimal elements for minimizing morbidity, mortality, and cost, while maximizing the potential for neurological recovery and functional independence. The systems approach is based on a continuity of care from the accident scene through the acute and rehabilitative periods and on through the lifelong outpatient programs for paralysis victims. One of the basic tenets of a systems approach is the availability of a multidisciplinary team of physicians, nurses, and allied health care professionals who are committed to the treatment of individuals with a relatively rare and devastating injury. Part of the underlying philosophy on which the systems approach was founded was that seeing a large number of patients with a similar diagnosis ("volume experience") results in a better understanding of the disease and ultimately in improved care delivery and patient outcome (Green and Eismont, 1984).

The first phase of the systems approach to SCI involves prehospital management programs. Prehospital management comes under the direction of Emergency Medical Services and is divided into three major components: communication, transportation, and education (Hall et al., 1976). Of all the clinical care phases in the systems approach, the prehos-

Neural Regeneration and Transplantation, pages 171–182

pital management has impacted the most on the early survival and improved prognosis of SCI victims today, a change that can be attributed directly to the sophistication of first responders, trained paramedics who have replaced inexperienced police and ambulance drivers. Such paramedics (usually fire rescue personnel) are trained in immobilization, extrication, and spinal and systemic evaluation and stabilization.

There is little doubt among clinicians that paramedics have reduced the morbidity, mortality, and neurological consequence of spinal cord injury. They are skilled in establishing an airway, maintaining circulation, immobilizing the spinal column, and preventing secondary spinal cord injury from systemic complications such as hypoxia, shock, or vertebral column instability. The prehospital phase represents the first phase of the laboratory/clinical interface for spinal cord parenchymal protection or regeneration.

The second phase of care in the systems approach is the acute inhospital program. Although a goal of the prehospital phase must be the limitation of parenchymal damage and although paramedics can deliver intravenous medications such as neuropeptides or steroids, the acute inhospital care phase represents the first opportunity to conduct a controlled clinical trial of laboratory/clinical interface (with invasive or surgical strategy) for the enhancement of spinal cord regeneration. The acute inhospital phase starts with the emergency room triage by a multidisciplinary team of physicians, nurses, and allied health professionals. Priorities are similar to those at the accident scene, including stabilization of physiological parameters and immobilization of the spinal column. The majority of spinal cord-injured persons have associated multisystem injuries; stabilization of these injuries becomes a significant priority, since they increase morbidity, mortality, and length of care, translating into increased costs.

Once a SCI patient has been stabilized and evaluated in the emergency room, depending on the level and type of injury and other organ involvement, he/she is either taken to the SCI Intensive Care Unit (ICU) or directly to the operating room. Patients taken to the ICU are most often those with cervical and thoracic in-juries above T12 or patients with spinal column injury without neurological deficit. The cervical injuries are directed into an aggressive program of reduction and realignment of their spinal column dislocations.

Patients taken immediately to the operating room include those with life-threatening penetrating wounds and those with thoracolumbar junction or lumbar fractures, as well as those with the rare cervical burst fractures, herniated discs, or intractable locked facets. Major indications for surgery are: intractable neural element compression or severe spinal column instability refractory to standard immobilization techniques.

Penetrating wounds of the spinal cord or cauda equina are treated differently than the closed injuries. In the penetrating wound the priority is life saving, especially when it involves the neck, chest, or abdomen, with associated viscera. Exploratory surgery is usually emergent, and neurological injury becomes a secondary priority. In certain cases, such as the complete lesions from thoracic gunshot wounds, surgical intervention only increases the morbidity, without changing the outcome. In contrast, the thoracolumbar junction or lumbar penetrating injury surgery can result in a significant decrease in pain and recovery of neurological function, especially in incompletely paralyzed patients (Green and Eismont, 1984; Green and Magana, 1987).

The third phase of the systems approach is rehabilitation. Although the rehabilitation phase actually begins when the patient first arrives in the ICU, formal rehabilitation begins when the patient is transferred to the SCI rehabilitation center. The average rehabilitation time for a paraplegic is 3 to 4 months and for a quadriplegic 4 to 6 months. However, like the acute care phase, the length of rehabilitation is directly related to the level of injury, the age of the patient, the severity of the injury, and systemic injuries or complications. The obvious goal of rehabilitation is to return paralyzed or partially paralyzed individuals back to their families and to society in a condition as independent as possible, physically and financially. The process not only focuses on teaching SCI patients how to get in and out of wheelchairs and building up their residual muscles, but includes bowel and bladder training. In addition to the conventional therapy and resistive exercises utilized around the world, rehabilitative engineering has made some computerized modalities available, including multichannel electromyography (EMG) biofeedback and closed loop functional electrical stimulation, which are presently being utilized by at least some of the impatient rehabilitation population. In the future they will be increasingly integrated into the early acute care and rehabilitation center programs. Good physical rehabilitation is a crucial factor in providing an optimal candidate for the application of a SCI regeneration protocol that might be instituted beyond the acute stage of injury (Green and Eismont, 1984).

Lifelong follow-up care constitutes the fourth phase of the systems approach. Once the SCI patient completes the rehabilitation phase of care and is discharged from initial hospitalization, lifelong follow-up care begins. The patient is instructed to return to the rehabilitation center semiannually for an outpatient examination to evaluate patient compliance with programs taught during the rehabilitation phase, and for an assessment of the patient's health status. The patient is evaluated by the same multidisciplinary specialists who treated her/him in the rehabilitation phase. In addition to the regularly scheduled evaluation appointments, patients are encouraged to visit the center as problems arise. This care phase of a systems approach is vital to the preservation of viable candidates for a regeneration approach for chronically paralyzed persons (Green and Eismont, 1984).

CLINICAL RESEARCH CONSIDERATIONS

Animal laboratory research permits the investigator to select subjects on the basis of age, weight, sex, and a countless number of other variables. Starting with a homogeneous group, an equivalent injury is produced in each animal, using a standardized method. The subjects are then divided into two or more groups, with one group serving as the control or placebo group, while the other groups receive the experimental interventions that are being tested. A simple comparison of group outcomes usually yields the information necessary to determine the effectiveness, if any, of the intervention. Clinical SCI research, on the

other hand, cannot easily assemble equivalent preintervention groups. This problem can be overcome with the use of sophisticated statistical design and analysis techniques, provided the investigator can identify the potential concomitant and/or intervening variables (e.g., initial severity, extent of injury, etc.) that may influence outcomes.

Essential to the development of a productive clinical research strategy is the ability to classify spinal cord injuries according to severity, on a number of dimensions, and an awareness of other factors that may influence outcome. A lack of appreciation that the potential for a functional recovery is related to the velocity and the anatomical level of the insult to the spinal cord as well as the age of the individual and other preexisting factors may have contributed to the failure of many previously implemented clinical trials to demonstrate a differential outcome as a result of treatments. This failure is in part attributable to the absence of a comprehensive body of knowledge on some of the subtleties of long-term changes in neurological function following injury. It is essential to create a historical data bank on a sufficient number of SCI victims who are objectively evaluated in a prospective reliable fashion using quantifiable assessments. These assessments must be performed frequently and serially, beginning at the accident scene through long-term follow up, and can be used to identify factors that contribute to outcome.

Neuro-Spinal Index of Function

The medical literature is sparse in regard to the quantification and classification of neurological function in spinal man, which is essential for documentation of successful clinical intervention. Equally lacking is the natural history of recovery or loss of function. The University of Miami Neuro-Spinal Index (UMNI) was developed to serve as a quantitative measure of degree of spinal cord function that could be used to follow patients' neurological progress (Klose et al., 1980; Green et al., 1985). The degree of spinal cord function is assessed using standard techniques, but an overall score is computed by summing the values of the individual item scores. The test contains both a motor and sensory evaluation, which can be reviewed jointly or separately. The entire range of overall scores can vary between 0 and 460, where 0 represents no detectable function, and 460 characterizes normal neurological function. To ensure standardization of assessment (i.e., valid and reliable measures), trained physical therapists are assigned to conduct the test. The motor and sensory scoring procedure is as follows:

MOTOR FUNCTION

The scale scores are obtained through standard manual muscle test techniques. The muscle groups chosen for the test were selected on the basis of functional significance as correlated to the level of injury. Twenty-two separate muscle groups are assessed bilaterally, so that 44 individual tests are performed with each individual muscle group scored on a 1–5 scale where:

0 = No function.
1 = There is a visible or palpable flicker of contraction, but no resultant movement of limb or joint.
2 = The muscle can only make its normal movement when the limb is so positioned that gravity is eliminated.
3 = The muscle is able to make its normal movement against gravity but not against additional resistance.
4 = The muscle, although able to make its full normal movement, is overcome by resistance.
5 = Normal power.

Since 44 muscle groups are tested on a 5-point basis, the total motor score ranges from 0 to 220.

SENSORY FUNCTION

The sensory scale score provides an estimate of total body sensation. Two sensory modalities were chosen for testing, based on ease of testing and their anatomical separation within the spinal cord. The lateral spinothalamic tracts are assessed with pin prick, while the dorsal columns are assessed with vibration using a tuning fork. This differential sensory exam provides a more sensitive measure of completeness of injury. Since different skin areas or dermatomes of the body are innervated by specific levels of the spinal cord, this test

also determines level of injury for that modality.

Each stimulus is presented bilaterally to each of the dermatome areas innervated by the 30 levels of the spinal cord. Item scores are assigned as follows: 0 = absent; 1 = present, but abnormal; 2 = normal. Sensory indices range from 0 = no detectable sensation to 240 = total normal body sensation.

An abbreviated form of the UMNI scale has been prepared for paramedical use in the accident scene assessment, which will be essential to any clinical trials utilizing accident-scene therapies and interventions. The results of a study performed almost 10 years ago using the UMNI showed for the first time what many took for granted but had never documented in a quantified manner, namely, that open injuries do not do as well as closed injuries, complete lesions do not do as well as incomplete lesions, and high-velocity injuries do not do as well as low-velocity injuries. That study also showed that older patients had a higher morbidity and mortality than younger patients; the initial level of injury was also important in prognosis. Additionally, results of the study indicated that a more accurate prognosis can be made a day or a week after injury than in the first minutes or hours.

Other Quantitative Indices

A quantifiable classification of SCI with regard to parenchymal damage should include not only a neurological examination utilizing an objective scale such as the UMNI, but also physiological monitoring in the form of evoked responses. Somatosensory-evoked responses are well developed and widely accepted, but they only monitor a single modality of sensory function, specifically the dorsal columns, and therefore provide limited information on spinal cord integrity. At the present time and undoubtedly in the future, inclusion of motor-evoked responses using electromagnetic stimulators can be combined with somatosensory-evoked responses to yield a more comprehensive multimodality computerized monitoring system of both the efferent and afferent pathways.

Another important consideration for the conduction of clinical trials is the inclusion of imaging techniques utilizing objective scales of severity for spinal cord and spinal column disruption. Properly assessing SCI patients and studying the effectiveness of clinical interventions as they relate to quantifiable severity levels of spinal cord parenchymal and bony spinal column damage demands the inclusion of imaging techniques. With the advent of magnetic resonance imaging (MRI) technology, parenchymal component analysis becomes a feasible goal, and with the use of computerized tomography (CT) scanning in conjunction with conventional plain X-rays, developing scales for severity of spinal column disruption also becomes a feasible goal (Green et al., 1981). In addition, factors such as preinjury spinal canal dimensions play an important role; for example, athletes with congenitally small canals are more likely to become paralyzed than those with congenitally large canals experiencing similar bony injuries. It is only logical and reasonable that the availability of such information should precede clinical trials of any medical or surgical treatment of SCI victims, including regeneration strategies.

Level and Completeness of Injury

An important variable that must be considered when planning strategies for the study of spinal cord regeneration is level of injury. The spinal cord is strikingly different in circuitry and other anatomical and physiological factors, not only within the confines of the cervical-thoracic, thoracic-lumbar, and sacral spinal cord segments, but also within different levels of these segments. Each area has unique characteristics of blood supply and architecture that must be considered when planning a reasonable strategy for treatment. For example, the vascularity of the spinal cord is grossly different at the various spinal levels and even within the major spinal divisions, such as cervical, thoracic, and lumbosacral. Where the cervical area has a rich blood supply supported by the anterior spinal artery, the caudal portion of the cord has its blood supply supported by the artery of Adamkiewicz. There is a watershed zone between the two in the upper and midthoracic area that would call for additional perfusion considerations, as one develops treatment strategies. An injury to the thoracolumbar junction or below involves not purely upper motor neuron damage, as seen in cervical and thoracic injuries, but a lower motor neuron-cauda equina component that would require at least partially, if not totally, different treatment strategies (Green et al., 1981). The spinal column at different levels also has distinct biomechanical characteristics that must also be taken into consideration when planning any significant invasive or surgical treatments. Patients who manifest a neurological deficit are divided into two major categories of injury, namely, quadriplegic and paraplegic. More accurately, the division should include quadriparetic and paraparetic as well as quadriplegic and paraplegic categories. Quadriplegics are individuals with some degree of paralysis of all four extremities, associated with a cervical spinal cord injury; they usually have an associated spinal column injury. Paraplegics have some degree of paralysis of both lower extremities, usually associated with thoracic and/or lumbar level spinal column injuries. Both categories have some degree of bowel, bladder, and sexual dysfunction, if not total loss of function. The terms quadriplegic and paraplegic are more commonly associated with what is called complete injuries; the terms quadriparetic and paraparetic are more properly associated with what are considered incomplete injuries.

The injuries of SCI patients are categorized as complete or incomplete lesions, relating to the degree of neurological function (or the lack thereof) below the level of injury. In a complete lesion, there is no motor or sensory function distal to the site of injury. Most often paraplegics and quadriplegics who have complete lesions have some local preservation of function for one, two, or three levels, either at or below the level of injury. The key for differentiating between complete and incomplete is any *distal* preservation of motor or sensory function. Some authors include reflexes in their definition, i.e., motor, sensory, or reflex function. However, we find that reflexes are the least reliable component of the neurological examination and should not be depended upon for diagnosis, prognosis, or complete or incomplete categorization. Such reflexes include the cremasteric and bulbocavernous and other superficial and even deep tendon reflexes. The rectal examination is an essential part of the neurological assessment of the paralyzed or partially paralyzed person, since this area again is innervated by the most peripheral portion of the cord. In spite of the fact that the force causing most spinal cord injuries is directly applied to the periphery of the spinal cord, the relatively soft central gray matter is more susceptible to injury. Hemorrhage and edema migrate out in a centrifugal fashion toward the periphery. Therefore patients who are complete with regard to motor and sensory examination of their extremities and trunk should still be evaluated for what is termed sacral sparing. This means that there is some evidence of voluntary motor control of the anal sphincter or of sensory perception, i.e., pain, temperature, or touch sensation in the anal or perianal area. By their presence, these functions classify SCI victims as incomplete, despite the lack of extremity or trunk motor or sensory function, and give them a totally different prognosis, since the majority of incomplete patients have a significant degree of neurological recovery (Green and Klose, 1981).

Type of Injury

In addition to the neurological classifications based on level and completeness, another form of categorization is based on the presence of spinal shock and a number of neurological patterns termed syndromes. Spinal shock is a physiological transection of the spinal cord that may be associated with a grossly normal-appearing spinal cord or, in other cases, with significant parenchymal damage. The spinal shock patient is flaccid, with no motor, sensory, or reflex function and with a lower motor neuron status of bowel and bladder. Many clinicians incorrectly tell their patients that they cannot assess whether they are complete or incomplete until they resolve their spinal shock. This resolution occurs in humans at 6 to 16 weeks. The resolution of spinal shock is heralded by a transformation into an upper motor neuron status, including hyperreflexia of the trunk and extremities and spasticity of the bowel and bladder. The confusion lies in the fact that spinal shock has nothing to do with prognosis. In fact, by definition, any patient in spinal shock is a complete injury with only a few percentage points chance of spontaneous recovery, i.e., there is no motor or sensory sparing below the level of injury; the resolu-

tion of spinal shock does not change that prognosis or diagnosis.

Another physiological state is neurogenic shock or the acute cervical spinal cord syndrome (Schneider et al., 1958). This syndrome, like spinal shock, is poorly understood, but is most often associated with cervical or upper thoracic injuries and at times can be found with brainstem injuries. Such patients manifest a triad of low blood pressure, low pulse, and low temperature, associated with a sympathectomy-like clinical picture. The typical manifestation in the emergency room may be a blood pressure of 90/60, a pulse in the 40s or 50s, and a temperature in the mid or low 90s. These patients should only be treated symptomatically in the emergency room (e.g., with intravenous atropine) and should not be treated with cardiogenic drugs, pacemakers, etc. unless an assessment with a Swans Ganz catheter reveals that they do not have adequate cardiac perfusion. For some reason, the majority of these patients seem to convert spontaneously out of the neurogenic shock state within the first 1 to 2 weeks of injury. Many authors attribute the significant morbidity and mortality of surgery, especially during the first week following spinal cord injury, to neurogenic shock syndrome. In most cases, it does not require treatment. The neurogenic shock syndrome, like the spinal shock syndrome, is in our experience only seen in complete injuries.

A relatively common example of misdiagnosis of completeness with regard to prognosis is the anterior cord syndrome (Schneider, 1955). Patients with this syndrome most often have a flexion type of spinal column injury. The neurological deficit is usually attributed to damage to the anterior spinal artery system, which results in the loss of motor, pain, and temperature function (i.e., no evidence of lateral column function), but with preservation of touch, position sense, and vibration (i.e., preservation of the dorsal columns). Patients with this syndrome are categorized as incomplete, when in fact there is no evidence of any improvement in motor, pain, or temperature function observable in this patient group, probably because there are separate circulation systems for the posterior columns (i.e., the posterior spinal artery system vs. the anterior spinal artery system). Anterior spinal cord syndrome patients do not have a good prognosis for recovery of motor, pain, and temperature function. However, they are much better off than complete patients because their preservation of crude touch and position sense allows them to do much better with regard to independence and transfer; since they perceive pressure, they are better able to prevent decubitus ulcers.

The central cord syndrome, which is usually seen in middle-aged or elderly males who have often had a hyperextension injury of the cervical spine, is rarely associated with bony disruption. Such patients most often have a pre-existing spondylosis and stenosis, and the injury to the spinal cord frequently occurs at the middle or lower cervical segments, where the greatest degree of spinal column mobility exists. Central cord syndrome patients have severe quadriparesis, with the deficit in the upper extremities greater than the lower. The most significant degree of deficit is noted in the distal upper extremities, especially the hands and fingers, which are weak and numb, but they also experience burning dysesthesias and usually have partial loss of bowel, bladder, and sexual function. Most of these patients improve spontaneously.

The Brown-Sequard syndrome describes a physiological hemisection of the spinal cord associated with ipsilateral loss of touch, vibration, position sense, and motor function and contralateral loss of pain and temperature sensation. Such cases may be associated with brachial plexus injuries. Brown-Sequard patients often have significant neurological recovery, including walking, with a major residual deficit in the ipsilateral upper extremity. This syndrome is commonly associated with rotational injuries or penetrating wounds to the spinal canal. Although most patients improve significantly, a small percentage may actually deteriorate and can become quadriplegic.

The posterior cord syndrome is an extremely rare entity seen in patients with selective loss of the dorsal columns associated with a penetrating wound or a laterally directed closed injury that selectively injures the dorsal columns. Such patients, although they have preservation of pain and temperature sensation, are devastated functionally because of their loss of position sense. This is an ex-

tremely rare lesion and represents less than 1% of the SCI population.

Although there are several classical incomplete syndromes, most patients fall into what is called the "mixed motor and sensory group," meaning a combination of all the above syndromes.

In addition to the "pure" spinal cord injuries we have described up to this point, the researcher must be cognizant of certain types of injuries that also include peripheral or lower motor neuron damage. The second most mobile segment of the spinal column is the thoracolumbar junction. This level is unique with regard to neurological deficit because most often it contains the conus medullaris, i.e., the termination of the cord and beginning of the cauda equina. Injury to this area is usually associated with a mixed conus/cauda equina syndrome, which is a combination of upper and lower motor neuron injuries. In our opinion these injuries should not be treated conservatively when they arrive initially in the emergency room (i.e., in the same fashion we treat the cervical injuries, by a closed realignment of the spinal column), but should be given, in most cases, emergency surgery to decompress the neural elements. We are very aggressive with these injuries, even if they remain a complete conus injury, i.e., with loss of bowel, bladder, and sexual function and saddle anesthesia. If such patients are decompressed early and adequately, they usually become ambulatory, through restoration and/or preservation of lumbar root function. They often ambulate with only the assistance of ankle splints and Canadian crutches. This is a much more preferable status than that of a flaccid paraplegic with intractable local pain from an unreduced dislocation at the thoracolumbar junction. Lumbar injuries fall into the same surgical consideration category, since they are pure lower motor neuron injuries and obviously should be treated aggressively to optimize the potential of neurological recovery. This is in contrast to the injuries below T1 and above T12 that usually manifest as complete injuries. Because of the poor blood supply of this area, it is most unlikely for patients to have complete thoracic injuries and then make a significant neurological recovery. Most of the complete patients who fall into the category of the 3–7% that become incomplete and significantly improve actually are from cervical or thoracolumbar junction injuries (Green et al., 1985; Green and Magana, 1987).

Velocity and Force of Injury

One of the potential confounding factors relating to functional outcome that these authors have identified is the velocity and force of the causal insult. On this basis we have divided spinal cord injuries into three categories, based on velocity and force of injury. The first category is the high-velocity injury, which includes, for example, a high-speed car or motorcycle crash or a bullet driving into and through the spinal column. This type of injury may completely crush the spinal cord, so that there is no possibility for restoration of its original shape and configuration. This fact may in part explain why clinical trials of steroids, etc. have not been as successful as the animal studies preceding them (Green et al., 1980; Bracken et al., 1984); the human study groups included subjects with this type of injury as well as subjects with less severe parenchymal damage. It is possible that some interventions may only be beneficial for certain subsets of the SCI population. However, even in high-velocity injuries, when developing a strategy for regeneration, one must attempt to act aggressively to limit the parenchymal damage. This strategy includes utilizing sophisticated systemic treatment protocols and reestablishing what we have termed "physiological homeostasis." Not only must one normalize oxygenation and perfusion to the CNS as well as to the rest of the body, but one must also establish relative normalization of the spinal column by rapidly realigning it to remove any significant extrinsic pressure from the contained CNS tissue. Unfortunately, spinal column realignment is not totally safe in the prehospital phase because of the lack of imaging capability. Applying traction without radiological control can result in actual worsening of the neurological condition. For the present, with our level of technology, we must settle for moving the patient into a neutral supine position and immobilizing the spinal column until arrival at the hospital.

The second category is the moderate-velocity injury. One might consider certain diving accidents, low-speed vehicle accidents, falls, and sporting accidents as falling into this group. These injuries are significant enough to create major neurological functional deficits, often initially indiscernible from the high-velocity injuries described above. However, if one examines the spinal cord grossly and microscopically, a significant difference appears between the high- and moderate-velocity insults. In some cases, as evidenced by recent sophisticated MRI scanning and in animal models, the spinal cord can appear intact in spite of the initial complete and severe paralysis. There are many biochemical and vascular theories and explanations for this state of physiological disconnection without concomitant physical disruption (Hagushi et al., 1984). This group of patients, with moderate-velocity injuries, has the most to gain from an aggressive clinical treatment program directed mainly toward physiological and spinal column homeostasis, but also including pharmacological interventions such as neuropeptides, etc. In most major SCI centers, from 3–7% of what appear initially to be complete lesions evolves into incomplete lesions with a totally different and more favorable prognosis. In our experience the moderate-velocity group can also go the other way (i.e., lesions remain complete and paralysis permanent) without such aggressive and sophisticated triage and treatment.

The third category, low-velocity injuries, are associated with short-distance falls or very low-velocity vehicle or sports accidents, and are most often associated with minor degrees of deficit that are often transitory. One example is a spinal cord concussion. The patient has a significant deficit that usually resolves within the first minutes and hours of injury (maximum time period 24 hr); it is often associated with little or no spinal column disruption or no MRI evidence of parenchymal damage. In general, the lower velocity injuries often respond to appropriate systemic supportive care; if some deficit exists, they would be the most likely of the three categories to benefit from pharmacological intervention such as neuropeptides or steroids, as discussed above. Although most low-velocity injuries improve almost in spite of the treatment provided, one must remember that a small percentage of patients who show no deficit initially deteriorate later and may become complete and irreversible. Some of these individuals deteriorate neurologically as a result of systemic problems such as hypoxia, hypotension, or sepsis; others fail because of spinal malalignment and extrinsic compression or intra- or extraparenchymal hemorrhage.

One must also include in the low-velocity group patients who have spinal column injury without spinal cord injury. They represent about three to four times as many patients as those who have neurological deficits and, if treated properly, in most cases will remain without deficit (Green et al., 1981). However, one must recognize that without proper treatment, some of these patients are at extremely high risk for developing a deficit, especially in cases of severe spinal column disruption. They must be handled very carefully in order to keep them out of the spinal cord-injured ranks (Green et al., 1980a; Green and Klose, 1981).

DEVELOPMENT OF TREATMENT STRATEGIES

When establishing strategies of treatment of acute, subacute, and chronic SCI victims, one must take into consideration both the clinical realities as described in some detail above and the state of the art of laboratory and applied research. As in the systems approach, where it makes more sense to prevent an injury than to treat one, an equally obvious statement would be that it makes more sense to preserve as much spinal cord parenchyma as possible and to limit tissue damage than to replace it, i.e., with transplantation, nerve grafting, etc. It is well known clinically that very few patients with paralysis have actual physical severance of the spinal cord. As a matter of fact, the number is probably less than 3%. Reviewing a large number of MRIs of chronically injured SCI patients anywhere from weeks to months to years after injury, one must appreciate that in many cases there is a poor correlation between the actual appearance of the spinal cord and the degree of deficit, i.e., patients with a highly atrophic cord may be ambulatory with minimal deficit, and other patients with a grossly normal-appearing cord may have complete lesions. Most patients with SCI injury, therefore, have significant residual cord tissue, and we know from the animal literature (Eidelberg,

1983) that it takes only about 10% preservation of the spinal cord parenchyma to allow ambulation. Therefore a major strategic approach to the treatment of SCI victims must be to initiate an aggressive program to preserve whatever parenchyma is not irreversibly lost at the initial moment of impact by minimizing secondary injury, whether it be physical or metabolic. Many of the injury characteristics that have been observed and documented in the laboratory also exist in humans with SCI. One of the authors has personally observed the spinal cords of humans severed from 50–70% by gunshot or stab wounds. Some of these patients could walk with a slight limp at most on one side and exhibited good control of bowel, bladder, and sexual function. These activities require only unilateral preservation of whatever tissue is not irreversibly damaged by the primary injury, emphasizing the need to prevent secondary physical and metabolic damage. As scientific clinicians we must strive to develop a means for evaluating the status of the residual spinal cord parenchyma. It is this tissue that may be alive, i.e., viable but nonfunctional, and if identified could potentially be utilized as a much more feasible source of additional functional improvement then a transplant or bypass. In neurology and neurosurgery we observe patients almost on a daily basis who have neurological tissue that is viable and nonfunctional. Recently one of the authors surgically released a congenitally tethered spinal cord of an 11-year-old child who had never had feeling or movement in his toes on one foot; he woke up postoperatively with movement and feeling in those toes. This procedure obviously did not regenerate his spinal cord, but the release of a small degree of pressure or traction on his nervous system converted tissue from a viable nonfunctional to a viable functional state. There are many similar examples: the central cord syndrome patient who, after plateauing neurologically, suddenly improves with regard to pain, sensation, and strength in his hands following a decompression; the spinal cord-injured patient who, years after injury, manifests significant residual cord compression and a discrepancy between his motor and sensory levels and improves locally following a delayed decompression. Are these examples of CNS regeneration?

Doubtful! The more likely explanation is the phenomenon described above. Therefore a logical approach to the restoration of function for some SCI victims must include identifying viable but nonfunctioning neural tissue and determining a means to activate and use it. Utilization may be enhanced through technologies such as computerized multichannel EMG biofeedback. There are thousands of fibers and tracts in the spinal cord that are not necessarily utilized to perform normal functional activities. Techniques like biofeedback can be useful in that they provide the individual with cognitive cues not otherwise available to perform a function. It is possible within the CNS to locate and utilize alternate pathways or detours in order to restore function. A good example of this type of function transfer can be seen in the neurosurgical procedure in which an injured 7th cranial nerve is anastomosed to the 11th or 12th and then, through visual learning (i.e., a form of biofeedback), the patient learns to smile symmetrically by shrugging a shoulder or moving the tongue. The same principle could be utilized with fetal cell transplants or nerve grafting to establish new spinal cord connections. Many SCI patients who appear to have functionally complete lesions may in reality have incomplete ones; we may simply lack the knowledge of how to identify and activate these pathways.

Rehabilitative engineering in the form of computerized closed loop or open loop functional electrical stimulation (FES), with or without orthotics, can be utilized to enhance functional activity. One reasonable scenario might be the combination of computerized biofeedback and FES in combination with the patient's own residual muscle tissue to convert him/her to a functional ambulator. Another (for an anterior cord syndrome with proprioceptive sparing) could utilize such a hybrid biofeedback/FES system with braces, i.e., taking advantage of the function that is preserved combined with engineering technology to produce a functional ambulator.

A major treatment strategy for the development of SCI regeneration or restoration of functional integrity could be the development of a method to effect reconnection in the CNS, just as one would splice a wire or telephone cable. This approach might include fetal cell trans-plants, nerve grafts, or peripheral nerve bypasses that could be used to bridge areas with actual physical separations. Peripheral nerve grafts would be available as autografts from sources such as the sural nerve, but fetal cell transplants present a more complex challenge. Issues include safety, morality, sterility, viability, and many other logistical considerations. Molecular biologists could potentially develop cell lines that might eliminate the majority of these obstacles (Gage and Buzsaki, Chapter 13, this volume).

Establishing a CNS reconnection that will restore communication lines is a complex challenge, in contrast to Parkinson's disease, Alzheimer's disease, or movement disorders in which we may be dealing primarily with neurotransmitter depletion. A successful therapy for the latter diseases may simply involve transplanting cells capable of providing a continuous source of the depleted neurotransmitters. In contrast, in SCI, stroke, or head injury, we must deal with complex circuitry and establish reconnections. All patients with spinal cord injuries have a cystic lesion area at the injury site, but only 5–10% of these cysts progress in their rostral and caudal extent. However, even these small cystic areas create a barrier impeding physical or functional reconnection. Even if fetal cell transplants or peripheral nerve grafts could bridge or bypass an area of cystic degeneration, the challenge is to make these connections functional, an overwhelming task if one assumes that it is necessary to actually connect fiber A to fiber A and fiber B to fiber B. However, considering peripheral nerve anastomosis procedures that result in functional recovery without end-to-end matching, one can imagine that a useful communication could be established between proximal and distal fibers even though it may not be a replication of the preexisting network. This fundamental connection might provide a functional neuromuscular interface whose activity could be refined with biofeedback, electrical stimulation, etc. to produce the desired functional activity.

Each of the major strategies presently being utilized in regeneration research, i.e., fetal cell transplantation, nerve grafting (peripheral nerve bypass), neurotrophic factors, and electrical fields, has potential. However, a major strategic error has perhaps been to search for a simple solution to a very complex problem, i.e., a one-operation, one-drug, or one-modality approach. A more feasible therapeutic scenario might be fetal cell transplantation and/or peripheral nerve graft, supported metabolically and environmentally by an infusion of growth factors with a miniosmotic pump as the fiber growth is directed and possibly stimulated by an implanted electrical field generator. This type of integrated multimodality strategy makes more sense than to continue searching for the simple or quick solution. In the same way that the multidisciplinary team approach to SCI patient care has produced a better outcome, the multidisciplinary and multimodality approach in the basic laboratory to create and refine therapy strategies might be more productive.

While the basic sciences are developing the building blocks to create clinical treatments, clinical scientists must simultaneously develop applied research approaches or strategies to utilize the information and implement programs to test the applicability of those treatments. Applied research in spinal cord injury is quite broad in its scope and involves research programs in almost every component of the care system. Prehospital research includes the development of more sophisticated monitoring systems, especially wireless telemetry systems. Direct spinal cord monitoring with evoked responses could be utilized in the same manner we monitor the cardiac function with wireless telemetry today. The development of better immobilization devices and of portable imaging equipment would permit fracture reduction at the accident scene. Medical treatment is no doubt improving as a result of applied research, with the mortality in most major centers dropping from 10% to less than 5% over the last decade. Improvement has also been extended into the rehabilitation and lifelong follow-up phase of care, where the average spinal cord injury patient who survives the first year has a relatively normal life expectancy and is more likely to die of cancer, stroke, or heart disease than the traditional renal failure or decubitus ulcers (Mesard et al., 1978).

Research has advanced most rapidly in the rehabilitation and outpatient phases, in which the marriage of engineering and medicine in the form of biomedical or rehabilitation engineering has produced rapidly evolving progress in rehabilitation. One such advance is the construction of computerized multichannel EMG biofeedback equipment utilizing visual and auditory feedback in conjunction with sensitive-surface electrodes and a rapid-processing computer developed to enhance patient function. This technology can also identify and monitor viable but nonfunctional CNS tissue and can be used to help control spasms, especially in partially innervated muscles. The technician can mount electrodes on the flexors and extensors of the elbow, for example, and teach the patient in a very short time to relax the extensors while activating the flexors, and vice versa, for a more fluid effective movement in the spastic extremity. Electromyography is invaluable in helping to identify the presence of motor units. Patients may have a C6 motor function but no C7 motor function and at the same time display good C7 sensation. If the EMG biofeedback unit is able to identify motor unit activity in C7, then the patient is much more likely to respond to a delayed decompression with recovery of C7 motor function.

Another rehabilitative engineering advance has been the development of sophisticated FES devices. Closed loop systems combined with computer technology are presently available and in one instance have been used in lower extremity bicycle ergometry exercise protocols that have proved this method effective in reversing muscle atrophy and cardiopulmonary deconditioning, especially in quadriplegics. Open loop FES is commonly applied to upper extremity muscles and, in some cases, lower extremities for maintaining range of motion, decreasing spasticity, and strengthening incompletely paralyzed muscles. Another promising area of biomedical engineering is the development of an implantable stimulator system for evacuation of the bladder and bowels. Active clinical trials are in progress, and these systems are becoming more sophisticated and functional. Implantable electrodes, or in some cases surface electrodes, have been used for stimulation of lower extremity muscles of paraplegics and quadriplegics to allow mobilization with or without braces. The most practical strategy involves a combination of surface electrical stimulation along with a light-weight externally worn orthosis. This nononinvasive combination has proved so effective that a complete paraplegic recently walked 7 miles in the Honolulu Marathon at a rate of 1 1/2 miles an hour. This is a much safer technique than the use of implantable electrodes, which are not yet refined enough for long-term safety and function.

Another area of applied research that has advanced dramatically is sexuality and reproduction. It is now appreciated that most spinal cord-injured men and women can have their own children. Special implantable and nonimplantable devices are available to provide erections in males and, by alkalinizing the urine and using electroejaculation stimulators and bladder suction techniques, a spinal cord injured-male's own sperm can be used to fertilize a woman's ova. Quadriplegic and paraplegic women are capable of bearing children, with some electing to do so with natural childbirth techniques.

Technology developed for high quadriplegics includes sophisticated environmental control systems designed to allow persons with absolutely no movement in their arms or legs to perform tasks such as opening and closing doors and windows, turning on or adjusting radio or television sets, raising and lowering beds, etc. Vans are available with equally sophisticated control systems.

Close basic science and applied interaction is necessary for practical treatments to evolve. Basic scientists should appreciate the clinical realities, limitations, and problems, and clinicians should be fully aware of the state of the art of basic science research strategies, including transplantation, electrical fields, nerve grafting and application of nerve growth factors. As the basic neurosciences have literally exploded over the past decade, so has the clinical applied research field. Important lessons remain for clinicians to learn from basic scientists, including experimental design, statistical analysis, and a more scientific methodology in the approach to clinical problems. On the other hand, there are important lessons for basic scientists to learn from clinicians regarding the realities of spinal cord injury in humans, including logistical considerations, systemic consequences, and the feasibility of various strategies that are now being evaluated in test tubes or Petri dishes and that will hopefully-someday become available for human beings.

REFERENCES

Bracken MB, Collins WF, Freeman DF, Shepard MJ, Wagner FW, Silten RM, Hellen KG, Ransohoff J, Hunt WE, Perot PL, Gross RG, Green BA, Eisenberg HM, Rifkinson N, Goodman JH, Meagher JN, Fischer B, Clifton GL, Flamm ES, Rawe SE (1984): Efficacy of methylprednisolone in acute spinal cord injury. JAMA 251:45–52.

Eidelberg E (1983): Loss and recovery of locomotor function after spinal cord lesions in cats and monkeys. In Seil FJ (ed): "Nerve, Organ, and Tissue Regeneration: Research Perspectives." New York: Academic Press, pp 231–242.

Green BA, Klose KJ (1981): Acute spinal cord injury, part I. In Sheinberg P (ed): "Neurology and Neurosurgery Update Series," vol II, Lesson 27.

Green BA, Eismont FJ (1984): Acute spinal cord injury: A systems approach. CNS Trauma 1:173–195.

Green BA, Magana IA (1987): Spinal cord trauma: Clinical aspects. In Davidoff M (ed): "Handbook of the Spinal Cord," vols IV and V. New York: Marcel Dekker, pp 63–92.

Green BA, Green KL, Klose KJ (1980a): Kinetic nursing for acute spinal cord injury patients. Paraplegia 18:181–186.

Green BA, Khan T, Klose KJ (1980b): A comparative study of steroid therapy in acute experimental spinal cord injury. Surg Neurol 13:91–97.

Green BA, Callahan RA, Klose KJ, De La Torre J (1981): Acute spinal cord injury: Current concepts. Clin Orthop 154:125–135.

Green BA, Klose KJ, Goldberg ML (1985): Clinical and research considerations in spinal cord injury. In Becker DP, Povlishock JT (eds): "Central Nervous System Trauma Status Report." Bethesda: NINCDS, NIH, pp 341–368.

Hall WJ, Green BA, Colodonato JP (1976): Spinal cord injury: Emergency management. Emer Med Serv 5:28–36.

Hayashi N, Green BA, Veraa RP (1984): Local spinal cord blood flow and oxygen metabolism. In Davidoff M (ed): "Handbook of the Spinal Cord," vols. II and III. New York: Marcel Dekker, pp 817–827.

Klose KJ, Green BA, Smith RS, Adkins RH, MacDonald AM (1980): University of Miami Neuro-Spinal Index (UMNI): A quantitative method for determining spinal cord function. Paraplegia 18:331–336.

Mesard L, Carmody A, Mannarino E, Ruge D (1978): Survival after spinal cord trauma. Arch Neurol 35:78–83.

Schneider RC (1955): The syndrome of acute anterior spinal cord injury. J Neurosurg 12:95.

Schneider RC, Thompson JM, Bebin J (1958): The syndrome of acute central cervical spinal cord injury. J Neurol Neurosurg Psychiatry 21:216–227.

Stover SL, Fine PR (ed) (1986): "Spinal Cord Injury: The Facts and Figures." Birmingham: University of Alabama at Birmingham.

Young JS, Northrup NE (1979): Statistical information pertaining to some of the most commonly asked questions about spinal cord injury. Science Digest 1:11.

12

Reactive Astrocyte and Axonal Outgrowth in the Injured CNS: Is Gliosis Really an Impediment to Regeneration?

PAUL J. REIER, PhD, LAWRENCE F. ENG, PhD, AND LYN JAKEMAN

Deparments of Neurological Surgery and Neuroscience, University of Florida College of Medicine, Gainesville, Florida 32610 (P.J.R., L.J.); Department of Pathology, Veterans Administration Medical Center, and Stanford University School of Medicine, Palo Alto, California 94304 (L.F.E.)

Scar formation represents one of the hallmark histopathological features of the injured central nervous system (CNS). This cellular response to neural tissue damage is most commonly attributed to the astrocyte, one of the major supporting (i.e., neuroglial) cell types of the nervous system. Although other neural and nonneural cells can also contribute to the development of scar tissue, considerable attention has been directed to the astrocyte over the years, given the prevalence of its so-called reactive form in the injured CNS and the multiple roles that the astrocyte is now recognized to play under normal conditions (Fedoroff and Vernadakis, 1986a, b, c). Accordingly, numerous studies have been directed at characterizing the cellular dynamics (e.g., proliferative, metabolic, growth) that contribute to the development of astrocytic scars following trauma to the brain and spinal cord.

What has become generally appreciated is that gliosis represents the product of a rather aggressive cellular reaction that is at least partly directed at tissue repair. The astrocyte may thereby play a major role in restoring some degree of structural and physiological integrity at the site of injury, as well as at more distant levels where substantial loss of neuronal processes and/or cell bodies has occurred.

On the other hand, this process also seems to entail a contradiction in that the matrix of an astrocytic scar has been thought to be capable of thwarting spontaneous regeneration. However, while this view has been embedded in the literature for many years, it has not been uniformly accepted. Various lines of more recent in vivo and in vitro experimentation have also suggested that astrocytes in the mature CNS may produce neuronotrophic and neurite-promoting factors that are actually beneficial to neuronal survival and the outgrowth of neuritic processes (Lindsay, 1986; Manthorpe et al., 1986). Lastly, there is a new line of developing evidence indicating that other CNS cellular constituents may also have an adverse effect on axonal outgrowth.

Thus the significance of astrocytic reactivity and scar formation in relation to axonal regeneration has been challenged from a number of different perspectives. What has emerged is a far more complex picture of the role played by astrocytes and of the overall consequences of gliosis in the injured CNS than previously conjectured from conventional histopathological analyses.

In this chapter, the problem of gliosis and regeneration is reviewed by first addressing what a glial scar is from histological and histophysiological perspectives, and then moving to a discussion of some observations that have prompted further consideration of the original view that gliosis prevents regeneration by forming physical barriers to growing nerve fibers. Experimental models are then described that have been used to reevaluate the impact of

Neural Regeneration and Transplantation, pages 183–209

scar formation on regeneration with contemporary techniques. Finally, various cellular mechanisms related to scarring are outlined that have been proposed to account for limited regeneration in the CNS. It should be noted that the purpose of this chapter is to highlight some of the more essential issues related to this subject rather than to provide an exhaustive survey of the literature. More comprehensive discussions have been presented in other recent reviews (Reier et al., 1983a, 1988; Wells and Bernstein, 1985; Lindsay, 1986; Reier, 1986; Eng et al., 1987; Reier and Houlé, 1988).

HISTOLOGY AND HISTOPATHOLOGY OF THE GLIAL SCAR

Various configurations of glial scar tissue, as seen in different regions of the CNS with light and electron microscopy, have been recently described (Bignami et al., 1980; Nathaniel and Nathaniel, 1981; Reier, 1986). Therefore, only a general summary will be provided here to establish a point of reference for subsequent discussion of the cellular make-up of the glial scar and of mechanisms that may be affecting axonal growth in the presence of an astroglial matrix.

Fundamentally, gliosis in the injured CNS, as in many other types of neuropathology, entails proliferation. This process primarily reflects an increase in the number of astrocytes, though the term is also frequently used by neuropathologists in reference to an amplification in the number of glial cytoplasmic processes. Hypertrophy represents a second major component of the glial response, as evidenced by substantial changes in the volume of astroglial cell bodies and processes.

While at the histological level the expression of both of these cellular responses can be qualitatively appreciated with a number of classical staining methods (e.g., Cajal's gold mercuric chloride, Del Rio Hortega silver carbonate, eosin and hematoxylin), one of the more contemporary approaches involves the immunocytochemical demonstration of astrocytic cell bodies and cytoplasmic processes (Eng, 1985; Dahl et al., 1986). For example, by using an antibody to glial fibrillary acidic protein (GFAP), a major protein subunit of glial intermediate filaments (Eng, 1985), astrocytes can be detected in normal tissue, and changes in their number, size, and distribution of cytoplasmic processes can often be visualized by striking differences in staining intensity in areas of scar formation (Figs. 12–1, 12–2). The augmented staining intensity observed in sections exposed to GFAP antiserum is consistent with the increased intermediate filament content of astrocytes and elevated density of astrocytic processes typically seen in electron micrographs of gliotic areas (Fig. 12–3).

Generally, gliosis, as earmarked by proliferation and hypertrophy, occurs in response to axonal degeneration. Thus a dense astroglial meshwork is usually formed in areas of white matter where the majority of fibers have undergone Wallerian degeneration (Fig. 12–2). Often the glial scars in fiber tracts consist not only of astrocytes, but also of numerous macrophages, microglia, oligodendrocytes, and myelin debris (Fig. 12–4). Reactive astrocytes also form scars in gray matter as a result of fiber or terminal degeneration, as well as the retrograde loss of neuronal cell bodies. Gliosis in gray matter tends to be variable in density, depending upon the extent of degeneration that has occurred. It should be noted that astrocytic reactivity can also be precipitated in gray matter by peripheral nerve lesions (Graeber and Kreutzberg, 1986).

In addition to proliferation and hypertrophy, glial scarring can involve an encapsulation process (Matthews et al., 1979; Bernstein, 1983; Reier et al., 1983a), which forms the basic tissue setting that the majority of experimental studies of gliosis and regeneration have addressed. To appreciate this component of the glial response, it is worth recalling that astrocytes normally partition the CNS from surrounding non-CNS tissue (e.g., meningeal layers, perivascular connective tissue) by forming a limiting membrane (i.e., external glial-limiting membrane [EGLM], glia limitans) (Fig. 12–5). At the surface of the brain, spinal cord, or optic nerve, as well as around blood vessels, this membrane (as seen with the electron microscope), consists of a relatively smooth layer of closely apposed cytoplasmic endfeet of astrocytic processes with a continuous basal lamina intervening between this limiting membrane and the overlying pia (Peters, et al., 1976).

When the interior of the CNS is breached, a

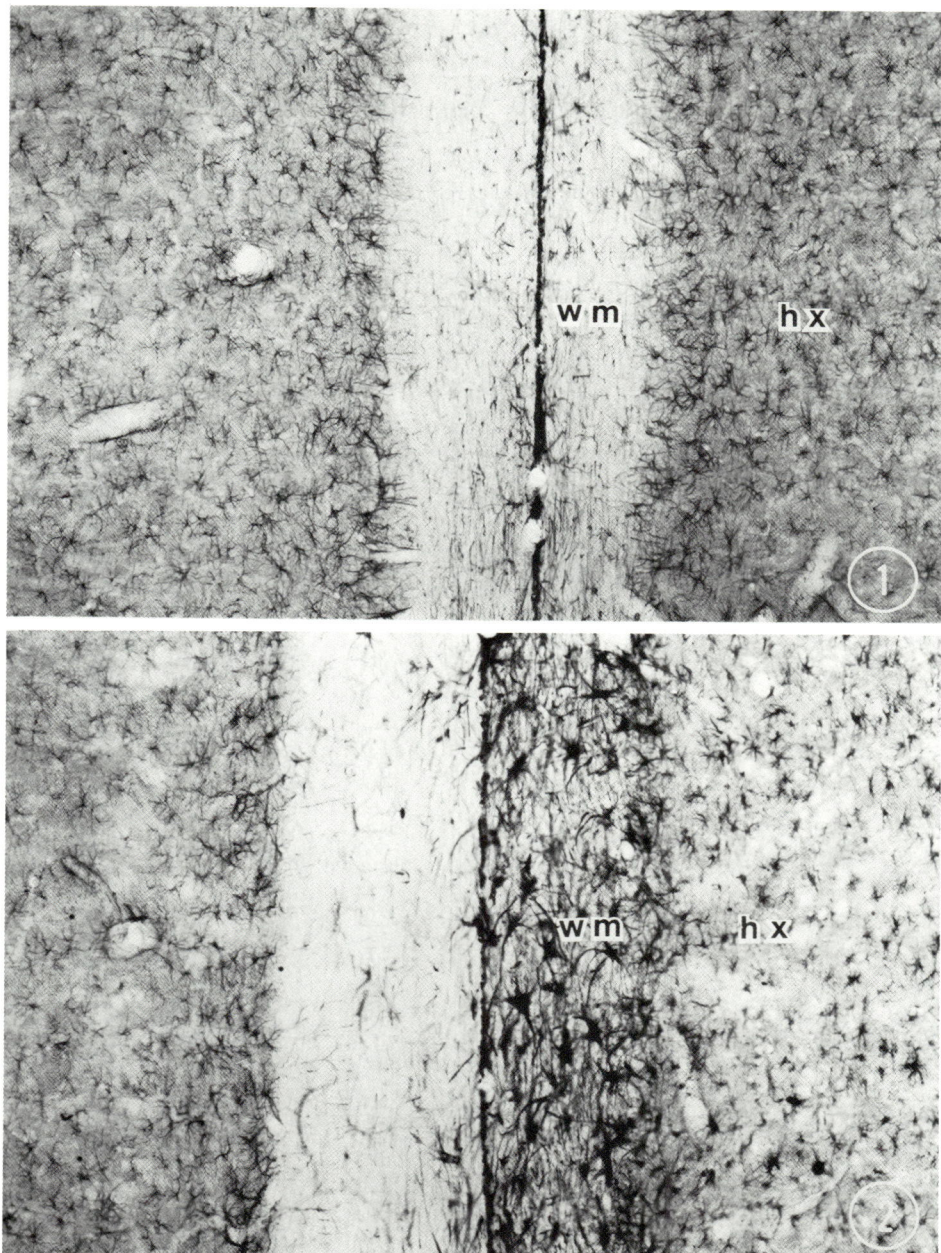

Figure 12–1. Horizontal section of the adult rat spinal cord stained with the antibody to glial fibrillary acidic protein (GFAP). This field shows the distribution of astrocytes in gray (hx) and white matter (wm) rostral and both ipsi- and contralateral to a hemisection lesion. The hemisected side is indicated by the label "hx." × 100.

Figure 12–2. A photograph of the same section used for Figure 12–1, but showing a field two spinal segments caudal to the hemisection lesion. Note that the astrocytes stained with anti-GFAP in the gray matter ipsilateral to the lesion (hx) are slightly more prominent than the astroglia seen contralateral to the injury. An especially dramatic degree of gliosis is seen in the injured white matter (wm). × 100.

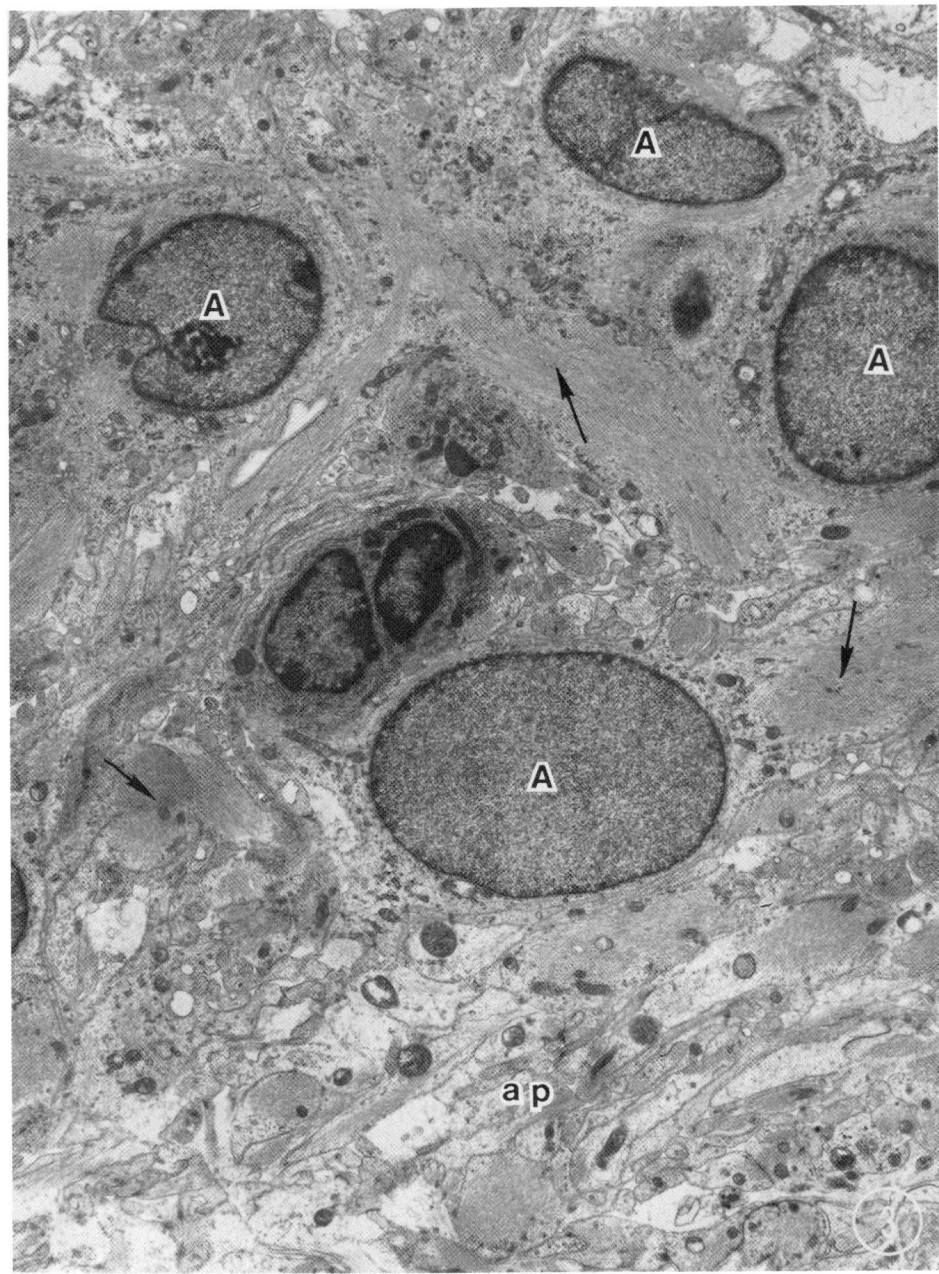

Figure 12–3. An electron micrograph of an area of glial scar formation in the injured spinal cord of the adult rat. The nuclei of several astrocytes (A) are shown surrounded in some instances by cytoplasm containing dense bundles of intermediate filaments (arrows). Astrocytic processes (ap) are also seen in the lower portion of the field forming a complex protoplasmic matrix. ×7,200.

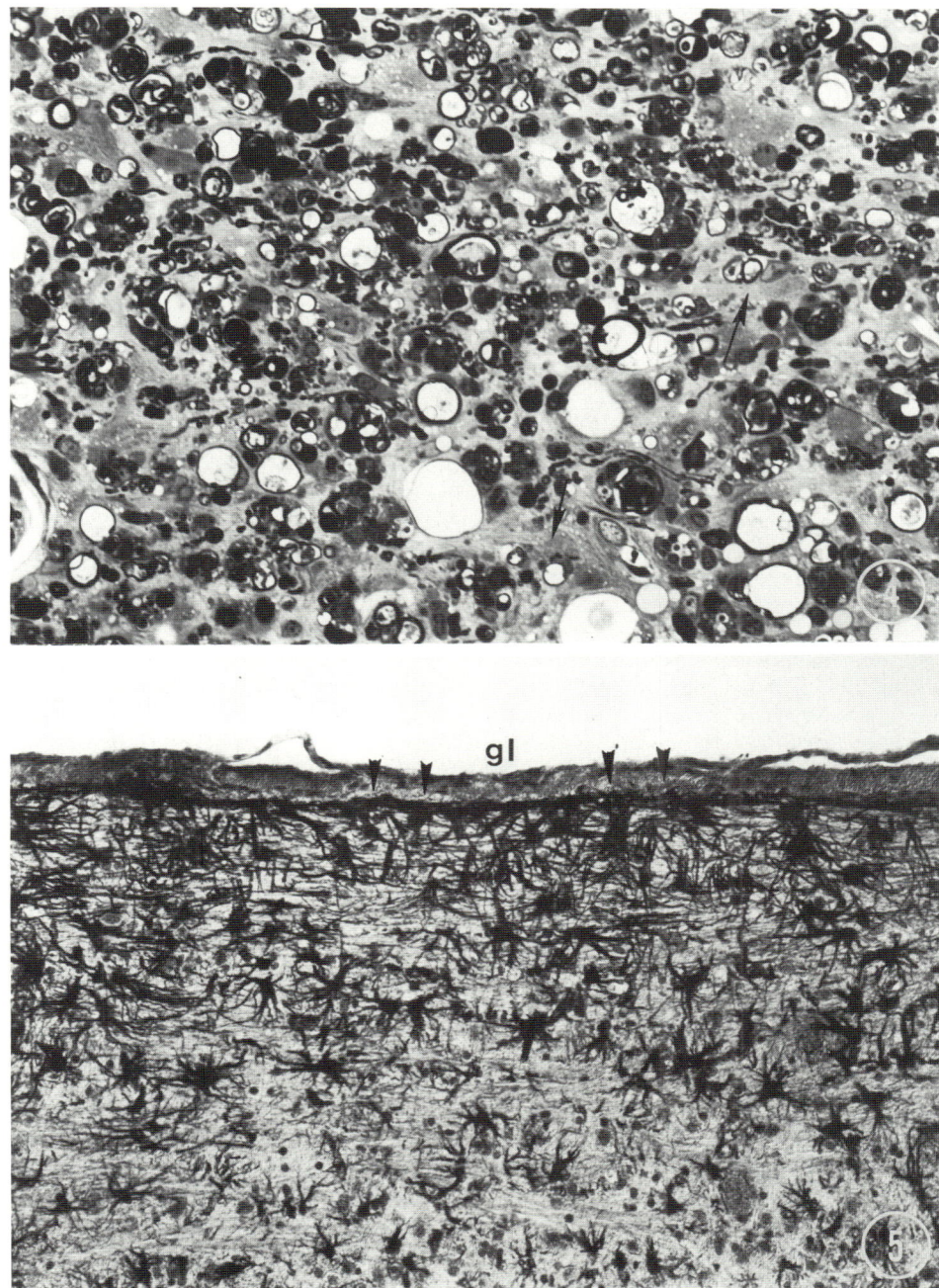

Figure 12–4. The development of a glial scar in a region of degenerating white matter. Note the darkly stained myelin ovoids and macrophages embedded in a lightly stained astrocytic matrix (arrows). ×390.

Figure 12–5. Horizontal section of a normal adult rat spinal cord. The glia limitans (i.e., external glial limiting membrane, gl) is indicated by arrowheads pointing to the darkly stained astrocytic margin of this section stained with anti-GFAP. ×190.

glial capsule is eventually formed over the exposed neuropil. For example, studies of neocortical stab lesions in the rodent have demonstrated that a new EGLM is established by 20 days postinjury (Berry et al., 1983; Mathewson and Berry, 1985). Likewise, an accumulation of astrocytes occurs at the margin of the lesion in the injured adult rat spinal cord by 1 week, and a glial scar (Figs. 12–6, 12–7) is formed by 2 weeks along the damaged rostral and caudal surfaces (Barrett et al., 1981).

In contrast to the EGLM of the normal CNS, the reconstituted astrocytic boundary is generally much thicker, because of the presence of multiple layers of either flattened or hypertrophied cytoplasmic processes (Figs. 12–8—12–10). The restored EGLM often exhibits a more tortuous configuration as a result of the convoluted interdigitation of astrocytes and non-CNS elements. Consequently, the reconstituted EGLM can extend into the depths of the CNS parenchyma near the edge of a transection lesion.

That mesodermal elements exert a major influence over this glial reaction to injury has been suggested by various lines of evidence derived from tissue culture studies (reviewed in Reier and Houlé, 1988). In addition, astrocytic encapsulation does not occur in neonatal animals in which CNS lesions are characterized by less fibroblastic and macrophagic invasion of the wound (Berry et al., 1983).

In summary, the extent of gliosis induced by trauma depends upon the nature of the injury (e.g., invasive or noninvasive), the severity of injury as reflected by the degree of tissue degeneration (retrograde and Wallerian), and the distance from the lesion site. The cellular composition of the scar can vary also. For example, when the CNS neuropil becomes externalized to the peripheral interstitial tissue environment, a fibroglial scar consisting of astrocytes, fibroblasts, and dense collagenous accumulations, among other mesodermal tissue constituents, forms along the damaged surfaces of the CNS. On the other hand, as a product of Wallerian degeneration or axonal die-back, gliosis also occurs at more distant levels from the lesion. In the more extreme instances, such areas of scarring can be seen as a complex mosaic of interdigitating, tightly packed astrocytic processes (Figs. 12–8, 12–10). In those areas, the scar is predominantly composed of astrocytes; however, microglia, oligodendrocytes, myelin debris, and macrophages are also frequently present.

As noted above, such expressions of glial reactivity can be regarded as being part of a repair process. On one hand, encapsulation appears to be directed at reestablishing the normal anatomical separation of CNS and non-CNS tissue microenvironments. On the other hand, glial scarring in gray or white matter at more distant levels from the lesion site seems to be directed at filling expanded domains of extracellular space resulting from neuronal degeneration. While the overall benefits of glial reactivity leading to scar formation are not fully known, it would appear as a matter of pure conjecture that the astrocyte may be playing an important role in restoring some degree of physiological homeostasis in the injured CNS.

GLIOSIS AS A BARRIER TO AXONAL REGENERATION
The "Scar" Hypothesis

At the same time, however, this cellular response has been thought to create a milieu responsible for the inhibition of axonal elongation. Many of the earlier histological reports described an abortive regeneration characterized by axons terminating in scar tissue (Penfield, 1927; Ramón y Cajal, 1928; Sugar and Gerard, 1940). This point was amplified by subsequent studies performed by Windle and his associates (Windle and Chambers, 1950; Windle et al., 1952a, b, 1953). In those experiments, some stimulation of axonal growth could be promoted through an intraspinal lesion by preventing the formation of glial and collagenous scars (i.e., by interfering with the astroglial-fibroblastic encapsulation process) with a pyrogenic bacterial polysaccharide or corticosteroids. Therefore one of the more traditional hypotheses explaining the failure of any sustained spontaneous axonal regrowth in the CNS has been that scar tissue imposes a physical barrier to growing axons (Penfield, 1927; Ramón y Cajal, 1928; Clemente, 1955, 1964; Windle, 1956). This view was further supported by some electron microscopic investigations (Lampert and Cressman, 1964; Kao et al., 1977), which showed axons either

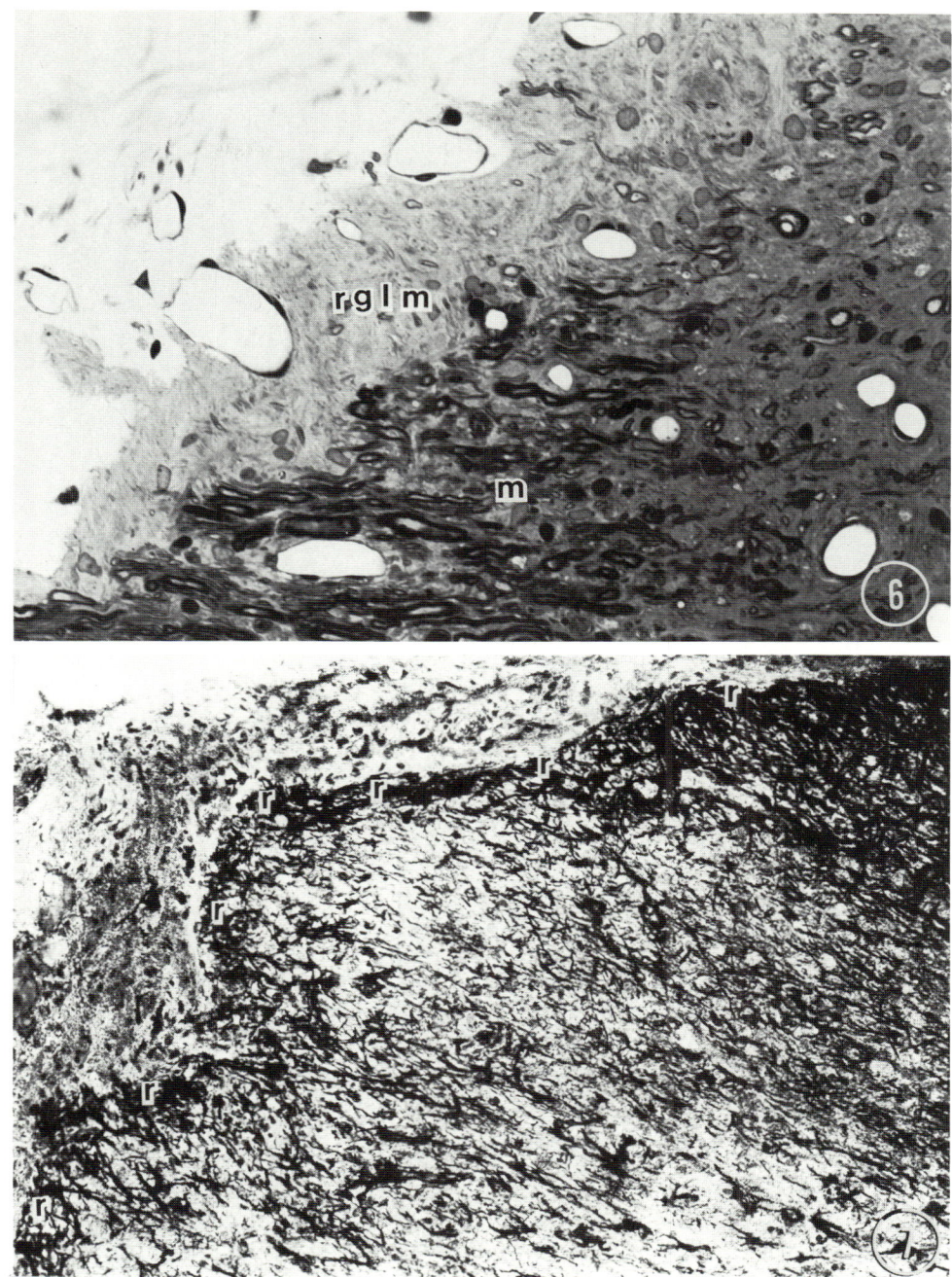

Figure 12–6. A section of tissue from the injured adult rat spinal cord that was embedded in plastic and cut at 2 μm in thickness. The field shows the damaged surface of the spinal cord resulting from transection. Note that a reconstituted glial-limiting membrane (rglm) has formed and that few of the longitudinally sectioned myelinated (m) axons (dark profiles) appear to have penetrated this glial scar. ×390.

Figure 12–7. A paraffin section of the injured rat spinal cord stained with anti-GFAP. Note the reconstituted glial-limiting membrane (r). External (i.e., toward the left) to this scar is a zone consisting of collagenous scar tissue. ×190.

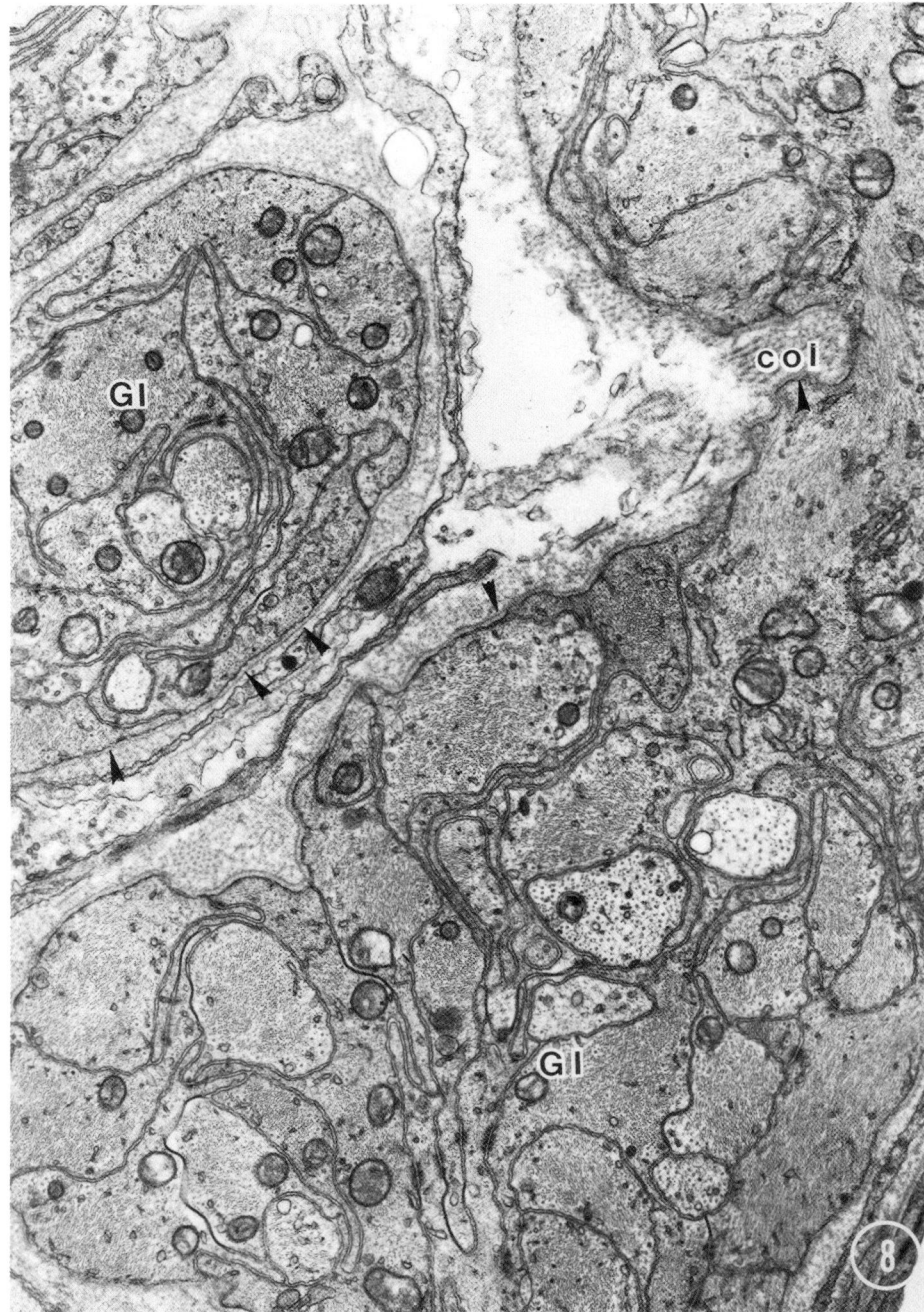

Figure 12–8.   An electron micrograph showing a region of the reconstituted glial-limiting membrane (Gl). A dense accumulation of hypertrophic astrocytic processes is indicated. The astrocytic scar is bounded by a basal lamina (arrowheads) and collagen (col). × 16,800.

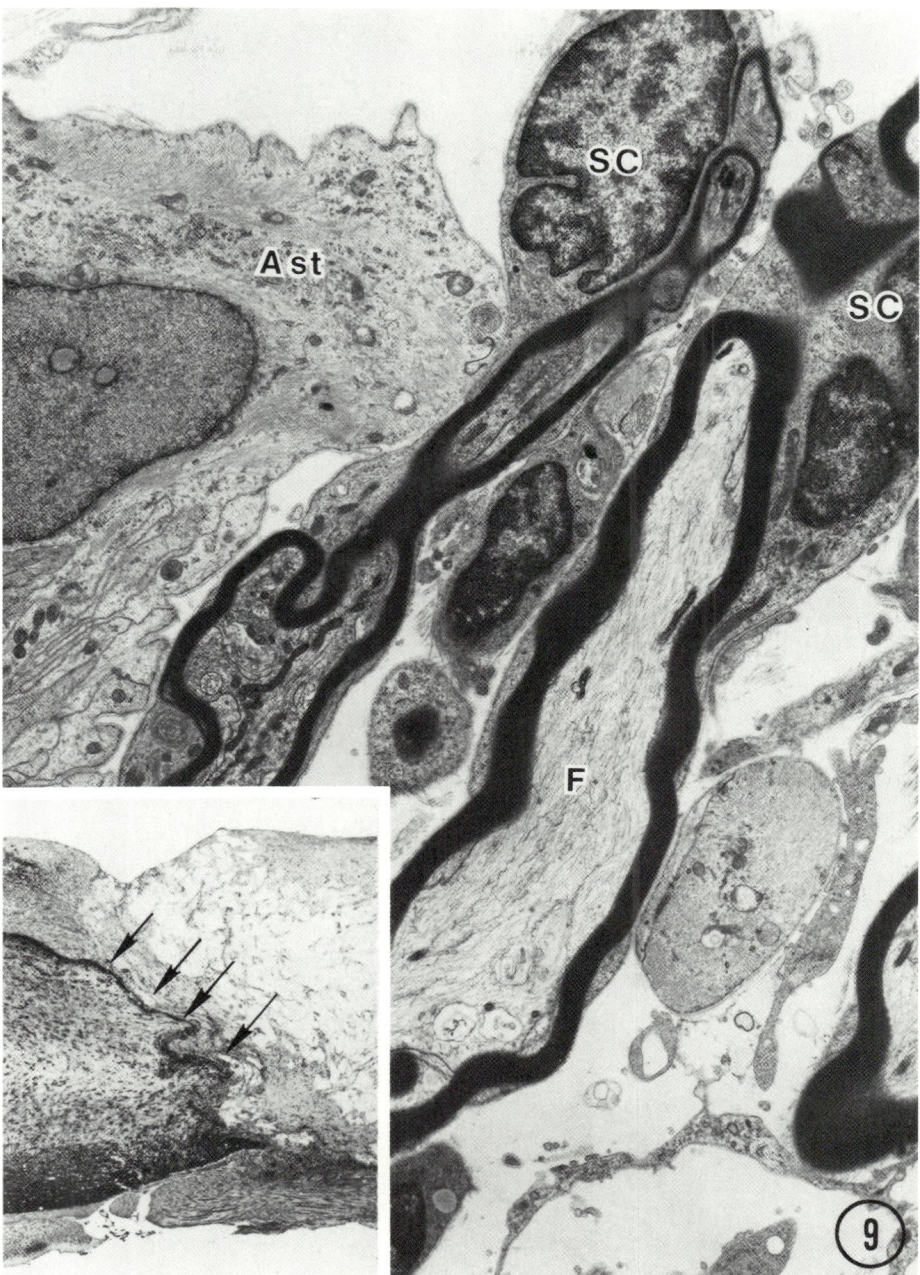

Figure 12–9. An electron micrograph showing another view of a glial capsule formed along the injured surface of a transected spinal cord in the adult rat (see inset for general orientation). The astrocytic scar is seen to the left (Ast); to the right, axons (F) are seen surrounded by Schwann cells (SC). ×4,800. **Inset:** A low-magnification light microscopic view of the glial capsule (revealed by anti-GFAP staining) formed along the injured surface (arrows) of the adult rat spinal cord after transection of the spinal cord. Although not readily apparent in this micrograph, some axons of dorsal root origin are coursing adjacent to the outer surface of the glial capsule. This light microscopic image corresponds to the more detailed companion electron micrograph. ×25.

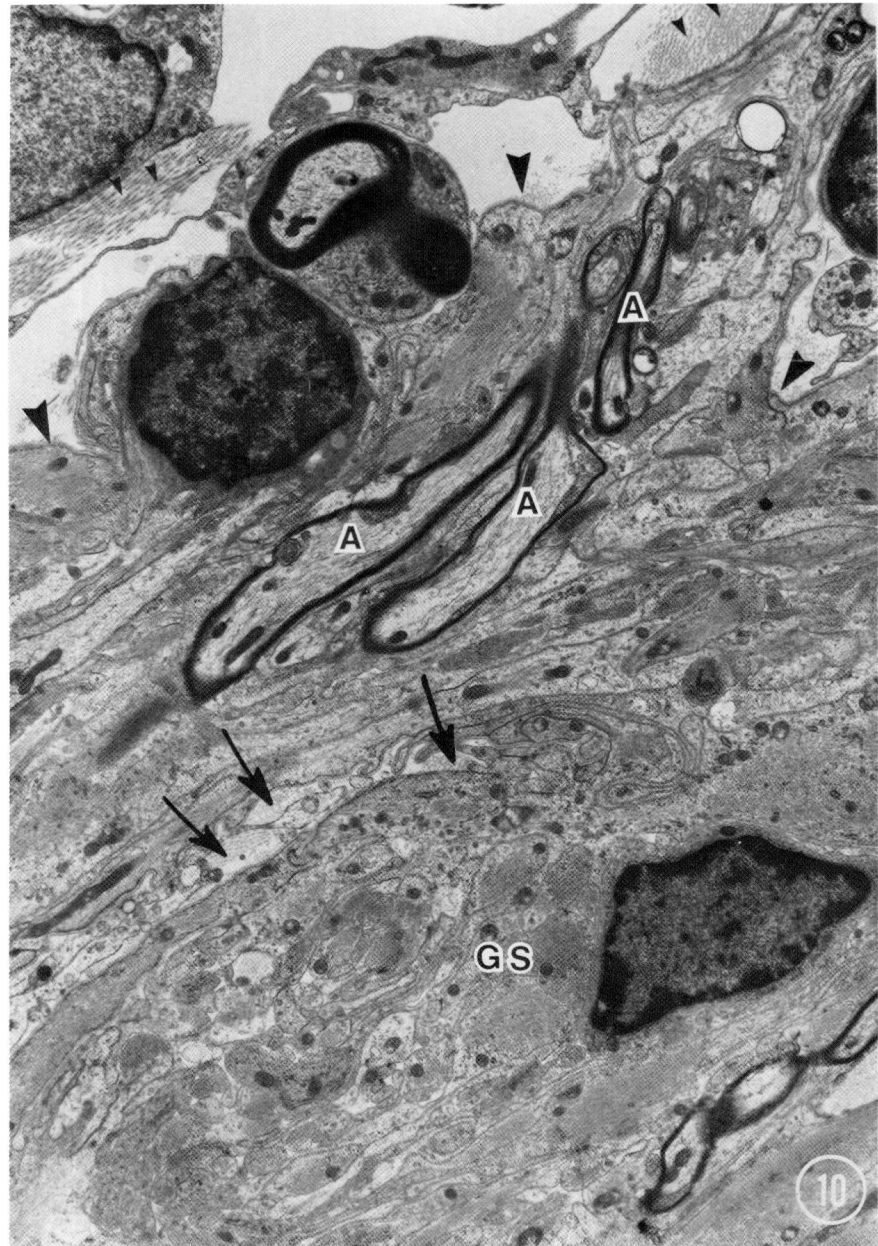

Figure 12–10. The convoluted nature of the reconstituted glial-limiting membrane along a spinal cord lesion is illustrated in this electron micrograph. The arrows point to pockets of collagen that are present in a fold of the glial capsule. Large arrowheads indicate the basal lamina formed along the outermost layer of astrocytic processes, and small arrowheads note other clusters of collagen. A few myelinated axons (A) appear to have penetrated the edge of the glial capsule. A more compact astrocytic scar (GS), consisting of densely packed cytoplasmic processes, is seen deeper within this glial envelope. ×7,200.

being deflected or ending blindly as they encountered a glial scar.

Challenges to the Glial Scar Hypothesis

More recently, however, it has been asked whether astrocytic scarring is a problem at all or whether the idea that the formation of a physical obstacle to growing axons actually represents a mechanism whereby astrocytes influence axonal outgrowth (Berry, 1979; Kiernan, 1979; Barron, 1983; Mathewson and Berry, 1985). It has also been argued that gliosis does not appear to be a primary determinant of the failure of regeneration, as robust axonal outgrowth was not seen in some cases even when glial reactivity was absent (Gilson and Stensaas, 1974; Goldberg and Frank, 1980; Guth et al., 1981).

Ultrastructural studies of the injured spinal cord have also yielded observations inconsistent with the barrier concept. For example, instances have been noted wherein some axons appeared to have penetrated the reconstituted glial capsule (e.g., Fig. 12–10) at the injured surfaces of the transected spinal cord (Matthews et al., 1979; Reier et al., 1983a; Reier, 1986). Another major challenge stems from reports of the successful regeneration of certain neuronal populations, notably the regrowth of monoaminergic (Björklund and Steneve, 1979) and neurohypophyseal axons (Dellman, 1973; Berry, 1979; Kiernan, 1979).

Each of these arguments, however, can be tempered by other points of view. The fact that gliosis may not be a primary factor in determining the success of regeneration does not necessarily preclude it from having a major impact on axonal elongation. With regard to contradictory ultrastructural findings, it should not be overlooked that while some fibers may appear to have negotiated a seemingly formidable glial terrain, it is often difficult to be certain that they actually traversed a gliotic area after rather than before the establishment of the scar. Concerning specific neuronal populations, the regeneration of monoaminergic fibers is more consistently linked with chemically induced axotomies rather than mechanical (i.e., transection) lesions. The quality and extent of the glial response undoubtedly differ in these two situations. In fact, while monoaminergic fibers exhibit slow, but rather extensive, regrowth after chemical axotomy, some observations indicate that similar fiber systems regenerate less successfully when confronted by a scar resulting from trauma (Björklund et al., 1971; Nygren et al., 1971). The regeneration of neurohypophyseal axons also appears to be dependent upon the nature of the surrounding cellular microenvironment. While capable of regenerating after being severed in the neurohypophysis, these fibers are unable to do so when axotomy occurs in the hypothalamus, where a more typical astrocytic environment exists (see Discussion in Dellman, 1986).

EXPERIMENTAL SUPPORT OF THE GLIAL SCAR HYPOTHESIS

As these considerations illustrate, many settings are not readily amenable to a rigorous evaluation of axonal growth in the presence of a gliotic microenvironment. It has been possible, however, to examine the interactions between regenerating axons and astroglial microenvironments in greater depth using a number of more suitable experimental models in conjunction with a variety of contemporary neuranatomical methodologies.

Regeneration at the Dorsal Root Entry Zone

A compelling example of an astrocytic matrix being incompatible with axonal regeneration derives from studies of the regrowth of injured dorsal root fibers at the level of the dorsal root entry zone (DREZ) (Stensaas et al., 1979, 1987; Reier et al., 1983a; Bignami et al., 1984; Reier and Houlé, 1988). When primary afferent fibers are damaged (e.g., by crush) between the dorsal root ganglion and spinal cord, they respond by exhibiting a robust outgrowth that is maintained within the peripheral portion of the dorsal root. However, upon reaching the peripheral nervous system (PNS)-CNS transition region (i.e., DREZ), the majority of these fibers are unable to advance further and thus fail to reenter the spinal cord (Fig. 12–13A).

The cellular organization of the DREZ before (Berthold and Carlstedt, 1977; Reier, 1986) and after (Stensaas et al., 1987) dorsal root damage has been extensively described elsewhere. In brief, the DREZ entails a transition between endoneurial cellular components of the peripheral nerve portion of the root and a dome or fringe of astrocytic processes at the surface of the spinal cord that can extend for a short distance into the root (Fig. 12–11) (Schlaepfer et al., 1979). Thus the DREZ is essentially an interface of a few hundred microns between the peripheral environment of the dorsal root and CNS environment of the superficial dorsal horn.

After crush injury of the dorsal root, the astrocytic fringe often becomes enlarged as a result of astroglial hypertrophy (Fig. 12–12). Eventually, finger-like islands of densely packed astrocytic processes, collectively surrounded by a basal lamina, extend further peripherally and interdigitate with components of the root endoneurium. In principle, the cellular architecture of this modified dorsal root entry zone assumes many of the features characteristic of a reconstituted glia limitans (e.g., as seen in relation to spinal cord transection or neocortical stab wounds) but without many of the secondary histophathological changes (e.g., fibroblastic and collagenous scarring) that often complicate defining astrocytic effects on axonal regeneration.

After contacting the "reactive" glial dome, only a very small number of regenerating dorsal root fibers seem capable of traversing the DREZ (Liuzzi and Lasek, 1987b). The majority of these axons are either deflected back toward the ganglion or form abortive terminal enlargements (Stensaas et al., 1979, 1987; Liuzzi and Lasek, 1987a). The latter are also referred to as "arrested end-bulbs" and are characterized by large accumulations of organelles. Such profiles are usually indicative of the cessation of axonal outgrowth and have been observed within the astroglial matrix for up to at least 2 years after the initial dorsal root lesion (Stensaas et al., 1979, 1987).

While in most cases the failure of axons to reenter the spinal cord was associated with the presence of a thick scar, Stensaas et al. (1979) found that axonal growth also ceased at the PNS-CNS transition zone even when regeneration was initiated well in advance of an obvious glial reaction. As other investigations have shown, even a single layer of astrocytes appears capable of discouraging axonal growth into the spinal cord (Carlstedt, 1985a).

That the cellular microenvironment at the PNS-CNS transition zone of the DREZ influences regeneration has been further supported by recent transplantation studies. Using an intraspinal transplantation procedure developed in this laboratory (Reier et al., 1986), transected dorsal roots were juxtaposed to grafts of embryonic spinal cord tissue placed into lesions of the adult rat spinal cord (Tessler et al., 1988). Under these conditions, injured, mature primary afferent fibers were able to reinnervate fetal CNS tissue, including regions of the grafts resembling the normal superficial dorsal horn (Fig. 12–14). In another investigation, Carlstedt et al. (1986) observed that crushed dorsal root fibers were able to reenter the intact spinal cords of neonatal rats. Such regrowth, however, was limited to the first week of postnatal life.

Some change must therefore be occurring (either at the DREZ or within the spinal cord during early postnatal life in the rat) that progressively renders the microenvironment less favorable to axonal elongation. These results are consistent with other studies showing that regenerative axonal elongation is also limited to the early postnatal period in the rodent in other parts of the CNS (Grafe and Shoenfeld, 1982, Sijbesma and Leonard, 1986; Smith et al., 1986).

Nerve Anastomosis Experiments

A variation of the DREZ experimental model has also been used to test whether the arrested regrowth of dorsal root axons at the PNS-CNS transition zone was merely due to some inherent metabolic limitation on the part of the dorsal root ganglion cell. This possibility has been entertained (Lasek et al., 1981) on the basis of a report by Barnes and Worrall (1968) noting that motoneuron fibers could penetrate the DREZ when the cut proximal stumps of ventral roots were coapted with the severed central ends of dorsal roots. Furthermore, higher regenerative rates for motor, as compared with sensory, axons have been described (Takano, 1976; Meier and Sollmann, 1977; Risling et al., 1983), and Wujek and Lasek (1983) have noted that the central processes of dorsal root ganglion cells regenerate more slowly than their peripheral branches.

Repetitions of the Barnes and Worrall experiment, however, have led to disparate results.

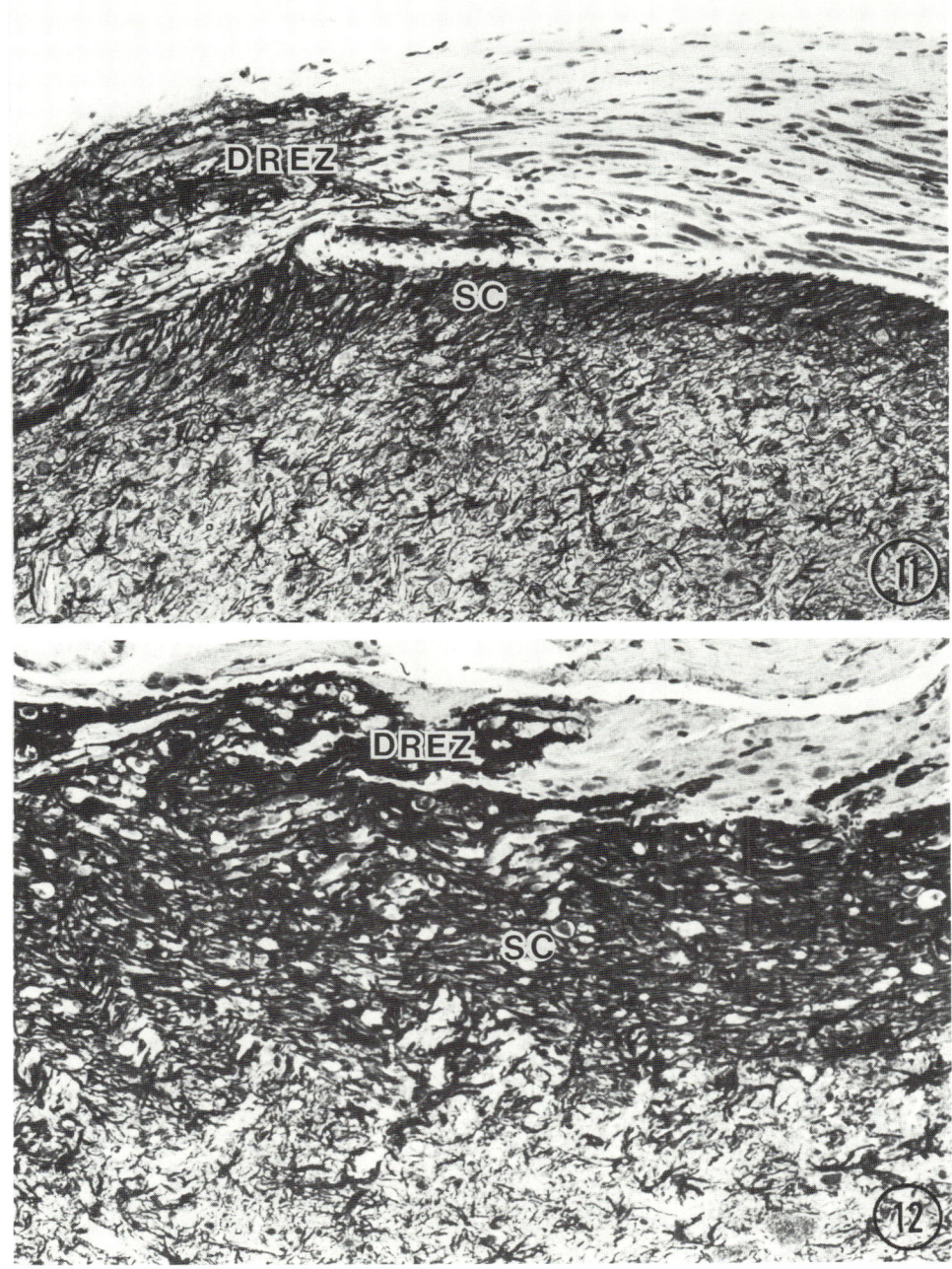

Figure 12–11. A longitudinal section of the rat spinal cord (SC) stained with antibodies to GFAP (i.e., to show astroglia) and neurofilament protein (i.e., to reveal axons). The anti-GFAP shows the distribution of astrocytic processes at the dorsal root entry zone (DREZ) of a normal dorsal root. Longitudinal axonal profiles are seen at the right of the DREZ. × 190.

Figure 12–12. Another longitudinal section of the adult rat spinal cord (SC) stained as described for Figure 12–11. In this case, the dorsal root had been cut, and the DREZ is now seen to be more deeply stained than that shown in the previous figure. This difference in staining can be attributed to hypertrophy and closer aggregation of astrocytic processes (similar to that depicted in Fig. 12–8). Note also the more intense glial staining at the periphery of the spinal cord. × 190.

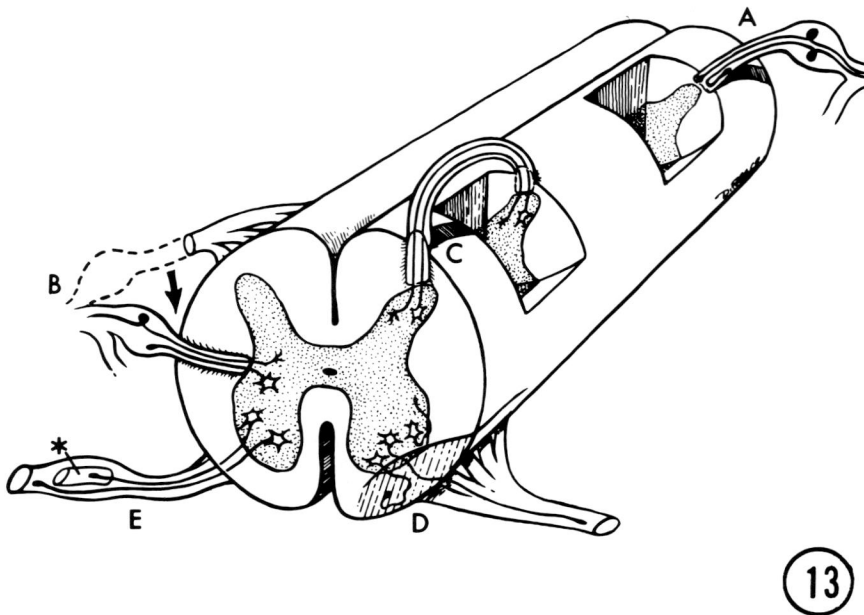

Figure 12–13.   A diagram summarizing various experimental models that have been used to study the influence of reactive astrocytes on axonal regeneration: **A:** The dorsal root entry zone. **B:** Insertion of the proximal cut end of the dorsal root into the spinal cord (this is also comparable to the introduction of the regenerating stump of a damaged peripheral nerve into the CNS). **C:** PNS-to-CNS grafts. **D:** Growth of motoneuron axons (cut within the spinal cord) toward the ventral roots. **E:** Grafting of optic nerve tissue (asterisk) between the cut ends of a peripheral nerve. See text for more details. (Reproduced from Reier and Houlé, 1988, by permission of the publisher.)

On one hand, Carlstedt (1983) was unable to demonstrate any regrowth of ventral root fibers into the spinal cord, whereas Kingsley et al. (1984) reported that some axons did indeed cross the PNS-CNS transition zone and distribute within the dorsal horn. The documentation provided in the latter study, however, suggests that at best only a small number of fibers had traversed the DREZ. In that regard, the extent of regeneration noted by Kingsley et al. does not appear to differ dramatically with the apparently modest ingrowth that has been seen after dorsal root crushes, using a similar neuroanatomical tracing method (Liuzzi and Lasek, 1987b).

That differences in the growth capacities of some neuronal populations may enable growth to occur despite the presence of an astroglial matrix was also suggested in relation, for example, to monoaminergic and neurohypophyseal axons (see above). It is thus interesting that no regeneration of catecholaminergic fibers was observed into the spinal cord when the proximal stump of the hypogastric nerve was coapted with the central portion of severed dorsal roots (Carlstedt, 1985b). Taken together, these recent observations strongly indicate that at least at the DREZ, astroglia are able to impede the elongation of the vast majority of axons advancing toward the spinal cord irrespective of any potential or demonstrated differences in the intrinsic growth capacities of the parent neurons.

Insertion of Regenerating Peripheral Nerve Stumps Into the CNS

The results of the DREZ experiments have also been mirrored to a considerable extent by studies in which the regenerating proximal stump of a peripheral nerve was introduced into the substance of the CNS (LeGros Clark, 1943; Windle et al., 1952b; Clemente, 1958). In

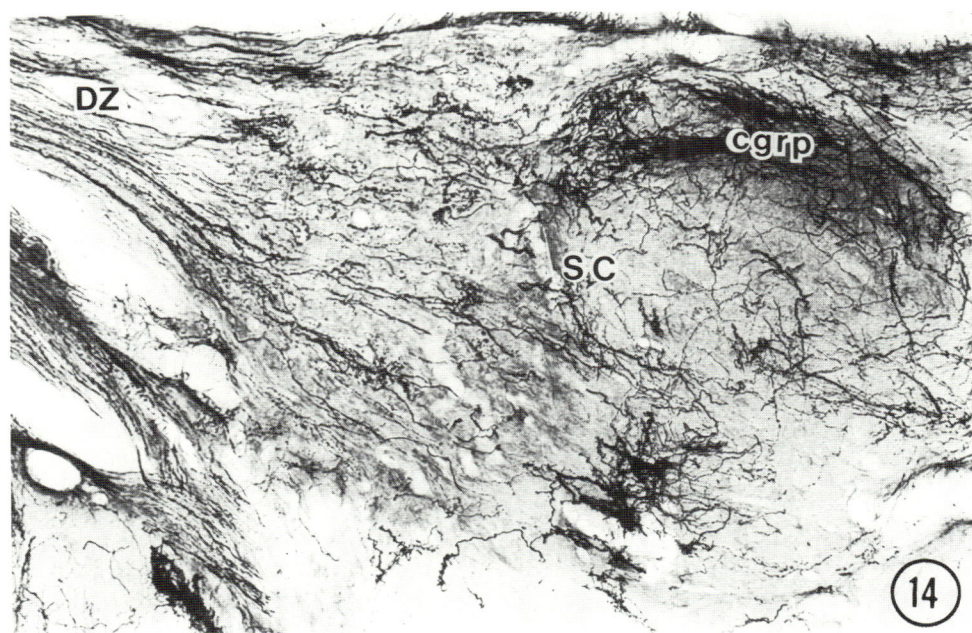

Figure 12–14. Ingrowth of primary afferent fibers into a fetal spinal cord graft (SC). In this experiment, the dorsal root (DZ) was cut, and the segment proximal to the spinal ganglion was placed adjacent to a piece of fetal tissue that had been introduced into a lesion of the adult rat spinal cord. In this case, primary afferent fibers containing the antigen calcitonin gene-related peptide (cgrp) were stained with an antibody to that substance. For more details, refer to Tessler et al. (1988). × 390.

some cases, neuromas were formed at the insertion site, whereas in others fibers either extended parallel to the scar or made U-turns back toward the peripheral nerve stump.

More recently, Carlstedt (1985a) reported that sensory axons were still unable to advance centrally following the insertion of dorsal roots into ectopic regions of the spinal cord (Fig. 12–13B). It is interesting that this ingrowth was absent even though only a minimal astroglial matrix developed at the insertion site. This result contrasts sharply with an earlier report (Turbes and Freeman, 1958) and suggests that failure of axons to grow past the DREZ is not due to some unique property of that region of the nervous system.

Grafting of CNS Tissue Into Regenerating Peripheral Nerves

The incompatibility of a CNS glial environment with axonal regeneration has also been demonstrated by a cable grafting procedure. In

a group of independent investigations, mature autologous optic nerve segments were introduced between the proximal and distal stumps of a peripheral nerve (Fig. 12–13E) (Aguayo et al., 1978, Weinberg and Spencer, 1979; Anderson and Turmaine, 1986; Hall and Kent, 1987). Later histological evaluations of the grafts revealed that only a few fibers had entered. It could not be determined from these experiments, however, whether myelin and axonal debris resulting from Wallerian degeneration initiated in the CNS tissue at the beginning of the experiments, rather than the astroglial population itself, was responsible for the limited axonal penetration of these grafts.

To address this issue (P. J. Reier, L. Guth, D. Johnson, and P. A. Trimmer, unpublished observations; results illustrated in Reier et al., 1983a), an optic nerve graft was prepared in which gliosis was first induced in situ by enucleating early postnatal rats at a time when gliogenesis is primarily being directed toward the production of astrocytes, and myelination has not yet been initiated. Thirty days later, a relatively homogeneous astrocytic scar was formed that was then grafted into the rat sciatic nerve as in the experiments cited above. Despite the absence of degenerating myelin and axonal material, only a modest ingrowth of peripheral nerve fibers was seen in these scars. The majority of fibers grew around the perimeter of the grafts, and none of those few fibers that had gained access to the scar advanced the full length of the graft ($\sim$ 5 mm). These results do not discount that other factors present in the degenerating optic nerve grafts of the original experiments could have had an inhibitory effect on axonal elongation. They do, however, suggest that either an astroglial environment is in itself incompatible with the outgrowth of nerve fibers or that the environment provided by PNS cellular elements was more attractive.

Grafts of Fetal CNS Tissue Into the Adult CNS

As noted earlier, it has been suggested that some neuronal populations may have greater metabolic capacities for extending their regenerating axons through an astroglial matrix than others. This has been contested, however, by the experiments described thus far in that even vigorously regenerating peripheral nerve fibers are generally unable to traverse an astrocytic scar. A similar result has been obtained in other recent studies involving transplants of fetal CNS tissue into the adult CNS. In brief, it was noted that when a scar is present, axons from the transplant are unable to cross the host-donor interface despite the fact that they are arising from developing neurons with, presumably, optimal growth properties (Reier and Houlé, 1988).

PNS Tissue Grafts Into the CNS

Another demonstration of the impact that the glial microenvironment of the CNS can exert on regeneration has derived from studies in which segments of peripheral nerve tissue were grafted to either the brain or spinal cord (reviewed in Aguayo, 1985; see also Chapter 5, this volume). Neurons that are intrinsic to the CNS can extend their axons for long distances in the presence of PNS tissue (Fig. 12–13C). In

contrast, no axonal penetration of optic nerve scars (as described above) is seen when such grafts are made to the CNS using the same procedures (Reier, unpublished observation).

The ability of CNS neurons to sustain exuberant axonal growth in PNS tissue rapidly subsides as axons reach the opposite end of these grafts. Thus CNS axons fail to grow for more than 1–2 mm past the PNS graft-CNS junction. Why this happens is not specifically known, though it may be related to the development of an encapsulating glial scar at the graft-CNS junction (Chi and Dahl, 1983; Fishman et al., 1983). Thus, when axons initially enter PNS grafts, there is usually an absence of extensive glial reactivity at the interface. At that stage, astrocytes might even facilitate axonal elongation into the PNS grafts (Weinberg and Raine, 1980). By the time axons have progressed to the other end, however, it appears that a more advanced scar is present that could limit the exit of these fibers (Fig. 12–13C).

In Vitro Studies

The results obtained with PNS-to-CNS and CNS-to-PNS grafts have been paralleled by recent in vitro studies. For example, Schwab and Thoenen (1985) have studied the behavior of neurites extending from peripheral neurons that were cocultured with segments of sciatic and optic nerve tissue. Neuritic outgrowth occurred preferentially toward the PNS substratum, whereas the CNS microenvironment was avoided.

Sandrock and Matthew (1987a,b,c) and Carbonetto et al. (1987) have examined axonal outgrowth from sensory and superior cervical ganglionic explants in the presence of CNS and PNS substrata prepared by affixing frozen sections of optic nerve, adult spinal cord, or sciatic nerve to coverslips or plastic dishes. Preferential neuritic elongation and greater attachment was observed in relation to PNS tissue, whereas axonal outgrowth was not sustained by mature CNS substrata.

FACTORS THAT MAY ACCOUNT FOR THE POOR GROWTH OF AXONS IN THE MICROENVIRONMENT OF A GLIAL SCAR

While most of the evidence cited in the preceding section focuses on the astrocyte as having a rather singular, adverse influence on axonal elongation, it needs to be emphasized, as at the beginning of this chapter, that many cell types can contribute to scar formation in the CNS. Accordingly, more than a single factor or cell type may be operational in preventing regeneration in the CNS. This does not, however, contest the potential of reactive astroglia to suppress regeneration as robust axonal elongation through the matrix of a scar, consisting predominantly of astrocytic elements, is more the exception (Risling et al., 1983) than the rule. Therefore the issue is not whether astrocytes alone or in conjunction with other cell types can prejudice regeneration, but rather, what is it about the overall glial scar microenvironment that renders it unfavorable to axonal elongation.

Concerning the original "barrier" hypothesis, it is easy to appreciate how static histological preparations revealing neuroma formation (Sung, 1981; Risling et al., 1983), recurrent axonal elongation (Ramón y Cajal, 1928; Lampert and Cressman, 1964), and blindly ending axonal profiles (Stensaas et al., 1987) in the presence of a complex and tightly knit arrangement of astrocytic processes, can lead one to envision the glial scar as being a physical obstacle to growing neuritic processes. Other mechanisms, however, could yield the same picture. In this regard, a shift has taken place in recent years toward consideration of newer molecular perspectives that could account for the inability of astrocytes and other cells in the injured CNS to provide a favorable microenvironment for sustained axonal elongation. Several of these hypotheses are based upon contrasting chemical features of PNS and CNS tissues, as well as on differences between immature and adult glia. In general, most of the hypotheses assert either that mature or reactive neuroglia are unable to synthesize the appropriate diffusible neurotrophic and surface-associated, neurite-promoting molecules or that they produce growth-inhibiting factors and/or cell surface constituents.

Astrocytes Do Not Provide the Necessary Tropic and/or Trophic Support For Axonal Regeneration

This is a view, rooted in the classical studies of degeneration and regeneration, that has gained considerable emphasis in more recent years (Varon, 1977; see also Chapter 7, this volume). In particular, Ramón y Cajal (1928) originally noted the paradoxical fact that axons in the PNS were unable to enter the CNS (e.g., at the DREZ), whereas some fibers in CNS white matter were able to penetrate peripheral nerve segments inserted into the brain.

Such findings have essentially been confirmed and extended with contemporary techniques, as discussed in the previous section, and suggest that whether or not axonal elongation is affected by astroglia may be dependent upon the direction of outgrowth relative to PNS and CNS domains. Thus, in the studies of 1) dorsal root regeneration; 2) PNS grafts to the CNS; and 3) CNS grafts to the PNS, the failure of axons within peripheral nerve environments to exhibit vigorous growth into and through an astrocytic interface could be a result of the stronger trophic and/or tropic influence of PNS tissue. Likewise, this finding could explain why some ultrastructural studies (Matthews et al., 1979; Reier et al., 1983a; Reier, 1986) have suggested that axons may have penetrated encapsulating scars (Fig. 12–10). If this view is correct, then it seems unlikely that an astrocytic scar could act as an absolute physical barrier in only one direction.

An interesting illustration of these points also derives from an experiment reported by Risling et al. (1983). Intramedullary segments of motoneuron axons were lesioned central to the CNS-PNS transition zone of the L7 ventral root in the cat spinal cord (Fig. 12–13D). An astroglial scar then developed, and the ventral root was completely denervated. By directly injecting into motoneurons a tracer that could be subsequently visualized histologically in the cell bodies and processes of these cells, it was possible to demonstrate that some motoneurons had eventually extended their regenerating axons through the glial scar, then past the CNS-PNS transitional region of the ventral root, and finally into the L7 root itself. These findings are particularly noteworthy in light of the fact that motoneurons are generally unable to grow through the PNS-CNS transition zone of the DREZ following dorsal-ventral root anastomosis.

The possible trophic and tropic differences between CNS and PNS tissue that bear upon the present discussion extend well beyond the scope of this chapter (for recent reviews see Cotman and Nieto-Sampedro, 1984; Lindsay, 1986; Manthorpe et al., 1986; Varon et al., 1988a, and Chapter 7, this volume). In general, it appears that injured peripheral nerve tissue may contain a variety of neurotrophic factors (Lundborg et al., 1982; Longo et al., 1983a, b; Williams et al., 1984; see also Reier and Houlé, 1988), including nerve growth factor (NGF) (Richardson and Ebendal, 1982; Rush, 1984; Heumann et al., 1987). There is evidence indicating that normal and reactive astrocytes are also capable of producing factors both in vivo and in vitro that can enhance neuronal survival and axonal elongation (Unsicker et al., 1984; Nieto-Sampedro et al., 1983; Lindsay, 1986). Many of these glial-derived factors, however, have not been characterized in great detail, and, in the majority of cases, their detection has involved bioassays using embryonic neurons in tissue culture. Thus it is still uncertain whether mature injured neurons can respond to such substances.

It is also possible that the factors most vital to regeneration in the injured CNS are not being produced (Hadani et al., 1984; Schwartz et al., 1985) or that their synthesis and release does not coincide with the period during which damaged neurons would be most responsive to them (Lindsay, 1986). Limited regeneration in vivo may also occur because such factors are simply not produced in sufficient amounts. What is manufactured may only be adequate for inducing short-distance extension of fibers, and it is possible that glial-derived factors in the adult CNS may exert a more profound regulatory effect upon collateral sprouting and reactive synaptogenesis (see Chapter 8, this volume) than upon long distance axonal growth.

Glial Scars Lack the
Appropriate Surface Properties

The absence of appropriate trophic factors, however, does not appear to be the full explanation for why astrocytes or other glia in CNS scar tissue seem unable to support axonal outgrowth. For a number of years, it has been speculated that either the plasma membranes of central glial cells lack components necessary for axonal outgrowth or that molecular constituents are present that may inhibit fiber elonga-

tion (for more detailed discussion, see Reier and Houlé, 1988). The importance of surface properties to neuron-glial interactions (Edelman, 1986) is underscored by the fact that there are at least six different types of molecules associated with neuronal and glial membranes in developing CNS tissue both in vivo and in vitro that mediate neuron-glial adhesion (Edmondson et al., 1988; Grumet and Edelman, 1988). Much remains to be done, however, to determine whether these are preserved into adulthood on central glia or expressed on reactive astrocytes and other scar-related cells. Whether the distribution of these molecules and mechanisms of cell-cell interaction (Bock et al., 1988; Rutishauser et al., 1988) are the same in adult glia as those seen in their immature counterparts must also be explored.

In relation to the previous discussion of trophic factors, the surfaces of CNS glial cells may also lack the necessary receptors for the substances produced. For example, in the PNS, Schwann cells distal to a lesion express the receptor for NGF on their plasma membranes (Taniuchi et al., 1986, 1988; Raivich and Kreutzberg, 1987). As noted above, the Schwann cell also produces NGF after nerve damage. It has been proposed (Taniuchi et al., 1986; Johnson et al., 1988) that this is a mechanism whereby NGF can become bound to a cellular substratum that is well known for being conducive to axonal regeneration. In this way, NGF can act to promote axonal elongation of some peripheral fiber populations both as a trophic, as well as tropic (i.e., neurite-promoting) agent (Sandrock and Matthew, 1987c). A similar mechanism could apply to other trophic and/or tropic substances and their target neurons. While NGF and other factors are produced in the CNS, it is interesting in regard to NGF that neither astrocytes nor oligodendrocytes produce NGF receptors.

Given these considerations, one could speculate that a population of NGF-dependent neurons in the CNS could be stimulated to regenerate if provided with a cellular environment that could facilitate the delivery of necessary trophic factor(s) to the neuronal cell body. This view is supported by an example seen in the septohippocampal system in which the retrograde death of axotomized cholinergic neurons in the medial septum and vertical diagonal

band nuclei can be prevented with exogenously administered NGF (reviewed in Varon
et al., 1988b). Kromer et al. (1981) have also
shown that regeneration of this fimbria-fornix
tract can be stimulated with transplants of fetal
hippocampal tissue. More recently, Kromer
and Cornbrooks (1985) have reported that reinnervation of the hippocampus can also be promoted by encouraging regeneration with implants of cultured Schwann cells. Both of these
graft preparations may thus contribute to regeneration through the delivery of NGF and,
possibly, other neuronotrophic factors as well.

Glia In the CNS Do Not Synthesize the Extracellular Matrix Molecules That Are Conducive to Axonal Outgrowth

The results obtained with grafts placed into
the septohippocampal system are not necessarily explained by trophic factors alone. For
example, the experiment of Kromer and Cornbrooks (1985) also suggests that the grafts of
cultured Schwann cells provided neurite-
promoting molecules (see Chapter 7, this volume), which are necessary for the adhesion
and progressive migration of growth cones
during axonal elongation and which, in some
cases, can amplify the effects of neuronotrophic factors (Edgar, 1985). Davis et al. (1987)
have also found that some regeneration could
be promoted in this neuronal system with
grafts of human placenta enriched in regard to
one such factor (i.e., laminin). These and many
other experimental findings underscore another view about scar tissue in the CNS, viz.,
that positive effectors of axonal elongation in
the PNS and in vitro are either absent or
present in insufficient quantities (for more extensive review, see Reier and Houlé, 1988).

By definition, neurite-promoting factors are
"special proteins conferring to the surfaces to
which they bind a particular ability to stimulate neuritic extension" (Manthorpe et al.,
1986). One such class of molecules is composed of extracellular matrix (ECM) substances
that have been shown to play a number of roles
in various organ systems (Hawkes and Wang,
1982). One function of ECMs in particular is
that they can promote the migration of cells
during, for example, development and tumor
formation. ECMs, such as type II collagen, fibronectin, and laminin have also been shown

to be capable of potentiating axonal outgrowth
in tissue culture (Lander et al., 1985; Manthorpe et al., 1986).

Reactive astroglia are capable of synthesizing laminin to a limited extent (Liesi et al.,
1984; Liesi, 1985), and when present, laminin
in an astrocytic matrix can support axonal
growth for at least a short distance (Kromer
and Cornbrooks, 1985). Apart from this limited
production of laminin, however, mature CNS
tissue otherwise appears to be generally deficient in this substance, along with fibronectin
and another ECM, heparan sulfate proteoglycan (HeSPG) (Carbonetto, 1984; Carbonetto et
al., 1987). Furthermore, recent evidence suggests that a laminin-HeSPG complex is a physiological substratum for axonal outgrowth in
the PNS that is absent in the CNS (Chiu et al.,
1986; Sandrock and Matthews, 1987a, b).

Whether ECMs are present in the CNS that
are actually inhibitors of axonal outgrowth has
also been recently considered. Bignami et al.
(1987) have reported that astrocytes in white
matter produce a substance that appears to be
closely related to a brain-specific hyaluronec-
tin that blocks neurite outgrowth in vitro (see
also Dahl et al., 1986).

Astrocytes and/or Other Constituents of Glial Scars Do Not Have the Appropriate Proteolytic Mechanisms

For regeneration to occur, it is likely that the
ECM surrounding growth cones needs to be
continuously restructured, such as occurs in
the case of neoplastic cells (Reich, 1978). One
way in which this can be achieved is through
the action of proteolytic enzymes, and recent
studies have indicated that an imbalance between proteases and protease inhibitors (Guenther et al., 1985; Monard, 1985, 1988; Kalderon, 1986; Kalderon et al., 1988) may account
for the limited outgrowth in most astroglial
matrices. Kalderon, for instance, has reported
that plasminogen activator (PA), which gener-
ates the protease plasmin, is low in mature
astroglial populations and cultured oligodendrocytes, but is high in the immature astrocyte
and in Schwann cells. In contrast, protease inhibitory activity is a major feature of mature
and reactive astrocytes. Addition of the inhibitor to injured peripheral nerves can impair regeneration.

Likewise, Guenther et al. (1985) have presented evidence for the existence of a glia-derived factor that inhibits thrombin, and urokinase- and PA-dependent caseinolysis or fibrinolysis (for review, see Monard et al., 1988). While this or a homologous protein is produced in the injured PNS, a comparable substance has not been detected in the CNS after injury (Patterson, 1985).

Astrocytes Induce the Formation of Presynaptic Terminals

The formation of vesicle filled terminal bulbs, resembling synaptic endings, in the midst of an astrocytic scar matrix has been reported in a description of axonal responses to optic nerve injury (Richardson et al., 1982). A similar result was subsequently reported by Carlstedt (1985c), who observed the development of axonal terminals containing accumulations of vesicles and neurotransmitter within the glial matrix of the DREZ during the regeneration of cholinergic and catecholaminergic nerves that had been coapted with the central stumps of severed dorsal roots. Carlstedt proposed that astrocytes may block elongation by inducing axons to form presynaptic terminals. This finding has been more recently amplified in a study by Liuzzi and Lasek (1987b), who proposed that the arrest of axonal elongation under such circumstances could entail the activation of intraaxonal proteolytic processes and subsequent degradation of cytoskeletal proteins (neurofilament constituents in particular) that in part are necessary for sustained axonal outgrowth (see Chapter 3, this volume).

While the specific reason for axons undergoing such changes in the presence of astroglia has not been established, it is conceivable that astrocytes may act as pseudoneuronal targets. This is a reasonable possibility, given that a number of tissue culture studies have indicated that mammalian astrocytes possess many neuron-like characteristics, including for example, process-bearing morphology, affinity for some markers that were once thought to be neuron-specific, and biophysical and electrophysiological properties that are also comparable with those exhibited by neurons (Bevan and Raff, 1985). Furthermore, these cells show both uptake of, and receptors for, a variety of neurotransmitters (Hosli et al., 1986;

Kimelberg, 1986; Lauder and McCarthy, 1986; Massarelli et al., 1986).

CAN THE SCARRING RESPONSE BE MANIPULATED?

In light of this discussion of the effect of gliosis on axonal outgrowth and some of the potential underlying mechanisms, the natural question arises of whether scarring can be eventually controlled in any way or (in the case of chronic lesions) modified so as to promote a more dynamic regenerative response that could potentially lead to some degree of functional return.

As far as the control of gliosis is concerned, numerous efforts have and continue to be directed toward gaining a better understanding of the metabolic, growth, proliferative, and migratory dynamics of scar-associated cells, in particular the astrocyte, following CNS trauma (Reier, 1986; Eng et al., 1987; Reier and Houlé, 1988). For example, a variety of substances have been identified in recent years having putative mitogenic and growth-promoting effects on astroglia (Nieto-Sampedro, 1988), and some progress has also been made in defining how other cell types (e.g., macrophages and/or microglia) may be involved in promoting scar formation (Giulian, 1988; Nieto-Sampedro, 1988).

Other clues suggesting that it may be possible to suppress, at least in part, a glial response have emerged from recent transplantation studies. As discussed elsewhere in this volume (Chapters 13 and 14), many experiments in the past several years have shown that grafts of embryonic neural tissue can ameliorate some functional deficits in animals with various experimental neurological disorders. In addition, several investigations have shown that such transplants, when placed into acute lesions, can fuse directly with host tissue without the formation of intervening glial scars (Kromer, 1980; Reier et al., 1983b, 1986; Zimmer and Sunde, 1984; Kruger et al., 1986). Recent findings also suggest that embryonic tissue may be able to stimulate some regression of an existing scar after transplantation into chronic injury sites (Houlé and Reier, 1988).

How fetal grafts can affect the development or maintenance of a glial scar remains to be elucidated. On one hand, it is possible that in acute lesions the grafts may have physically prevented the infiltration of cellular elements that promote the development of a glial-limiting membrane (Reier et al., 1983b). On the other hand, immature CNS tissue may have molecular properties that can influence the responses of mature glial elements to injury or stimulate partial regression of existing scars.

The latter consideration is reinforced by some findings indicating that immature non-neuronal elements have a capacity for modulating glial and other cellular responses to trauma in the CNS. These observations have derived from studies of transplants of enriched populations of astroglial cells obtained from either tissue culture (Kesslak et al., 1986) or by harvesting young atrocytes that attach to artificial membranes placed into lesions of immature brains (Silver and Ogawa, 1983; Smith et al., 1986). For instance, in a pair of recent publications (Smith et al., 1986; Smith and Silver, 1988), it was reported that immature glia caused a reduction of gliosis, bleeding, and secondary necrosis. Kliot et al. (1988) have more recently seen immature astrocytes as capable of augmenting the regeneration of crushed dorsal root axons past the DREZ in adult rats. After entering the spinal cord, these axons formed terminal arborizations within the spinal gray matter.

The modulation of glial scars by immature CNS tissue via a molecular mechanism has also been suggested by the work of Hadani et al. (1984). These authors showed that substances released by neonatal rabbit optic nerve into tissue culture medium can lead to a stimulation of regeneration in the mature rabbit visual system. This process may occur through activation or modification of the biosynthetic activities of scar-forming astrocytes (Schwartz et al., 1988).

ARE ASTROCYTES THE ONLY CNS COMPONENT AFFECTING AXONAL ELONGATION?

Up to this point, discussion has largely centered upon the rather singular involvement of the astrocyte in defining the extent to which neuritic growth can be achieved in the CNS. As noted earlier, however, the glial scar consists of other cellular elements that may also play a role, as suggested by the results of a tissue cul-

ture study in which dissociated sympathetic or sensory neurons were grown in NGF-supplemented medium and cocultured with explants of optic and sciatic nerve (Schwab and Thoenen, 1985). While axons from these neurons actively invaded the PNS explants, they did not enter the optic nerve segment, even though the survival and growth of these NGF-dependent neurons was maintained with NGF. Furthermore, the same situation obtained even when the test substrata were frozen (see also Carbonetto et al., 1987). Therefore the failure of axons to grow within a CNS environment in this tissue culture preparation did not seem to be entirely due to the absence of appropriate trophic factors. It was thus suggested that myelin proteins and the membrane constituents of myelin-producing oligodendrocytes may be inhibitors of fiber outgrowth (Schwab and Caroni, 1988). This finding has since been extended by experiments showing that myelin extracts obtained from spinal cord white matter can represent a highly nonpermissive substratum for axonal elongation (Caroni and Schwab, 1988a). In these experiments, minor protein fractions of Mr 35 and 250 kD associated with CNS myelin were found to exert a nonpermissive effect on axonal elongation. Proteases could abolish this nonpermissive action, as did extraction of these protein fractions from myelin. On the other hand, the addition of these fractions to an otherwise permissive substratum resulted in diminished neuritic outgrowth, as well as of spreading of murine 3T3 cells. Specific blocking antibodies have also recently been shown to neutralize the nonpermissive properties of CNS myelin membranes and of living oligodendrocytes in vitro (Caroni and Schwab, 1988b). As yet the underlying mechanisms of this effect by myelin-associated proteins on axonal outgrowth are unknown. Also, it is not clear why gray matter appears to be more conducive to axonal elongation than white matter (see discussion in Caroni and Schwab, 1988a), as myelin is present in the former. Nevertheless, these findings suggest that oligodendrocytes and myelin debris could contribute to some extent to the inhibitory influence that glial scars in degenerated white matter seem to exert on regeneration (see also, Kao et al., 1977).

The study by Caroni and Schwab (1988a)

also showed that myelin in the chick CNS is nonpermissive to axonal outgrowth. In contrast, myelin from lower vertebrates (e.g., fishes and frogs) was comparable with PNS myelin in that it did not impede neuritic elongation. The latter is consistent with an extensive literature documenting regenerative growth in various amphibian species and the goldfish (for reviews see Reier et al., 1983a; Reier, 1986), even when extensive gliosis is present (Reier, 1979). The story, however, is not completely clear. For example, Stensaas (1983) reported the absence of axonal regeneration in the dorsal columns of the newt spinal cord. Interestingly, degeneration of white matter was noted as being very slow in comparison with other CNS areas (e.g., optic nerve), where dramatic regeneration is typically observed.

CONCLUSIONS

Over the last decade or so, there has been a growing sense of optimism concerning the potential for achieving some degree of CNS functional repair. While the intrinsic ability of mature CNS neurons to survive axotomy and metabolically support a vigorous regrowth of their injured axons is still a major issue (see Chapters 3 and 6, this volume), it is now recognized that neurons within the CNS have the potential for regeneration and that the cellular microenvironment surrounding the preserved proximal ends of injured axons can define the extent to which this capacity is expressed (see Chapter 5, this volume). In this light, although scar formation is not a primary determinant of the outcome of any spontaneous effort at fiber regrowth, there are many lines of evidence, as this review has shown, indicating that gliosis can govern the general success of regeneration by establishing a cellular matrix that in some way discourages axonal elongation. Thus any surgical or pharmacological strategy directed toward creating an optimum setting for regeneration and functional recovery in either the brain or spinal cord must take into account the extent to which scar formation could bear upon the success of the approach being tested (Eng et al., 1986; Reier and Houlé, 1988).

While the idea that scar formation is a physical barrier to regenerating axons can be challenged, the hypothesis has been useful in stimulating a new conceptual framework about cellular mechanisms in the injured CNS that can influence the outcome of regeneration. Accordingly, further progress in regeneration and neural plasticity clearly demands a better understanding of the cellular biology and synthetic properties of cells contributing to scar formation (Eng et al., 1986). This is already exemplified by the fact that with regard to the astrocyte, this cell can no longer be viewed as a purely adverse element in the damaged CNS.

While scarring represents only one part of a complex problem, it is nonetheless apparent that such fresh perspectives can ultimately be instrumental in defining future therapeutic approaches. For example, an ideal strategy might be one designed to modulate the astrocyte's response to injury so as to gain from its potential neurotrophic effect while at the same time tempering its scarring response.

That such a manuever could become a reality is suggested by studies showing that some glial responses in the mature nonregenerating CNS can be altered by grafts of fetal CNS tissue and that axonal regeneration may be enhanced through the transplantation of immature astroglia or the introduction of chemical substances obtained from developing mammalian and regenerating nonmammalian CNS tissue. Such approaches to the problem serve to indicate the existence of molecules that can be studied in greater depth by virtue of the steady advances being made in different fields of biotechnology (e.g., manipulation of gene expression) that are now being used to resolve various issues in basic and clinical neurobiology, as well as in many other areas of biomedical science. Through the combination of new hypotheses and technical developments, it is no longer a matter of wild speculation that methods may be developed some day that can permit mature central glia to express axonal growth-promoting substances elaborated by their counterparts in the immature CNS. Alternatively, it may be possible to suppress the expression of scar-promoting or regeneration-inhibiting biosynthetic products.

While considerable work quite obviously still needs to be done, progress in CNS regeneration research is moving more rapidly, and such gains help to give a flavor of encouragement to an area of clinical and basic science that has been largely clouded by a sense of pessimism.

ACKNOWLEDGMENTS

The author's investigations described in this review were supported by NIH Grants NS 13836, NS 22316, The Paralyzed Veterans of America, and The American Paralysis Association.

REFERENCES

Aguayo AJ (1985): Axonal regeneration from injured neurons in the adult mammalian central nervous system. In Cotman CW (ed): "Synaptic Plasticity." New York: Guilford Press, pp 457–483.

Aguayo AJ, Dickson R, Trecarten J, Attiwell M, Bray GM, Richardson P (1978): Ensheathment and myelination of regenerating PNS fibres by transplanted optic nerve glia. Neurosci Lett 9:97–104.

Anderson PN, Turmaine M (1986): Axonal regeneration through living and freeze-dried CNS tissue. Neuropathol Appl Neurobiol 12:389–399.

Barnes CD, Worrall N (1968): Reinnervation of spinal cord by cholinergic neurons. J Neurophysiol 13:689–694.

Barrett CP, Guth L, Donati EJ, Krikorian JG (1981): Astroglial reaction in the gray matter of lumbar segments after midthoracic transection of the adult rat spinal cord. Exp Neurol 73:365–377.

Barron KD (1983): Axon reaction and central nervous system regeneration. In Seil FJ (ed): "Nerve, Organ and Tissue Regeneration: Research Perspectives." New York: Academic Press, pp 3–34.

Bernstein JJ (1983): During glial scar formation and cavitation necrosis after injury the spinal cord regenerates neuronal cell processes. In Seil FJ (ed): "Nerve, Organ and Tissue Regeneration: Research Perspectives." New York: Academic Press, pp 215–230.

Berry M (1979): Regeneration in the central nervous system. In Smith WT, Cavanagh JB (eds): "Recent Advances in Neuropathology," no. 1. Edinburgh: Churchill Livingstone, pp 67–111.

Berry M, Maxwell WL, Logan A, Mathewson A, McConnell P, Ashhurst DE, Thomas GH (1983): Deposition of scar tissue in the central nervous system. Acta Neurochir [Suppl] (Wien) 32:31–53.

Berthold CH, Carlstedt T (1977): General organization of the transitional region in S$_1$ dorsal rootlets. Acta Physiol Scand [Suppl] 446:23–42.

Bevan S, Raff M (1985): Voltage-dependent potassium currents in cultured astrocytes. Nature 315:1–3.

Bignami A, Dahl D, Rueger DC (1980): Glial fibrillary acidic protein (GFA) in normal neural cells and in pathological conditions. Adv Cell Neurobiol 1:285–310.

Bignami A, Chi NH, Dahl D (1984): Regenerating dorsal roots and the nerve entry zone: An immunofluorescence study with neurofilament and laminin antisera. Exp Neurol 85:426–436.

Bignami A, Dahl D, Gilad V, Gilad G (1987): White matter astrocytes. Do they produce a non-permissive substrate for axonal growth. Soc Neurosci Abstr 13:1040.

Björklund A, Stenevi U (1979): Regeneration of monoaminergic and cholinergic neurons in the central nervous system. Physiol Rev 59:62–100.

Björklund A, Katzman R, Stenevi U, West KA (1971): Development and growth of axonal sprouts from noradrenaline and 5-hydroxytryptamine neurones in the rat spinal cord. Brain Res 31:21–33.

Bock E, Nybroe O, Linnemann E (1988): Developmental regulation of expression of the neural cell adhesion molecules NCAM and L1. In Reier PJ, Bunge RP, Seil FJ (eds): "Current Issues in Neural Regeneration Research." New York: Alan R. Liss, Inc., pp 237–242.

Carbonetto S (1984): The extracellular matrix of the nervous system. Trends Neurosci 7:382–387.

Carbonetto S, Evans D, Cochard P (1987): Nerve fiber growth in culture on tissue substrata from central and peripheral nervous systems. J Neurosci 7:610–620.

Carlstedt T (1983): Regrowth of anastomosed ventral root nerve fibers in the dorsal root of rats. Brain Res 272:162–165.

Carlstedt T (1985a): Regenerating axons form nerve terminals at astrocytes. Brain Res 347:188–191.

Carlstedt T (1985b): Regrowth of cholinergic and catecholaminergic neurons along a peripheral and central nervous pathway. Neurosci 15:507–518.

Carlstedt T (1985c): Dorsal root innervation of spinal cord neurons after dorsal root implantation into the spinal cord of adult rats. Neurosci Lett 55:343–348.

Carlstedt T, Dalsgaard C-J, Molander C (1986): Regrowth of lesioned dorsal root nerve fibers into the spinal cord of neonatal rats. Neurosci Lett 74:14–18.

Caroni P, Schwab ME (1988a): Two membrane protein fractions from rat central myelin with inhibitory properties for neurite growth and fibroblast spreading. J Cell Biol 106:1281–1288.

Caroni P, Schwab ME (1988b): Antibody against myelin-associated inhibitor of neurite growth neutralizes non-permissive substrate properties of CNS white matter. Neuron 1:85–96.

Chi NH, Dahl D (1983): Autologous peripheral nerve grafting into murine brain as a model for studies of regeneration in the central nervous system. Exp Neurol 79:245–264.

Chiu AY, Matthew WD, Patterson PH (1986): A monoclonal antibody that blocks the activity of a neurite regeneration-promoting factor: Studies on the binding site and its localization in vivo. J Cell Biol 103:1383–1398.

Clemente CD (1955): Structural regeneration in the mammalian central nervous system and the role of neuroglia and connective tissue. In Windle WF (ed): "Regeneration in the Central Nervous System." Springfield Ill: Charles C Thomas, pp 147–161.

Clemente CD (1958): The regeneration of peripheral nerves inserted into the cerebral cortex and the healing of cerebral lesions. J Comp Neurol 109:123–151.

Clemente CD (1964): Regeneration in the vertebrate central nervous system. Int Rev Neurobiol 6:257–301.

Cotman CW, Nieto-Sampedro M (1984): Cell biology of synaptic plasticity. Science 225:1287–1294.

Dahl D, Björklund H, Bignami A (1986): Immunological markers in astrocytes. In Fedoroff S, Vernadakis A (eds): "Astrocytes, Vol. 3: Cell Biology and Pathology of Astrocytes." San Diego: Academic Press, pp 1–26.

Davis GE, Blaker SN, Engvall E, Varon S, Manthorpe M, Gage FH (1987): Human amnion membrane serves as a substratum for growing axons in vitro and in vivo. Science 236:1106–1109.

Dellmann, H-D (1973): Degeneration and regeneration of neurosecretory systems. Int Rev Cytol 36:215–315.

Dellman, H-D (1986): Peptidergic neurosecretory axons regenerate into sciatic nerve autografts in the rat hypothalamus. Neuroendocrinology 44:292–298.

Edelman G (1986): Cell adhesion molecules in the regulation of animal form and tissue pattern. Annu Rev Cell Biol 2:81–116.

Edgar D (1985): Nerve growth factors and molecules of the extracellular matrix in neuronal development. J Cell Sci Suppl 3:107–113.

Edmondson JC, Liem RKH, Kuster JE, Hatten ME (1988): Astrotactin: A novel neuronal surface antigen that mediates neuron-astroglial interactions in cerebellar microculture. J Cell Biol 106:505–517.

Eng LF (1985): Glial fibrillary acidic protein: The major protein of glial intermediate filaments in differentiated astrocytes. J Neuroimmunol 8:203–214.

Eng LF, Reier PJ, Houlé JD (1986): Astrocyte activation and fibrous gliosis: Glial fibrillary acidic protein immunostaining of astrocytes following intraspinal cord grafting of fetal CNS tissue. In Seil FJ, Herbert E, Carlson BM (eds): "Neural Regeneration. Progress in Brain Research," vol. 71. Amsterdam: Elsevier, pp 439–455.

Fedoroff S, Vernadakis A (1986a) "Astrocytes, Vol. 1: Development, Morphology, and Regional Specialization of Astrocytes." San Diego: Academic Press.

Fedoroff S, Vernadakis A (1986b): "Astrocytes, Vol. 2: Biochemistry, Physiology, and Pharmacology of Astrocytes." San Diego: Academic Press.

Fedoroff S, Vernadakis A (1986c): "Astrocytes, Vol. 3: Cell Biology and Pathology of Astrocytes." San Diego: Academic Press.

Fishman PS, Nilaver G, Kelly JP (1983): Astrogliosis limits the integration of peripheral nerve grafts into the spinal cord. Brain Res 277:175–180.

Gilson BC, Stensaas LJ (1974): Early axonal changes following lesions of the dorsal columns in rats. Cell Tissue Res 149:1–20.

Giulian D (1988): Immunosuppression as a treatment for acute injury of the central nervous system. In Reier PJ, Bunge RP, Seil FJ (eds): "Current Issues in Neural Regeneration Research." New York: Alan R. Liss, Inc., pp 281–290.

Goldberg S, Frank B (1980): Will central nervous systems in the adult mammal regenerate after bypassing a lesion? A study in the mouse and chick visual systems. Exp Neurol 70:675–689.

Graeber MB, Kreutzberg GW (1986): Astrocytes increase in glial fibrillary acidic protein during retrograde changes of facial motor neurons. J Neurocytol 15:363–373.

Grafe MR, Schoenfeld TA (1982): Radial glial cells in the postnatal olfactory tubercle of hamsters. Brain Res 4:115–118.

Grumet M, Edelman GE (1988): Neuron-glia adhesion molecule interacts with neurons and astroglia via different binding mechanisms. J Cell Biol 106:487–503.

Guenther J, Hanspeter N, Monard D (1985): A glia-derived neurite-promoting factor with protease inhibitory activity. EMBO J 4:1963–1966.

Guth L, Barrett CP, Donati EJ, Deshpande SS, Albuquerque, EX (1981): Histopathological reactions and axonal regeneration in the transected spinal cord of hibernating squirrels. J Comp Neurol 203:297–308.

Hadani M, Harel A, Solomon A, Belkin M, Lavie V, Schwartz M (1984): Substances originating from the optic nerve of neonatal rabbit induce regeneration-associated response in the injured optic nerve of adult rabbit. Proc Natl Acad Sci USA 81:7965–7969.

Hall SM, Kent AP (1987): The response of regenerating peripheral neurites to a grafted optic nerve. J Neurocytol 16:317–331.

Hawkes S, Wang JL (1982): "Extracellular Matrix." New York: Academic Press.

Heumann R, Korsching S, Bandtlow C, Thoenen H (1987): Changes in nerve growth factor synthesis in nonneuronal cells in response to sciatic nerve transection. J Cell Biol 104:1623–1631.

Hösli E, Schousboe A, Hösli L (1986): Amino acid uptake. In Fedoroff S, Vernadakis A (eds): "Astrocytes, Vol. 2: Biochemistry, Physiology, and Pharmacology of Astrocytes." San Diego: Academic Press, pp 133–150.

Houlé JD, Reier PJ (1988): Transplantation of fetal spinal cord into the chronically injured adult rat spinal cord. J Comp Neurol, In Press.

Johnson, EM Jr, Clark HB, Schweitzer JB, Taniuchi M (1988): Expression of nerve growth factor receptors on Schwann cells after axonal injury. In Reier PJ, Bunge RP, Seil FJ (eds): "Current Issues in Neural Regeneration Research." New York: Alan R. Liss, Inc., pp 179–186.

Kalderon N (1986): The astrocyte and the failure of CNS neural regeneration: A study of inoculated astrocytes in a PNS regenerating model system. In Björklund A, Azmitia E (eds): "Cell and Tissue Transplantation into the Adult Brain." New York: Ann NY Acad Sciences 495:722–725.

Kalderon N, Ahonen K, Juhasz A, Kirk JP, Fedoroff S (1988): Astroglia and plasminogen activator activity: Differential activity level in the immature, mature and "reactive"astrocytes. In Reier PJ, Bunge RP, Seil FJ (eds): "Current Issues in Neural Regeneration Research." New York: Alan R. Liss, Inc., pp 271–280.

Kao CC, Chang LW, Bloodworth JMB Jr (1977): Axonal regeneration across transected mammalian spinal cords: An electron microscopic study of delayed microsurgical nerve grafting. Exp Neurol 54:591–615.

Kesslak JP, Nieto-Sampedro M, Globus J, Cotman CW (1986): Transplants of purified astrocytes promote behavioral recovery after frontal cortex ablation. Exp Neurol 92:377–390.

Kiernan JA (1979): Hypotheses concerned with axonal regeneration in the mammalian nervous sytem. Biol Rev 54:153–197.

Kimelberg HK (1986): Catecholamine and serotonin uptake in astrocytes. In Fedoroff S, Vernadakis A (eds):

"Astrocytes, Vol. 2: Biochemistry, Physiology, and Pharmacology of Astrocytes." San Diego: Academic Press, pp 107–132.

Kingsley RE, Messenger KK, Seall RH (1984): Long-term survival of peripheral axons that have reinnervated the spinal cord. Exp Neurol 84:347–357.

Kliot M, Smith GM, Siegal J, Tyrrell S, Silver J (1988): Induced regeneration of dorsal root fibers into the adult mammalian spinal cord. In Reier PJ, Bunge RP, Seil FJ (eds): "Current Issues in Neural Regeneration Research." New York: Alan R. Liss, Inc., pp 311–328.

Kromer LF (1980): Glial scar formation in the brain of adult rats is inhibited by implants of embryonic CNS tissue. Soc Neurosci Abst 6:688.

Kromer LF, Cornbrooks, CJ (1985): Transplants of Schwann cell cultures promote axonal regeneration in the adult mammalian brain. Proc Natl Acad Sci USA 82:6330–6334.

Kromer LF, Björklund A, Stenevi U (1981): Regeneration of the septohippocampal pathways in adult rats is promoted by utilizing embryonic hippocampal implants as bridges. Brain Res 210:173–200.

Kruger S, Sievers J, Hansen C, Sadler M, Berry M (1986): Three morphologically distinct types of interface develop between adult host and fetal brain transplants: Implications for scar formation in the adult central nervous sytem. J Comp Neurol 249:103–116.

Lampert P, Cressman M (1964): Axonal regeneration in the dorsal columns of the spinal cord of adult rats. Lab Invest 13:825–839.

Lander AD, Fujii DK, Reichardt LF (1985): Purification of a factor that promotes neurite outgrowth: Isolation of laminin and associated molecules. J Cell Biol 101:898–913.

Lasek RJ, McQuarrie IG, Wujek JR (1981): The central nervous system regeneration problem: Neuron and environment. In Millesi H, Mingrino S, Gorio A (eds): "Post-Traumatic Peripheral Nerve Regeneration: Experimental Basis and Clinical Implications." New York: Raven Press, pp 59–70.

Lauder J, McCarthy K (1986): Neuron-glial interactions. In Fedoroff S, Vernadakis A (eds): "Astrocytes, Vol. 2: Biochemistry, Physiology, and Pharmacology of Astrocytes." San Diego: Academic Press, pp 295–314.

LeGros Clark WE (1943): The problem of neuronal regeneration in the central nervous system. II. The insertion of peripheral nerve stumps into the brain. J Anat 77:251–259.

Liesi P (1985): Laminin-immunoreactive glia distinguish regenerative adult CNS systems from non-regenerative ones. EMBO J 4:2505–2511.

Liesi P, Kaakkola S, Dahl D, Vaheri A (1984): Laminin is induced in astrocytes of adult brain by injury. EMBO J 3:683–686.

Lindsay RM (1986): Reactive gliosis. In Fedoroff S, Vernadakis A (eds): "Astrocytes, Vol. 3: Cell Biology and Pathology of Astrocytes." San Diego: Academic Press, pp 231–262.

Liuzzi FJ, Lasek RJ (1987a): Some dorsal root axons regenerate into the adult rat spinal cord. An HRP study. Soc Neurosci Abstr 13:395.

Liuzzi FJ, Lasek RJ (1987b): Astrocytes block axonal regeneration in mammals by activating the physiological stop pathway. Science 237:642.

Longo FM, Manthorpe M, Skaper SD, Lundborg G, Varon S (1983a): Neuronotrophic activities accumulate in vivo within silicone nerve regeneration chambers. Brain Res 261:109–117.

Longo FM, Skaper SD, Manthorpe M, Williams LR, Lundborg G, Varon S (1983b): Temporal changes in neuronotrophic activities accumulating in vivo within nerve regeneration chambers. Exp Neurol 81:756–769.

Lundborg G, Dahlin LB, Danielsen N, Gelberman RH, Longo FM, Powell HC, Varon S (1982): Nerve regeneration in silicone chambers: Influence of gap length and of distal stump components. Exp Neurol 76:361–375.

Manthorpe M, Rudge JS, Varon S (1986): Astroglial cell contributions to neuronal survival and neuritic growth. In Fedoroff S Vernadakis A (eds): "Astrocytes, Vol. 2: Biochemistry, Physiology, and Pharmacology of Astrocytes." San Diego: Academic Press 2:315–376.

Massarelli R, Mykita S, Sorrentino (1986): The supply of choline to glial cells. In Fedoroff S, Vernadakis A (eds): "Astrocytes, Vol. 2: Biochemistry, Physiology, and Pharmacology of Astrocytes." San Diego: Academic Press, pp 155–174.

Mathewson AJ, Berry M (1985): Observations on the astrocyte response to a cerebral stab wound in adult rats. Brain Res 327:61–69.

Matthews MA, St. Onge MF, Faciane CL, Geldred JB (1979): Axon sprouting into segments of rat spinal cord adjacent to the site of a previous transection. Neuropathol Appl Neurobiol 5:181–196.

Meier C, Sollmann H (1977): Regeneration of cauda equina fibres after transection and end-to-end suture. Light and electron microscopic study in the pig. J Neurol 215:81–90.

Monard D (1985): Implications of proteases and protease inhibitors in neurite outgrowth. In Hamprecht B Neuhoff V (eds): "Neurobiochemistry, Selected Topics." Colloquium-Mosbach, Berlin: Springer-Verlag 36:7–12.

Monard D (1988): Glia-derived nexins and neurite outgrowth. In Reier PJ, Bunge RP, Seil FJ (eds): "Current Issues in Neural Regeneration Research." New York: Alan R. Liss, Inc., pp 159–166.

Nathaniel EJH, Nathaniel DR (1981): The reactive astrocyte. Adv Cell Neurobiol 2:249–301.

Nieto-Sampedro M (1988): The control of astrocyte populations in rat brain. In Reier PJ, Bunge RP, Seil FJ (eds): "Current Issues in Neural Regeneration Research." New York: Alan R. Liss, Inc., pp 301–310.

Nieto-Sampedro M, Manthorpe M, Barbin G, Varon S, Cotman CW (1983): Injury-induced neuronotrophic activity in adult rat brain: Correlation with survival of delayed implants in the wound cavity. J Neurosci 3:2219–2229.

Nygren L-G, Olson L, Seiger A (1971): Regeneration of monoamine-containing axons in the developing and adult spinal cord of the rat following intraspinal 6-OH-dopamine injections or transections. Histochemie 28:1–15.

Patterson PH (1985): On the role of proteases, their inhibitors and the extracellular matrix in promoting neurite outgrowth. J Physiol [Paris] 80:207–211.

Penfield W (1927): The mechanisms of cicatricial contraction in the brain. Brain 50:499–517.

Peters A, Palay SL, Webster H deF (1976): "The Fine Structure of the Nervous System: The Neurons and Supporting Cells." Philadelphia: WB Saunders.

Raivich G, Kreutzberg GW (1987): Expression of growth factor receptors in injured nervous tissue. I. Axotomy leads to a shift in the cellular distribution of specific β-nerve growth factor binding in the injured and regenerating PNS. J Neurocytol 16:689–700.

Ramón y Cajal S (1928): "Degeneration and Regeneration of the Nervous System," translated and edited by RH May. New York: Hafner.

Reich E (1978): Activation of plasminogen: A general mechanism for producing localized extracellular porteolysis. In Berlin RD, Herrmann H, Lepow IH, Tanzer JM (eds.): "Molecular Basis of Biological Degradative Processes." New York: Academic Press pp 155–169.

Reier PJ (1979): Penetration of grafted astrocytic scars by optic nerve axons in Xenopus tadpoles. Brain Res. 164:61–68.

Reier PJ (1986): Astrocytic scar formation following CNS injury: Its microanatomy and effects on axonal elongation. In Fedoroff S, Vernadakis A (eds): "Astrocytes, Vol. 3: Cell Biology and Pathology of Astrocytes." New York: Academic Press, pp 263–324.

Reier PJ, Houlé JD (1988): The glial scar: Its bearing on axonal elongation and transplantation approaches to CNS repair. In Waxman SG (ed): "Functional Recovery in Neurological Disease." New York: Raven Press, pp 87–138.

Reier PJ, Stensaas LJ, Guth L (1983a): The astrocytic scar as an impediment to regeneration in the central nervous system. In Kao CC, Bunge RP, Reier PJ (eds): "Spinal Cord Reconstruction." New York: Raven Press, pp 163–196.

Reier PJ, Perlow MJ, Guth L (1983b): Development of embryonic spinal cord transplants in the rat. Dev Brain Res 10:201–219.

Reier PJ, Bregman BS, Wujek Jr (1986): Intraspinal transplantation of embryonic spinal cord tissue in neonatal and adult rats. J Comp Neurol 247:275–296.

Richardson PM, Ebendal T (1982): Nerve growth activities in rat peripheral nerve. Brain Res 246:57–64.

Richardson PM, Issa VMK, Shemie S (1982): Regeneration and retrograde degeneration of axons in the rat optic nerve. J Neurocytol 11:949–966.

Risling M, Cullheim S, Hildebrand C (1983): Reinnervation of the ventral root L7 from ventral horn neurons following intramedullary axotomy in adult cats. Brain Res 280:15–23.

Rush RA (1984): Immunohistochemical localization of endogenous nerve growth factor. Nature 312:364–367.

Rutishauser U, Acheson A, Hall AK, Mann DM, Sunshine J (1988): NCAM as a general regulator of cell contact. In Reier PJ, Bunge RP, Seil FJ (eds): "Current Issues in Neural Regeneration Research." New York: Alan R. Liss, Inc., pp 229–236.

Sandrock AW, Matthew WD (1987a): An in vitro neurite-promoting antigen functions in axonal regeneration in vivo. Science 237:1605–1608.

Sandrock AW, Matthew WD (1987b): Identification of a peripheral nerve neurite growth-promoting activity by development and use of an in vitro bioassay. Proc Natl Acad Sci USA 84:6934–6938.

Sandrock AW, Matthew WD (1987c): Substrate-bound nerve growth factor promotes neurite growth in peripheral nerve. Brain Res 425:360–363.

Schlaepfer WW, Freeman LA, Eng LF (1979): Studies of human and bovine spinal nerve roots and the outgrowth of CNS tissues into the nerve root entry zone. Brain Res 177:219–229.

Schwab ME, Thoenen H (1985): Dissociated neurons regenerate into sciatic but not optic nerve explants in culture irrespective of neurotrophic factors. J Neurosci 5:2415–2423.

Schwab ME, Caroni P (1988): Oligodendrocytes and CNS myelin are non-permissive substrates for neurite growth and fibroblast spreading in vitro. J. Neurosci. In Press.

Schwartz M, Belkin M, Harel A, Solomon A, Lavie V, Hadani M, Rachailovich I, Stein-Izsak C (1985): Regenerating fish optic nerves and a regeneration-like response in injured optic nerves of adult rabbits. Science 228:601–603.

Schwartz M, Harel A, Cohen A, Stein-Izsak C, Fainaru M, Rubinstein M, Belkin M, Solomon A (1988): Glial-derived substances associated with CNS regeneration. In DeVellis J, Gorio A, Haber B, Perez-Polo R (eds): "Cellular and Molecular Aspects of Neural Development and Regeneration." Heidelberg: Springer-Verlag, in press.

Sijbesma H, Leonard CM (1986): Developmental changes in the astrocytic response to lateral olfactory tract section. Anat Rec 215:374–382.

Silver J, Ogawa MY (1983): Postnatally induced formation of the corpus callosum in acallosal mice on glia-coated cellulose bridges. Science 220:1067–1069.

Smith GM, Silver J (1988): Transplantation of immature and mature astrocytes and their effect on scar formation in the lesioned CNS. Prog Brain Res: (In Press).

Smith GM, Miller RH, Silver J (1986): The changing role of forebrain astrocytes during development, regeneration failure, and induced regeneration upon transplantation. J Comp Neurol 251:23–43.

Stensaas LJ (1983): Regeneration in the spinal cord of the newt Notopthalmus (Triturus) pyrrhogaster. In Kao CC, Bunge RP, Reier PJ (eds): "Spinal Cord Reconstruction." New York: Raven Press, pp 121–149.

Stensaas LJ, Burgess PR, Horch KW (1979): Regenerating dorsal root axons are blocked by spinal cord astrocytes. Soc Neurosci Abstr 5:684.

Stensaas LJ, Partlow LM, Burgess PR, Horch KW (1987): Inhibition of regeneration: The ultrastructure of reactive astrocytes and abortive axon terminals in the transition zone of the dorsal root. In Seil FJ, Herbert E, Carlson BM (eds): "Neural Regeneration." Progress in Brain Research," vol. 71. Amsterdam: Elsevier, pp 457–468.

Sugar O, Gerard RW (1940): Spinal cord regeneration in the rat. J Neurophysiol 3:1–19.

Sung JH (1981): Tangled masses of regenerated central nerve fibers (non-myelinated central neuromas) in the central nervous system. J Neuropathol Exp Neurol 40:645–657.

Takano K (1976): Absence of the r-spindle loop in the reinnervated hind leg muscles of the cat: "Alpha muscle." Exp Brain Res 26:343–354.

Taniuchi M, Clark HB, Johnson EM Jr (1986): Induction of nerve growth factor receptor in Schwann cells after axotomy. Proc Natl Acad Sci USA 83:4094–4098.

Taniuchi M, Clark HB, Schweitzer JB, Johnson EM Jr (1988): Expression of nerve growth factor receptors by Schwann cells of axotomized peripheral nerves: Ultrastructural localization, suppression by axonal contact, and binding properties. J Neurosci, In Press.

Tessler A, Himes BT, Houle, Reier PJ (1988): Regeneration of adult dorsal root axons into transplants of embryonic spinal cord. J Comp Neurol: 270:537–548.

Turbes CC, Freeman LW (1958): Peripheral nerve-spinal cord anastomosis for experimental cord transection. Neurol 8:857–861.

Unsicker K, Vey J, Hofmann, H-D, Muller TH, Wilson AJ (1984): C6 glioma cell-conditioned medium induced neurite outgrowth and survival of rat chromaffin cells in vitro: Comparison with the effects of nerve growth factor. Proc Natl Acad Sci USA 81:2242–2246.

Varon S (1977) Neural growth and regeneration: A cellular perspective. Exp Neurol 54:1–6.

Varon S, Manthorpe M, Davis GE, Williams LR, Skaper SD (1988a): Growth factors. In Waxman SG (ed.): "Functional Recovery in Neurological Disease. Advances in Neurology," vol. 47. New York: Raven Press, pp 493–521.

Varon S, Hagg T, Manthorpe M (1988b): Neuronal rescue in CNS lesions. In Reier PJ, Bunge RP, Seil FJ (eds): "Current Issues in Neural Regeneration Research." New York: Alan R. Liss, Inc., pp 67–74.

Weinberg EL, Spencer PS (1979): Studies on the control of myelinogenesis. 3. Signalling of oligodendrocyte myelination by regenerating peripheral axons. Brain Res 162:273–279.

Weinberg EL, Raine CS (1980): Reinnervation of periph-eral nerve segments implanted into the rat central nervous system. Brain Res 198:1–11.

Wells MR, Bernstein JJ (1985): Scar formation and the barrier hypothesis in failure of mammalian central nervous system regeneration. In Dacey RG (ed): "Trauma of the Central Nervous System." New York: Raven Press, pp 245–257.

Williams LR, Powell HC, Lundborg G, Varon S (1984): Competence of nerve tissue as distal insert promoting nerve regeneration in a silicone chamber. Brain Res 293:201–211.

Windle WF (1956): Regeneration of axons in the vertebrate central nervous system. Physiol Rev 36:427–439.

Windle WF, Chambers WW (1950): Spinal cord regeneration associated with a cellular reaction induced by administration of a purified bacterial pyrogen. In: Fifth International Anatomy Congress, Oxford, p 196.

Windle WF, Clement CD, Chambers WW (1952a): Inhibition of formation of a glial barrier as a means of permitting a peripheral nerve to grow into the brain. J Comp Neurol 96:359–369.

Windle WF, Clemente CD, Scott D Jr, Chambers WW (1952b): Induction of neuronal regeneration in central nervous system of animals. Trans Am Neurol Assoc 77:164.

Windle WF, Clemente CD, Scott D Jr., Chambers WW (1953): Induction of neuronal regeneration in central nervous system of animals. Trans Am Neurol Assoc 77:164.

Wujek JR, Lasek RJ (1983): Correlation of axonal regeneration and slow component "b" in two branches of a single axon. J Neurosci 3:243–251.

Zimmer J, Sunde N (1984): Neuropeptides and astroglia in intracerebral hippocampal transplants: An immunohistochemical study in the rat. J Comp Neurol 227:331–347.

13

CNS Grafting: Potential Mechanisms of Action

FRED H. GAGE, PhD, AND GYÖRGY BUZSÁKI, MD

Department of Neurosciences, University of California at San Diego, La Jolla, California 92093

Damage to the central nervous system results in neuronal cell death or permanent functional changes that cause behavioral deficits, due to the loss or severe damage of the cells required to carry out important functions. Neuronal grafting is a powerful approach to studying the reestablishment of severed connections and the substitution of lost cells and pathways in the adult mammalian brain. Substantial evidence has emerged over the last decade that intracerebral grafting may be a useful technique for the restoration of function; at least some of these connections may help behavioral recovery of animals and humans with experimental or disease-related lesions. (Sladek and Gash, 1984; Björklund and Stenevi 1985).

In this chapter we will review the various possible mechanisms of graft action and attempt to distinguish among them.

MECHANISMS OF GRAFT ACTION

Grafts to the central nervous system do not all act by a common mechanism in each model system used. A thorough examination of graft-host interactions with each model system will provide the most useful information regarding the mechanism of action and potential applications and limitations of intracerebral grafting. In some cases replacement of a class of cells capable of delivering the appropriate neurotransmitter or other humoral substances may be sufficient, whereas in other cases restoration of lost connectivity or repacement of neuronal computations seems essential. Converse-

ly, survival, growth, and maturation of the grafted tissue are influenced by the type of brain lesion. In the following discussions, schematic diagrams will be used to illustrate different mechanisms through which grafts can function. The schematics are based on the simple system seen in Fig. 13–1 and deal with one-way trafficking of information from the cell source through an axonal substrate to a neuronal target. Fig. 13–2 illustrates the disconnection of the source cells from the target, which results in functional disruption. The subsequent modifications of this schematic represent the variety of ways grafts can be used to potentiate or induce recovery of function.

Neurotrophic Mechanism

In the simplest case, specific neuronal connections may not be required. The transplanted tissue (neurons, glia, or other cell types) may secrete neurotrophic factors that may save the axotomized, deafferented, or otherwise damaged host neurons from secondary death, thus reducing the damaging consequences of the lesion (Fig. 13–3). In addition, the supply of trophic factors may facilitate axon sprouting from the surviving neurons, resulting in a more complete reinnervation. Furthermore, cells in the transplant may remove excitotoxic amino acids (Meldrum, 1985) or extracellular Ca^{2+} liberated after anoxia, epilepsy, or injury. These alternative or additive modes of graft action are illustrated by experiments in which behavioral recovery after frontal cortex lesions in rats was equally facilitated by fetal cortex grafts, cultured purified astrocytes, or gelfoam derived from a brain wound (Kesslak et al., 1986). Such experiments may

Neural Regeneration and Transplantation, pages 211–226
© 1989 Alan R. Liss, Inc.

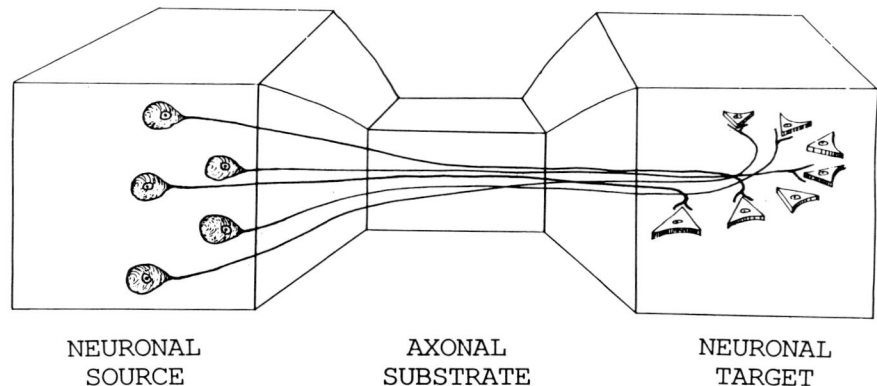

NEURONAL   AXONAL   NEURONAL
SOURCE   SUBSTRATE   TARGET

Figure 13–1.   Schematic drawing of the simple one-synapse axonal pathway, indicating the oval cells of origin (left) and the axonal substrate (center) in which the axons of the neurons reach the target structure (right), with its pyramid-shaped cells. This is the intact model on which all subsequent drawings are based.

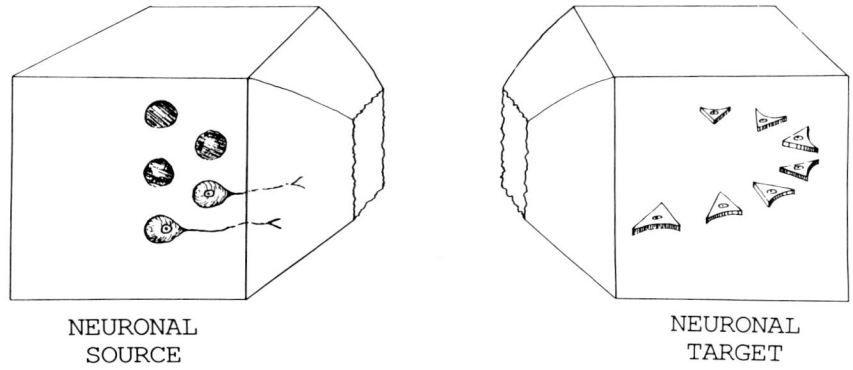

NEURONAL   NEURONAL
SOURCE   TARGET

Figure 13–2.   The lesion. Transection or damage to the axonal substratum results in the loss of terminals in the target tissue and a degeneration of the cells that have been axotomized.

isolate the critical cellular and/or humoral factors responsible for the graft-induced improvement of neuronal function.

Nonregulated Neuronal Grafts

The functional changes seen with transplants placed into one of the cerebral ventricles may be most parsimoniously explained by relatively constant release of humoral factors into the host cerebrospinal fluid (CSF) or adjacent structures (Freed et al., 1980; Gash et al., 1980, Perlow et al., 1980). Such an effect of the graft resembles the therapeutic effects of drug-releasing infusion pumps. A mechanism of action of this kind is exemplified by a recent study (Freund et al., 1985) in which no host afferents to nigral grafts were detected, despite the fact that the grafts had themselves formed extensive dopaminergic connections with the host brain and had produced behavioral improvement (Fig. 13–4). Another case of nonregulated graft action is exemplified by experiments involving fetal raphe neurons placed into the hippocampus of adult rats. The grafted serotonergic neurons displayed their characteristic pacemaker-like discharge pattern; however, they showed no significant behavioral change in activity across the sleep-

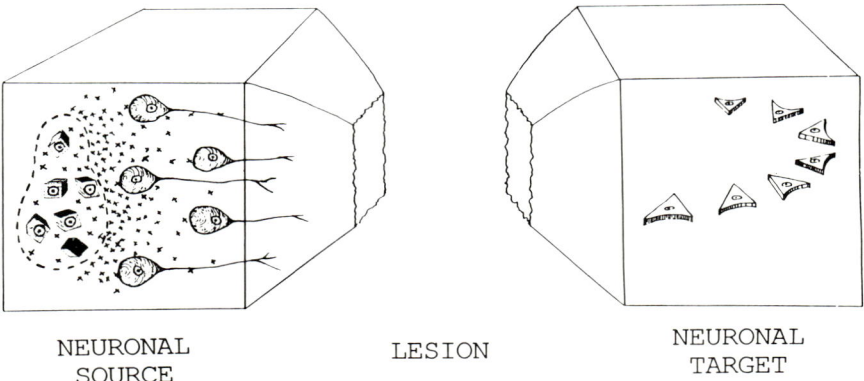

NEURONAL
SOURCE

LESION

NEURONAL
TARGET

Figure 13–3. Neurotrophic mechanism. Implantation of cells in the vicinity of the axotomized cells that can secrete neuronotrophic factors could support and maintain the survival and function of those denervated cells.

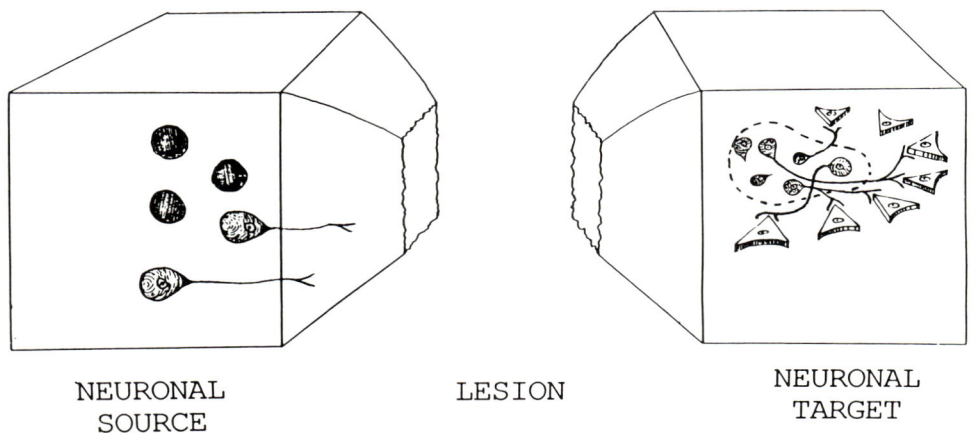

NEURONAL
SOURCE

LESION

NEURONAL
TARGET

Figure 13–4. Nonregulated neuronal grafts. Implantation of fetal cells from the same region of the fetal brain from which the adult cells originate can result in the innervation of the denervated target cells by the axons from these new cells. However, these cells are still disconnected from the inputs that may normally innervate them on the proximal side of the damage.

waking cycle (Trulson et al., 1986). The benevolent effect of the graft in this category may be explained by the enabling or permissive action of a graft released substance. The diffuse release of an active amine or neuromodulator may gate the action of other neurotransmitters tonically (Schwartz et al., 1978; Brown and Arbuthnott, 1983; Nicoll, 1985; Gage and Björklund, 1986a). The degree of "level setting" may be regulated by nonneuronal mechanisms (e.g., hormones, drugs, temperature) and the size of the graft.

Regulated Graft Mechanisms

A further step in the graft-host integration is the establishment of host-graft interconnections. Provided that the newly formed afferents to the transplant are functionally relevant, the host brain may effectively regulate the activity of the graft neurons. In cases in which the graft action is based on the release of diffusible substances, the host-brain feedback mechanism will provide an efficient regulatory mechanism whose therapeutic effect can supersede any ex-

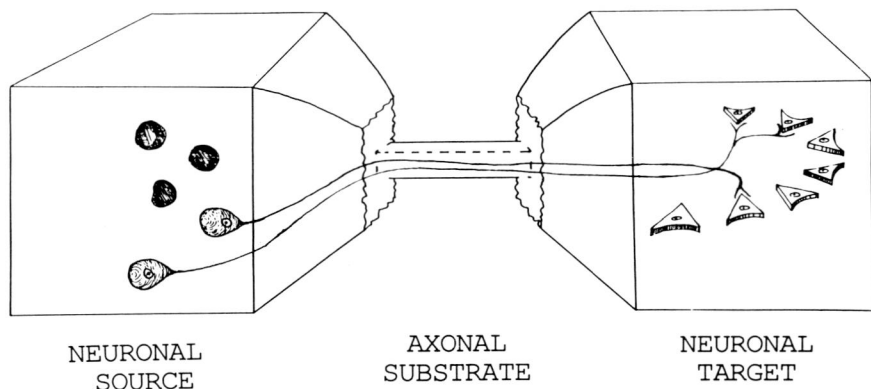

NEURONAL
SOURCE

AXONAL
SUBSTRATE

NEURONAL
TARGET

Figure 13–5. Passive bridge. Placement of nonneuronal or neuronal (see Figure13–7B) material in the cavity between the cells of origin and target can promote axonal regeneration if the substrate contains the appropriate neurite-promoting molecules. In some systems this can also promote survival of the cells of origin by giving them trophic support, but in many cases the factors important for neurite promotion are different from those required for cell survival.

ternal diffusion pump systems. With functional graft-host synapses, the host-graft feedback loop will offer a precisely tuned modulating system. Evidence for the existence of a regulated host-graft-host mechanism will be shown below.

Nonregulated Nonneuronal Grafts

If one takes for granted that in some conditions nonregulated release of neurotransmitter or perhaps trophic factor may be sufficient to allow for functional recovery, then nonneural tissue, which by its nature does not synaptically release transmitter, can be used as donor tissue and chosen for its intrinsic properties, or for the properties it can be modified to express. Attempts to use culture cells include the use of tumor cell lines, such as the IMR-32 (Kordower et al., 1987), PC 12 cells (Hefti et al., 1985b; Jeager, 1987), or primary glia (Gumpel et al., 1987; Smith et al., 1987) based on their ability in culture to synthesize certain desirable molecules. Another approach that is undertaken in our laboratory is to take primary glia cells, fibroblasts, or other cell lines as donor cells, and genetically modify them by using retroviruses to insert a new or "transgene" into the genome of the donor cells. These genetically modified cells are then transplanted to the brain of a host animal (Gage et al., 1987). This allows for direct control of the number of cells expressing

the gene product, the type of cell expressing the gene product, and the type of gene desired. Future work in this area of genetically modified cells will indeed focus on the regulated release of the transgene product, by either intrinsic or extrinsic regulatory factors.

"Passive" Neuronal or Nonneuronal Bridges

When septal or hippocampal grafts are placed in the fimbria-fornix cavity, fibers from the septum and other brainstem areas have been reported to regrow into the host hippocampus (Kromer et al., 1981; Buzsáki et al., 1987a,b) (Fig. 13–5). In a similar manner, hippocampal projection neurons may be able to grow back through the graft to their original septal and diencephalic targets. According to this "passive" bridge model, the fetal tissue merely serves as a scaffold to induce and guide regeneration of the severed host connections (Aguayo, 1985). This "bridging" function of the graft may be dissociated experimentally from its trophic action by implanting the fetal grafts at various intervals after the brain damage. Trophic factors should be made available to the host brain immediately after injury prior to cell death. Success with delayed grafting indicates factors other than mere detoxicating or trophic effects of graft function are involved. In

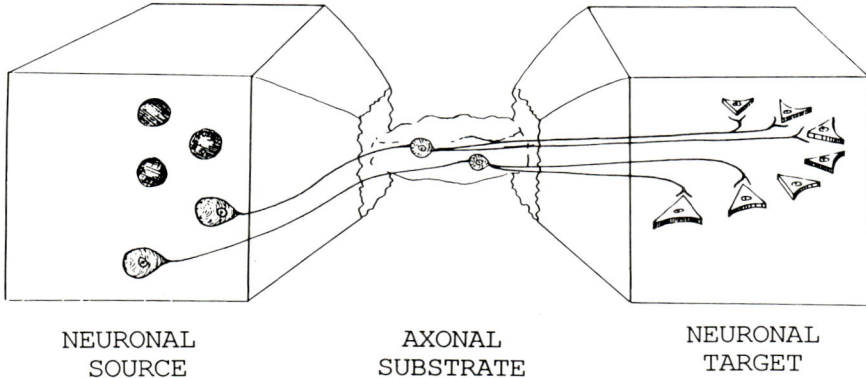

NEURONAL   AXONAL   NEURONAL
SOURCE   SUBSTRATE   TARGET

Figure 13–6.   Active bridge. When cells from the same region of the fetal brain as the cells of origin are placed in the lesion cavity, these cells can by themselves reinnervate the denervated cavity, but they can also act as a bridge between the cells of origin and the target.

addition to the use of fetal neuronal tissue as bridging material, it is reasonable to consider the use of nonneuronal tissue that contains or can produce or sequester the important elements from the environment to induce the directed growth of host axons. This possibility has emerged as a result of the characterization of molecules in the extracellular matrix, particularly in the basement membrane, which are important in axonal elongation and neurite promotion. This has been accomplished with some success by Aguayo and colleagues (Chapter 5, this volume). In addition, cultured extracellular matrix molecule producing Schwann cells have been employed to produce a bridge between the septum and hippocampus following a fimbria-fornix transection (Kromer and Cornbrooks, 1987). Recently, we have used a human placental membrane as a bridge material in the septohippocampal system (Davis et al., 1987; Gage et al., 1988). This material has real advantages in that it is acellular, does not induce an inflammatory response in the host brain, and yet can act as a bridge to allow or induce damaged axons to regrow toward their target area. In the future other more direct methods will involve the direct presentation of these isolated molecules on synthetic or other artificial surfaces that can be easily and economically reproduced.

"Active" Neural Bridge

An "active" version of the bridge model assumes that by establishing both afferent and efferent connections with the host brain, the graft may become part of a one-way (e.g., subcortical input-graft-hippocampus) circuitry (Fig. 13–6). In such a model the main function of the graft is to actively relay the information from the host afferents to the host targets (Lund and Simons, 1985). This model will be elaborated further below.

The passive and active versions of graft bridges may be distinguished experimentally by destroying the neurons of the graft bridge by, e.g., ibotenic acid lesions after the reestablishment of the host-host or host-graft-host circuitries. If neurons of the graft are actively participating in relaying information, the restored function will be severed after destruction of the graft neurons.

Neuronal Replacement

In cases of regulation and nonregulated control, as discussed above, the graft tissue is not, in most cases, placed into the location of the cell loss or dysfunction, but rather in the target area, where synaptic contacts are made. For example, the fetal substantia nigra is implanted in the striatum, not the host substantia nigra, and the cholinergic basal forebrain is implanted in the hippocampus, not the host basal forebrain. This is not to say that regulated release of transmitter does not occur or that correct synaptic contacts are not made, but the complete restoration of normal circuitry is unlikely under these conditions. However, several graft models allow for the analysis of neuronal replacement. One of these is an animal model of Huntington's disease (Deckel et al., 1983; Isacson et al., 1984, 1985). In this model neurotoxic lesions of the striatum result in a near total depletion of all striatal cells, and the challenge of the model is to replace the striatal cells by grafting fetal striatum directly to the adult damaged striatum. Recent evidence suggests that many of the normal cells and their afferent and efferent connections develop correctly, and some types of functional recovery have been observed (Deckel et al., 1986; Isacson et al., 1987). In another model system, Sotelo and colleagues (1987) have shown that in specific rodent genetic mutations, selective cell populations are absent, and wild-type fetal neuronal grafting to the developing brain of these mutants can allow or promote migration of cells previously missing to their appropriate laminar locations, where several of the appropriate connections can be made.

Deleterious Actions of Brain Grafts

The growing volume of grafted tissue placed into the ventricular system may obstruct the free flow of the cerebrospinal fluid, resulting in hydrocephalus. Similarly, the fast growing graft may destroy the host brain by compression or other means.

The nervous system has long been considered an immunologically privileged site. Indeed, cells expressing major histocompatibility complex antigens are not found in the CNS. Brain grafts, however, may alter the protective blood-brain barrier, thus increasing the entrance of patrolling lymphocytes into the CNS (Rosenstein, 1987). The inflammatory interface may exert an inadvertent influence on the activity of neighboring host neurons.

Surgical removal of microscopic areas from the brain of an embryo is not an easy task. In order to harvest a sufficient number of cholinergic or other monoaminergic precursor cells, relatively large areas must be excised. It is estimated that in suspension grafts less than 5% of the transplanted tissue contains the required cell types (Gage and Björklund, 1986b). The remaining majority of neurons may thus set up undesired connections with the host or may retard the formation of the expected connections.

As will be discussed below, the probability of new synapse formation among the graft neurons is higher than between the host afferents and graft cells. In certain conditions, undesirable reverberatory excitatory circuits may result, with consequent epileptic discharges in the graft, which occasionally may spread to the host as well (Buzsáki et al., 1987b). These and other unexpected complications must be considered in search of the restorative abilities of brain grafts.

MODEL: SEPTOHIPPOCAMPAL SYSTEM

An important prerequisite for successful and credible studying of intracerebral grafting is the use of well defined animal models of brain damage and consequent demonstration of functional reinstitution.

The septohippocampal system has been employed with considerable success in studies of intracerebral grafting. There are four main reasons:

1. The chemical neuroanatomical organization is well established, specifically, the cholinergic cells of origin in the septal-diagonal band region and their routes of passage, as well as the characteristic pattern of terminal lamination within the hippocampal formation are well described (Storm-Mathiesen, 1979; Armstrong et al., 1983; Gage et al., 1983; Mesulam et al., 1983; Amaral and Kurz, 1985).

2. The principal and most characteristic electrophysiological property of the hippocampus (rhythmic slow activity or theta activity) is dependent on the anatomical and cholinergic integrity of the septohippocampal circuitry (Buzsáki et al., 1983).

3. The hippocampal formation has long been associated with learning and memory, and substantial evidence supports the importance of the cholinergic system in the mechanism by which the hippocampus may influence learning and memory (O'Keefe and Nadel, 1978; Olton et al., 1979).

4. The septohippocampal system can be nearly completely disconnected by surgically transecting the major pathways connecting the septal area and the hippocampus via the fimbria-fornix (Björklund and Stenevi, 1977; Gage et al., 1983). This bilateral surgical transection results in a nearly complete elimination of the cholinergic contribution to the hippocampus, the elimination of the theta ac-

tivity, and a severe and long-lasting disruption of learning and memory in rats.

Together these components of the cholinergic septohippocampal system have provided an experimental model within which to investigate the anatomical, biochemical, electrophysiological, and behavioral effects of graft-host interactions.

The Lesion

The septohippocampal cholinergic pathway has been lesioned uni- or bilaterally with an aspirative lesion of the fornix-fimbria and the overlying cingulate cortex. This so-called fimbria-fornix lesion transects all dorsal routes of cholinergic axons from the septal-diagonal band area innervating the hippocampal formation (as well as the posterior cingulate cortex) running in the fimbria, the dorsal fornix, and the supracallosal striae. The lesion removes about 90% of the cholinergic innervation of the entire hippocampal formation. The residual innervation reaches the hippocampus via the so-called ventral route (through the amygdaloid-piriform lobe); it is confined entirely to the ventral (temporal) tip of the hippocampal formation (Gage et al., 1984; Milner and Amaral, 1984). The aspirative fimbria-fornix lesion is nonselective and removes, in addition to the cholinergic afferents, a range of other afferent and efferent connections of the hippocampus and the medial neocortex as well. The fimbria-fornix lesion is made under visual control, and thus the completeness of the lesion with respect to its cholinergic denervating effect can reliably be assessed under the operating microscope.

Grafting Procedures

Two principal techniques have been used to graft tissue to the previously denervated hippocampal regions. The first involves the transplantation of solid pieces of tissue to a surgically prepared transplantation cavity in which the graft is placed in direct contact with the denervated hippocampus (Figs. 13–5, 13–6). In this procedure good graft survival is ensured by preparing the cavity in such a way that the graft can be placed on a richly vascularized surface (e.g., the pia in the choroidal fissure) that can serve as a "culturing bed" for the grafts (Stenevi et al., 1976). The vessel-rich

ventral surface of the fimbria-fornix lesion provides such a "culuring bed." This cavity is in direct communication with the lateral ventricle, which may allow the CSF to circulate through the graft cavity and thus probably help the graft to survive, particularly during the early postoperative period.

The second technique we have used involves injection of dissociated cell suspensions into the depth of the brain (Björklund et al., 1980, 1983c; Schmidt et al., 1981). Pieces of cultured cells of fetal tissue are trypsinized or mechanically dissociated, and small volumes of the suspension can then be stereotaxically injected into the desired site using a microsyringe (Figs. 13–3, 13–4). A major advantage of this technique is that it allows precise and multiple placements of the cells. The technique also makes possible accurate monitoring of the number of cells injected by counting the density of cells in the suspension (Brundin et al., 1985).

Graft Survival and Axonal Growth

Solid pieces of the embryonic septal-diagonal band area have been found to be capable of providing a new cholinergic innervation of the cholinergically denervated hippocampal formation in fimbria-fornix–lesioned young rats. With such solid grafts the reinnervation process is protracted over several months. With cell suspension grafts of the septal-diagonal band region, injected directly into the denervated hippocampus, we have been able to increase the rate of reinnervation of the denervated hippocampus as well as to increase the total area of the denervated hippocampus that is reinnervated by the acetylcholinesterase (AChE)-positive fibers growing out from the grafted cells (Björklund et al., 1983a).

The septal cell suspension grafts are found as several cellular aggregates or tissue masses within the hippocampal or choroidal fissures, within the overlying ventricle, or embedded in the host hippocampal tissue. It has been estimated that the implanted tissue grows to about twice its initial volume and that approximately 60% of the potential number of cholinergic neurons survive, provided the implants are made into a cholinergically denervated (i.e., fimbria-fornix–lesioned) hippocampus (Björklund et al., 1983b).

A new AChE-positive innervation is established from the grafts, starting between 1 and 3 weeks after implantation. By 3 months the entire hippocampal formation was reached by the ingrowing fibers, with a terminal density approaching that of the normal hippocampus (Björklund et al., 1983b).

The laminar pattern established by the newly formed AChE-positive terminal networks was remarkably similar to that of the normal AChE-positive innervation, even with respect to finer details. This finding suggests that the distribution of the ingrowing fibers from the graft was highly specific. Other experiments, using grafts of various types of monoaminergic neurons, have shown that the patterning of the ingrowing axons is characteristic for each neuron type, and that it is greatly dependent on both graft placement and the presence or absence of the intrinsic cholinergic innervation (Björklund et al., 1976, 1979).

Electron microscopy, using choline acetyltransferase (ChAT) immunocytochemistry, has shown that the ingrowing cholinergic axons from the grafts form abundant synaptic contacts with neuronal elements in the host dentate gyrus in both the fimbria-fornix–lesioned young rats and the nondenervated aged rats (Clark and Dunnett, 1986; Clarke et al., 1986). Although the graft-derived synapses in the aged rats were remarkably similar to normal synapses qualitatively, some abnormalities were found in the fimbria-fornix–lesioned young rats with respect to the relative distribution of contacts or dendrites and neuronal perikarya.

Biochemical Measures of Graft Function

The activity of the cholinergic innervation of the denervated hippocampus, derived from solid or suspension grafts of the septal-diagonal band area, has been monitored biochemically by measurement of the acetylcholine-synthesizing enzyme ChAT and of acetylcholine synthesis in vitro (Björklund et al., 1983c). The synthetic enzyme ChAT is specifically localized in cholinergic neurons and is a good marker for cholinergic neurotransmission. ChAT activity has therefore been used to measure the time course and magnitude of fiber outgrowth from both solid and suspended septal grafts. Graft-derived ChAT activity was barely detectable by 10 days after the implantation of cell suspension grafts, but it sharply increased between 10 days and 1 month in the region of the host hippocampus close to the grafts. By 6 months, ChAT activity was restored to near normal levels in all segments of the previously denervated hippocampal formation. When comparing the total ChAT activity derived from the solid grafts and the cell suspension grafts, the cell suspension grafts appeared to be about twice as effective as the solid grafts, although the amount of tissue grafted was about the same in each case.

The functional activity of the septal grafts was further assessed by measurements of [^{14}C]acetylcholine synthesis from [^{14}C]glucose in vitro in fimbria-fornix–lesioned rats with septal suspensions implanted into the depth of the denervated hippocampus (Björklund et al., 1983c). The overall hippocampal [^{14}C]acetylcholine synthesis was restored to normal levels in the grafted animals, and estimates of acetylcholine turnover rate suggested that the transmitter machinery of the newly established septohippocampal connections operated at a rate similar to that of the intrinsic septohippocampal pathway. Thus these septal cell suspensions seem capable of maintaining function at a near normal level despite their abnormal position.

The magnitude of lesion-induced functional alterations in different regions of the hippocampal formation is reflected in the local rates of [^{14}C]2-deoxyglucose (2-DG) utilization. A measure of recovery is the degree to which this index of functional activity can be normalized following reinnervation by solid septal grafts (Kelly et al., 1985). Transection of the septohippocampal pathway by a unilateral fimbria-fornix lesion resulted in a 30–50% reduction in 2-DG utilization throughout the ipsilateral hippocampal formation, and this depressed metabolism persisted 6 months after the lesion. Interestingly, the areas of depressed 2-DG utilization within the lesioned hemisphere were largely coextensive with the areas of the cingulate cortex and the hippocampal formation that had been substantially cholinergically denervated as a consequence of the fimbria-fornix transection. Fimbria-fornix–lesioned rats that had received solid septal grafts displayed a significant recovery in hippocampal 2-DG utilization compared with the rats with lesion alone. The graft-induced recovery in 2-DG utilization was significantly correlated with the graft-induced recovery in AChE staining density in adjacent sections from the same brains, thus suggesting a relation between the cholinergic reinnervation from the septal grafts and the restoration of functional glucose utilization. Indeed, the area of the host hippocampus and dentate gyrus that showed a complete restoration of AChE-positive innervation in these grafted animals was normalized with respect to the 2-DG utilization rate, whereas the area with only partial AChE-positive reinnervation showed a partial but incomplete recovery of 2-DG use. Together with the biochemical data cited above, these results strongly suggest that the cholinergic component of the grafts is functional at the biochemical level and influences, or normalizes, the overall functional performance of the deafferented hippocampal formation.

Graft Induced Amelioration of Learning and Memory Impairment

The hippocampus has a special role in learning and memory, and bilateral fimbria-fornix or medial septal lesions in rats are known to result in severe impairment in both working memory and spatial memory (O'Keefe and Nadel, 1978; Olton et al., 1979). These lesions disrupt several major afferent and efferent connection systems of the hippocampal formation. Nevertheless, because similar (but less pronounced) effects are obtained by pharmacological blockade of cholinergic transmission (Whitshaw, 1985; Whitshaw et al., 1985), it appears that damage to the cholinergic septohippocampal pathway contributes greatly to the memory impairments seen after fimbria-fornix or medial septal lesions.

In the eight-arm radial maze (Low et al., 1982), rats with solid septal grafts (7 months after transplantation) showed a positive linear trend in maze performance over days of testing, but overall did not differ significantly from nongrafted rats with lesions. However, potentiation of cholinergic transmission by pretreatment with the AChE inhibitor physostigmine produced significant enhancement of maze performance in the grafted group, but not in the lesioned control group, and in some cases the grafted rats performed as well as the nonlesioned control animals. In a more recent study on intrahippocampal grafts of septal cell suspensions in rats with medial septal lesions, Pallage and co-workers (1986) obtained significant graft-induced recovery of radial maze performance, also in the absence of AChE inhibition.

In a study using a T-maze forced choice alternation test (performed 6 months after transplantation), Dunnett and colleagues (1982) reported that seven of nine rats with solid septal grafts and four of five rats with septal suspension grafts were able to learn the task, some of them up to the level of control rats. The remaining rats with septal grafts and a separate group of rats with control grafts taken from the brainstem locus coeruleus region performed at chance level, similar to the rats that received only the fimbria-fornix lesion. The subsequent microscopic analysis showed a significant correlation between performance of the grafted rats and the amount of graft-derived AChE-positive staining in the previously denervated hippocampus.

Nilsson et al. (1987) tested the ability of septal suspension or solid grafts to improve spatial reference and working memory in the Morris (1981) water maze task in rats with bilateral fimbria-fornix lesions. Of the grafted rats, 60–80% showed significant recovery of spatial memory. This observation was seen in rats that had been pretrained in the task prior to lesion and grafting, and in rats that had not been exposed to the water maze prior to lesion and transplantation. In the pretrained rats, the bilateral fimbria-fornix lesion completely abolished the acquired performance. Whereas the lesioned, nongrafted rats could relearn the task partially using nonspatial strategies, the lesioned rats with septal grafts were capable of reacquiring a spatial memory of the platform site. Interestingly, central muscarinic receptor blockade by atropine (50 mg/kg) completely abolished the reacquired spatial memory in the grafted animals. This atropine effect was also seen in the normal control rats but to a lesser extent. Peripheral receptor blockade induced by atropine methylbromide, which passes the blood-brain barrier poorly, had no effect. Segal and coinvestigators (1987) have reported similar results on intrahippocampal septal suspension grafts in rats with medial septal lesions.

Electrophysiological Studies of Intact and Lesioned Hippocampus

The most characteristic hippocampal electroencephalographic (EEG) pattern is the rhythmical slow activity (RSA or theta rhythm) which, in the rat, occurs during exploratory behaviors (walking, running, rearing, sniffing) and the paradoxical phase of sleep (Vanderwolf, 1969). The sources of rhythmicity are the cholinergic and possibly noncholinergic "pacemaker" cells of the medial septum and the nucleus of the diagonal band of Broca. Cells in these regions fire rhythmically following various deafferentations and in the in vitro slice preparation (Petsche et al., 1962; Vinogradova et al., 1985).

Another pattern of spontaneous hippocampal activity is the irregularly occurring sharp wave (SPW) of 40–120 ms duration. SPWs never occur during behaviors accompanied by RSA waves (Buzsáki et al., 1983; Buzsáki, 1986). SPWs are observed in order of frequency during slow wave sleep, immobility, drinking, eating, face washing, and body grooming (0.1–6 Hz). SPWs occur synchronously in both hippocampi either in isolation or in groups of two to seven spikes, and reflect near simultaneous depolarizations of the pyramidal cells in CA1, CA3, and subiculum and granule cells in the dentate gyrus.

Hippocampal SPWs are invariably correlated with the synchronous discharge of a great number of pyramidal cells, granule cells and, interneurons. In between the bursts of SPW, the activity of the neurons is suppressed (Buzsáki, 1986). SPWs are controlled by two pharmacologically and anatomically distinct systems, each of which alone is capable of inhibiting the generation of SPWs. One is a cholinergic-muscarinergic path coursing in the fimbria-fornix. The other input is atropine-resistant, and its fibers run above the corpus callosum. The two SPW-suppressive mechanisms may be identical or concurrently operative with the two RSA systems (Buzsáki et al., 1983). It is hypothesized that SPWs are triggered by a population burst of CA3 pyramidal

cells as a result of temporary disinhibition from afferent control. Indeed, mono- and multisynaptic evoked responses show a several-fold increase during the SPWs.

Surgical subcortical deafferentation of the hippocampus, such as used in transplant studies, results in marked and permanent changes of the hippocampal electrical patterns. RSA is absent completely and is replaced by low-amplitude fast activity during exploratory behaviors.

The incidence and amplitude of SPWs may be increased following fimbria-fornix transection and can occur during behaviors normally associated with RSA, although at a lower probability. SPWs in the two hippocampi occur asynchronously and at different frequencies. Population spikes in the dentate gyrus evoked by stimulation of the entorhinal input (perforant path) may be as large as 20 mV, while in the normally behaving rat they rarely exceed 10 mV. Similarly, the trisynaptic response in CA1 is also exaggerated. Large, multiple population spikes may be present. Occasionally, two or three responses with 15–25 ms intervals may be observed in response to single pulses, indicating reverberation in the entorhinal-hippocampal-entorhinal cortex circuitry. Not infrequently, strong pulses can evoke seizure activity, which is never seen in the intact rat in response to single volleys.

In short, the surgical removal of the inhibitory or feed-forward inhibitory subcortical inputs will result in a highly excitable, seizure-susceptible hippocampal system that is not only malfunctional, but via its remaining afferents may deteriorate the function of its targets as well.

Electrophysiological Studies of Grafts to the Lesioned Hippocampus

In unilaterally lesioned animals we studied the electrophysiological changes in the host hippocampus by solid septal and hippocampal grafts and by dissociated suspensions of septal, locus coeruleus, and hippocampal neurons in an attempt to explain the behavioral improvements observed in bilaterally lesioned and grafted animals (Low et al., 1982; Gage et al., 1983; Nilsson et al., 1987).

The most striking reparative change we observed was the reappearance of hippocampal

RSA in some rats with septal and hippocampal bridges. Concurrent with RSA, granule cells and interneurons in the host hippocampus fired rhythmically, phase-locked to RSA. Cross-correlation of RSA from the transplanted and the intact hippocampi revealed that hippocampal EEG was modulated by the same "pacemaker." As in normal rats, RSA was present only during running and walking and absent during drinking and immobility. The depth profile and the septo-temporal distribution of the power of RSA correlated with the density and distribution of the graft-mediated AChE-positive reinnervation of the host hippocampus (Buzsáki et al., 1987a). Considerably better restoration was found with septal than with hippocampal bridges. In several rats with hippocampal grafts, RSA was not present at all or occurred in brief (0.5–2 s) rhythmic bursts during walking-running transitions. Instead, large-amplitude SPWs frequently occurred, at a higher rate closer to the hippocampal transplant.

Suspension grafts did not restore context-specific RSA in the host hippocampus. Rhythmic EEG waves and phase-locked unit firing for up to several seconds were occasionally observed in the rats of the septal suspension group, but only during immobility (Buzsáki et al., 1988).

Like the rats with solid hippocampal grafts, rats with fetal hippocampal cell suspensions seemed more prone to seizures. In a subgroup of rats with bilateral fimbria-fornix lesions and unilaterally transplanted hippocampal cell suspensions, the enhanced excitability of the grafted hippocampus was obvious. Some of these rats also displayed spontaneous behavioral seizures. Such preparations (bilateral fimbria-fornix transections and unilateral graft placement) thus provide an excellent model for studying the epilepsy enhancing/suppressing effects of brain tissue transplants.

The above findings led us to suggest that at least a minor portion of the RSA "pacemaker" cells of the host septum survives the transection of the fimbria-fornix (Gage et al., 1986) and that a graft of fetal septal or hippocampal tissue implanted into the lesion cavity may be capable of transmitting the rhythmic activity of the host hippocampus. Since both septal and hippocampal tissues were able to restore RSA

in the host hippocampus, the findings support the "passive bridge" model of graft action (Fig. 13–5). The less successful recovery with hippocampal bridges may be explained by assuming that the hippocampal graft used up a good portion of the regenerating septal axons, thus resulting in less complete reinnervation of the host hippocampus. Alternatively, the better restoration of RSA with solid septal tissue may be due to the participation of grafted septal neurons. If we accept this "active bridge" model (Fig. 13–6), we have to assume that the pacemaker cells of the graft were controlled by the same subcortical mechanisms that control the pacemaker cells in the intact septum. Recording neuronal activity from the septal graft in behaving rats may resolve this issue.

Physiological Mechanisms of Behavioral Improvements by Grafts in the Denervated Hippocampus

Grafts restoring the subcortical control of the hippocampus appear ideal for behavioral recovery. Thus the nearly perfect reappearance of the electrical activity of the host hippocampus in some animals with solid grafts could be taken to indicate that the "bridging" technique may be more efficient than suspension grafts in attempts to restore behavioral deficits. Indeed, behavioral deficits in different types of spatial tasks in fimbria-fornix–damaged rats were significantly improved by solid septal grafts placed into the lesion cavity (Low et al., 1982; Nilsson et al., 1987). Cell suspensions of fetal septal tissue injected directly into the deafferented hippocampus were similarly effective in improving performance (Dunnett et al., 1982), although subcortical afferents were not restored in these animals, and the electrophysiological consequences of septal graft bridges and suspension injections, as shown above, are very different.

In rats with suspension grafts of septal tissue at two or three levels along the septotemporal axis of the hippocampus, subcortical control is not reestablished, but reinnervation of the host hippocampus by AChE-positive fibers is nearly complete (Björklund et al., 1983). It is possible that the nonregulated cholinergic and/or GABA-ergic cells of the graft suppressed the deleterious amplifying action of the host hippocampus (Fig. 13–4). Furthermore, it is possible that the axons of the host hippocampus contacted the grafted septal cells, thereby establishing a regulatory feedback circuitry between the host and graft. Direct recording from the transplanted septal cells may determine the regulated or nonregulated nature of the suspension graft cells.

It should be emphasized that reinnervation and restoration of RSA from graft bridges were restricted to the septal pole of the host hippocampus. Thus, even if normal function reappeared completely in some lamellae of the host hippocampus, the physiological activity of the major portion of the structure remained similar to that of fimbria-fornix–lesioned animals. The reason for this lack of complete reinnervation may be explained below, and strategies to overcome it will be explored.

Attempts to Reconstruct Normal Circuitry

Following a complete lesion of the fimbria-fornix, cells in the medial septum and the diagonal band of Broca undergo severe morphological changes, including shrinkage and complete atrophy (Daitz and Powell, 1954; Gage et al., 1986). Cell death after the axotomy occurs in both AChE-positive and other cells. The greatest cell loss was observed in the medial septum (65%) and the vertical limb of the nucleus of the diagonal band (55%). A portion of the surviving AChE-positive neurons shrank by about 20%. A similar cell loss was demonstrable in the medial septum (50%) and the diagonal band (50%) in cresyl violet-stained sections. Since AChE-positive cells account for only about one-third of the cell population in medial septum, the above figures indicate that noncholinergic neurons also degenerate as a result of fimbria-fornix transection. It is known that both GABA-ergic and substance-P neurons of the septal area project to the hippocampus via the fimbria-fornix (Kohler et al., 1984; Shults et al., 1984; Amaral and Kurz, 1985; Wainer et al., 1985). These neurons are also affected by the fimbria-fornix lesion (Petersen et al., 1987).

In preliminary experiments we found that the presence of fetal hippocampal tissue placed into the fimbria-fornix cavity was not able to reduce the percentage of cell loss in the septal area (unpublished findings). Thus our electrophysiological findings, namely the re-

turn of RSA in the host hippocampus and the rhythmic firing of the neurons in the grafted hippocampus, must be attributed to the survival of a relatively minor population of septal pacemaker cells. We hypothesize that the physiological recovery would have been more complete had the majority of the neurons in the medial septum-diagonal band survived.

Several neurotrophic factors have been detected in the hippocampus and retrogradely transported specifically to neurons of the basal forebrain (Schwab et al., 1979; Seiler and Schwab, 1984). Moreover, exogenous nerve growth factor (NGF) has been shown in vivo and in vitro to stimulate ChAT activity of these cells in both developing and adult animals (Gnahn et al., 1983; Hefti, 1986; Mobley et al., 1986). In addition, it has been reported recently that intermittent or continuous infusion of NGF through an intraventricular cannula device promoted the survival of neurons in the medial septum and the nucleus of the diagonal band after partial (Hefti, 1986) or complete (Williams et al., 1986; Kromer, 1987) transection of the fimbria-fornix.

Following complete damage to the fimbria-fornix, NGF treatment resulted in the survival of 100% of both cholinergic and noncholinergic neurons in the vertical limb of the diagonal band. In the medial septum NGF infusion lead to a sparing of 60% of the cholinergic neurons and 50% of the total neurons (Nissl sections) relative to the brains with surgical lesions only (Williams et al., 1986). These findings thus demonstrate that intraventricular infusion of NGF leads to a substantial protection of neurons of the septal region following axotomy and support the hypothesis that death of the transected neurons is due to the loss of target-derived endogenous neurotrophic factors.

Fetal hippocampus placed into the fimbria-fornix cavity did not promote survival of the neurons in either the medial septum or the diagonal band. Percentage of cell loss in the transplanted rats was essentially similar to those with fimbria-fornix lesion only (our unpublished findings). The failure to protect the septal area cell loss by fetal hippocampal implants may be accounted for by a recent finding that the NGF and NGF messenger-RNA content of the hippocampus is very low at birth and begins to increase significantly only

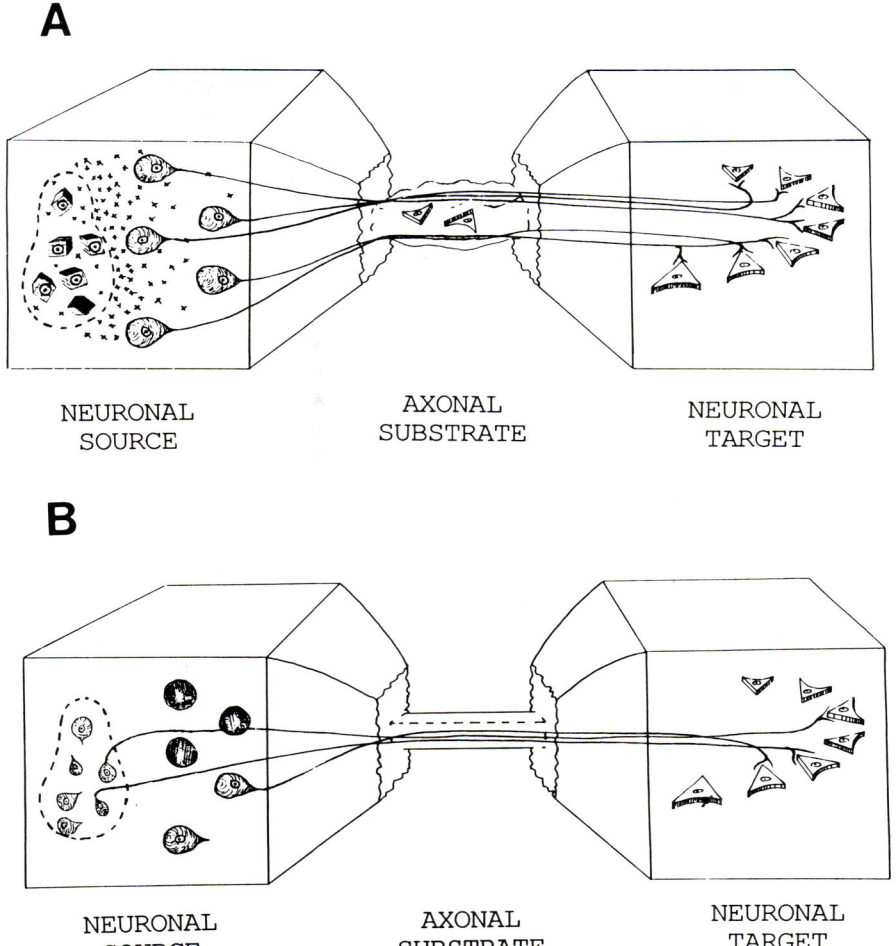

A

NEURONAL
SOURCE

AXONAL
SUBSTRATE

NEURONAL
TARGET

B

NEURONAL
SOURCE

AXONAL
SUBSTRATE

NEURONAL
TARGET

Figure 13–7. Neuronal reconstruction. **A:** A similar reconstruction can be made combining the neurotrophic mechanism with the passive bridge. The fetal brain-derived target cells in the illustrated passive neuronal bridge do not contribute fibers that connect with the host target cells. **B:** Attempts can be made to reconstruct the damaged brain by neuronal replacement of the cells of origin in the appropriate location, combined with an active or passive bridge in the lesion cavity.

during the second postnatal week (Large et al., 1986). The low NGF level in the transplanted hippocampus during the first 1 or 2 weeks after transplantation may explain its inability to protect the neurons from dying in the septal area. We propose that the combination of fetal hippocampal transplantation and transient NGF treatment may result in a permanent survival of the neurons in the septal area following their axotomy. In this way a reconstruction of appropriate neural circuitry can be estab-lished, which is more like that of the intact organism (Fig. 13–7). Under these conditions, we expect a more complete restoration of nor-mal structure and function, both electrophys-iologically and behaviorally.

ACKNOWLEDGMENTS

We thank Sheryl Christenson and Jan Ber-glund for typing, drawing, and photography. This research was supported by grants from the J.D. French Foundation and NIA AG6088, and the Office of Naval Research, and California State DHHS.

REFERENCES

Aguayo AJ (1985): Axonal regeneration from injured neurons in the adult mammalian central nervous system. In Cotman CW (ed): "Synaptic Plasticity." New York: Guilford Press, pp 457–484.

Amaral DG, Kurz J (1985): An analysis of the origins of the cholinergic and noncholinergic septal projections to the hippocampal formation of the rat. J Comp Neurol 240:37–59.

Armstrong DM, Saper CB, Levey AI, Wainer BH, Terry RD (1983): Distribution of cholinergic neurons in rat brain demonstrated by the immunocytochemical localization of choline acetyltransferase. J Comp Neurol 216:53–68.

Björklund A, Stenevi U (1977): Reformation of the severed septohippocampal cholinergic pathway in the adult rat by transplanted septal neurons. Cell Tissue Res 185:289–302.

Björklund A, Stenevi U (1985): "Neural Grafting in the Mammalian CNS." Amsterdam: Elsevier.

Björklund A, Stenevi U, Svendgaard N-A (1976): Growth of transplanted monoaminergic neurons into the adult hippocampus along the perforant path. Nature 262:787–790.

Björklund A, Kromer LF, Stenevi U (1979): Cholinergic reinnervation of the rat hippocampus by septal implants is stimulated by perforant path lesion. Brain Res 173:57–64.

Björklund A, Schmidt RH, Stenevi U (1980): Functional reinnervation of the neostriatum in the adult rat by use of intraparenchymal grafting of dissociated cell suspensions from the substantia nigra. Cell Tissue Res 212:39–45.

Björklund A, Gage FH, Schmidt RH, Stenevi U, Dunnett SH (1983a): Intracerebral grafting of neuronal cell suspensions. VII. Recovery of choline acetyltransferase activity and acetylcholine synthesis in the denervated hippocampus reinnervated by septal suspension implants. Acta Physiol Scand [Suppl] 522:59–66.

Björklund A, Gage FH, Stenevi U, Dunnett SB (1983b): Intracerebral grafting of neuronal cell suspensions. VI. Survival and growth of intrahippocampal implants of septal cell suspensions. Acta Physiol Scand [Suppl] 522:48–58.

Björklund A, Stenevi U, Schmidt RH, Dunnett SB, Gage FH (1983c): Intracerebral grafting of neuronal cell suspensions. I. Introduction and general methods of preparation. Acta Physiol Scand [Suppl] 522:1–10.

Brown JR, Arbuthnott GW (1983): The electrophysiology of dopamine (D2) receptors: A study of the actions of dopamine on corticostriatal transmission. Neuroscience 10:349–355.

Brundin P, Isacson O, Björklund A (1985): Monitoring of cell viability in suspensions of embryonic CNS tissue and its criterion for intracerebral graft survival. Brain Res 331:251–259.

Buzsáki G (1986): Hippocampal sharp-waves: Their origin and significance. Brain Res 398:242–252.

Buzsáki G, Leung LS, Vanderwolf CH (1983): Cellular basis of hippocampal EEG in the behaving rat. Brain Res Rev 6:139–171.

Buzsáki G, Gage FH, Czopf J, Björklund A (1987a): Restoration of rhythmic slow activity in the subcortically denervated hippocampus by fetal CNS transplants. Brain Res 400:334–347.

Buzsáki G, Gage FH, Kellenyi L, Björklund A (1987b): Behavioral dependence of the electrical activity of intracerebrally transplanted fetal hippocampus. Brain Res 400:321–333.

Buzsáki G, Czopf J, Kondakor I, Björklund A, Gage FH (1988): Cellular activity of intracerebrally transplanted fetal hippocampus during behavior. Neuroscience, 22:871–883.

Clarke DJ, Dunnett SB (1986): Formation of cholinergic synapses by intrahippocampal septal grafts as revealed by choline acetyltransferase immunocytochemistry. Brain Res 369:151–162.

Clarke DJ, Gage FH, Nilsson OG, Björklund A (1986): Grafted septal neurons form synaptic connections in the dentate gyrus of behaviorally impaired aged rats. J Comp Neurol 252:483–492.

Daitz HM, Powell TPS (1954): Studies of the connexions of the fornix system. J Neurol Neurosurg Psychiatry 17:75–82.

Davis GE, Blaker SN, Engvall E, Varon S, Manthorpe M, Gage FH (1987): Human amnion membrane serves as a substratum for growing axons in vitro and in vivo. Science 233:1106–1109.

Deckel AW, Robinson RG, Coyle JT, Sanberg PR (1983): Reversal of long-term locomotor abnormalities in the kainic acid model of Huntington's disease by day 18 fetal striatal implants. Eur J Pharmacol 93:287–288.

Deckel AW, Moran TH, Coyle JT, Sanberg PR, Robinson RG (1986): Anatomical predictors of behavioral recovery following fetal striatal transplants. Brain Res 365:249–258.

Dunnett SB, Low WC, Iversen SD, Stenevi U, Björklund A (1982): Septal transplants restore maze learning in rats with fornix-fimbria lesions. Brain Res 251:335–348.

Freed WJ, Perlow MJ, Karoum F, Seiger A, Olson L, Seiger A, Wyatt RJ (1980): Restoration of dopaminergic function by grafting of fetal rat substantia nigra to the caudate nucleus: Long-term behavioral, biochemical, and histochemical studies. Ann Neurol 8:510–519.

Freund TF, Bolam JP, Björklund A, Stenevi U, Dunnett SB, Smith AD (1985): Efferent synaptic connections of grafted dopaminergic neurons reinnervating the host neostriatum: A tyrosine hydroxylase immunocytochemical study. J Neurosci 3:603–616.

Gage FH, Björklund A (1986a): Neural grafting in the aged brain. Annu Rev Physiol 48:447–459.

Gage FH, Björklund A (1986b): Enhanced graft survival in the hippocampus following selective denervation. Neuroscience 17:89–98.

Gage FH, Björklund A, Stenevi U (1983): Reinnervation of the partially deafferented hippocampus by compensatory collateral sprouting from spared cholinergic and noradrenergic afferents. Brain Res 268:27–37.

Gage FH, Björklund A, Stenevi U (1984): Cells of origin of the ventral cholinergic septohippocampal pathway undergoing compensatory collateral sprouting following fimbria-fornix transection. Neurosci Lett 4:211–216.

Gage FH, Wictorin K, Fisher W, Williams LR, Varon S, Björklund A (1986): Retrograde cell changes in medial septum and diagonal band following fimbria-fornix transection: Quantitative temporal analysis. Neuroscience 19:241–255.

Gage FH, Wolff JA, Rosenberg MB, Xu L, Yee J-K, Shults C, Friedmann T (1987): Grafting genetically modified cells to the brain: Possibilities for the future. Neuroscience, in press.

Gage FH, Blaker SN, Davis GE, Engvall E, Varon S, Manthorpe M (1988): Human amnion membrane matrix as a substratum for axonal regeneration in the central nervous system. Exp Brain Res, in press.

Gash DM, Sladek JR, Jr., Sladek CD (1980): Functional development of grafted vasopressin neurons. Science 210:1367–1369.

Gnahn H, Hefti F, Heumann R, Schwab ME, Thoenen H (1983): NGF-mediated increase of choline acetyltransferase (ChAT) in the neonatal rat forebrain: Evidence for a physiological role of NGF in the brain? Dev Brain Res 9:45–52.

Gumpel M, Lachapelle F, Gansmuller A, Baulac M, Baron van Evercooren A (1987): Transplantation of human embryonic oligodendrocytes into shiverer brain. In Azmitia EC, Björklund A (eds): "Cell and Tissue Transplantation into the Adult Brain." New York: New York Academy of Science, pp 71–86.

Hefti F (1986): Nerve growth factor (NGF) promotes survival of septal cholinergic neurons after fimbrial transection. J Neurosci 6:2155–2162.

Hefti F, Hartikka JJ, Eckenstein F, Gnahn H, Heumann R, Schwab M (1985a): Nerve growth factor increases choline acetyltransferase but not survival or fiber outgrowth of cultured fetal septal cholinergic neurons. Neuroscience 14:55–68.

Heft F, Hartikka JJ, Schlumpf M (1985b): Implantation of PC12 cells into the corpus striatum of rats with lesions of the dopaminergic nigrostriatal neurons. Brain Res 348:283–288.

Isacson O, Brundin P, Kelly PAT, Gage FH, Björklund A (1984): Functional neuronal replacement by grafted striatal neurones in the ibotenic acid-lesioned rat striatum. Nature 311:458–460.

Isacson O, Brundin P, Gage FH, Björklund A (1985): Neural grafting in a rat model of Huntington's disease. Progressive neurochemical changes following striatal ibotenic acid lesions and striatal tissue grafting. Neuroscience 16:799–817.

Isacson O, Pritzel M, Dawbarn D, Brundin P, Kelly PAT, Wiklund L, Emson PC, Gage FH, Dunnett SB, Björklund A (1987): Striatal neural transplants in the ibotenic acid-lesioned rat neostriatum: Cellular and functional aspects. In Azmitia EC, Björklund A (eds): "Cell and Tissue Transplantation into the Adult Brain." New York: New York Academy of Science, pp 537–556.

Jaeger CB (1987): Morphological and immunocytochemical characteristics of PC12 cell grafts in rat brain. In Azmitia EC, Björklund A (eds): "Cell and Tissue Transplantation Into the Adult Brain." New York: New York Academy of Science, pp 334–351.

Kelly PAT, Gage FH, Ingvar M, Lindvall O, Stenevi U, Björklund A (1985): Functional reactivation of the deafferented hippocampus by embryonic septal grafts as assessed by measurements of local glucose utilization. Exp Brain Res 58:570–579.

Kesslak JP, Nieto-Sampedro M, Globus J, Cotman C (1986): Transplants of purified astrocytes promote behavioral recovery after frontal cortex ablation. Exp Neurol 92:377–390.

Kohler C, Chan-Palay V, Wu JY (1984): Septal neurons containing glutamic acid decarboxylase immunoreactivity project to the hippocampal region in the rat brain. Anat Embryol 169:41–44.

Kordower JH, Notter MFD, Yeh HH, Gash DM (1987): An in vivo and in vitro assessment of differentiated neuroblastoma cells as a source of donor tissue for transplantation. In Azmitia EC, Björklund A (eds): "Cell and Tissue Transplantation Into the Adult Brain." New York: New York Academy of Science, pp 606–623.

Kromer LF, Björklund A, Stenevi U (1981): Regeneration of the Septo-hippocampal pathways in adult rats is promoted by utilizing embryonic hoppocampal implants as bridges. Brain Res. 210:173–200.

Kromer LF (1987): Nerve growth factor treatment after brain injury prevents neuronal death. Science 235:214–217.

Kromer LF, Cornbrooks CJ (1987): Identification of trophic factors and transplanted cellular environments that promote CNS axonal regeneration. In Azmitia EC, Björklund A (eds): "Cell and Tissue Transplantation Into the Adult Brain." New York: New York Academy of Science, pp 207–225.

Large TH, Bodary SC, Clegg DO, Weskamp G, Otte U, Reichardt LF (1986): Nerve growth factor gene expression in the developing rat brain. Science 234:352–355.

Low WC, Lewis PR, Bunch ST, Dunnett SB, Thomas SR, Iversen SD, Björklund A, Stenevi U (1982): Functional recovery following neural transplantation of embryonic septal nuclei in adult rats with septohippocampal lesions. Nature 300:260–262.

Lund RD, Simons DJ (1985): Retinal transplants: Structural and functional interrelations with the host brain. In Björklund A, Stenevi U (ed): "Neural Grafting in the Mammalian CNS." Elsevier: Amsterdam, pp 345–354.

Meldrum B (1985): Possible therapeutic applications of antagonists of excitatory amino acid neurotransmitters. Clin Sci 68:113–122.

Mesulam MM, Mufson EJ, Wainer BH, Levey AI (1983): Central cholinergic pathways in the rat: An overview based on an alternative nomenclature (Ch1–Ch6). Neuroscience 10:1185–1201.

Milner TA, Amaral DG (1984): Evidence for a ventral septal projection to the hippocampal formation of the rat. Exp Brain Res 55:579–585.

Mobley WC, Rutkowski JL, Tennekoon GI, Gemski J, Buchanan K, Johnston MV (1986): Nerve growth factor increases choline acetyltransferase activity in developing basal forebrain neurons. Mol Brain Res 1:53–62.

Morris RGM (1981): Spatial localization does not require the presence of local cues. Learn Motiv 12:239–260.

Nicoll RA (1985): The septo-hippocampal projection: A model of cholinergic pathways. Trends Neurosci 533–536.

Nilsson OG, Shapiro ML, Gage FH, Björklund A (1987): Spatial learning and memory following fimbria-fornix transection and grafting of fetal septal neurons to the hippocampus. Exp Brain Res 67:195–215.

O'Keefe J, Nadel L (1978): "The Hippocampus as a Cognitive Map." Oxford: Clarendon Press.

Olton DS, Becker JT, Handelman GE (1979): Hippocampus, space and memory. Behav Brain Sci 2:313–365.

Pallage V, Toniolo G, Will B, Hefti F (1986): Long-term effects of nerve growth factor and neural transplants on behavior of rats with medial septal lesions. Brain Res 386:197–208.

Perlow MJ, Kumakura K, Guidiotti A (1980): Prolonged survival of bovine adrenal chromaffin cells in rat cerebral ventricle. Proc Natl Acad Sci USA 77:5278–5281.

Peterson G, Williams LR, Varon S, Gage FH (1987): Loss of GABAergic neurons in medial septum after fimbria-fornix transection. Neurosci Lett 76:140–144.

Petsche H, Stumpf C, Gogolak G (1962): The significance of the rabbit's septum as a relay station between the midbrain and the hippocampus. The control of hippocampal arousal activity by septum cells. Electroencephalogr Clin Neurophysiol 14:202–211.

Rosenstein JM (1987): Neocortical transplants in the mammalian brain lack a blood-brain barrier to macromolecules. Science 235:772–774.

Schmidt RA, Björklund A, Stenevi U (1981): Intracerebral grafting of dissociated CNS tissue suspensions: A new approach for neuronal transplantation to deep brain sites. Brain Res 218:347–356.

Schwab ME, Otten U, Agid Y, Thoenen H (1979): Nerve Growth Factor (NGF) in rat CNS: Absence of specific retrograde axonal transport and tyrosine hydroxylase induction in locus coeruleus and substantia nigra. Brain Res 168:473–483.

Schwartz R, Creese J, Coyle JT, Snyder SH (1978): Dopamine receptors localized on cerebral cortical afferents to rat corpus striatum. Nature 271:766–768.

Segal M, Greenberger V, Milgram HW (1987): A functional analysis of connections between grafted septal neurons and a host hippocampus. Prog Brain Res 71:349–357.

Seiler M, Schwab ME (1984): Specific retrograde transport of nerve growth factor (NGF) from neocortex to nucleus basalis in the rat. Brain Res 300:33–39.

Shults CW, Quirion R, Chronwall B, Chase TN, O'Donohue TL (1984): A comparison of the anatomical distribution of substance P and substance P receptors in the rat central nervous system. Peptides 5:1097–1128.

Sladek JR Jr, Gash DM (1984): "Neural transplants: Development and Function." New York: Plenum Press.

Smith GM, Miller RH, Silver J (1987): Astrocyte transplantation induces callosal regeneration in postnatal acallosal mice. In Azmitia EC, Björklund A (eds): "Cell and Tissue Transplantation into the Adult Brain." New York: New York Academy of Science, pp 185–207.

Sotelo C, Alvarado-Mallart RM (1987): Cerebellar transplantations in adult mice with heredodegenerative ataxia. In Azmitia EC, Björklund A (eds): "Cell and Tissue Transplantation Into the Adult Brain." New York: New York Academy of Science, pp 242–268.

Stenevi U, Björklund A, Svendgaard N-A (1976): Transplantation of central and peripheral monoamine neurons to the adult rat brain: Techniques and conditions for survival. Brain Res 114:1–20.

Storm-Mathisen J (1979): Localization of transmitter candidates in the brain: The hippocampal formation as a model. Prog Neurobiol 8:351–388.

Trulson ME, Hosseini A, Trulson TJ (1986): Serotonin neuron transplants: Electrophysiological unit activity of intrahippocampal raphe grafts in freely moving cats. Brain Res Bull 17:461–468.

Vanderwolf CH (1969): Hippocampal electrical activity and voluntary movement in the rat. Electroencephalogr Clin Neurophysiol 26:407–418.

Vinogradova OS, Bragin AG, Kitchigina VF (1985): Spontaneous and evoked activity of neurons in intrabrain allo- and xenografts of the hippocampus and septum. In Björklund A, Stenevi U (eds): "Neural Grafting in the Mammalian CNS." Amsterdam: Elsevier, pp 409–420.

Wainer BH, Levey AI, Rye DB, Mesulam M, Mufson EJ (1985): Cholinergic and non-cholinergic septohippocampal pathways. Neurosci Lett 54:45–52.

Whishaw IQ (1985): Cholinergic receptor blockade impairs local but not taxon strategies for place navigation in a swimming pool. Behav Neurosci 99:979–1005.

Whishaw IQ, O'Connor WT, Dunnett SB (1985): Disruption of central cholinergic systems in the rat by basal forebrain lesions of atropine: Effects on feeding, sensorimotor behaviour, locomotor activity and spatial navigation. Behav Brain Res 17:103–115.

Williams LR, Varon S, Peterson GM, Wictorin K, Fischer W, Björklund A, Gage FH (1986): Continuous infusion of nerve growth factor prevents basal forebrain neuronal death after fimbria-fornix transection. Proc Natl Acad Sci USA 83:9231–9235.

14

Transplantation in Parkinson's Disease: Experimental and Clinical Trials

A.-C. GRANHOLM, PhD, **I. STRÖMBERG**, PhD, **G.A. GERHARDT**, PhD, **Å. SEIGER**, MD, PhD, **L. OLSON**, MD, PhD, AND **B.J. HOFFER**, MD, PhD

Departments of Pharmacology (A.-C.G., G.A.G., B.J.H.) and Psychiatry (G.A.G.), University of Colorado Health Sciences Center, Denver, Colorado 80262; Department of Histology and Neurobiology, Karolinska Institute, Stockholm, Sweden (I.S., L.O.); and Department of Neurological Surgery, Research Laboratories, University of Miami School of Medicine, Miami, Florida 33101 (Å.S.)

While there has been a recent surge of interest in transplantation of neurohumoral elements to ameliorate such diverse conditions as Huntington's disease, spinal cord injury, and Alzheimer's disease, it is only with Parkinson's disease that such speculations have approached reality. The etiology of Parkinson's disease is not known, and the disease results in structural damage to the neurons in the mesencephalic nucleus substantia nigra, which causes a degeneration of the nigrostriatal dopaminergic pathway leading to severe disturbances of motor function (Hornykiewicz, 1966; Rinne et al., 1980). Effective control of parkinsonian symptoms can be achieved in a large number of patients by the use of dopaminergic agents (Yahr, 1984). However, after a longer period, efficacy diminishes with reemergence of parkinsonian symptoms, as well as a number of untoward responses, such as dyskinesia (Yahr, 1984).

During postnatal maturation of the human nervous system, many neurons in the peripheral nervous system will retain their ability to regenerate and to reform specific synaptic contacts in the target area. This regenerative potential is, however, lacking within the central nervous system (CNS), despite the reported ability of uninjured CNS axons to undergo some sprouting and synaptogenesis (Bernstein and Bernstein, 1971, 1973; Prendergast and Stelzner, 1976). Thus, lesions or degenerative diseases of the adult mammalian CNS result in

permanent loss of function in the injured region as well as the target areas to which this region projects.

Despite the fact that regeneration of severed neuronal connections in the mammalian CNS has been the focus of intensive anatomical and physiological investigation during the past 3 decades, relatively little success has been achieved. Although it is extremely difficult to promote CNS nerve regeneration (Clemente and Windle, 1954; Puchala and Windle, 1977), recent experiments with transplantation techniques have begun to provide insight into cellular reactions that may influence cell survival, axonal growth, and synaptogenesis in the mammalian CNS. Transplantation techniques have evolved in several laboratories throughout the world (Olson and Seiger, 1972; Murphy and Sturm, 1975; Björklund and Stenevi, 1979; Das et al., 1979; Lund and Harvey, 1981; Olson et al., 1983, 1984; Stenevi et al., 1985). The adult CNS can "host" either with peripheral tissues, especially of neural crest origin, or with embryonic CNS tissues provided by donor fetuses. In the case of fetal implants, the adult CNS host will be exposed to developing presynaptic elements that are capable of extensive growth and synaptogenesis. Numerous investigators have suggested that transplantation may prove an important approach in treating neurodegenerative disorders. Recently, much excitement has been generated by reports of improvement of Parkinson's disease symptoms after intracranial placement of autografts of adrenal medulla

Neural Regeneration and Transplantation, pages 227–237
© 1989 Alan R. Liss, Inc.

(Madrazo et al., 1986; Olson et al., 1986; Lindvall et al., 1987; Drucker-Colin et al., 1988; Jiao et al., 1988). The results as well as techniques have varied extensively between the groups, but the data presented so far should lead to further studies in a number of hospitals all over the world. The present chapter attempts to provide an introduction to clinical and preclinical studies of transplantation in parkinsonism along with a general discussion of the medical and ethical issues raised in this context.

ANIMAL MODELS OF PARKINSONISM

Parkinson's disease does not occur spontaneously in animals. An animal model for parkinsonism has been developed in which animals are subjected to neurotoxin-induced nigrostriatal lesions using injections of either 6-hydroxydopamine (6-OHDA) (Ungerstedt, 1968, 1971a) or, more recently, N-methyl-4-phenyl-1,2,3,6-tetrahydropyridine (MPTP) (Davis et al., 1979; Langston et al., 1983; Hallman et al., 1985; Sundström et al., 1987). A bilateral stereotaxic injection of 6-OHDA into the ascending nigrostriatal tract causes a specific degeneration of dopamine-containing neurons, resulting in severe akinesia, adipsia, and aphagia (Ungerstedt, 1971b). This supports the theory that the nigrostriatal dopamine pathway (Fig. 14–1) is responsible for the control of motor behavior and probably also for sensorimotor integration (Ungerstedt 1971b; Krauthamer, 1975). The nigrostriatal pathway is essentially uncrossed and monosynaptic (Andén et al., 1964, 1966a, b; Hökfelt and Ungerstedt, 1969, 1973; Ungerstedt, 1971a). A unilateral depletion of dopamine in the rat results in asymmetry of posture and movements (Andén et al., 1966a, 1967; Herrera-Marschitz et al., 1985). The direction of asymmetry reflects the dominance of the depleted or the intact dopamine pathway. Stimulation of unilaterally denervated rats with amphetamine results in strong ipsilateral rotational behavior (Ungerstedt and Arbuthnott, 1970; Ungerstedt, 1971d), while the dopamine receptor agonist apomorphine causes contralateral rotation (Andén et al., 1967; Ernst, 1967), as a result of an activation of supersensitive striatal dopamine receptors on the denervated side (Ungerstedt, 1971c). This animal model of parkinsonism has been used extensively during the past 2 decades, with the unlesioned side serving as an internal control. In addition, some years ago it was accidentally discovered in young addicts that the drug MPTP produces severe motor deficits that greatly resemble those of Parkinson's disease (Davis et al., 1979; Burns et al., 1983; Langston et al., 1983; Jenner et al., 1984). Extensive studies in both rodents and primates have shown that the drug selectively damages the nigrostriatal dopamine pathway (Langston et al., 1983; Hallman et al., 1985; Redmond et al., 1986), but that this damage is, in some species, transient (Backay et al., 1985; Hallman et al., 1985; Peroutka et al., 1985).

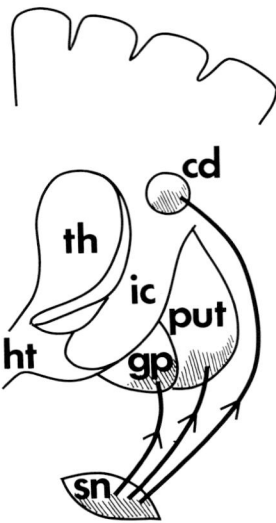

Figure 14–1. Schematic diagram showing the nigrostriatal pathway. cd, caudate nucleus; put, putamen; gp, globus pallidus; th, thalamus; sn, substantia nigra; ht, hypothalamus; ic, internal capsule.

Transplantation of Chromaffin Cells

Adrenal medullary chromaffin cells are of neural crest origin and have been shown to form varicose processes (Olson, 1970) and transform into neuron-like cells (Strömberg et al., 1988b) when separated from the adrenal cortex and placed into the anterior chamber of the eye. Such cells have been grafted into the striatum of 6-OHDA-lesioned rats in an attempt to restore motor function (Freed et al.,

1981, 1983b; Herrera-Marschitz et al., 1984; Strömberg et al., 1984, 1985a; Olson, 1985). Soon after transplantation, the surviving chromaffin cells produced large amounts of catecholamines that diffused through the denervated host striatum and stimulated supersensitive host dopamine receptors, resulting in a pronounced rotational response (Herrera-Marschitz et al., 1984). Initially, the catecholamines released from the transplanted chromaffin cells were norepinephrine and small amounts of dopamine, with very small amounts of epinephrine. Interestingly, the dopamine-to-norepinephrine ratio increased significantly with time (Freed et al., 1983a). This alteration of catecholamine content is possibly due to separation of the medulla from cortical tissue. The transplanted chromaffin cells rarely formed catecholamine-containing fibers (Strömberg et al., 1984). The partial reversal of apomorphine-induced rotations caused by such grafts for several months after grafting was therefore probably due to a diffuse release of catecholamines from the cell bodies.

Striatum is a brain area with particularly low endogenous levels of nerve growth factor (NGF) (Whittemore et al., 1985). A more significant and longer lasting behavioral effect of intrastriatal chromaffin grafts was seen after administration of NGF to the host animal (Strömberg et al., 1985a). The presence of NGF increased the number of cells surviving the grafting procedure as well as the amount of nerve processes formed by the grafted chromaffin cells. When a dialysis fiber in the host striatum was used to supply NGF continuously during the first month after transplantation, catecholamine-containing fibers were seen leaving the graft and extending toward the source of NGF (Strömberg et al., 1985a). The conclusion drawn from these experiments in the rat model of Parkinson's disease is that adult homologous transplants of adrenal medullary tissues can, at least partially, substitute for the missing nigral dopaminergic innervation of striatum if NGF is given after transplantation. However, Bohn and coworkers (1987) have recently suggested that transplantation of adult adrenal medullary tissue into MPTP-lesioned mice can enhance recovery of endogenous dopamine neurons. Moreover, Bankiewicz and coworkers (1988) found a similar increase in endogenous sprouting in striatum after sham transplantation of cerebellar tissue to MPTP-lesioned monkeys, suggesting a nonspecific sprouting effect of brain tissue transplants on the denervated nigrostriatal pathway. Such endogenous sprouting may account for some of the increased motor function reported after adrenal medullary transplantation to MPTP-treated animals.

Transplants of Fetal Neuroblasts

It was first shown in 1979 (Björklund and Stenevi, 1979; Perlow et al., 1979) that fetal dopaminergic neuroblasts from the substantia nigra grafted into contact with the denervated striatum in rats could reverse the motor asymmetries induced by unilateral nigrostriatal lesions. These studies have since been successfully repeated with transplants of fetal mesencephalic tissue from a number of species, including man (Björklund et al., 1980a, b; Freed et al., 1980, 1983b; Schmidt et al., 1982, 1983; Dunnett et al., 1983a, b; Brundin et al., 1985, 1986; Olson et al., 1986; Strömberg et al., 1986). Recently, similar effects have been reported after transplantation of dopamine-producing neurons to the striatum of monkeys with MPTP-induced parkinsonism (Backay et al., 1985; Redmond et al., 1986).

Intracranial implantation of fetal neural tissue may provide the adult host brain with a number of beneficial factors, including reconstruction of the circuitry, neurotransmitters, and trophic factors. However, it is of great importance that a thorough evaluation of temporal and regional developmental properties be performed. Thus transplants of optimal origin and donor age can be adequately prepared and implanted into the lesioned brain, leading to substantial improvement of the motor deficits described above. Several critical parameters concerning the optimal dissecting techniques as well as donor stages have been developed using the introcular transplantation technique (Olson et al., 1983, 1984). The substantia nigra region is prepared from the ventromedial part of the fetal mesencephalon (Seiger and Olson, 1977). Good survival of rat dopamine neuroblasts is obtained with donors of gestational days 14 to 17. Dissected material can either be grafted as small pieces (1–2 mm^3) or in the form of a cell suspension (Björklund et al.,

1980b, 1983a, b). Solid pieces can be transplanted to striatum facing the lateral ventricle, to artificially made surfaces in the bottom of previously prepared cavities (Björklund and Stenevi, 1979; Mahalik et al., 1985; Stenevi et al., 1985; Strömberg et al., 1985b), or to intraparenchymal sites (Schmidt et al., 1982). In all cases, grafted dopaminergic neurons will eventually provide the adjacent host striatum with an extensive innervation of dopaminergic terminals.

The effects of nigral grafting have now been thoroughly characterized. Fetal substantia nigra neurons will survive grafting to the host striatum and send processes into the surrounding brain (Björklund and Stenevi, 1979; Perlow et al., 1979; Björklund et al., 1980a, b, 1983a, b; Freed et al., 1980; Strömberg et al., 1985b). Graft-to-host as well as host-to-graft synapses are formed (Freund et al., 1985a, b; Mahalik et al., 1985), and the levels as well as turnover of dopamine in the lesioned striatum approach normal (Freed et al., 1980; Schmidt et al., 1982, 1983). The postural asymmetry recovers significantly (Björklund and Stenevi, 1979; Perlow et al., 1979; Björklund et al., 1980; Freed et al., 1980; Dunnett et al., 1983b).

Recently, the endogenous release of dopamine from grafted dopamine-containing neurons has been demonstrated with electrochemical techniques in rats (Hoffer et al,. 1985; Rose et al., 1985). Potassium-induced releases were recorded using rigid assemblies of K^+-filled pipettes attached to nafion-coated graphite epoxy capillary electrochemical working electrodes (Gerhardt et al., 1984). The assembly was stereotaxically lowered into the rat brain to measure dopamine release in the striatum of transplant-reinnervated animals. The contralateral side was used as a control for normal dopamine release in an intact striatum. The release values were then correlated with immunohistochemistry for tyrosine hydroxylase and placements adjacent to transplant sites. Within 1 mm of the transplants, the releases were almost of normal magnitude, while they were markedly reduced more distal from the transplants.

Moreover, electrophysiological studies have shown that dopaminergic neurons in intrastriatal grafts are tonically active and appear to induce normal excitability in host caudate cells (Wuerthele et al., 1981). Furthermore, dopamine receptor supersensitivity after 6-OHDA denervation of the striatum is normalized by nigral transplants, as evidenced by receptor autoradiography and computer-assisted image analysis (Freed et al., 1983b). Thus it has been convincingly demonstrated by a number of techniques that syngeneic grafts of fetal substantia nigra can provide the dopamine-denervated striatum with a functionally appropriate reinnervation.

Transplants of Human Fetal Neuroblasts Into Rodents

In terms of ongoing and future clinical transplantation trials, one important issue has recently been raised: Can fetal human neuroblasts survive transplantation and provide an appropriate substitute for the lesioned nigrostriatal pathway of the host? The donor age seems to be critical for the success of transplantation of dopamine-containing neurons, both in rodents (see Olson et al., 1983, 1984) and in man (Brundin et al., 1986), although when tissue fragments of human fetal substantia nigra rather than cell suspensions are used, a relatively wide spectrum of donor stages (up to 12 weeks) survives grafting to rodent recipients (Strömberg et al., 1986). Based on the prenatal development of human monoamine neurons (Olson et al., 1973), extensive studies must be undertaken in an animal model to determine the optimal donor age, size of the tissue to be grafted, and viability of these cells in an adult brain before human fetal neuroblasts can be used for clinical purposes. As an initial approach to answer these questions, xenogeneic transplantation of human fetal brain tissues has been performed in immunocompromised rodents (Brundin et al., 1986; Strömberg et al., 1986; Bickford et al., 1987; Olson et al., 1987). These initial studies have shown that human fetal brain tissue will survive and continue to develop when transplanted to the anterior chamber of the eye (Bickford et al., 1987; Olson et al., 1987) or to the dopamine-denervated striatum (Brundin et al., 1986; Strömberg et al., 1986). The human brain tissue in our experiments was obtained following termination of first-trimester pregnancies. Healthy women with an apparently normal pregnancy in the 6th to 12th week of gestation,

TABLE 14–1. Rotational Behavior and Density of Dopamine Reinnervation of Striatum in Rats That Received Human Fetal Substantia Nigra (SN) Grafts (Apomorphine (0.05 mg/kg) was used to induce rotational behavior. Tyrosine hydroxylase immunohistochemistry was used to estimate dopamine nerve terminal density on a 0–6 scale, where 6 represents normal density)*

Rat no.	Gest. age of human SN graft (weeks)	Average pregraft rotations (turns in 1 hr)	Time of last rotation (days post-grafting)	Decrease of rota-tions (% of pre-grafting)	Time of sacrifice (days post-grafting)	Density of tyrosine hydroxylase innervation (semiquant. estimates)
1	9–10	670	41	59	59	+ +
2	12	592	62	60	80	(+)
3	9	867	81	26	88	+ + +
4	12	833	109	19	116	+ + + +
5	9–12	1,097	131	15	140	+ + +
6	12	649	152	51	165	+ + + +

*Reproduced from Strömberg et al., 1986, by permission of the publisher.

admitted to the hospital for elective abortion, were informed both orally and in writing about the aim of the study and the procedure to be used and gave their consent. Anonymity was strictly maintained. The abortion was performed using paracervical blockade following premedication. After routine dilation of the cervical canal, the conceptions were removed by vacuum aspiration. The fetal tissue was collected and kept in isotonic saline until further processing. The study was approved by the Regional Ethical Committee of the Karolinska Hospital. All experiments conformed to guidelines of the Swedish Medical Research Council and the U.S. Public Health Service. Cyclosporin-treated albino rats (Sprague-Dawley), initially used as hosts, were 6-OHDA-lesioned unilaterally and received three to six pieces of human fetal substantia nigra placed at the bottom of a cavity on top of the striatum (Strömberg et al., 1986). Two to four months after transplantation, all six animals had viable grafts (see Table 14–1) that had grown to fill much of the cavities. Moderate-to-large numbers of tyrosine hydroxylase-positive cell bodies were found, with numerous thick, tyrosine hydroxylase-positive processes (Fig. 14–2) extending into the host brain. The apomorphine-induced rotations were decreased in the grafted animals with moderate effects after 2 months and more pronounced effects after 3–5

months (Table 14–1). Recently, fetal human nigral cells have also been grafted to the striatum of athymic nude rats (Strömberg et al., 1988a). The nude rats (rNu, Harlan Laboratories) have been shown to lack T-cell function (Festing et al., 1978; Vos et al., 1980) and can be used for xenogeneic grafting experiments without cyclosporin treatment, eliminating any systemic effects of immunosuppressive agents. We have recently demonstrated potassium-induced monoamine release from these human xenografts. The transplants of human mesencephalic tissue contain numerous positive cell bodies and neurites, extending into the rodent host striatum. No signs of rejection have been found in any of these transplants to athymic rats. The fetal human brain tissue appears to develop according to a human maturation schedule rather than to that of the rodent host. These initial studies suggest that it is possible to study the development of human CNS using an animal model. In addition, these data demonstrate that human fetal substantia nigra dopamine cells can reinnervate a denervated striatum and reduce the motor deficits caused by nigrostriatal damage.

CLINICAL TRIALS OF ADRENAL MEDULLARY GRAFTS

When the adrenal medullary transplants in animal models (Freed et al., 1981) proved ca-

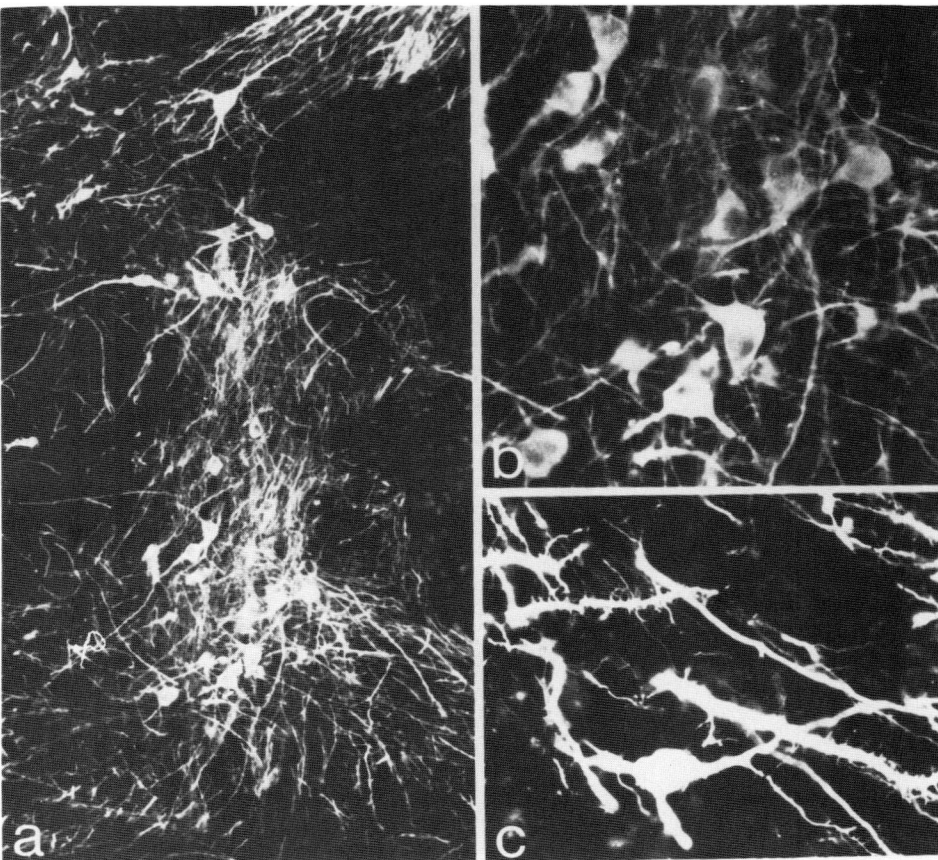

Figure 14–2. Tyrosine hydroxylase-like immunoreactivity in a human substantia nigra transplant after 4 months in a cortical cavity of a rat host. **a:** Tyrosine hydroxylase-positive cell bodies and processes in the graft. × 120. **b:** Higher magnification of cells in the lower portion of the graft shown in a. Cells have a mature appearance with multiple dendritic processes. × 300. **c:** Detail of dendritic and axonal processes in graft neuropil. Several processes have a spiny appearance suggestive of dendrites, while others are smooth, suggestive of axons. × 300. (Reproduced from Strömberg et al., 1986, by permission of the publisher.)

pable of partially reversing symptoms of experimental parkinsonism, the first clinical trials of chromaffin autografts were initiated on four severely affected Swedish Parkinson patients (Backlund et al., 1985; Olson et al., 1986; Lindvall et al., 1987). In the first two patients, small pieces of the patients' own adrenal medullae were transplanted using a stereotaxic cannula to the interior of the caudate nucleus (Fig. 14–3) (Backlund et al., 1985). No significant deleterious effects of the operation were observed in either of these two patients. However, adre-

nal medullary grafts placed in the caudate nucleus seemed to affect the severe motor symptoms to a minor degree and only for a short period of time. A similar intraparenchymal transplantation was used in a second pair of patients, but this time the grafts were placed in the putamen, since recent studies had suggested that the putamen is more involved in motor control than the caudate nucleus (DeLong and Georgopoulos, 1981; Nyberg et al., 1983). Two implantations of 15–20 1–2-mm^3 sized adrenal medullary tissue pieces were

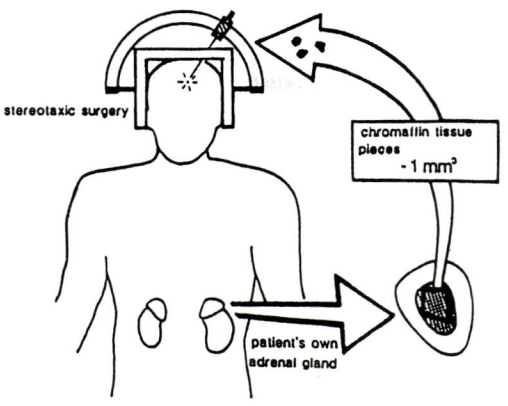

Figure 14–3. Schematic illustration of the chromaffin autografting procedure used in parkinsonian patients in Sweden. (Reproduced from Olson et al., 1986, by permission of the publisher.)

made close to each other centrally in the right putamen. The stereotaxic technique has been previously described (Leksell and Jernberg, 1980). The first patient in this study exhibited a transient improvement of motor performance in the limbs contralateral to the implantation site (Lindvall et al., 1987). In addition, the patient exhibited longer episodes of normal function for about 2 months. The second patient reported a minor improvement of balance and gait, again lasting about 2 months. Electrophysiological studies of motor readiness and auditory-evoked potentials were consistent with increased catecholaminergic activity in the basal ganglia after transplantation in both patients. Immediately after grafting, one of the patients showed signs of sympathetic hyperactivity, perhaps due to a release of catecholamines into the blood stream. Taken together, these initial trials of adrenal medullary transplantations have shown transient positive effects on the motor deficits associated with idiopathic Parkinson's disease.

Groups in Mexico and China have attempted similar clinical approaches with much greater reported success. Madrazo and coworkers in Mexico City (Madrazo et al., 1986; Drucker-Colin et al., 1988) claim a significant amelioration of most clinical signs of Parkinson's disease after open microsurgical implantation of adrenal medullary autografts. These studies included 20 patients, ranging from 35 to 59 years in age, who had severe rigidity, tremor, and akinesia. A 3-mm^3 cavity was made unilaterally in the head of the caudate nucleus after exposure through the third ventricle. The cavity was filled with four to six fragments of adrenal medullary tissue. The transplants were supported by two or more stainless steel staples and were in contact with the caudate nucleus and the cerebrospinal fluid. The onset of improvement of parkinsonian symptoms ranged from almost immediately (2–4 days) to 15–30 days postoperatively. Almost all clinical manifestations, such as independent walking, self-feeding, articulation, and writing, were reported to be improved up to 50%; some patients were even reported to have returned to work shortly after surgery. It was concluded by the Mexican group that transplantation of adrenal medullary tissue to the caudate nucleus ameliorates the symptoms of Parkinson's disease. Three of the 20 reported cases have since died. Jiao and coworkers (1988) have reported similar amelioration of motor deficits in parkinsonian patients after adrenal medullary autografts. The patients treated by Jiao were 46 to 57 years old. Four cases have recently been documented by this group. The grafts were placed in metal holders and inserted stereotaxically into the head of the right caudate nucleus in each case. This approach was similar to the procedure reported by Backlund and coworkers (1985). The patients were given amantidine and herbal "tonics" postoperatively. Improvement of facial mobility and the ability to walk was reported in all four cases 3 months postoperatively, with a slow increase in recovery up to 6 months after surgery. Dopamine levels in the cerebrospinal fluid showed a two- to threefold increase after grafting. Allen and coworkers (1988) have reported slight improvement of motor function 6–12 weeks after surgery in six patients with Parkinson's disease; they received implants of adrenal medullary tissue according to the procedure described by Madrazo and coworkers (1986). During 1987, several other neurosurgical teams in the United States initiated similar transplant procedures for Parkinson's disease.

The work that has been presented so far in this field leaves some key questions unanswered: What was the range of symptoms in the parkinsonian patients before surgery? Were the patients always evaluated at the same time of the day before and after surgery, and during nonmedication intervals? How can the patients express bilateral improvement of the motor function when only a unilateral implant was performed? Why were the transplants placed in the caudate when several studies have shown that motor regulation is controlled primarily from the putamen? How could the patients in Mexico recover so completely after transplantation? Recent data indicating an endogenous fiber sprouting effect after transplantation may be significant in this context (Bohn et al., 1987; Bankiewicz et al., 1988). Perhaps an injury to the brain produced by the grafting or some trophic factors in the transplant itself stimulate sprouting of the remaining nigrostriatal fibers. Further studies should be undertaken to clarify the exact mechanisms whereby adrenal medullary transplants alter symptoms in Parkinson's disease.

CONCLUSIONS

In conclusion, fetal nigral neurons or NGF-treated adrenal chromaffin cells can successfully reinnervate and ameliorate parkinson-like symptoms in animal models. In terms of ongoing and future clinical trials, there are some practical questions to be resolved:

1. What are the selection criteria for patients to be implanted?

2. Do adrenal medullary autografts survive and produce dopamine or other catecholamines in patients?

3. Which surgical procedure is most suitable for the implants and how should this procedure be standardized?

4. How can graft function be measured non-invasively other than behaviorally?

5. Is it ethically reasonable and medically beneficial to implant human fetal brain tissue into the brains of parkinsonian patients?
As answers to these questions are obtained, the evolution of brain cell transplantation from promise to reality may provide an exciting new neurology for the next decade.

ACKNOWLEDGMENTS

This work was supported by grants from the Swedish Medical Research Council (04X-3874, 14X-03185, 14X-06555, 25P-6326) and US Government grant NS 09199.

REFERENCES

Allen GS, Burns RS, Tulipan NB (1988): Human adrenal autografts as a potential therapy for Parkinson's disease. In: "Progress in Brain Research," vol 74. Amsterdam: Elsevier, in press.

Andén N-E, Carlsson A, Dahlström A, Fuxe K, Hillarp N-A, Larsson K (1964): Demonstration and mapping of nigro-striatal dopamine neurons. Life Sci 3:523–530.

Andén N-E, Dahlström A, Fuxe K, Larsson K (1966a): Functional role of the nigro-neostriatal dopamine neurons. Acta Pharmacol Toxicol 24:264–274.

Andén N-E, Dahlström A, Fuxe K, Larsson K, Olson L, Ungerstedt U (1966b): Ascending monoamine neurons to the telencephalon and diencephalon. Acta Physiol Scand 67:313–326.

Andén N-E, Rubenson A, Fuxe K, Hökfelt T (1967): Evidence for dopamine receptor stimulation by apomorphine. J Pharm Pharmacol 19:627–629.

Backay RAE, Fiandaca MS, Barrow DL, Schiff A, Collins DC (1985): Preliminary report on the use of fetal tissue transplantation to correct MPTP-induced Parkinson-like syndrome in primates. Appl Neurophysiol 48:358–361.

Backlund E-O, Granberg PO, Hamberger B, Knutsson E, Mårtenson A, Sedvall G, Seiger Å, Olson L (1985): Transplantation of adrenal medullary tissue to striatum in Parkinsonism. First clinical trials. J Neurosurg 62:169–173.

Bankiewicz KS, Plunkett RJ, Oldfield EH, Jacobowitz DM, Porrino LJ, Vaidya U, DiPorzio U, Schuette WH, Markowitz A, London WT, Kopin IJ (1988): Transient and longterm functional improvement by adrenal and fetal mesencephalic implants into caudate nuclei of MPTP parkinsonian monkeys. In: "Progress in Brain Research," vol 74. Amsterdam: Elsevier, in press.

Bernstein JJ, Bernstein ME (1971): Axonal regeneration and formation of synapses proximal to the site of lesion following hemisection of the rat spinal cord. Exp Neurol 30:336–351.

Bernstein ME, Bernstein JJ (1973): Regeneration of axons and synaptic complex formation rostral to the site of hemisection in the spinal cord of the monkey. Int J Neurosci 5:15–26.

Bickford-Wimer P, Granholm A-C, Bygdeman M, Seiger Å, Olson L, Hoffer BJ, Strömberg I (1987): Human fetal neuroblasts transplanted to the anterior eye chamber of athymic rats: Electrophysiological and structural studies. Proc Natl Acad Sci USA 84:5957–5961.

Björklund A, Stenevi U (1979): Reconstruction of the nigrostriatal dopamine pathway by intracerebral nigral transplants. Brain Res 177:555–560.

Björklund A, Dunnett SB, Stenevi U, Lewis ME, Iversen SD (1980a): Reinnervation of the denervated striatum by substantia nigra transplants: Functional consequences as revealed by pharmacological and sensori-motor testing. Brain Res 199:307–333.

Björklund A, Schmidt RH, Stenevi U (1980b): Functional reinnervation of the neostriatum in the adult rat by use of intraparenchymal grafting of dissociated cell suspensions from the substantia nigra. Cell Tissue Res 212:39–45.

Björklund A, Stenevi U, Schmidt RH, Dunnett SB, Gage FH (1983a): Intracerebral grafting of neuronal cell suspensions. I. Introduction and general methods of preparation. Acta Physiol Scand [Suppl] 522:1–7.

Björklund A, Stenevi U, Schmidt RH, Dunnett SB, Gage FH (1983b): Intracerebral grafting of neuronal cell suspensions. II. Survival and growth of nigral cell suspensions implanted in different brain sites. Acta Physiol Scand [Suppl] 522:9–18.

Bohn MC, Cupit L, Marciano F, Gash DM (1987): Adrenal medulla grafts enhance recovery of striatal dopaminergic fibers. Science 237:913–916.

Brundin P, Nilsson OG, Gage FH, Björklund A (1985): Cyclosporin A increases survival of cross-species intrastriatal grafts of embryonic dopamine-containing neurons. Exp Brain Res 60:204–208.

Brundin P, Nilsson OG, Strecker RE, Lindvall O, Åstedt B, Björklund A (1986): Behavioural effects of human fetal dopamine neurons grafted in a rat model of Parkinson's disease. Exp Brain Res 65:235–240.

Burns RS, Chiueh CC, Markey SP, Ebert MH, Jacobowitz DM, Kopin IJ (1983): A primate model of parkinsonism: selective destruction of dopaminergic neurons in the pars compacta of the substantia nigra by N-methyl-4-phenyl-1,2,3,6-tetrahydropyridine. Proc Natl Acad Sci USA 80:4546–4550.

Clemente CD, Windle WF (1954): Regeneration of severed nerve fibers in the spinal cord of the adult cat. J Comp Neurol 101:691–731.

Das GD, Hallas BH, Das KG (1979): Transplantation of neural tissues in the brains of laboratory mammals: Technical details and comments. Experientia 35:143–153.

Davis GC, Williams AC, Markey SP, Ebert MH, Caine ED, Reichert CM, Kopin IJ (1979): Chronic parkinsonism secondary to intravenous injection of meperidine analogues. Psychiatry Res 1:249–254.

DeLong MR, Georgopoulos AP (1981): Motor functions of the basal ganglia. In: Brooks V (ed): "Handbook of Physiology: The Nervous System, vol II: Motor Control." Bethesda: American Physiological Society, pp 1017–1061.

Drucker-Colin R, Madrazo I, Shkurovich M, Ostrosky-Solis F and Torres C (1988): Open microsurgical autograft of adrenal medulla to caudate nucleus of patients with Parkinson's disease. In: "Progress in Brain Research," vol 74. Amsterdam: Elsevier, in press.

Dunnett SB, Björklund A, Schmidt RH, Stenevi U, Iversen SD (1983a): Intracerebral grafting of neuronal cell suspensions. IV. Behavioral recovery in rats with unilateral implants of nigral cell suspensions in different forebrain sites. Acta Physiol Scand [Suppl] 522:29–37.

Dunnett SB, Björklund A, Stenevi U (1983b): Transplant induced recovery from brain lesions: A review of the nigrostriatal model. In Wallace RB, Das GO (eds): "Neural Tissue Transplantation Research." New York: Springer Verlag, pp 191–216.

Ernst AM (1967): Mode of action of apomorphine and dexamphetamine on gnawing compulsions in rats. Psychopharmacologica 10:316–323.

Festing MW, May D, Connors TA, Lovell D, Sparrow S (1978): An athymic nude mutation in the rat. Nature 274:365–366.

Freed W, Perlow M, Karoum F, Seiger Å, Olson L, Hoffer B, Wyatt R (1980): Restoration of dopaminergic function by grafting of fetal rat substantia nigra to the caudate nucleus: Long-term behavioral, biochemical and histochemical studies. Ann Neurol 8:510–519.

Freed W, Morihisa J, Spoor E, Hoffer B, Olson L, Seiger Å, Wyatt R (1981): Transplanted adrenal chromaffin cells in rat brain reduce lesion-induced rotational behavior. Nature 292:351–352.

Freed W, Karoum F, Spoor HE, Morihisa JM, Olson L, Wyatt RJ (1983a): Catecholamine content of intracerebral adrenal medulla grafts. Brain Res 269:184–189.

Freed W, Ko G, Niehoff D, Kuhar M, Hoffer BJ, Olson L, Spoor E, Morihisa J, Wyatt R (1983b): Normalization of spiroperidol binding in the denervated rat striatum by homologous substantia nigra transplants. Science 222:937–939.

Freund TF, Bolam JP, Björklund A, Stenevi U, Dunnett SB, Powell JF, Smith AD (1985a): Efferent synaptic connections of grafted dopaminergic neurons reinnervating the host neostriatum: A tyrosine hydroxylase immunocytochemical study. J Neurosci 5:603–616.

Freund TF, Bolam JP, Björklund A, Dunnett SB, Smith AD (1985b): Synaptic connections of grafted dopaminergic neurons that reinnervate the neostriatum: A tyrosine hydroxylase immunohistochemical study. In Björklund A, Stenevi U (eds): "Neural Grafting in the Mammalian CNS." Amsterdam: Elsevier, pp 529–537.

Gerhardt GA, Oke AF, Nagy G, Moghaddam B, Adams RN (1984): Nafion-coated electrodes with high selectivity for CNS electrochemistry. Brain Res 290:390–395.

Hallman H, Lange J, Olson L, Strömberg I, Jonsson G (1985): Neurochemical and histochemical characterization of neurotoxic effects of N-methyl-4-phenyl-1,2,3,6-tetrahydropyridine (MPTP) on brain catecholamine neurons in the mouse. J Neurochem 44:117–127.

Herrera-Marschitz M, Strömberg I, Olson L, Ungerstedt U (1984): Adrenal medullary implants in the dopamine-denervated rat striatum. II. Rotational behavior during the first seven hours as a function of graft amount and location and its modulation by neuroleptics. Brain Res 297:53–61.

Herrera-Marschitz M, Forster C, Ungerstedt U (1985): Rotational behaviour elicited by intracerebral injections of apomorphine and pergolide in 6-hydroxy-dopamine-lesioned rats. II. The striatum of the rat is heterogeneously organized for rotational behaviour. Acta Physiol Scand 125:529–535.

Hoffer BJ, Rose G, Gerhardt G, Strömberg I, Olson L (1985): Demonstration of monoamine release from transplant-reinnervated caudate nucleus by in vivo electrochemical detection. In Björklund A, Stenevi U (eds): "Neural Grafting in the Mammalian CNS." Amsterdam: Elsevier, pp 437–447.

Hökfelt T, Ungerstedt U (1969): Electron and fluorescence microscopical studies on the nucleus caudatus putamen of the rat after unilateral lesions of ascending nigro-neostriatal dopamine neurons. Acta Physiol Scand 76:415–426.

Hökfelt T, Ungerstedt U (1973): Specificity of 6-hydroxydopamine induced degeneration of central monoamine neurons: An electron and fluorescence microscopic study with special reference to intracerebral injection on the nigrostriatal dopamine system. Brain Res 60:269–297.

Hornykiewicz O (1966): Dopamine (3-hydroxytyramine) and brain function. Pharmacol Rev 18:925–964.

Jenner P, Rupniak NMJ, Rose S, Kelly E, Kilpatrick G, Lees A, Marsden CD (1984): 1-Methyl-4-phenyl-1,2,3,6-tetrahydropyridine-induced parkinsonism in the common marmoset. Neurosci Lett 50:85–90.

Jiao SS, Zhang WC, Ding MC, Sun JB (1988): The clinical study of adrenal medullary tissue transplantation to striatum in parkinsonism. In: "Progress in Brain Research," vol 74. Amsterdam: Elsevier, in press.

Krauthamer GM (1975): Catecholamines in behavior and sensorimotor integration: the neostriatal system. In Friedhoffer AJ (ed): "Catecholamines and behaviour 1. Basic Neurobiology" New York: Plenum Press, pp 59–87.

Langston JW, Ballard P, Tetrud JW, Irwine I (1983): Chronic parkinsonism in humans due to a product of meperidine-analog synthesis. Science 219:979–980.

Leksell L, Jernberg B (1980): Stereotaxis and tomography. A technical note. Acta Neurochir (Wien) 52:1–7.

Lindvall O, Backlund E-O, Farde L, Sedvall G, Freedman R, Hoffer B, Nobin A, Seiger Å, Olson L (1987): Transplantation in Parkinson's disease: Two cases of adrenal medullary grafts to putamen. Ann Neurol 22:457–468.

Lund RD, Harvey AR (1981): Transplantation of tectal tissue in rats. I. Organization of transplants and pattern of distribution of host afferents within them. J Comp Neurol 201:191–209.

Madrazo I, Drucker-Colin R, Diaz V, Martinez-Mata J, Torres C, Becerril JJ (1986): Open microsurgical autograft of adrenal medulla to the right caudate nucleus in two patients with intractable Parkinson's disease. New Engl J Med 316:831–834.

Mahalik T, Finger T, Strömberg I, Olson L (1985): Substantia nigra transplants into denervated striatum of the rat: Ultrastructure of graft and host interconnections. J Comp Neurol 240:60–70.

Murphy JE, Sturm E (1975): Conditions determining the transplantability of tissues in the brain. J Exp Med 38:183–197.

Nyberg P, Nordberg A, Wester P, Winblad B (1983): Dopaminergic deficiency is more pronounced in putamen than in nucleus caudatus in Parkinson's disease. Neurochem Pathol 1:193–202.

Olson L (1970): Fluorescence histochemical evidence for axonal growth and secretion from transplanted adrenal medullary tissue. Histochemie 22:1–7.

Olson L (1985): On the use of transplants to counteract the symptoms of Parkinson's disease: Background, experimental models and possible clinical applications. In Cotman CW (ed): "Synaptic Plasticity." New York: Guilford Press, pp 485–505.

Olson L, Backlund E-O, Gerhardt G, Hoffer BJ, Lindvall O, Rose G, Seiger Å, Stromberg I (1986): Nigral and adrenal grafts in parkinsonism: Recent basic and clinical studies. In Yahr MD, Bergmann KJ (eds): "Advances in Neurology," vol 45. New York: Raven Press, pp 85–94.

Olson L, Björklund H, Hoffer BJ (1984): Camera bulbi anterior: New vistas on a classical locus for neural tissue transplantation. In Sladek JR, Gesh DM (eds): "Neural Transplants, Development and Function." New York: Plenum Press, pp 125–166.

Olson L, Boreus LO, Seiger Å (1973): Histochemical demonstration and mapping of 5-hydroxytryptamine-and catecholamine-containing neuron systems in the human fetal brain. Z Anat Entwickl Gesch 139:259–282

Olson L, Seiger Å (1972): Brain tissue transplanted to the anterior chamber of the eye: 1. Fluorescence histochemistry of immature catecholamine and 5-hydroxytryptamine neurons reinnervating the rat iris. Z Zellforsch 135:175–194.

Olson L, Seiger Å, Strömberg I (1983): Intraocular transplantation in rodents. A detailed account of the procedure and examples of its use in neurobiology with special reference to brain tissue grafting. In Fedoroff S, Hertz L (eds): "Advances in Cellular Neurobiology" vol 4. New York: Academic Press, pp 407–442.

Olson L, Strömberg I, Bygdeman M, Granholm A-C, Hoffer BJ, Freedman R, Seiger Å (1987): Human fetal tissues grafted to rodent hosts: Structural and functional observations of brain, adrenal and heart tissues in oculo. Exp Brain Res 67:163–178.

Perlow M, Freed W, Hoffer BJ, Seiger Å, Olson L, Wyatt R (1979): Brain grafts reduce motor abnormalities produced by CNS damage. Science 204:643–647.

Peroutka SJ, DeLanney L, Irwin I, Ison PJ, Ricaurte G, Schegel JR, Langston JW (1985): 1-Methyl-4-phenyl-1,2,3,6-tetrahydropyridine (MPTP) induced dopamine D_2-receptor hypersensitivity in the mouse is transient. Res Commun Chem Pathol Pharmacol 48:163–171..

Prendergast J, Stelzner DJ (1976): Increases in collateral axonal growth rostral to a thoracic hemisection in neonatal and weanling rats. J Comp Neurol 166:145–162.

Puchala E, Windle WF (1977): The possibility of structural and functional restitution after spinal cord injury. A review. Exp Neurol 55:1–42.

Redmond DE, Sladek JR, Roth RH, Collier TJ, Elsworth JD, Deutch AY, Haber S (1986): Fetal neuronal grafts in monkeys given methylphenyltetrahydropyridine. Lancet 1:1125–1127.

Rinne UK, Klinger M, Stamm G (1980): "Parkinson's Disease: Current Progress, Problems and Management." Amsterdam: Elsevier.

Rose G, Gerhardt G, Strömberg I, Olson L, Hoffer B (1985): Monoamine release from rat caudate nucleus reinnervated by substantia nigra grafts: An in vivo electrochemical study. Brain Res 341:92–100.

Schmidt RH, Ingvar M, Lindvall O, Stenevi U, Björklund A (1982): Functional activity of substantia nigra grafts reinnervating the striatum: Neurotransmitter metabolism and (^{14}C)-2-deoxy-D-glucose autoradiography. J Neurochem 38:737–748.

Schmidt RH, Björklund A, Stenevi U, Dunnett SB, Gage FH (1983): Intracerebral grafting of neuronal cell suspensions. III. Activity of intrastriatal nigral suspension implants as assessed by measurements of dopamine synthesis and metabolism. Acta Physiol Scand [Suppl] 522:19–28.

Seiger Å, Olson L (1977): Quantitation of fiber growth in transplanted central monoamine neurons. Cell Tissue Res 179:285–316.

Stenevi U, Kromer LF, Gage FH, Björklund A (1985): Solid neural grafts in intracerebral transplantation cavities. In Björklund A, Stenevi U (eds): "Grafting in the Mammalian CNS." Amsterdam: Elsevier, pp 41–49.

Strömberg I, Almquist P, Bygdeman M, Finger TE, Gerhardt GA, Granholm A-C, Mahalik TJ, Seiger Å, Hoffer BJ, Olson L (1988a): Intracerebral xenografts of human mesencephalic tissue into athymic rats: Histochemical and in vivo electrochemical studies. Nature Proc Nat Acad Sci USA, in press.

Strömberg I, Bygdeman M, Goldstein M, Seiger Å, Olson L (1986): Human fetal substantia nigra grafted to the dopamine-denervated striatum of immunosuppressed rats: Evidence for functional reinnervation. Neurosci Lett 71:271–276.

Strömberg I, Herrera-Marschitz M, Hultgren L, Ungerstedt U, Olson L (1984): Adrenal medullary implants in the dopamine-denervated rat striatum. I. Acute catecholamine levels in grafts and host caudate as determined by HPLC-electrochemistry and fluorescence histochemical image analysis. Brain Res 297:41–51.

Strömberg I, Herrera-Marschitz M, Ungerstedt U, Ebendal T, Olson L (1985a): Chronic implants of chromaffin tissue into the dopamine-denervated striatum. Effects of NGF on survival, fiber growth and rotational behaviour. Exp Brain Res 128:2–15..

Strömberg I, Hultgårdh-Nilsson A, Hedin U, Ebendal T (1988b): Short- and longterm fate of intraocular chromaffin cell suspensions with and without initial NGF support. Cell Tissue Res (submitted).

Strömberg I, Johnson S, Hoffer BJ, Olson L (1985b): Reinnervation of dopamine-denervated striatum by substantia nigra transplants: Immunohistochemical and electrophysiological correlates. Neuroscience 14:981–990

Sundström E, Strömberg I, Tsutsumi T, Olson L, Jonsson G (1987): Studies on the effect of 1-methyl-4-phenyl-1-2-3-6-tetrahydropyridine (MPTP) on central catecholamine neurons in C57 BL/6 mice. Comparison with three other strains of mice. Brain Res 405:26–38.

Ungerstedt U (1968): 6-hydroxy-dopamine induced degeneration of central monoamine neurons. Eur J Pharmacol 5:107–110.

Ungerstedt U (1971a): Stereotaxic mapping of the monoamine pathway in the rat brain. Acta Physiol Scand [Suppl] 367:1–48.

Ungerstedt U (1971b): Adipsia and aphagia after 6-hydroxydopamine induced degeneration of the nigrostriatal dopamine system. Acta Physiol Scand [Suppl] 367:95–122.

Ungerstedt U (1971c): Postsynaptic supersensitivity after 6-hydroxydopamine induced degeneration of the nigrostriatal dopamine system. Acta Physiol Scand [Suppl] 367:69–93.

Ungerstedt U (1971d): Striatal dopamine release after amphetamine or nerve degeneration revealed by rotational behaviour. Acta Physiol Scand [Suppl] 367:49–68.

Ungerstedt U, Arbuthnott GW (1970): Quantitative recording of rotational behavior in rats after 6-hydroxydopamine lesions of the nigrostriatal dopamine systems. Brain Res 24:485–493.

Vos JG, Kreeftenberg JG, Kruijt BC, Kruizinga W, Steerenberg P (1980): The athymic nude rat. II. Immunological characteristics. Clin Immunol Immunopathol 15:229–237.

Whittemore SR, Ebendal T, Lärkfors L, Olson L, Seiger Å, Strömberg I, Persson H (1985): Developmental, regional and post-lesion expression of nerve growth actor (NGF) and NGF mRNA in rat brain. Soc Neurosci Abstr 11:660.

Wuerthele SM, Freed WJ, Olson L, Morihisa J, Spoor L, Wyatt RJ, Hoffer BJ (1981): Effect of dopamine agonists and antagonists on the electrical activity of substantia nigra neurons transplanted into the lateral ventricle of the rat. Exp Brain Res 44:1–10.

Yahr MB (1984): The limitations of long-term use of anti-Parkinson drugs. Can J Neurol Sci 11:191–194.

15

Immunologic Considerations in Transplantation to the Central Nervous System

MARTIN K. NICHOLAS, PhD, AND **BARRY G.W. ARNASON,** MD

Department of Neurology and The Brain Research Institute, The University of Chicago, Chicago, Illinois 60637

In this chapter we will consider the role of immune mechanisms in the acceptance or rejection of tissue implants into the central nervous system (CNS). Recent work has suggested that the neurologic deficits of Parkinson's disease in man can be reversed, at least in part, by implanting autologous (self) adrenal medulla (Madrazo et al., 1987) or allogeneic (nonself but the same species) fetal substantia nigra or adrenal medulla (Madrazo et al., 1988) into the caudate nucleus. A considerable body of work in experimental animals has indicated that allogeneic, and to a lesser extent xenogeneic (different species), implants of neural and nonneural tissues into the brain can similarly correct defective function, at least for a time (reviewed in Björklund and Stenevi, 1985; Nottenbohm, 1985; Sladek and Gash, 1986; Azmitia and Björklund, 1987). These successes have prompted proposals that allogeneic tissue implants to the brain might be used to treat a wide range of human diseases. Foreign tissues are usually rejected by the host into which they are placed; it is important therefore to know whether, and, if so, to what extent, rejection mechanisms that apply to transplants into or onto other sites apply to implants into the brain as well. At a first consideration, grafts into brain appear to behave differently from grafts into or onto other sites. This has led to the view that the brain is *immunologically privileged,* a concept that will be discussed here in some detail.

Many investigators have reported success with the transplanting of foreign tissues to the CNS. Others, ourselves included, have encountered considerable variability. We have observed the universal rejection of xenogeneic neural tissues exchanged between immunocompetent rats and mice. Neocortical tissue obtained from fetal mice, when placed into the cerebral cortex of adult rats, is rejected within the first few weeks of transplantation. Fetal rat neocortex transplanted to the cerebral cortex of adult mice is similarly rejected (Fig. 15–1). In our hands, allogeneic grafts of fetal neocortical mouse tissue placed into the lateral ventricle of genetically dissimilar host mice have, in many instances, also been rejected, albeit at a considerably slower rate than for between-species grafts (Fig. 15–2). These studies and those of several others, demonstrating either histologic signs of rejection or evidence for host sensitization following neural transplantation, suggest that the degree of genetic disparity (histoincompatibility) between donor and host tissues is a critical determinant of the fate of tissues transplanted to the CNS (Mason et al., 1986; Nicholas et al., 1987; Sloan and Charlton, 1988; Widner et al., 1988). The immunologic privilege of the CNS is far from absolute. Tissues placed within the CNS can be recognized and destroyed by cells of the host immune system.

It is also critical to know whether CNS implants can sensitize the host to antigens shared by implant and host with generation of immune responses against both. Were this the

Neural Regeneration and Transplantation, pages 239–284
© 1989 Alan R. Liss, Inc.

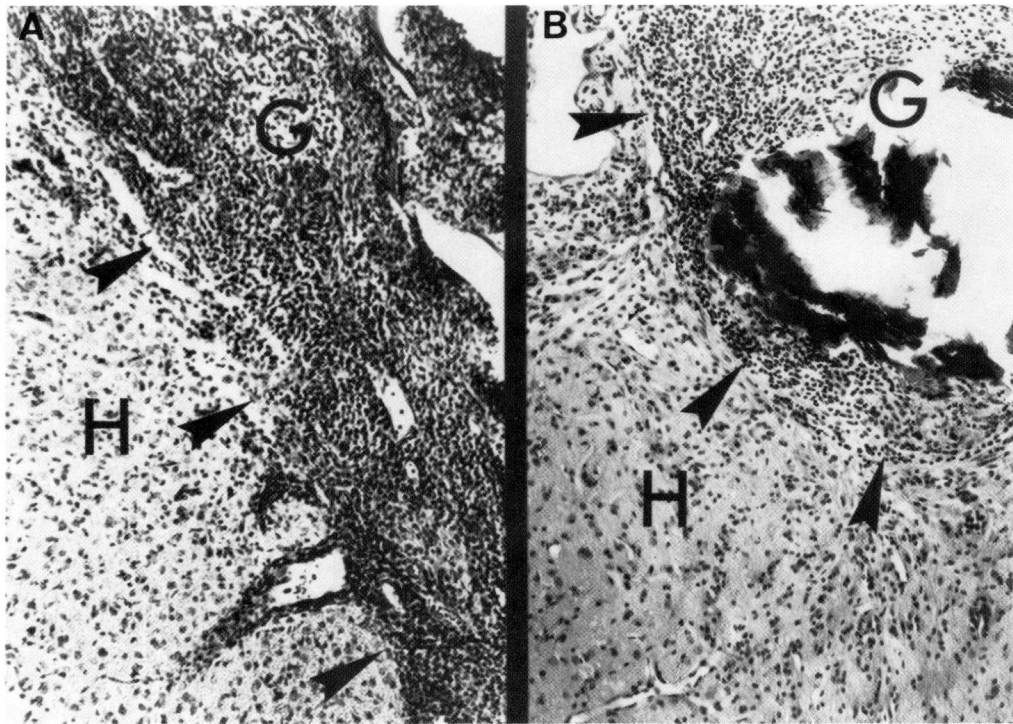

Figure 15–1.   Representative sections from formalin-fixed, paraffin-embedded intracerebral neural xenografts 2 weeks after transplantation, stained with hematoxylin and eosin. Note the heavy mononuclear cell infiltrate and necrosis in the grafted tissues (arrowheads). The transplants have been rejected in both cases. **A:** Fetal mouse neocortex (gestational age at implanting, 16 days) transplanted to the cerebral cortex of an adult rat. **B:** Fetal rat neocortex (gestational age at implanting, 16 days) transplanted to the cerebral cortex of an adult mouse. G, grafts; H, host. × 100.

case, then foreign brain implants might not merely fail in terms of therapy of disease because of their rejection by the host, but might also be directly deleterious to the host.

As recently as January, 1982, 24 multiple sclerosis (MS) patients received transplants of porcine brain fragments to their subcutaneous abdominal fat (Bauer, 1983). The initiator of this project, a Yugoslav surgeon, could provide no cogent rationale for its implementation. He did, however claim to have had 25 years of undocumented success in treating MS with swine brain implants. None of the 24 patients improved after transplantation. In fact, neurologic complications occurred in at least five patients leading, in one instance, to death. An immunologic process was shown to underlie these complications in the one case where evidence for it was sought (Knorr-Held et al., 1986). This patient developed a severe polyradiculoneuritis 11 days after swine brain implantation. He was shown to have an immune response directed against gangliosides shared by the neural implant and his own tissues.

That neuroimmunologic complications might follow peripheral implanting of swine brain was hardly surprising. Neuroparalytic accidents have been known to follow the administration of brain-derived rabies vaccines since the late 19th century, and an immunologic etiology has long been held responsible for these accidents (Arnason, 1987). Indeed, both humoral and cellular immune responses to CNS antigens have now been demonstrated in patients suffering neuroparalytic complications of rabies vaccination, the initiating

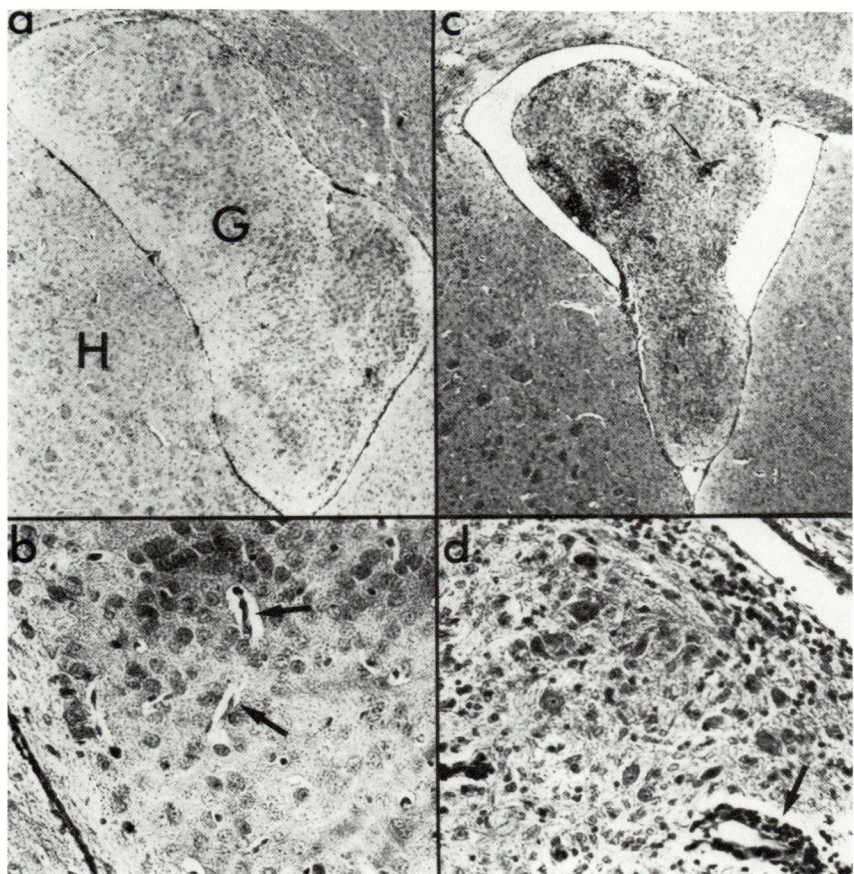

Figure 15–2.   Representative sections from formalin-fixed, paraffin-embedded intraventricular neural implants 4 weeks after transplantation, stained with hematoxtlin and eosin. **a:** Murine fetal neocortical isograft (gestational age at implanting, 16 days). G, graft; H, host. ×40. **b:** Higher power view of the isograft shown in a. Note the well-developed neuropil and the absence of mononuclear cell infiltrates. Arrows point to blood vessels devoid of any associated inflammation and are typical of those found in neural isografts. ×200. **c:** Murine fetal neocortical allograft (gestational age at implanting, 16 days). Donor and host differ at both class I and class II MHC loci and at multiple minor histocompatibility (mH) loci (see text). Note the number of inflammatory cells present, especially in perivascular cuffs (arrow) ×40. **d:** Higher power view of the allograft shown in c. Note the looseness of the neuropil and the mononuclear cell infiltrates (arrow). ×200.

agent(s) being nervous tissue components of the vaccine preparations (Uchimura and Shiraki, 1957; Hemachuda et al., 1987). Neuroparalytic accidents following administration of brain-derived rabies vaccine occur in 1 in 100 to 1 in 1,000 vaccinees. The results of the porcine brain implant fiasco described above suggest that when the stimulus is sufficiently strong, 20% of individuals, perhaps more, may develop this complication. Furthermore, systemic administration of CNS tissue to experimental animals has long been known to result in experimental allergic encephalomyelitis (EAE), a T-cell mediated inflammatory disease in which CNS myelin is destroyed. The specter therefore looms that transplants of CNS tissue to the CNS could be followed by neuroparalytic accidents within host CNS.

TABLE 15.1. Transplantation Terminology

Transplant between	Current terminology	Older terminolgy
Self to self	Autograft	Autograft
Genetically identical members of the same species (inbred animals)	Isograft (syngeneic graft)	Homograft
Genetically dissimilar members of the same species	Allograft	Homograft
Different species	Xenograft	Heterograft

While the implanting of porcine brain to the subcutaneous fat was not the first application of neural transplantation to man (Woolsey et al., 1944), it was among the more dramatic in terms of negative results. Moreover, these results were a direct consequence of immunologic processes. As such, this experiment serves as a cautionary tale—an appropriate introduction to immunologic considerations in neural transplantation. Clinical applications of CNS transplantation currently being proposed, and in some instances implemented, represent a new approach to an old problem: the restoration of function after disease or injury. However, transplantation to the CNS brings problems of its own to the field of neuroscience and to transplantation immunology.

A BRIEF OVERVIEW

Transplantation Terminology and Immunologic Principles

The immunologist Niels Jerne (1985) has popularized the concept of a grammar of the immune system. Appropriately, the grammatical dictum "to every rule there is an exception" applies particularly well to transplantation immunology within the CNS. The brain's status as an immunologically privileged site (see below) already makes it an exception to many of the general rules of transplantation biology. With further research in CNS transplantation, additional exceptions may follow. Nevertheless, to understand the implications of results in neural transplantation the reader must have some knowledge of the basic principles that govern transplant acceptance or rejection in other tissues. Significant conceptual changes and refinements have occured in immunology since the first transplant papers were written, and this is reflected inevitably by changes in terminology. Thus papers written 20 years ago bear little resemblance to those written today. These changes make the review of transplantation papers somewhat difficult. A brief overview of the terminology currently used in describing donor/host transplantation relationships is outlined below.

The act of transplanting a tissue from one site on an individual to another site on the same individual is known as autografting and the transplant itself as an autologous graft or autograft. In principle, this is no different from isografting; that is, the transplantation of tissues between genetically identical members of the same species. (Note that isografts, also known as syngeneic grafts, could differ from the host to which they are transplanted because of viral infection, oncogenesis, or some other alteration of donor tissue.) Transplants between genetically dissimilar members of the same species are known as allografts. These are the most common transplants used in clinical medicine today. Allografts are usually rejected because of disparities between the graft and the host unless the immune system of the host is suppressed. Allograft disparities can vary from single amino acid substitutions (point mutations) on a single cell surface protein to multiple substitutions on one or more proteins. Note that even point mutations in single cell surface molecules can lead to vigorous allograft rejection (Isakov and Bach, 1983). Lastly, the exchange of tissues between members of different species is known as xenografting and the transplant itself as a xenogeneic graft, or xenograft. A comparison of these terms with some older, less frequently used synonyms, is given in Table 15.1. For the sake of clarity we will restrict ourselves to current terminology here, even when discussing older papers. Additional immunologic definitions, concepts, and principles will be introduced where relevant to the material under discussion.

Early Tranplantation Studies and the Discovery of Histocompatibility

Autologous transplants of many types, including the reattachment of severed noses and ears and skin grafting, were often successful in the hands of European surgeons in the 18th and 19th centuries. The ability of these tissues to survive after reattachment to their original hosts demonstrated that nonimmunologic barriers to graft survival could be overcome. Similar attempts to exchange tissues between genetically dissimilar individuals (allografts) met with uniform failure. Prior to the 1930s, however, theories advanced to explain the failure of allografts were vague and unsatisfying. In 1931, Karl Landsteiner suggested that the success or failure of a transplanted tissue might be governed by principles similar to those recently shown by him to govern the success or failure of blood transfusions. In 1933, based upon observations of workers in the field of mouse genetics, (who were encountering variability in survival of tumors transplanted between inbred strains of mice), J.B.S. Haldane suggested that immunologic mechanisms might be operative. Three years later, Peter Gorer (1936) discovered "antigen II," and a connection between genetically determined cell surface proteins and the acceptance or rejection of transplants was made.

Gorer's pioneering work established that mice of strains that were identical at antigen II loci would accept allografts for prolonged periods, whereas grafts that differed from the host at antigen II loci were rejected promptly because of an immune response of the host against foreign forms of antigen II. From these studies emerged the concept that a single discrete family of antigens was paramount in determining whether an allograft would succeed or fail. The genetic loci encoding antigen II on mouse cells became known as H-2 (H for histocompatibility). It became clear from a large body of subsequent work that the H-2 system was comprised of several discrete regions all aligned on chromosome 17 of the mouse but separated one from the next, and that there was great polymorphism at each region of the complex. In outbred animals this polymorphism

suffices to render each individual uniquely different from all other members of the same species so that allografts between outbred animals are almost always rejected because of H-2 differences between them. Later, other loci encoding histocompatibility antigens distinct from H-2 were discovered when it was noted that grafts between H-2 identical mice were sometimes rejected after delays that could vary from weeks to months. Because the antigens responsible appeared to have a less immediate effect on the success or failure of a transplanted tissue than did H-2 molecules, the family of H-2 antigens came to be designated as the major histocompatibility complex (MHC) and all the others as minor histocompatibility (mH) loci. It soon became evident that similar families of molecules exist in all mammalian species, so that man, like the mouse, has an MHC (located on human chromosome 6), as well as numerous mH loci.

Few discoveries have had as great an impact on immunology as that of the MHC. A review of its many properties lies beyond the scope of this discussion. Interested readers should consult Klein (1986). Several features of the MHC critical to an understanding of graft rejection will, however, be introduced below and developed later in this chapter.

Response of the host to MHC antigens is usually the principal determinant of allograft acceptance or rejection, and MHC molecules constitute the classic "transplantation antigens." Yet foreign grafts constitute an artificial rather than a natural situation, and for this reason the major natural biologic role of the MHC is likely to lie elsewhere. Zinkernagel and Dougherty (1974) showed that cytotoxic T cells (see below for a fuller description) primed to respond to lymphocytic choriomeningitis (LCM) virus would kill virus-infected cells, but with an important restriction. Killing would only occur if the infected cells shared MHC molecules with the cytotoxic T cells. That is to say, cytotoxic T cells would recognize and lyse cells bearing viral antigens on their surface only if the infected cells also expressed self-encoded MHC molecules. T cells primed to LCM virus would not kill LCM-infected cells that expressed foreign rather than self MHC antigens. From this and much subsequent work emerged the concept that one of the major functions of the MHC is as a presenter of antigens to T cells so that a self-encoded MHC molecule in association with a foreign antigen is recognized as altered self.

Note the potential paradox here. Graft rejection requires recognition of and response to foreign MHC, yet for response to more usually encountered foreign antigens (e.g., viruses) host MHC must present the antigen. In the latter case, the T cell fails to recognize and be primed by viral antigen presented together with foreign MHC, nor will primed T cells destroy cells bearing viral antigen unless they express self MHC. One possible explanation for this apparent paradox, and one for which there is good evidence, as discussed in greater detail below, is that a subpopulation of T cells recognizes and is primed directly by foreign MHC molecules. This subpopulation, once primed, may respond directly to cells bearing foreign MHC and kill them (Sprent and Schaefer, 1985, 1986; Warrack and Kappler, 1987). Other T cells may require that degraded (see below) foreign MHC components be presented to them together with self-encoded MHC before they can respond. Regardless of the way in which foreign MHC antigens are recognized, those T cells capable of doing so comprise 5–10% of the total T cell population (Lindahl and Wilson, 1977).

With regard to mH antigens, whose role in allogeneic brain graft rejection may belie their denigratory designation (see below), there are data pointing to self (i.e., host) MHC restrictions for presentation of antigen (Loveland and Simpson, 1986) and for priming. On the other hand, once priming has occurred, foreign mH-reactive T cells (after cloning) recognize foreign mH determinants on third-party allogeneic stimulator cells directly, i.e., a mH antigen will be recognized on a cell carrying a never before encountered foreign MHC complex (Hunig and Bevan 1982).

Molecules encoded by the MHC are divided into several classes based on both structural and functional criteria. Those most important in graft rejecton are the class I and II MHC molecules, which belong to a family of proteins known collectively as the immunoglobulin gene superfamily (Williams, 1982, 1987). Members of this family share functional and structural features, and many are of critical importance in regulating immune processes. Their shared functional role is the mediation of cell-cell adhesion interactions. Structurally, they are characterized by the presence of domains: peptide loops of approximately 110 amino acids created by intrapeptide disulfide linkages. This shared feature has led to the theory that the different members of the immunoglobulin gene superfamily evolved from duplications of the same progenitor gene. Molecules of the immunoglobulin gene superfamily of particular interest to this discussion include, in addition to the class I and II MHC molecules, immunoglobulin itself (both membrane-bound and secreted), T cell receptors for antigen, and the CD3, CD4, and CD8 molecules found on T cells. These molecules are depicted schematically in Fig 15–3. References to each of these proteins will be made throughout this chapter. Their properties will be further clarified as the discussion evolves.

Class I molecules consist of an α chain (encoded in the MHC) that is noncovalently linked with B-2 microglobulin (not encoded in the MHC). In man, there are three class I loci, known as A, B, and C. Each person expresses two A, two B, and two C molecules, inheriting one of each pair from each of his parents. Class II molecules consist of an α and a β chain, both of which are encoded in the MHC. There are three class II families of loci in man known as DP, DQ, and DR. With respect to DR, most individuals express two forms, the same α chain being linked with either a β1 or β2 chain. Thus, each individual expresses eight class II molecules, four from each parent. Graft rejection responses are directed against both class I and class II molecules, but under some circumstances response against class I antigens is of greater importance than for others. For example, allografts of skin to mice that differ from the donor at only class I MHC loci are rejected within several weeks of grafting. Allografts of heart and thyroid tissue in the same donor-host combinations are not rejected (Isakov et al., 1979). Data obtained from thousands of human renal transplant recipients indicate that histocompatibility between donor and host at MHC class II loci (especially HLA-DR) is a better predictor of graft survival than donor-host histocompatibility at class I MHC loci (Grounewoud, 1987; Opelz, 1987). Similar findings are

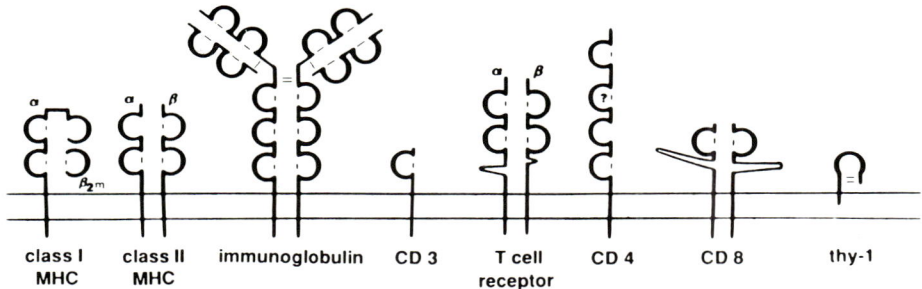

class I   class II   immunoglobulin   CD 3   T cell   CD 4   CD 8   thy-1
MHC   MHC   receptor

Figure 15–3. Structures of proteins belonging to the immunoglobulin gene superfamily referred to in this chapter. All are shown in their membrane-associated forms. The carboxyl and amino termini of each molecule are located on the cytoplasmic and extracellular sides of the plasma membrane, respectively. Loops indicate portions of the molecules that may form domains similar to those observed in immunoglobulin molecules, leading some to suggest that these molecules evolved from a common progenitor gene. The symbols represent putative intrachain and interchain disulphide bonds. Possible N-linked glycosylation sites (not shown) exist on all the molecules depicted here. The class I MHC molecules is composed of a membrane-spanning α chain containing three domains. In a functional class I molecule the α chain is noncovalently associated with β2-microglobulin (not encoded by the MHC). The class II MHC molecule is a heterodimer composed of α and β chains noncovalently bound. The β chain exhibits a much greater degree of polymorphism than the α chain. Immunoglobulion molecules are highly polymorphic, and five classes are recognized. Shown here is the basic immunoglobulin structure consisting of two identical light chains and two identical heavy chains. Disulphide bonds link each light chain to a heavy chain. The heavy chains are similarly linked to one another. Antigen-binding is associated with variable regions located in the domains at the amino end of the molecule. Immunoglobulin destined for secretion is differentially processed and does not contain a membrane-spanning sequence. Further modifications occur prior to secretion, but these modifications differ depending upon the class of immunoglobulin in question. CD3 is a multi-molecular nonpolymorphic molecule. The basic structure of its components is shown here. A functional CD3 molecule is characterized by the association of three different chains, γ, δ and ϵ, with the T-cell receptor for antigen. The T-cell receptor, like immunoglobulin, is highly polymorphic. Most T-cell receptors are composed of two covalently linked polypeptides, α and β. As mentioned above, in its functional form, the T-cell receptor is associated with the CD3 complex. As with immunoglobulin, variable regions of the T-cell receptor associated with antigen-binding are located in domains at the amino end of the molecule. CD4 is a nonpolymorphic molecule found on approximately two-thirds of mature T cells. CD4 expression is correlated with specificity for target cells that bear class II MHC molecules. The ? in the second domain indicates that this region of the molecule fulfills few of the criteria for inclusion as an immunoglobulin-like domain. CD8 is a nonpolymorphic molecule found on approximately one-third of mature T cells. CD8 expression is correlated with specificity for target cells that bear class I MHC molecules. Thy-1, among the simplest members of the immunoglobulin gene superfamily, does not span the cell membrane but is instead associated with it by a phosphoinositol linkage. Thy-1 is allelically expressed and is found on both lymphocytes and nervous tissues in some species.

emerging with regard to human heart transplants, but the number of cases analyzed remains relatively small (Pfeffer et al., 1987). For allografts of brain to brain there is some evidence to sugest that class II disparities between graft and host may be of greater import than class I disparities (Nicholas et al., 1988).

Class I and II molecules differ greatly in their tissue distribution. This may be particularly important with regard to graft rejection, since the degree to which a tissue expresses MHC molecules may relate to its acceptance or rejection (Matis et al., 1983; Halloran et al., 1986, Fabre et al., 1987). Class I proteins are expressed on virtually all nucleated cells (brain cells being a notable exception). The distribution of class II MHC products is, in health, far more restricted. These molecules are normally expressed on B cells, on monocytes and the macrophages that devolve from them, on dendritic cells (see below for a fuller description), and on so-called tissue-specific macrophages in both rodents and man. Class II products are also expressed by activated T cells in man, but not in rodents. Note that while virtually all nucleated cells express class I molecules at all times, the cells that ordinarily express class II MHC molecules all subserve immunologic functions. As we shall see, under normal conditions this differential distribution of MHC molecules can be viewed as a mechanism for the diversification and specialization of the immune response. In the context of graft rejection, however, this diversification can be viewed as a mechanism for increasing the number of potential antigens on grafted cells to which the host can react.

CHARACTERIZING THE BRAIN AS AN IMMUNOLOGICALLY PRIVILEGED SITE

The study of immune-mediated diseases of the nervous system and of brain-immune system interactions has a long history. Advances in immunology have aided considerably in forwarding our understanding in these areas. Although neural transplantation has been used to study nervous system development and to correct neural deficits, the major contribution of transplantation immunology to the study of the nervous system has been in characterizing the brain as an immunologically privileged site (Barker and Billingham, 1977; Head and Billingham, 1985). Although work in this area spans most of the 20th century, (the first report is dated 1914), it is neither rigorous nor exhaustive. Indeed, it is better characterized as sporadic and equivocal, With clinical trials in neural transplantation already underway, a critical evaluation of the work that has led to the characterization of the brain as a privileged site for transplantation is in order.

The CNS is one of several sites considered immunologically privileged. Others include the anterior chamber and cornea of the eye, the prostate and testes, and the bone marrow space, to name but some (Barker and Billingham, 1977; Head and Billingham, 1985). The word privilege implies a benefit, an advantage enjoyed because of a few special conditions. The benefit bestowed upon immunologically privi-

leged sites is *relative* isolation from the immune system, so that foreign tissues transplanted to these sites survive longer than the same tissues transplanted to nonprivileged sites. The conditions that interact to confer immunologic privilege to a given site are, to some extent, site-specific. Yet many immunologically privileged sites are characterized by shared anatomic peculiarities involving either the lymphatic or vascular sytems, or both. CNS immunologic privilege is probably related to both the absence of a well-developed lymphatic system within the CNS (but see below) and to the presence of the blood-brain barrier.

As mentioned previously, expression of MHC antigens varies between tissues. The absence of, or very low expression of, MHC encoded antigens, including class I antigens, by cells of the normal CNS may be of great importance in conferring immunologic privilege insofar as grafts of CNS to CNS are concerned (as opposed to grafts to the CNS of skin or endocrine tissues, which do express class I MHC antigens). These considerations, as well as others, will be discussed more fully after reviewing some of the basic principles underlying transplantation immunology and the early studies that led to the brain's characterization as an immunologically privileged site.

The CNS has been used as a transplant site by numerous investigators for the better part of the 20th century. A variety of allogeneic and xenogenic tissues, including tumors, skin, endocrine organs, and neural tissues have been implanted. Today, with the exception of skin, all of these tissues are being considered for therapeutic transplants to the human CNS. Many of the experiments carried out before the 1980s, however, were designed to study immunologic privilege with little or no thought given to potential therapeutic applications. Nevertheless, the information gathered in these earlier experiments bears upon present and future efforts and is worthy of review.

Although her work was not published until 1917, Elizabeth Dunn demonstrated as early as 1903 that neural tissue allografts transplanted between neonatal offspring of outbred rats were capable of surviving. The implications derived from her work, however, did not involve the CNS as a privileged site for transplantation so much as they demonstrated the feasibility of transplants to the CNS at all. As with the study of the MHC, systematic examination of the brain as an immunologically privileged site began with tumor studies. Prior to the development of in vitro tissue culture techniques, biologists interested in perpetuating tumor cells developed systems for passaging these cells in susceptible mice. In 1914 it was observed that allogeneic carcinomas placed in the CNS of mice survived longer than those transplanted subcutaneously (Ebeling, 1914). This finding was soon confirmed by others using a variety of allogeneic tumors and, by 1921, had been extended to xenogeneic tumors (Shirai, 1921). As early as 1923, however, it was apparent that survival of intra-CNS tumor transplants varied and that the outcome could be altered by manipulating experimental conditions (Murphy and Sturm, 1923). The fate of these transplants appeared to depend upon both host and donor factors. Although transplanted tumors did survive for longer periods in the CNS than elsewhere, mononuclear cells were found by most investigators within or around many of the surviving tumors, suggesting, even at this early stage, that immunologic privilege might be relative.

The next papers on tumor transplants to the brain did not appear for nearly 25 years, and it was not until 1964 that an experiment was undertaken to determine whether the fate of an allogeneic tumor differed when it was transplanted to the CNS of several strains of genetically defined mice (Scheinberg et al., 1964). In this study, intra-CNS tumor survival varied from strain to strain, but immunogenetic theory of the time could not readily explain the differences in survival. In all of these studies there are risks inherent in attempts to compare responses to tumor transplants with those to normal tissue transplants. Rapid growth of tumors and the elaboration by them of numerous factors, including some with immunosuppressive and angiogenic effects, might significantly alter the outcome of tumor transplant studies. Fortunately, investigations into the fates of other tissues transplanted to the brain were underway at the same time.

Although the transplantation of skin to the CNS has no therapeutic application, several experiments employing skin transplants to brain led to critical observations regarding immunologic privilege. As with tumors, it is clear that skin allografts transplanted to the CNS survive longer than when transplanted elsewhere. Indeed, success with intracerebral skin allografts appears to be as great as that with any other tissue, even though allogeneic skin placed orthotopically (that is, to a site that is the normal one for the transplanted tissue) leads to a vigorous immune response and rapid rejection. In 1948, Sir Peter Medawar, who was honored with a Nobel Prize for his work on transplantation immunology, demonstrated that intracerebral skin grafts in a population of outbred rabbits took in virgin animals but were rejected promptly if the animals had been presensitized with an orthotopic skin graft (Medawar, 1948). That is to say, if a piece of skin from rabbit A was transplanted to the brain of rabbit B, it survived for an extended period. On the other hand, if a piece of skin from rabbit A was first transplanted to the skin of rabbit B and allowed to reject, a second piece of skin from rabbit A, when placed in the CNS of rabbit B, was rejected. Because cells of a presensitized rabbit were capable of infiltrating and destroying intracerebral skin grafts, it was argued that immunologic privilege was simply the result of a failure of tissue transplanted to the CNS to sensitize the host. Subsequent studies with inbred rats confirmed the observation that allogeneic skin grafted intracerebrally survives longer than skin grafted to other sites, including other immunologically privileged sites (Raju and Grogan, 1977).

In 1966, Scheinberg et al. demonstrated accelerated rejection of orthotopic skin grafts in outbred rabbits that had received an intracerebral skin graft from the same donor prior to the placement of the orthotopic graft. This suggested that, contrary to Medawar's earlier conclusion, systemic sensitization of the host by an intracerebral allograft can occur, and in this instance did occur. These findings were later extended by Geyer and his collaborators (1979), who demonstrated systemic sensitization after the intracerebral transplantation of MHC class I disparate skin in inbred rats but not after the intracerebral transplantation of MHC class II disparate skin. As with the previously cited study, sensitization was determined by the ability of an animal with an intracerebral skin graft to reject a subsequently placed orthotopic skin graft in an accelerated manner. Interestingly, a single intracerebral skin graft was all that was needed to sensitize the host when donor-host combinations involved multiple mH antigen disparities in addition to a single MHC class I difference. In a subsequent study the authors demonstrated that if the donor-host combination involved a MHC class I disparity alone (no mH disparities), then a second intracerebral skin graft was needed after rejection of the first before host sensitization was observed (Geyer et al., 1985).

The transplantation of endocrine organs to the brain provided the first experiments in which the functional status of an intra-CNS transplant could be measured. A variety of tissues, including thyroid, pancreas, ovary, and adrenal gland have been placed in several allo- and xenogeneic hosts. Again, results have differed considerably between groups, with some claiming long-term acceptance and restoration of lost function (Pomerat et al., 1944) and others reporting varying degrees of rejection (Woodruff, 1960; Lance, 1967). An additional challenge to the notion that intracerebral grafts failed to sensitize their host was put forth when Lance (1967) demonstrated systemic sensitization following the placement of intracerebral thyroid allografts in dogs. As others had done with intracerebral skin grafts, Lance demonstrated accelerated rejection of orthotopic skin allografts in dogs that had received intracerebral allogeneic thyroid tissue prior to the placement of the skin graft. Skin and thyroid in this experiment were syngeneic with one another. Lance's finding, coupled with the observations of Scheinberg et al. (1966) and of Geyer and Gill (1979), demonstrated that some tissues placed intracerebrally were fully capable of sensitizing the host, thus creating a paradox. If intra-CNS allografts can sensitize the immune system of the host and if (as Medawar demonstrated) sensitized cells can destroy intra-CNS allografts, why do allogeneic tissues placed within the CNS ever survive? This question remains unanswered.

It is obvious from the results outlined above that the brain was characterized as a relatively privileged transplantation site years before anything was known about the specifics of immunologic responses to foreign antigens. Because few took an interest in therapeutic transplants to the CNS before the 1970s, little work was done using neural tissues to further characterize the brains' immunologically privileged status. As interest in the application of neural transplantation grew, it is fair to say that research into the immunologic mechanisms underlying the success or failure of transplants to the CNS lagged behind that in other areas such as study of functional recovery. Numerous transplant studies carried out in the 1970s involved the implanting of syngeneic tissues. Outbred animals were used in many others, limiting the information available regarding the degree of histoincompatibility between donor and host. Potential immunologic consequences were seldom considered in these experiments. Notable exceptions are found in the work of Hasek and Lodin and their collaborators (Hasek et al., 1977; Lodin et al., 1977) and of Zalewski et al. (1978). Both groups demonstrated, among other things, that survival of transplants to the CNS could be enhanced by first rendering animals unresponsive to allogeneic donor histocompatibility antigens. The process by which animals were made unresponsive to these alloantigens is known as tolerance induction. In the experiments described below, tolerance was induced by injecting large numbers of lymphocytes into newborn rats. The lymphocytes were obtained from adult animals of the strains to which the investigators wished to establish tolerance. Immunologic tolerance to antigens on these newly infused cells is thought to arise by the same mechanisms that lead to tolerance of self-encoded molecules early in life; that is, by the mechanisms that enable lymphocytes to discriminate between self and nonself.

Hasek et al. (1977) first demonstrated the extension of immunologic tolerance to the CNS in a tumor transplant model. Immunocompetent adult rats were able to resist the growth of allogeneic tumor cells injected into the brain, provided the dose was sufficiently low, i.e., the tumor was rejected. Animals rendered immunologically tolerant to histocompatibility antigens expressed by the tumor cells were unable to suppress tumor growth following intracranial tumor injection and eventually died of CNS tumor burden. Similarly, Zalewski et al. (1978) transplanted allogeneic vagal nodose ganglia and associated peripheral nerve trunks to the spinal cords of adult rats in several inbred strain combinations. They demonstrated reduced inflammation and extended survival of transplants placed in rats rendered unresponsive to donor histocompatibility antigens when compared with transplants in nontolerant animals. In addition, using appropriate donor-host strain combinations, they were able to demonstrate greater inflammation in transplants that differed from their hosts at both mH and MHC loci than in those that differed only at mH loci. This finding, recently confirmed by others (Mason et al., 1986) using allografts of fetal CNS to adult CNS, may be of particular importance in determining the fate of neural tissues transplanted to the CNS. That is to say, synergism of the immune responses directed against *both* allogeneic MHC and mH antigens may lead to intra-CNS allograft rejection, while immune responses directed against *either* MHC or mH alloantigens may not.

Lodin et al. (1977), using the same tumor transplant model described in the preceding paragraph, demonstrated the ability of sublethal doses of intracerebrally administered allogeneic tumor cells to sensitize the host, thus protecting it from subsequent challenges with otherwise lethal doses of the same tumor. They found that preimmunization by an intracerebral route was as effective as preimmunization by an intramuscular route. Furthermore, they found that the concentration of cytotoxic antibodies (directed against antigens expressed by the tumor) in the serum of preimmunized rats was greater in those animals that had received intracerebral injections than in those that had received intramuscular injections.

In summary, experiments conducted between 1914 and 1979 demonstrated that the CNS could serve as an immunologically privileged transplant site for numerous tissues. The variability in results, however, lead one to conclude that privilege is relative and likely to depend upon multiple factors. To better understand possible explanations for the relative protection afforded foreign tissues transplanted to the brain we will review, in general terms, the mechanisms underlying graft rejection when tissues are placed in nonprivileged sites.

GRAFT REJECTION

Graft rejection has received as much attention as any other area in the field of immunology. While much has been learned, many questions remain unanswered, and controversy still exists. Our understanding of the rejection process comes from the piecing together of data derived from a variety of in vivo and in vitro experimental models and from clinical transplantation in man. The different models used to study rejection can be viewed as variations on a theme. That is to say, although skin and kidney allografts may both undergo rejection, the mechanisms underlying these processes may differ, as already mentioned. Thus conclusions based on the study of skin graft rejection may or may not relate directly to the study of renal transplant rejection, let alone brain implants. Moreover, graft acceptance may reflect more than the inability of the host to mount an effective immune response against the graft. Graft acceptance may involve active suppression of the immune response (Kamada et al., 1980). Graft rejection is a dynamic process, and possible mechanisms leading to it can be easily conceptualized. Indeed, a number of methods for measuring the rejection response have been developed. On the other hand, graft acceptance, despite histoincompatibility, and the mechanisms underlying this phenomenon are more difficult to conceptualize and study. This important aspect of transplant immunology cannot be overlooked, however, when studying graft rejection, and particularly grafts of brain to brain.

The processes of graft rejection are divided by convention into two arms. The first is host sensitization, that is, the stimulation of the host immune system that leads to the generation of an immune response. The second is the effector phase, that is, the mounting of the immune response within the graft itself. These are often referred to as the afferent and efferent arms, respectively.

Sensitization takes place primarily in those lymph nodes to which lymph from the graft region flows. In grafts such as kidneys, in which vascular anastomoses are established surgically at the time of transplantation, considerable response may also occur in the spleen. Lymph node responses to antigens involve, for the greater part, the generation of primed T cells. Splenic responses are characterized by a proportionately greater B cell response (Waksman, 1980).

Sensitization requires presentation of antigen to the T and B cells. B cells have surface-bound immunoglobulin, and antigenic material binds to the immunoglobulin on those B cells that bear appropriate binding sites for that antigen (Fig. 15–3). Antigen recognized by B cells may be free-floating or presented to them on the surface of accessory cells such as macrophages. Presentation is not MHC-restricted. B cells recognize and respond to proteins, carbohydrates, lipids, and combinations among them, such as glycolipids. Antigen binding occurs in the immunoglobulin-variable region, located at the amino end of the molecule. Antigen binding to surface-bound immunoglobulin triggers B cell proliferation, followed by a reprogramming of those clones that have been expanded by contact with antigen to synthesize and release antibody. Reprogramming is facilitated by T cell help (see below). Circulating antibody can bind free-floating antigen or antigen on the surface of cells located at a distance from the antibody-producing cell.

T cells respond to antigen differently from B cells (Marrack and Kappler, 1987). The T cell receptor for antigen is at all times bound to the T cell (see Fig. 15–3). T cell receptors respond only to antigens that are bound to the surface of other cells, i.e., cell-to-cell contact is required, and short range effects are the rule. T cell receptors are further restricted in that they only recognize short peptide sequences, which for the most part are generated by intracellular processing of larger peptides. The system has its advantages; soluble antigen that might otherwise occlude T cell receptors and prevent an interaction with a target cell is ignored, thus improving efficiency.

The presentation of foreign graft antigens to host T cells can occur in several ways. Grafts usually contain at least some mobile cells, such as lymphocytes, macrophages, and dendritic cells (specialized cells of the monocyte/macrophage lineage that are extremely potent as antigen presenters) (Lechler and Batchelor, 1982). These cells normally move into and out of the tissues and can be viewed as passengers within

a graft. Once a graft has been placed, they move out of it and make their way via lymphatic channels to the regional lymph nodes and via the circulation to the spleen. Note that such motile cells are themselves immunocytes and as such carry both class I and class II antigens. They can function as direct presenters of foreign MHC antigen to a subpopulation of host T cells. The potency of dendritic cells as T cell activators may relate in part to the fact that they release interleukin-1 (Il-1), a potent monokine that aids in the activation of T cells presented with antigen. The role of passenger dendritic cells as sensitizers for graft rejection is considerable. Advantage has been taken of this fact in the following way: if tissues to be grafted are first maintained in tissue culture for a time prior to grafting, passenger lymphocytes and dendritic cells die off. A graft depleted of these elements is more likely to be accepted than one not so depleted (Lechler and Batchelor, 1982; Faustman et al., 1984).

Within brain implants, microglia are the prime candidates for the direct sensitization mechanism described above. Ameboid microglia express class I and II MHC antigens, clearly perform a phagocytic role akin to that of macrophages, often express surface macrophage-associated phenotypic markers, and when isolated from brain and grown in tissue culture synthesize and release Il-1 in the same way as activated macrophages and dendritic cells (Ting et al., 1983; Perry et al., 1985; Giulian et al., 1986; Hayes et al., 1987). All of the above is not surprising, since microglia are generally believed to be bone marrow-derived. While there is firm evidence that microglia traffic into brain, evidence that they traffic out is harder to come by. Ting et al. (1983) irradiated inbred mice with 1,000 R and reconstituted them with bone marrow cells of a different strain so as to create chimeras. MHC class II-positive cells in the brains were exclusively of donor bone marrow origin, indicating that MHC class II-bearing cells unique to the host disappeared after chimerization. The observation speaks for turnover of microglia. Microglia are radiation-resistant and the data, while indirect, are consistent with a bidirectional movement of microglia into and out of brain. Dendritic cells themselves have been sought in brain but not found (Hart and Fabre, 1981).

MHC products are continually shed. Host macrophages may scavenge antigenic fragments from the graft-host interface and transport them to the lymphoid tissues. Free antigen may also be swept into the circulation of the lymph and be carried to the spleen or lymph nodes. Circulating host T cells may come into direct contact with the graft, be primed by this contact, and then make their way back to the lymphoid organs. Lastly, circulating host T cells that come into contact with the graft may enter it and remain there instead of returning to a lymphoid organ. Provided the appropriate microenvironment for lymphocyte priming and proliferation exists within the graft, these newly resident cells may be able to become sensitized, to proliferate, and to exert their effector functions without leaving the grafted tissue. The process is sometimes known as peripheral sensitization, to distinguish it from the central sensitization that occurs in the lymphoid organs. Peripheral sensitization may be of particular importance in grafts to the CNS, since conventional lymphatic channels are probably absent from the CNS (see below).

In general, shed MHC material must be processed by host phagocytic cells, which ingest large peptides and convert them to small peptide fragments (Allen, 1987). These fragments are spit out by the phagocytic cells and bind to host MHC on antigen-presenting cells by a limited number (three or so) of interspersed amino acid residues known as an agretope. Single MHC molecules are quite promiscuous, in that they are able to bind a variety of different agretopes. The T cell receptor reacts with the "other face" of a processed peptide fragment. This also is comprised of interspersed amino acid residues and is known as an epitope. The T cell receptor for antigen is a heterodimer (Fig. 15–3), that is, it is composed of an α and a β chain (encoded in man by genes located on chromosomes 14 and 7, respectively). As with bound immunoglobulin on B cells, variable regions at the amino end of the α and β molecules are responsible for antigen binding.

The vast majority of mature T cells carry one of the pair of surface proteins known as CD4 and CD8; they never carry both (Fig. 15–3). In ways that are not fully understood, the CD4 molecule directs T cells that bear it to respond to antigenic epitopes presented by class II MHC molecules, whereas the CD8 molecule directs T cells bearing it to respond to epitopes presented by class I MHC molecules (Littman, 1987; Warrack and Kappler, 1987). There is reason to believe that the process requires direct adhesion of CD4 to self class II MHC molecules and of CD8 to self class I MHC molecules. There is also some evidence that the subpopulations of T cells capable of recognizing foreign MHC on graft cells are similarly restricted: CD4$^+$ host cells responding to foreign class II MHC antigens and CD8$^+$ host cells responding to foreign class I MHC molecules (Sprent and Schaefer, 1985, 1986; Rosenberg et al., 1986; Sprent et al., 1986; Marrack and Kappler, 1987).

Approximately two-thirds of mature T cells are CD4 + one-third CD8 +. Not only do CD4 + and CD8 + cells recognize antigen differently, but they also subserve, for the most part, discrete functions. The CD4 molecule is found primarily on T-helper cells and on the effectors of delayed-type hypersensitivity (DTH), whereas the CD8 molecule is found primarily on cytotoxic and on suppressor T cells. This is not invariable. For example, cytotoxic CD4 + cells are known (Kaplan et al., 1984), as are CD8 + cells that produce lymphokines normally associated with helper T cell function (Rosenberg et al., 1986). Nevertheless, the division of CD4 + and CD8 + cells into helper/DTH and cytotoxic/suppressor categories, respectively, remains a useful generalization.

As is the case with immunoglobulin, T cell receptors for antigen exhibit great diversity, so that only a small proportion of them are capable of recognizing any single epitope. Contact with foreign MHC on intact foreign cells, or of processed foreign MHC epitopes (and presumably mH antigen epitopes, as well) bound to self MHC on antigen-presenting host cells, triggers T cell proliferation of those clones capable of recognizing that foreign MHC. The T cell receptor is linked to a multimolecular complex of peptides known collectively as CD3 (Oettgen and Terhorst, 1987). The CD3 complex functions as a signal transducer to tell the T cell that its receptor for antigen has engaged antigen in an appropriate way. T cell proliferation is a major consequence of the CD3 mediated signal. This proliferative phase continues for several days and results in clonal expansion such that large numbers of specifically sensitized cells are generated. CD4 + T cells, if removed from the spleen or lymph nodes during this phase of the response, will proliferate when exposed in vitro to cells that share class II MHC antigens with the graft. This can be assessed by measuring their ability to incorporate tritiated thymidine [^{3}H]thymidine. In some circumstances CD8 + cells removed at the same time can be shown to be directly cytotoxic to target cells bearing class I MHC antigens of the graft.

While class I MHC antigens trigger responses of CD8 + cells and class II molecules trigger responses of CD4 + cells, the two responses are not totally independent. Antigen-driven CD4 + helper T cells release interleukin-2 (Il-2), a major lymphokine that helps the expansion of antigen-activated T cells. Most CD4 + and CD8 + antigen-driven T cells express Il-2 receptors, as do antigen driven B cells. Il-2 released by the CD4 + T cells favors proliferation of Il-2 receptor-bearing cells. Thus exposure to class II antigens augments the T cell response to class I antigens and presumably to mH antigens as well. It also augments B cell proliferation and antibody production by B cells, as already mentioned. In the same vein, if mH antigens trigger CD4 + T cells to release Il-2, they too may augment the response to MHC antigens. There is evidence that MHC class II does have a role as a restriction element for presentation of certain mH antigens, (including two known to exist in brain; see Scheid et al., 1972). Responses to mH antigens that are MHC class II-restricted would be expected to be confined to CD4 + T cells.

The stage is now set for the effector arm of the response. During the time that the afferent arm of the response is being generated, the graft becomes revascularized, except in those instances in which direct anastomoses between graft and host vessels were already made at the time of grafting. Host and graft vasculature make contact, and new channels form, so that blood flows through the graft. Sensitized cells, now ready to become effectors, leave the lymph nodes by the efferent lymph channels and enter the circulation. Sensitized cells leave the spleen to enter the circulation directly.

Effector cells are carried in the blood to the graft, which they enter and attack. Effector cells attach to graft endothelial cells, which they may destroy if graft MHC antigens are expressed by them. This may lead to infarction and thrombosis of the graft. Other cells traverse the endothelium to enter graft parenchyma, the cells of which may also be attacked and destroyed. CD8 + cells recognizing foreign class I MHC on the graft cells kill them by a cytotoxic process in which a product made by them punches holes in the target cell membrane so that extracellular fluid enters, and the cells swell and eventually lyse. A small population of CD4 + cells recognizing class II antigens on target cells kills their targets in a similar fashion. These are the class II-restricted cytotoxic T cells. Upon recognition of class II antigen on foreign cells, the majority of CD4 + cells react by releasing lymphokines, among them lymphotoxin, a product capable of directly damaging target cells. In addition, other lymphokines released by CD4 + cells arm macrophages, which have a considerable role as the final vectors of foreign tissue destruction (Duncan and Stepkowski, 1986).

It has already been pointed out that class II MHC molecules are ordinarily not expressed on cells other than those of the immune system. However, certain products released by effector T cells, notably γ-interferon, are capable of inducing class II MHC expression on cells of many types, including some in the brain (Wong et al., 1985). Gamma-interferon may convert otherwise innocuous graft cells into appropriate targets for CD4 + helper T cells. Gamma-interferon also up-regulates class I MHC antigen expression on target cells, again favoring their destruction by effector host CD8 + cytotoxic T cells.

Histologic inspection of grafted tissues undergoing rejection at non-CNS sites reveals infiltrating cells of many types (Lowry et al., 1986). These include, in addition to the T cell types already discussed, B cells, macrophages, dendritic cells, natural killer (NK) cells, basophils, and other granulocytes. All of these cell types circulate and are drawn into the graft by chemoattractants released by macrophages and by effector T cells. The roles of these other cells are not totally understood, though clearly they contribute to phagocytosis and to removal of the foreign tissue. Macrophages, basophils, and granulocytes lack antigenic specificity, but functional analysis of the T cell infiltrate within skin grafts undergoing rejection indicates that perhaps no more than half the invading T cells are specifically reactive with graft antigens (Binz et al., 1976). It follows that T cells reactive with foreign MHC products attract into the lesion T cells with *irrelevant* antigenic specificities, at least to the task at hand. Why this should occur is not known. Just as class I- and class II-responsive T cells act synergistically during the afferent arm of the immune response, so do they in the effector phase as well. Cross talk of this sort between T cells may extend beyond those T cells programmed to respond to foreign graft antigens and lead to attraction of other T cells into the inflammatory focus.

Up to this point the discussion of the effector phase has centered on T cell responses. Antibody may also contribute to the effector arm of graft rejection (Williams et al., 1968). In the process known as hyperacute rejection, preformed cytotoxic antibodies directed against donor tissue are present at the time of transplantation. This occurs, for example, if a second graft from the same donor is applied to a host that has rejected the first. It is also a common feature in the rejection of xenografts. Upon binding to donor antigens on target cells, cytotoxic antibodies can initiate activation of the complement system, leading to opsonization or lysis of the target. This is the only form of rejection in which antibodies are the primary mediators of the process. Antibodies may also damage grafted tissue through the process known as antibody-dependent cell-mediated cytotoxicity (ADCC) (Gailiunes et al., 1978). ADCC results from the formation of a ternary complex between a target cell, a cell with cytotoxic potential, and an antibody that links the target cell to the cytotoxic cell. Antibody serves the critical bridging role in this system. The killer cells involved in ADCC do not contain antigen-specific receptors that allow them to make direct contact with a target cell. Instead, they contain receptors (known as Fc receptors) for a portion of the constant region of the antibody. Cell lysis occurs once the antibody has bound its target and the killer cell has bound the antibody.

Finally, under some conditions, antibodies may actually enhance the survival of foreign grafts (Morris, 1980). Treatment of a graft recipient with antiserum prior to transplantation has long been known to prolong graft rejection, provided the antiserum contains antibodies directed against donor histocompatibility antigens. In vitro studies have shown that these antibodies, known as enhancing antibodies, interfere with the binding of host lymphocytes to target cells, thereby blocking effector function. Thus, depending upon the circumstances, antibodies can work for or against the survival of transplanted foreign tissues.

This, then, is the general schema of graft rejection. In terms of intra-CNS implants and their acceptance or rejection, several questions loom. Do antigens from implants make their way along with resorbed CSF through the arachnoid villi into the circulation and thence to the spleen? Does the brain have a lymphatic drainage, and if so, does sensitization to foreign MHC or mH occur in regional nodes? Does peripheral sensitization occur in the grafts themselves? Do CNS grafts, unlike normal brain tissue, express considerable amounts of MHC molecules, thus favoring sensitization and graft rejection? Does the blood-brain barrier impede access of effector cells to the graft? When intra-CNS grafts become revascularized, do graft vessels anastomose with those vessels or is the vasculature entirely of host origin? Is there a hierarchy of MHC antigen expression by brain cells with, for example, selective expression by glia rather than neurons? Does γ-interferon released by activated T cells induce MHC antigen expression by brain cells as it does cells in other organs? Is the cellular infiltrate seen in brain grafts that are undergoing rejection similar to that seen in other organs during rejection, or are there differences? What role, if any, do antibodies play in the rejection or acceptance of tissues transplanted in the brain? Are MHC antigens paramount in rejection of brain grafts, or are antigens that are considered minor ones in other tissues major ones in brain? In what follows, we will attempt to address these questions based on current knowledge.

TRANSPLANTS IN THE CNS

There are essentially two types of CNS transplants: tissue fragment grafts and cell suspension grafts (reviewed in Das, 1983; Gage and Buzsaki, Chapter 13, this volume). The size of the tissue fragments used varies considerably, ranging from single large areas of dissected fetal brain (or other tissue) to multiple small tissue fragments. It has been the general experience that grafts of fetal and neonatal brain tissue are more likely to survive than transplants of brain tissue from older animals. Fetal and neonatal brain grafts, provided they are accepted, enlarge and mature within the host brain. Why these grafts should do better than adult grafts may relate to their developmental status at the time of transplantation. For example, a functional vasculature may be more readily established in actively dividing tissues than in terminally differentiated (postmitotic) adult neural tissue. Developing neural tissue may also be more responsive to the trophic effects of any number of growth factors.

It is also possible that the antigenic potentials of fetal and adult tissues, and hence their ability to sensitize the host following transplantation, differ. For example, Thy-1 is a cell surface protein of the immunoglobulin gene superfamily (Fig. 15–3) found on neurons, lymphoid cells, and several other tissues, including skin in the mouse. Thy-1 expression by mouse brain is known to increase markedly as the brain matures. The expression of Thy-1 by various neuronal populations also changes considerably during embryologic development of the mouse (Morris, 1985). Thy-1 is allelically expressed, but the difference between alleles is not sufficiently antigenic to cause the rejection of skin grafts exchanged between mice that differ at the Thy-1 locus only. The importance of Thy-1 as a minor antigen in brain rather than skin, however, is unknown. Many molecules may, like Thy-1, be differentially expressed during neural embryogenesis or postnatal development. It is possible that one or more of these molecules might act as alloantigens in a transplant situation and that the antigenicity of fetal and adult neural tissues might differ accordingly.

Cell suspension grafts have included cultured cells of many types and cells derived from freshly isolated donor tissue that is enzymatically dissociated so as to provide single cell suspensions that can then be immediately implanted. Both tissue fragment and cell suspension grafts can be placed intraventricularly or intraparenchymally. Surgical anastamoses of donor and host vessels have never been attempted in transplants to the CNS; thus both types of transplants are initially nonvascularized. The rate at which a blood supply is reestablished in transplants to the CNS appears to depend upon the tissue being transplanted and possibly on the site where it is placed, details of which will be discussed below.

We are aware of only one study directly comparing cell suspension and tissue fragment grafts to brain in terms of their relative abilities to generate a host immune response and to be accepted or rejected (Tze and Tai, 1984). It is distinctly possible that graft type might influence host response. On theoretical grounds, one might predict better survival of cell suspension than of tissue fragment grafts for several reasons. First, a tissue fragment graft constitutes a *localized* nidus, thus providing the immune system with a more substantial target than that provided by scattered donor cells. Since an immune response in a grafted tissue requires a recruitment into it of circulating cells and since lymphokines released by invading cells up-regulate MHC antigen expression, the intensity of the response is likely to be greatest where the pool of foreign antigen is most concentrated. Second, tissue fragment grafts require the development of a vasculature in order to survive. Graft rejection often begins as an intra- and perivascular event and direct attack on endothelial cells may lead to necrosis because of vessel occlusion (Anderson et al., 1977; Dvorak et al., 1980). Thus an attack on a vessel cell can compromise many others. Third, cell suspensions are usually prepared with proteolytic enzymes, one effect of which is the cleavage of potential antigens from cell surfaces (Pichler et al., 1985). During the critical early days after grafting, the antigenic load per cell of a cell suspension graft is, for this reason, likely to be less than that of a tissue fragment graft. On the other hand, if motile cells (microglia?) play an important role as sensitizers of the host, then their injection into the brain already in suspension may facilitate their egress from the CNS.

Different cell types within a graft may be more or less susceptible to immune attack depending on the antigens they express. Neurons may be particularly hardy in this regard, glia less so (see later). In a tissue fragment, graft neurons may be caught up in the destructive response as *innocent bystanders*. In a suspension graft this is, perhaps, less likely. Sorting of cell suspensions to remove those cells most likely to invoke an immune response, endothelial cells and microglia for example, might further improve success rates with cell suspension grafts (Lopez-Lozano et al., 1987). Tze and Tai (1984) demonstrated that single cell suspensions of pancreatic endocrine cells survived considerably longer in the brains of allogeneic rat hosts than did tissue fragments of pancreatic islets transplanted to the same sites. Lymphocytic infiltrates were found in and around all tissue fragment grafts, whereas no infiltrating lymphocytes were seen in and around the cell suspensions. Blood vessels, passenger leukocytes, and perhaps resident macrophages were removed in the purification process, thus lowering the *antigenic load* at the time of transplantation.

In the discussion so far, it has been implied that cell suspensions remain as such after grafting. This is not altogether the case. Some reaggregation of grafted cells may occur, converting a suspension graft, in part, into an aggregate one, which then becomes vascularized. Indeed, in the study mentioned above, Tze and Tai (1984) observed the aggregation of dissociated cells into small vascularized clumps of tissue. Similar findings have also been reported for the transplantation of neural tissue cell suspensions to the CNS (Lindsay et al., 1987). For this reason the effect of removal of donor endothelial cells, replacing them with with host endothelial cells (from host veins for example) should, in our opinion, be tested experimentally.

There are inherent differences in the way tissue fragment and cell suspension grafts are evaluated histologically. These differences may bear upon the interpretation of results. When evaluating a tissue fragment graft, for example, localized inflammation and tissue destruction, if present, will be evident. The eval-

uation of cell suspension grafts may be more problematic. Cells are often injected at multiple discrete sites. Grafted cells (neurons have been looked for in most cases) are then localized enzymatically or immunohistochemically. If cells are differentially susceptible to immune attack, i.e., if neurons are relatively resistant, immune responses directed against one cell type (endothelial cells or glia, for example), with loss of these cells, may be missed unless attempts are made to find them after transplantation.

Following transplantation, there is also a hazard in equating functional recovery to graft survival or failure of recovery to graft rejection. Recovery may depend upon trophic factors released by the graft prior to its destruction. For example, grafted adrenal medullary tissue has been shown to favor sprouting of remaining host axons into a damaged area (Bohn et al., 1987). Positive effects on the host have sometimes been seen following transplantation, even when the transplanted tissue cannot be found. For example, Freeman, et al., (1987) noted behavioral recovery in rats receiving transplants of rabbit neural tissue in an experimental model of Parkinson's disease even when the transplant did not survive. In the obverse of the above, Lance (1967) noted that failure of function of thyroid allografts to brain often preceded histologic evidence of graft rejection and concluded that histologic evidence of survival per se is not adequate evidence of biologic acceptance.

Does the Site of Transplantation Within the CNS Affect the Immunologic Outcome?

Intra-CNS transplants can be placed in two anatomic compartments: intraventricularly, or intraparenchymally. While some transplantation techniques make use of a combination of the two sites, most use one or the other. Intraventricular transplants provide a convenient space for containing tissue without causing excessive damage to host brain. The use of this site in experimental models has the added advantage of easing the search for grafted tissues upon histologic evaluation. The ventricle also provides the transplant with a constant supply of cerebrospinal fluid (CSF), which may favor the survival and growth of transplanted neural tissues until such time as a vasculature is established in the graft. Transplants placed within brain parenchyma itself can take several forms. They can be directly inserted into brain tissue, or placed in surgically created cavities. Cavities can be prepared at the time of transplantation or at any time prior to transplantation. Although a considerable degree of scarring may occur around preformed cavities, a rich vascular network forms in the cavity wall with which subsequently transplanted tissues can interact. The creation of cavities may also stimulate the local accumulation of neurotrophic factors, which may enhance transplant growth and survival (Nieto-Sampedro and Cotman, 1985).

It is reasonable to anticipate that the site of transplantation within the CNS might affect functional outcome. One might predict better recovery when tissues are transplanted into or near those brain regions with which they must interact to restore function than when transplanted to more distant sites. This has been shown to be the case in several studies (Dunnett et al., 1981a,b). Few studies have compared the immunologic fates of tissues transplanted to various CNS compartments. As early as 1923, Murphy and Sturm (1923) observed that mouse sarcomas in xenogeneic hosts underwent rapid rejection if the tumor came into contact with the ependymal lining. They concluded that the ventricle was an inhospitable transplantation site. Since that time, however, other investigators have demonstrated good survival of allogeneic tissues transplanted to the ventricle (Freed, 1983; Mason et al., 1986; Sloan and Charlton, 1988).

An immunohistochemical analysis of rat brain prompted Head and Griffin (1985) to speculate that the ventricles and certain white matter areas might be less favorable as transplant sites than other intraparenchymal sites. They observed greater numbers of MHC class II+ cells in the choroid plexus and in white matter tracts than in cortical parenchyma. Because these class II+ cells might act as antigen-presenting cells (i.e., similarly to dendritic cells or the Langerhans cells found in skin), they speculated that immune responses directed against graft antigens might be more likely to occur in these sites. This will remain a matter for speculation until it is demon-strated whether or not these cells are effective at antigen presentation in vivo and whether antigen presentation by host cells in the graft surround is a critical event in brain graft rejection. In addition, graft take may be affected by patterns of vascularization in different brain regions. For example, white matter is less vascularized than gray matter, so that establishing a blood supply to a graft may be less readily achieved following grafting to white than to gray matter. There is also the possibility that drainage of antigenic material to the deep cervical nodes (see below) rather than to the systemic circulation may be greater from grafts placed rostrally within the brain than caudally. This could affect host immune response and, in consequence, graft fate. In order to determine whether or not differences in transplant survival are a function of the site of intra-CNS placement, carefully controlled comparative studies of transplants placed in multiple sites will have to be conducted.

Vascularization of Neural Transplants

The source of graft endothelium in transplants to the CNS has been a subject of debate for several years. Until recently, the only evidence supporting vascularization by donor and/or host was based upon morphologic assessment. A comparison of the results obtained by many investigators using numerous tissues indicates that the relative contributions of donor and host vascular elements to CNS transplants depend upon the type of tissue transplanted. Indeed, the degree to which donor vascular elements contribute to patent transplant vasculature may depend not only upon the type of tissue transplanted, but also upon its developmental stage at the time of transplantation. For example, Ausprunk and Folkman (1976) observed that endothelial cells in transplants of adult rat heart fragments to the chorioallantioc membrane of chickens degenerated within several days of transplantation, leading to disruption of vessels within the transplant. On the other hand, donor-derived endothelial cells were, for the most part, undamaged when embryonic heart fragments were used instead of adult heart fragments. A patent vasculature was established in the grafts within 3 days when embryonic tissues were used, the graft vessels apparently composed of donor-derived endothelial cells. This is not a trivial point from the immunologic point of view, as vessel cells of donor origin in direct contact with the circulation of the host are potential candidates for immunologic attack (Anderson et al., 1977; Dvorak et al., 1980). Vessel cells of host origin, on the other hand, would be capable of serving as antigen-presenting cells to host T cells in local immune responses, provided they expressed MHC antigens.

Some adult tissues transplanted to the CNS appear to retain a significant portion of their vasculature. Others appear to be replaced, for the most part, by ingrowing vessels of host origin. For example, Svengaard et al. (1975a) reported that autologous iris implants placed in the caudal diencephalon were primarily vascularized by ingrowing CNS vessels. They based their conclusion upon morphologic changes observed in graft vasculature over the course of several weeks. They did suggest that iris vessels contributed, at least in part, to a patent vascularization within the first days of transplantation. The iris vessels were, however, eventually replaced by ingrowing CNS vessels.

Rosenstein and Brightman (1983) argued that autonomic ganglia transplanted to the fourth ventricle of rats were vascularized, at least in part, by anastomoses of host vessels at the graft margins with vessels of the grafted ganglia themselves. They based their conclusion on the observations that blood flow was established in the graft within 24 hr of transplantation and that many of the vessels exhibited functional properties of donor-derived cells.

Stewart et al. (1984) reported that autologous skin transplanted to the cerebral cortex of chickens retained its vasculature, apparently anastomosing with host vessels shortly after transplantation. They argued, among other things, that the establishment of host-derived vasculature would result in the degeneration of vessels present in the tissue at the time of transplantation that they did not see. They further argued that were the vessels within the graft of CNS origin, then the endothelial cells in newly formed vessels within the graft would have characteristics of brain endothelium rather than of skin, an unlikely supposition.

They also argued that if graft vasculature were host-derived, then the time course of graft reperfusion would have to be consistent with the rate of new vessel growth. As with the autonomic ganglia transplants mentioned above, reperfusion of skin transplanted to the cerebral cortex was felt by these investigators to be too rapid (within 48 hr) to be ascribed to ingrowth of host vessels. The vessels within the graft were noted to have retained morphologic characteristics of skin-derived endothelium.

Two methods for determining the source of transplant vasculature with greater certainty than was possible heretofore have been applied recently. One makes use of monoclonal antibodies that recognize vascular elements of either donor or host origin, but not both. Results are interpreted immunohistochemically. The other method uses radioactively labeled nucleotides to determine patterns of angiogenesis. Here, autoradiography is used for analysis. The presence of donor-derived vessels in several types of intra-CNS transplants has been demonstrated by both methods.

Monoclonal antibodies that distinguish donor tissue from that of the host have been used to demonstrate the presence of chimeric vessels (those composed of both donor and host elements) in neonatal and fetal cortical allografts to the ventricles of rodents. Using an antibody directed against a class I MHC molecule expressed by donor but not host tissue, Baker et al. have demonstrated integration of donor and host vasculature in neonatal cortical transplants to the third ventricle of the rat (Belinda J. Baker, personal communication). The union of donor and host vessels was evident 10 days after transplantation, and graft vascularization appeared to be complete by 30 days. Host vessels growing into the grafts were demonstrated using the same antibody on tissue from the reciprocal transplant scheme. At no time were vessels of donor origin found growing out into the host. In other transplant models in other sites, donor-derived vascular cells are often replaced over time by those of the host. In the Baker study, donor-derived vessels were still apparent 4 months after transplantation. We have demonstrated a similar finding in fetal neocortical allografts to the lateral ventricle of the mouse (unpublished observations). Using a monoclonal antibody directed against a class II

MHC molecule of donor but not host tissue, vessels expressing antigen were found in donor but not host tissue. This is shown in Fig. 15–4. As mentioned earlier, the presence of MHC molecules on donor vasculature provides the host with a readily accessible antigenic stimulus.

Using radionucleotides, Krum and Rosenstein (1987) have demonstrated the presence of donor-derived vessels in transplants of both autonomic ganglia and adrenal medullary tissue to the CNS of the rat. In their experiments, [^{3}H]thymidine was administered to transplant hosts at various time points before transplantation so as to prelabel host endothelial cells, which, during mitosis, incorporate [^{3}H]thymidine. The [^{3}H]thymidine injection schedule was such that grafted tissue was not exposed directly to the radiolabel. By this method they could determine the extent to which prelabeled host endothelial cells grew into transplanted tissue. With both autonomic ganglia and adrenal medullary transplants, reestablishment of blood flow was observed within 24 hr of transplantation. Only occasionally was a labeled endothelial cell found within the transplanted tissue itself, and then only near graft-host interfaces. On the other hand, surrounding host vessels contained numerous labeled cells. The labeling intensity of individual endothelial cells diminished as the graft was approached. This directional dilution of radiolabel indicated regional proliferation of prelabeled host endothelial cells at the graft-host interface. This was found whether grafts were placed intraventricularly or intraparenchymally. The rapid rate of graft reperfusion and the small number of labeled cells within the grafts adds further strength to the argument that tissue fragments transplanted to the CNS retain their own vessels and that these vessels fuse with newly synthesized host vessels to form the graft vasculature.

Using the same technique, these investigators recently demonstrated similar findings using transplants of fetal CNS tissue (Krum and Rosenstein, 1988), thus corroborating the findings from the monoclonal antibody studies already discussed. This work also confirms that of Lindsay and Raisman (1984), who noted radiolabeled endothelial cells in hippocampal explants of fetal and neonatal rat tissue transplanted to the hippocampi of adult hosts. In their experiments, tissue explants were labelled in vitro with [^{3}H]thymidine before implantation.

The studies outlined above make use of tissue fragment grafts. In all cases, donor-derived vessels were present. It is reasonable to conclude that vessel constituents are transplanted in all the tissue fragment models discussed, and it is not surprising to find that graft vessels fuse with host vessels. In cell suspension grafts, in contrast, the presence of donor derived vessels has never been demonstrated, and one would only expect to find them if significant numbers of vascular cells were transplanted as part of the suspension. Obviously, if donor-derived endothelial cells prove to be a source of antigenic stimulus to the host, their removal from cell suspension grafts by cell sorting techniques may prove invaluable to the success of neural transplants in man. As mentioned above, if endothelial cells prove to be a necessary component in some transplant models, endothelial cells of host origin (derived from the saphenous or other veins) might be added at the time of transplantation. There is reason to believe that peripherally derived endothelial cells will, as they contribute to the new circulation in a CNS graft, develop brain-type barrier properties. Endothelial blood-brain barrier properties develop in response to some aspect of the neural environment, as shown convincingly in the elegant studies of Stewart and Wiley (1981).

The integrity of the blood-brain barrier may also be important in determining the fate of neural transplants. A functional blood-brain barrier is characterized by the presence of continuous tight junctions between endothelial cells. Additionally, gaps and channels traversing individual endothelial cells are lacking. The vast majority of circulating substances are excluded by this barrier. Exchange of essential nutrients occurs through specific transport systems. Although the barrier does not exist in several areas of the brain, it is postulated that breakdown of the blood-brain barrier in areas where it normally exists leads to degenerative changes. Using the iris implant model mentioned above, Svengaard et al. (1975b) noted that central axons growing into autologous intracerebral iris implants underwent degenera-

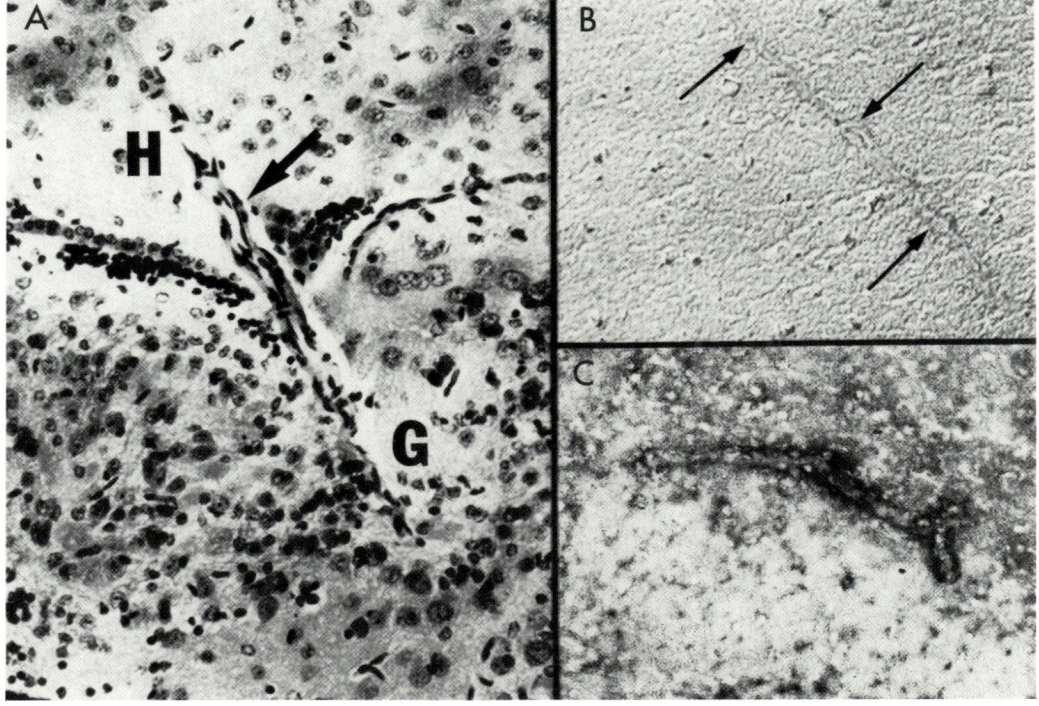

Figure 15–4.   Vascularization of intraventricular neural allografts. **A:** Section from a formalin-fixed, paraffin-embedded neural allograft 4 weeks after transplantation, stained with hematoxylin and eosin. The arrow points to a blood vessel traversing the graft-host interface. G, graft; H, host. ×200. **B:** A frozen section of host tissue surrounding a neural allograft 4 weeks after transplantation. **C:** A frozen section of a neural allograft 4 weeks after transplantation. B and C were both stained with a monoclonal antibody reactive with class I MHC molecules present on donor but not host tissues. The unstained vessel in B (arrows) is characteristic of all vessels in the host surround. Some vessels in the graft itself are reactive with the antibody, as shown in C. Thus at least some vessels within the graft appear to be of donor origin. Furthermore, they may express molecules associated with activation of the immune system.

tion 2 to 3 months after iris implantation. They suggested that these axons were insufficiently protected from damaging substances carried in the blood, because a blood-brain barrier had failed to develop in these transplants. This could have been due to the presence of iris derived vessels, although iris vessels in situ do exhibit barrier properties (Dernouchamps and Michiels, 1977). The original investigators argued that the vessels were brain-derived rather than iris-derived (see above). Additionally, the use of autologous implants required enucleation of the eye. Complications of enucleation must be considered potentially relevant in this study. Indeed, Rao et al. (1988) found accelerated rejection of intracerebral iris xenografts following enucleation of the host.

It has been demonstrated that the vasculature within non-CNS tissues transplanted to the CNS sometimes fails to develop a blood-brain barrier (Rosenstein and Brightman, 1983; Stewart et al., 1984). A question of greater controversy is whether or not transplanted CNS maintains its normal barrier properties. At least one investigator has suggested that fetal neocortical transplants fail to develop normal barrier properties when placed either in the ventricle or intraparenchymally (Rosenstein, 1987). Rosenstein used two compounds: horseradish peroxidase (MV $\sim$ 40,000), the standard by which blood-brain barrier integrity is measured, and fluoresceinetated immunoglobulin (MW $\sim$ 125,000), to demonstrate compromise of the blood-brain barrier. Neither of these substances will pass between the tight junctions of cerebral endothelial cells into the brain parenchyma when the blood-brain barrier is intact. Following their intravenous administration and using histochemical methods, he demonstrated the accumulation of both substances in and around the brain implants, suggesting compromise of the blood-brain barrier. Not all vessels demonstrated permeability to these substances, suggesting that normal barrier properties might be exhibited by some vessels. Because outbred rats were used in this study and because transplants were sometimes in contact with areas of host brain normally lacking a blood-brain barrier, it is impossible to determine whether or not the occasional breakdown in barrier properties observed in this study was the consequence of immunologi-

cally mediated events or the results of some intrinsic property of neovascularization. Using both isogeneic and allogeneic donor-host schemes, other investigators have argued in favor of an intact blood-brain barrier in CNS transplants to brain (Widner et al., 1988). Because allo- and xenogeneic tissues are the most likely sources of tissues for transplantation in man, resolution of this issue is of potential importance.

Disruption of the blood-brain barrier, or its failure to form, may or may not be of immunologic significance. If soluble factors such as lymphokines or immunoglobulins were allowed access to the CNS parenchyma, they could serve to initiate or enhance immunologic responses in and around grafted tissues. Gamma-interferon, if administered intravenously to normal animals, fails to induce MHC antigen expression in brain, but if injected directly into brain parnechyma, will do so (Wong et al., 1984). Additionally, antigens shed by grafted tissues might be provided easier access to the systemic circulation were the blood-brain barrier disrupted. It should be noted, however, that activated lymphocytes can gain access to CNS parnechyma in the presence of a blood-brain barrier. Thus immune responses can occur in the CNS without compromise of the barrier (Cutler et al., 1967). Problems in the maintainance of CNS homeostasis may be as important following compromise of the blood-brain barrier as potential immunologic consequences.

Does the Brain Have a Lymphatic Drainage?

The absence of lymphatic drainage is one of the principal features thought to contribute to the immunologic privilege of the CNS. A well-developed lymphatic system is critical to the maintenance of fluid homeostasis in most regions of the body. As much as 50% of the total circulating plasma proteins is returned to the systemic circulation by lymphatic routes. Accordingly, blockage of lymphatic flow results in edema distal to the site of blackade. Considered from the viewpoint of fluid homeostasis, the presumed absence of a need for CNS lymphatics can be explained by the presence of the blood-brain barrier. Because plasma proteins do not cross an intact blood-brain barrier, there should be no requirement for an extension of the lymphatic system to the CNS. However, blockage of cervical lymphatic drainage leads to lymphogenous encephalopathy, a condition characterized by cerebral and facial edema, apathy, and decreased seizure thresholds (Foldi, 1969). This disease state, which can arise as a result of pathologic conditions or as a complication of surgery in man, and for which an experimental animal model exists, demonstrates rather convincingly the presence of functional connections between the CNS and lymphatic systems at some level.

It has been known since 1869 that some portion of the CSF enters the nasal submucosa from the subarachnoid space, from whence it drains to the deep cervical lymph nodes (DCN) via lymphatic channels (Key and Retzius, 1875). This observation has since been substantiated by a number of investigators using a variety of experimental animals, including sheep, dogs, cats, rabbits, and rodents. Numerous substances, including dyes, radioactive isotopes, carbon and ink particles, or cells, have been injected both intracerebrally and intrathecally. In all cases, a portion of the tracer has been found in the DCN and, when looked for, in the submucosal space as well.

An intracerebrally injected tracer substance will find its way into the CSF within the ventricles and thence via normal routes of flow to the cortical subarachnoid space. Alternatively, or in addition, it may pass via the perivascular (Virchow-Robin) spaces directly to the subarachnoid space. It is generally agreed that the greatest proportion of CSF drains from the subarachnoid space directly to the venous circulation by way of the arachnoid villi. A significant amount, however, flows by an alternative path to the olfactory lobe and exits to the submucosal space via extensions of the subarachnoid space that extend through the cribiform plate. Recent ultrastructural studies indicate that the arachnoid merges with the perineurium on olfactory filaments and that dura on the cranial side of the cribiform plate is continuous with the periosteum on the nasal side (Erlich et al., 1986). At the level of the superficial nasal mucosa, the perineurium is composed of a single cell layer. In this region, numerous spaces resembling terminal lymphatic capillaries are seen, and it is at these sites that

the transfer of CSF from the CNS to the lymphatic system is thought to occur.

Several investigators have demonstrated the importance of CSF drainage to deep cervical lymphatic structures by blocking this route of passage. In one case, the cribiform plate was sealed with an acrylic glue (Bradbury et al., 1981). In another, the dura was lifted from the cribiform plate and the olfactory nerves removed by avulsion (Galkin, 1930). In the former instance, the flow of CSF through the cribiform plate to the olfactory submucosa was diminished by 90%; in the latter, accumulation of CSF in the DCN was prevented entirely.

In addition to drainage through the cribiform plate and nasal mucosa, it is generally agreed that small amounts of CSF may enter the lymphatic system via spinal nerve roots and the optic nerves. Of considerably greater controversy is the existence of lymphatics in the CNS proper. Foldi (1977) argues strongly for the presence of *prelymphatics* located in the adventitia of CNS vessels that connect directly with lymphatics in the adventitia of the extracranial carotid arteries. Such a pathway would allow for the passage of substances to the lymphatic system independent of the subarachnoid space and the CSF. This position is strengthened by the ultrastructural work of Prineas (1979), who has demonstrated the presence of thin-walled channels with lymphatic characteristics in the perivascular spaces of human brains. Bradbury and coworkers (1981) have argued, however, that the extracranial lymphatics associated with carotid vessels originate in the nasal submucosa.

Widner et al. (1985) have demonstrated immune reactivity in the DCN of the rat following the injection of antigen into the ventricular system and into the brain parenchyma itself. Using sheep red blood cells (SRBC) as a source of antigen, they observed increased weights of DCN in animals injected either intraventricularly or intraparenchymally. No increase in DCN weight was observed following intravenous injection. Interestingly, the intensity of the antibody response to SRBC was dependent upon the site of antigen administration. B cells producing anti-SRBC antibodies were found in the DCN 5 days after injection. The response was significantly greater when SRBC were injected intraparenchymally rather than intraventricularly. Tracer studies were carried out by Bradbury et al. (1981), who found more label in the DCN of rats injected intraparenchymally than in the DCN of those injected intraventricularly. Thus the greater B-cell response seen within the DCN after intraparenchymal antigen injection may reflect an increased antigenic load. Slow but sustained passage of antigen following its intracerebral injection could also be a factor, intrathecal antigen being quickly swept away along with the CSF into the general circulation and thence to the spleen. These considerations could bear on the fates of grafts placed intraparenchymally, as opposed to grafts placed in the ventricles.

Two standard in vitro correlates of the cell-mediated allograft response are the mixed lymphocyte reaction (MLR) and the ^{51}Cr release assay designed, in the experiments discussed here, to measure MHC class I-restricted cytolytic T-lymphocyte (CTL) activity. The MLR is a measure of lymphocyte proliferation in response to challenge with irradiated MHC class I and II antigen-bearing allogeneic or xenogeneic lymphocytes. The kinetics and intensity of these responses are commonly increased in cells derived from draining lymph nodes and spleen during and immediately following transplant rejection. If the CNS is functionally connected to the lymphatic system via the DCN, then in vitro assays of immune function using cells derived from these organs should bear this out.

We (Nicholas et al., 1987b) looked for enhanced MLR and CTL activity using cells obtained from the DCN and spleens of mice with allogeneic intraventricular neural implants, comparing them with those derived from mice with isogeneic implants. Lymphocytes from the DCN and spleens of transplant-bearing animals were stimulated in vitro with irradiated splenocytes obtained from mice that were histocompatible with the previously transplanted neural tissue. We reasoned that if mice bearing allogeneic neural implants had become sensitized to MHC alloantigens on the grafted cells, then, just as is seen with skin graft rejection, an enhanced proliferative response would be observed following in vitro challenge with relevant splenocytes. We were unable to detect a difference in cell proliferation of host DCN cells or of host splenocytes (as measured by [^{3}H]thymidine incorporation) when comparing the iso- and allograft groups both 1 and 2 months after neural transplantation. Similarly, no difference in cytotoxicity was observed when these same cells were used in a CTL assay, the target cells expressing high levels of the relevant class I MHC molecules. These findings suggest a lack of sufficient central (i.e., lymph node and spleen) sensitization to alloantigens following intraventricular neural transplantation to be detected by standard assay systems. Findings perhaps similar to ours were obtained by Widner, et al. (H. Widner, personal communication) following SRBC deposition in the brain. Although they were able to demonstrate reactivity by increased DCN weight and anti-SRBC antibody formation, proliferative assays and tests of CTL function were negative in their hands, as well. It will be of obvious interest to repeat work of this sort following placement of grafts intraparenchymally.

The transplanted neural tissue in the mice from which we obtained DCN and spleens for the studies described in the preceding paragraph did contain T cell infiltrates at the time the assays were performed. This finding suggests that recognition of the allogeneic graft by the host immune system had occurred, presumably at a level below the detection threshold of the in vitro assays used. Alternatively, sensitization within the grafts could be of the peripheral type, i.e., local trapping of nascent T cells with generation of an immune response entirely within the graft. That such a process is possible within brain is perhaps suggested by the work of Murphy and Sturm (1923). In their report they noted that mouse sarcomas grafted to the rat brain rarely grew if a small piece of autologous (i.e., host) spleen was transplanted along with the sarcoma. If the accompanying splenic tissue was of allogeneic origin, it had no inhibiting effect. Autologous lymphoid elements left the brain within 48 hr when they were injected alone. When given together with a mouse sarcoma, lymphoid elements persisted until the graft had been rejected.

Do Cells of the CNS Express MHC Antigens?

The tissues chosen for transplantation also play a role in determining the success or failure of a graft. As with immunologically privileged sites, might certain tissues also be immunologically innocuous? Upon transplantation, some tissues elicit brisker immune responses than others. This has led to the ranking of tissues according to their "immunogenicity." While it is not clear exactly what determines a tissue's overall immungenicity, the expression of both MHC and of mH antigens (responses to which, it will be recalled, may synergize) on a given tissue are of obvious importance (LaRosa and Talmadge, 1985). Where brain tissue fits into this hierarchy has yet to be determined. It is evident, however, that the ultimate fate of a tissue transplanted to any site is dependent upon both donor and host factors, and that the expression of histocompatibility antigens by donor tissues can be critical in determining graft survival.

Studies on the differential expression of MHC molecules by various tissues are complicated and controversial. A MHC molecule may be present on a given cell under normal physiologic conditions, or its expression may be induced in a variety of ways. The level of expression of a given molecule may vary greatly over time. For example, the expression of MHC molecules may vary during the course of development, as a result of aging, or during viral infection. In addition, numerous mediators of inflammatory and immune responses (e.g., prostaglandins and interferons) are known to alter the level of MHC expression. There may be species and strain differences in the degree to which particular molecules are expressed by a particular cell type. For example, class II MHC molecules are readily induced on astrocytes from mice of strains that are susceptible to experimental allergic encephalomyelitis (Massa et al., 1987). Induction of class II MHC molecules on astrocytes from EAE-resistant strains is less readily obtained. Additionally, MHC molecules may be passively acquired by cells. That is, molecules shed by one cell may become attached to another cell that does not normally express that MHC molecule.

The methods used to detect MHC molecules usually involve the use of antibodies (either monoclonal or polyclonal) directed against MHC products. These antibodies can be applied to tissue sections or to cultured cells and their binding studied by immunohistochemical techniques. Interpretation can be difficult. They can also be used in immunoabsorption studies in which various tissues (usually homogenized) are compared for their ability to bind antibodies directed against various MHC molecules. In all of these systems, purity and specificity of the antibodies are critical. Even monoclonal antibodies prepared as ascites fluid in mice can be contaminated with antiviral antibodies capable of cross-reacting with MHC molecules other than that against which the monoclonal immunoglobulin is directed, thus generating false positives (Klein 1986, page 153). When cultured cells are examined the conditions of culture may alter the outcome, since MHC expression may be up- or down-regulated, depending on the constituents of the medium. Of course, the finding of MHC products on cells in culture does not prove that cells of the same type express MHC products in vivo. It is always difficult to prove that a positive result in immunohistochemical staining does not reflect the passive acquisition of MHC molecules. In transplantation studies, the use of monoclonal antibodies that recognize either donor or host MHC products, but not both, can be of value in determining the source of a MHC molecule, but even these antibodies do not get around the problem of passive acquisition. The use of in situ hybridization and Northern blot analysis allows one to determine whether or not a given cell or cell population contains the mRNA for a given MHC molecule. These techniques depend upon the binding of radioactively labeled DNA that is complementary to the mRNA in question. The presence of the message, however, does not prove that its product is functionally expressed.

When evaluating the distribution of MHC molecules in CNS tissues, many cell types must be considered, including neurons, astrocytes, oligodendroglia, microglia, meningeal cells, cells of the choroid plexus and ependyma, and vessel-associated cells like endothelia, pericytes, and smooth muscle cells. Distinguishing these cell types from one another in histologic sections can be difficult, but the results are more likely to reflect the situation in vivo than those obtained with cultured cells. With these reservations in mind, we will now proceed with what is known of MHC molecule expression by the CNS under normal and pathologic conditions.

Very low or undetectable levels of both class I and II MHC molecules have been reported within the normal CNS of several species when immunoabsorption techniques have been used (Williams et al., 1980; Skoskiewicz et al., 1985). Here, the ability of homogenized CNS tissue to bind a known amount of antibody directed against a given MHC molecule is compared with that of other tissues. Using the binding of antibodies to a spleen preparation as an arbitrary measurement of 100% binding, one group found that normal human brain bound approximately 1% of an antibody directed against a class I MHC product (Williams et al., 1980). No binding whatsoever of antibodies directed against class II MHC products was observed. Note that 1% of the spleen cell level of binding on a homogenate of a tissue containing many cell types may reflect high levels of MHC antigen expression on a minor cell population such as microglia. Similarly, in a study of the normal mouse brain, another group was unable to detect any binding of antibodies directed against either class I or II molecules (Skoskiewicz et al., 1985). These investigators failed to detect binding in the CNS even after systemic administration of recombinant γ-interferon, a potent stimulator of MHC expression for many of the other tissues studied. The failure of γ-interferon to induce measurable levels of MHC molecules in the CNS was thought to be due to the blood-brain barrier, which prevents passage of γ-interferon to the CNS.

When examined histologically, very few cells in normal brain react with antibodies directed against MHC products, a finding consistent with the immunoabsorption studies. Several studies in both man and mouse suggest that fewer than 1% of the total cells in the normal CNS react with antibodies directed against class I or II MHC molecules (Nixon et al., 1982; Hauser et al., 1983). Reports of MHC molecule expression by brain greater than 1% have been published, but these findings were usually derived from *histologically normal* sections of otherwise diseased brain (DeTribolet et al., 1984; Lampson and Hickey, 1986). Whelan et al., (1986) recently reported the absence of class I MHC molecules on all cells except some blood vessels in areas of the brain lacking a blood-brain barrier. This finding suggests that the low or absent expression of these molecules is not due solely to the exclusion of circulating cytokines from CNS parenchyma. In normal brain, MHC class I molecules have been most consistently reported in association with cerebral blood vessels; however, even these reports are questionable (Lampson and Siegel, 1988). MHC class II reactivity has been described in choroid plexus (Head and Griffin, 1985), in white matter tracts (presumably in microglia) (Hauser et al., 1983), and in association with blood vessels (Lampson and Hickey, 1986). Ting et al. (1985) have presented evidence that many of the class II reactive cells found in brain originate in the bone marrow.

Various cells within the CNS can be induced to express either class I or II molecules. The readily demonstrated expression of class II molecules in the brains of animals with EAE and in patients with active MS suggests that induction of MHC molecules does occur in vivo in conjunction with immune responses in brain (Lassmann, 1983; Traugott et al., 1983). The same holds for brain implants already undergoing rejection (Nicholas et al., 1987a). What is not known is whether traumatized brain expresses MHC products to an abnormal extent. Obviously, brain implants are traumatized before and during the time they are implanted. Whether at such times or shortly thereafter (i.e., *after* grafting but *prior* to the onset of the host response) they, or for that matter traumatized host brain, express MHC antigens has never been, to our knowledge, addressed. Lampson and Siegel (1988) have remarked on the minimal expression of β2-microglobulin (noncovalently linked to class I MHC) in stab wounds in brain. Mason et al. (1986) found some syngeneic intraventricular fetal neural implants to be weakly reactive with antibodies directed against class I MHC molecules when evaluated 1 week after transplantation. Other grafts were unreactive. In our experience, syngeneic grafts, once established, do not express enough MHC to be detectable by standard techniques. It is possible that surgical trauma induces the production of cytokines by neural cells and immunocytes, which, in turn, enhance the expression of MHC molecules by grafted cells. Whether this holds for the first several days after grafting is simply not known. It would be of obvious interest to determine the extent to which MHC products are expressed in donor and host tissue following the trauma of tissue preparation and placement.

Once the rejection of a neural implant is underway, MHC antigens are vigorously expressed. Increased expression of MHC molecules by cells in orthotopically placed allogeneic grafts of many kinds, including kidney, liver, and pancreas, is also observed as these grafts are being rejected (Hall et al., 1984, Steiniger et al., 1985; So et al., 1987). This upregulation probably depends on the action of lymphokines such as γ-interferon released by invading cells. Injection of γ-interferon directly into the brains of mice, thus bypassing the blood-brain barrier, has been shown to induce MHC molecule expression by brain cells within 24 hr (Wong et al., 1984).

The bulk of the work involving induction of MHC molecules on CNS cells has involved cultured cells. As already mentioned, culture conditions do not always reflect the in vivo state. Lymphokines, including interferons α, β, and γ, have been shown to have variable effects on the expression of MHC molecules by cultured CNS cells. Using flow cytometric methods, Wong et al. (1985) demonstrated that the majority of cultured astrocytes, oligodendroglia, and microglia could be induced to express class I MHC products following stimulation with any of the three interferons. Gamma-interferon was 200 times as potent as α- or β-interferon. Gamma-interferon also stimulated the expression of class II products by these cells, while α- and β-interferon did not. Under the culture conditions employed by Wong et al., some neurons, perhaps 10%, were found to express class I but not class II molecules.

Fontana and coworkers (1984) have demonstrated the inducible expression of class II molecules on cultured astrocytes following incubation with γ-interferon. Furthermore, upon induction, the astrocytes proved capable of presenting myelin basic protein to encephalitogenic CD4+ T cells that proliferated in response to presented antigen, although a possible minor contamination with microglia was not formally excluded. Astrocytes not

induced with γ-interferon failed as antigen presenters.

Class I molecules can also be induced on astrocytes by stimulation with γ-interferon. Skias et al. (1987) demonstrated that γ-interferon treatment of cultured astrocytes led to a marked and sustained increase in class I molecule expression. Furthermore, these cells could be lysed by cytotoxic T cell clones specific for class I molecules. Lysis occurred even of astrocytes not induced by γ-interferon, in which case class I molecules could not be detected on them immunocytochemically. This lysis could be prevented by antibodies directed against the appropriate class I molecule. These findings are of potential importance when considering the fate of allogeneic and xenogeneic neural transplants. The expression of histocompatibility antigens by astrocytes makes them potential targets of T cell-mediated cytolysis, apparently even when the amount expressed is below the level of detection of standard immunohistochemical techniques.

As mentioned earlier, endothelial cells (and perhaps other vessel-associated cells) may play a critical role in mediating immune responses to transplanted tissues. Endothelial cells from many tissues, including those from the CNS, have been shown to subserve accessory cell functions. For example, McCarron et al. (1986) have shown that cultured murine cerebral endothelial cells derived from mice with EAE express class II MHC products. The levels of class II expression decrease with time unless the cells are repeatedly stimulated with γ-interferon. Similarly, cultured cerebral endothelial cells obtained from normal mice were found to express class II MHC products after stimulation with γ-interferon. These cells were shown to act as antigen-presenting cells to encephalitogenic T cell lines in vitro provided they had been induced to express class II molecules.

The importance of endothelial cells as primary stimulators of graft rejection was recently demonstrated by Ferry et al. (1987). As few as 10^4 endothelial cells, administered intravenously, sensitized rats to subsequent cardiac allografts, provided the endothelial cells shared class II MHC molecules with the grafted heart tissue. Host sensitization by endothelial cells was dependent upon their expression of class II MHC molecules at the time of injection. The expression of class II MHC molecules was readily induced on donor endothelial cells by culture with γ-interferon. It seems likely that endothelial cells exposed to γ-interferon also release lymphokines and that these lymphokines potentiate their capacity to serve as antigen-presenting cells (Wagner et al., 1985). Primed T cells reactive with class II MHC molecules (i.e., effectors of graft rejection) will respond to class II molecules alone. Virgin T cells require an additional signal such as that provided by Il-1 in order to become primed. Thus, in the efferent arm of the immune response, class II MHC molecule expression alone will suffice. For peripheral sensitization to be initiated in a graft, which we have already pointed out could well occur in brain grafts, a local source of lymphokine (i.e., Il-1) is required. Microglia or endothelial cells may provide this second signal (Wagner et al., 1985; Giulian et al., 1986).

Other vessel-associated cells are also capable of expressing MHC molecules. Using immunohistochemical methods, Wekerle et al. (1986) have shown that pericytes in the cerebral vessels of the rat are induced to express class II molecules during the course of EAE. Two other vessel-associated cells, vascular smooth muscle cells (Hart et al., 1987) and perithelial cells distinct from pericytes (Mato et al., 1986), have been said to express class II molecules in the normal rodent brain.

Few studies have been conducted on the expression of MHC molecules in neural transplants. Mason et al. (1986) demonstrated the presence of increased class I MHC molecules on cells in allo- and xenogeneic fetal neocortical transplants to the third ventricle in the rat (Nicholas et al. 1987a). We demonstrated similar findings for class II MHC molecules on neural allografts in the mouse. Figures 15–5 and 15–6 demonstrate the appearance of neural allografts transplanted to fully histoincompatible hosts (differing at all MHC and at multiple mH loci). In Fig. 15–5, the antibody used recognizes both donor and host MHC class II molecules, making it difficult (if not impossible) to determine the origin of the antibody-positive cells in the graft. It is interesting to note, however, that detectable levels of class II MHC antigens are being expressed by host cells in the areas surrounding the grafted tissue, and that the intensity of staining diminishes as the distance from the graft increases. This suggests a spillover of cytokines released by immunocytes within the rejecting graft to the host surround, with subsequent up-regulation of host MHC molecule expression. An alternative explanation would be passive acquisition of donor MHC antigens by host cells. Using a monoclonal antibody that recognizes only donor MHC molecules, we have demonstrated that reactivity is confined to blood vessels within the graft (Fig. 15–4) and to donor parenchymal cells (Fig. 15–6). This finding makes it unlikely that the MHC detected within vessels in the graft surround is acquired passively. In our own study, and that of Mason et al. (1986), the specific cell types reactive with the antibodies were not identified. Nevertheless, the expression of these molecules on transplanted cells provides the host with a potential immunologic target, which when present on other tissues in other sites, is associated with graft rejection.

Is There a Role for Minor Histocompatibility Antigens in Brain Implant Rejection?

In addition to MHC antigens, numerous mH antigens are known (Loveland and Simpson, 1986). Taken individually, most of these antigens have a limited effect of graft outcome, probably because the frequency of precursor cells for individual mH antigens is low relative to the frequency of precursors for MHC alleles (Bevan, 1975). Taken collectively, however, differences at multiple mH loci can have as powerful an effect on graft rejection as single MHC incompatibilities. Minor histocompatibility antigens are expressed on many tissues. The levels to which such antigens are expressed in brain has not been examined systematically. It is even possible that what is viewed as a minor antigen in skin or any other tissue could be a potent one in brain because of increased expression of it in brain. The obverse could hold as well; some mH antigens that are expressed throughout peripheral tissues may not be expressed in brain at all. It is known, for example, that the orders of *strength* of the mH antigens known as H-4, H-7, and H-8 differ, depending on the grafted tissue (brain was not

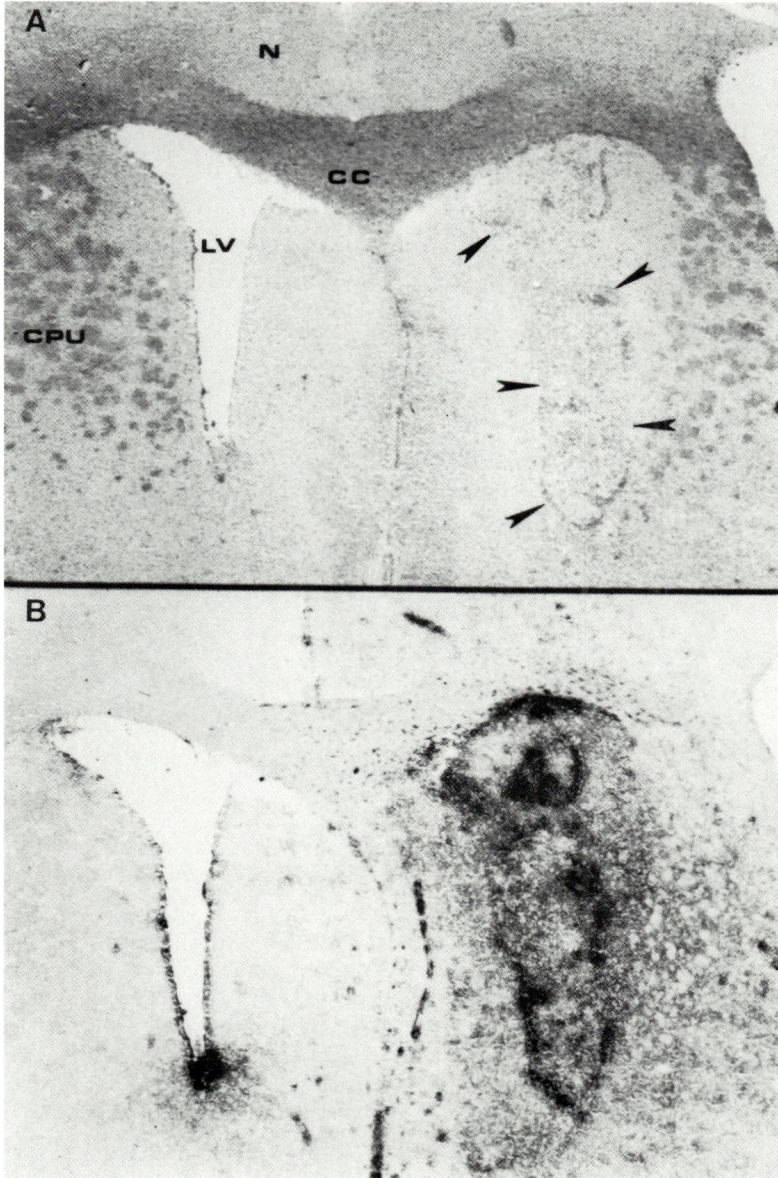

Figure 15–5.   Frozen sections of a murine intraventricular fetal neural allograft 4 weeks after transplantation. **A:** Staining with an irrelevant (isotype control) antibody. **B:** Staining of a serial section with a monoclonal antibody reactive with class II MHC molecules on both donor and host tissues. Arrowheads in A denote the graft-host interface. Note in B that class II MHC expression extends beyond the transplant itself and includes host blood vessels. N, neocortex; CC, corpus callosum; LV, lateral ventricle, CPU, caudate/putamen. ×30. (Photo courtesy of Alan R. Liss, Inc.)

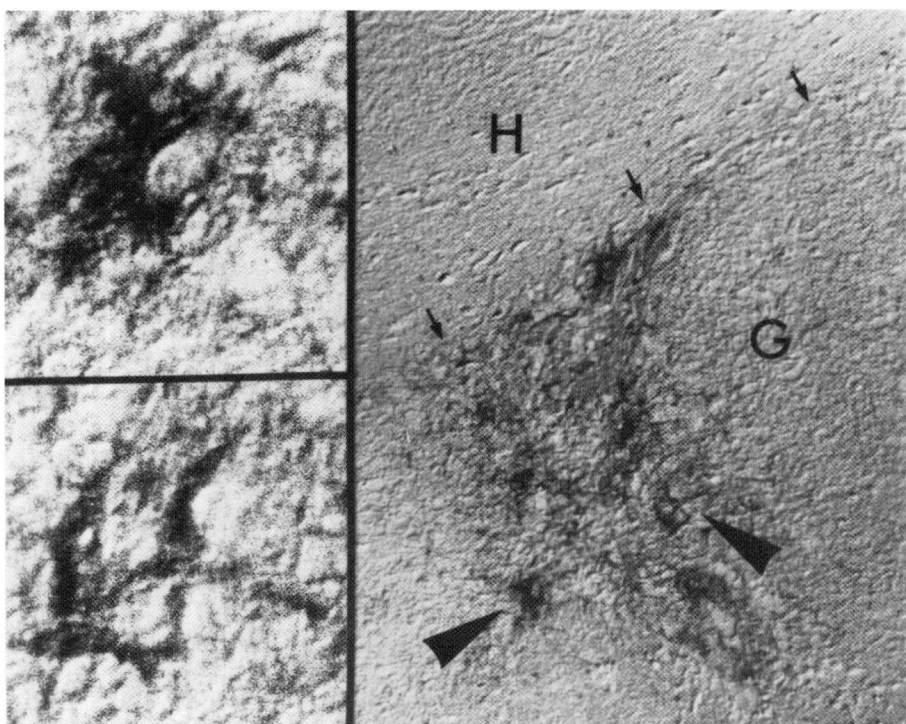

Figure 15–6.   Frozen sections of a murine intraventricular neural transplant 4 weeks after transplantation, stained with a monoclonal antibody reactive with donor but not with host class II MHC molecules. Note in the low-power view (large panel) that class II MHC expression is found in some areas of the transplant but not others. G, graft; H, host. Small arrows denote the graft-host interface. $\times 80$. Higher power views of cells indicated by arrowheads can be seen on the left. $\times 500$.

studied), suggesting that representation of a mH antigen may differ quantitatively among the tissues that express that mH antigen (Scheid et al., 1972). Most mH antigens have not been screened extensively for their degree of polymorphism, nor have any of them been characterized chemically to the present.

Included as mH antigens are the so-called tissue-specific or tissue-restricted antigens. One such antigen, Skn-1, is found on skin epidermal cells in some mouse strains but not in others (Fleming and Silvers, 1981; Steinmuller, 1983). Orthotopic skin grafts from Skn-1+ mice to Skn-1− mice are rejected, even when the donor and host are genetically identical at all histocompatibility loci except Skn-1. Interestingly, Skn-1 is present in brain and is also expressed by some neuroblastomas, although not by lymphoid cells. Note that skin

and brain are both derived from ectoderm, so that the presence of shared antigens not found in other tissues is not altogether unexpected. Skn-1 has not been demonstrated in nonneuronal tumors, nor has it been detected in thymus, lymph node, or spleen. Which brain cells express Skn-1, is, at present, unknown. The presence of this molecule on the mouse neuroblastoma, C-1300, suggests that neurons might express the Skn-1 antigen (Steinmuller, 1983). A second mH antigen, known as H-Y, is also expressed in brain. Whether additional tissue-restricted antigens exist on the cells of the DNS, and if so, to what extent, remains to be determined. One mH antigen, known as H-3, is noncovalently linked with β-2 microglobulin in the same fashion as the class I-MHC α chain. Since β-2 microglobulin is not expressed in normal brain, it is, in our opinion, unlikely that H-3 will be expressed in normal brain either (Rammensee et al., 1986). The fact that neural implants that differ at mH in addition to MHC loci are rejected more often and more rapidly than those that differ at the MHC alone argues in favor of expression of at least some mH antigens by brain (Mason et al., 1986).

Response to mH antigens is exclusively T cell-mediated and is invariably MHC-restricted. The H-Y antigen found on male cells, to which nulliparous female graft recipients respond, is MHC class II-restricted, as in all probability is Skn-1. Both, as noted above, are expressed in brain. In contrast, several other mH antigens (H-1, H-3, H-4, H-7, and H-25) are class I restricted. We have not been able to find data concerning their expression, or lack thereof, in brain.

Class I and class II MHC expression can be demonstrated once an immune response has been set in motion in a brain implant, though perhaps not before. It is distinctly possible that a response to one or more mH antigens expressed by brain may provide the spark that ignites class I and II MHC expression. This kindling process could then be followed by the generation of an immune response directed against donor MHC molecules.

Evidence continues to accumulate to suggest that mH antigens may have a greater role in graft rejection between MHC-incompatible hosts than was previously thought. For example, La Rosa and Talmadge (1985) found that cultured thyroid lobe allografts survived without inflammation in several donor-host combinations in which histoincompatibility was limited to the MHC. When histoincompatibilities were extended to include both the MHC and mH loci, significant inflammation and rejection occurred, suggesting synergism between major and minor histocompatibility antigens. Significant lymphocytic infiltrates were also seen in strain combinations in which donor-host disparities were limited to mH differences alone, suggesting a *major* role for *minor* antigens in the transplantation of thyroid glands in some donor-host combinations. Interestingly, we (Nicholas et al., 1987a) found more necrosis in intraventricular allogeneic brain implants if the host animal had received a subsequent skin graft that shared minor antigens (but no MHC antigens) with the transplanted neural tissue than we did in similar implants from animals that had received no skin grafts. This suggests that mH antigens might be similarly important in neural transplants.

Effects of Systemic Sensitization on Intra-CNS Transplants and Vice Versa

As mentioned earlier, Medawar (1948) demonstrated that skin transplanted to the brain was acutely rejected if the host animal had been previously sensitized with an orthotopic skin graft bearing the appropriate histocompatibility antigens. Since that time, several investigators have confirmed and extended these findings. The studies of Scheinberg et al. (1966) and Lance (1967) demonstrated the reverse phenomenon. That is, skin or thyroid transplanted to the brain led to accelerated rejection of subsequently placed orthotopic skin grafts. This suggested that skin or thyroid implanted to the CNS were capable of sensitizing the host to donor antigens.

William Freed (1983) extended the early findings of Medawar by assessing the effects of systemic host sensitization on intraventricular neural allografts. Freed demonstrated that placement of an orthotopic skin allograft on a rat bearing a neural transplant led to the rejection of both the skin and the neural tissue, provided the tissues were derived from genetically identical animals. He was working with an experimental model of Parkinson's disease for which behavioral tests of graft function exist. Any functional recovery displayed by animals after neural transplantation was abolished following systemic sensitization with orthotopic skin grafts.

Freed was unable to demonstrate systemic sensitization by intra-CNS allogeneic neural transplants. He found that rats with allogeneic neural implants rejected subsequent orthotopic skin grafts at the same tempo as control animals. In addition, no cytotoxic antibodies directed against donor alloantigens could be detected in the serum of animals with allogeneic brain implants. Comparison of these findings with those of Scheinberg and Lance outlined above suggests that allogeneic neural tissue transplanted to the CNS is less immunogenic than allogeneic skin similarly placed.

We have reproduced some of these findings in fetal neocortical transplants to the lateral ventricle of the mouse. In transplants between animals that differ completely at the MHC and at mH loci, inflammatory infiltrates are substantially increased following the placement of orthotopic skin grafts syngeneic with the transplanted neural tissue. The histologic picture obtained under these conditions is similar to that seen following the rejection of a neural xenograft (Fig. 15–1). Rejection of the orthotopic skin graft was no faster in mice that received intraventricular neural allografts than it was in control mice if only 2 weeks separated the placement of the neural transplants and the skin grafts. Thus it appears that rapid systemic sensitization does not occur following an intraventricular neural allograft. In contrast, accelerated rejection of orthotopic skin grafts has been observed if 4 months separate the grafting of the neural tissue and orthotopic skin (unpublished observations). This finding suggests, as with intracerebral skin grafts, that delayed host sensitization occurs following the placement of an intra-CNS neural allograft.

Widner et al. (1988) have also found evidence of systemic host sensitization following the intraparenchymal placement of allogeneic neural cell suspension grafts in the mouse. They demonstrated sensitization using a graft vs. host disease (GVHD) model. Splenocytes obtained from mice 6–7 weeks after allogeneic neural transplantation were compared with splenocytes from control mice for their ability to cause GVHD when injected into neonatal F_1 hybrid mice. The F_1 mice were obtained by mating the donor and host animals used in the neural transplantation scheme. This assay is a test of the ability of lymphocytes obtained from the recipient of an allograft to recognize and respond to cells of the donor. By using F_1 mice obtained from the breeding of donor and host in the original transplant scheme, splenocytes obtained from animals after neural transplantation will not be rejected by the host upon transfer to the F_1 mice, since they will not be perceived as foreign. However, if splenocytes in the transferred population have been primed by exposure to the intra-CNS transplant, then an immune response will be generated against cells of the F_1 animals that express donor antigens, that is, GVHD results.

There are many ways to assess GVHD. Widner et al. (1988) used the Simonsen assay. Briefly, the spleens of F_1 mice are removed 8 days after the intraperitoneal injection of 10^7 splenocytes obtained from either neural allograft recipients or control mice. If GVHD has occurred, the injected cells will have proliferated in the spleen, leading to an increase in its weight. Thus the weights of the spleens from the experimental and control groups are compared. If the ratio of experimental: control spleen weight exceeds 1.3, GVHD (i.e., sensitization) is said to have occurred. Widner and coworkers found evidence for systemic sensitization in four of five mice that had received intraparenchymal neural allografts in which the donor-host disparity involved both class I and II MHC loci. Five of eight animals were found to be sensitized when the donor-host disparity involved both MHC and mH loci.

Based upon the low level of MHC antigen expression by normal mammalian brain, one might predict enhanced survival of CNS-derived tissues transplanted to nonprivileged sites, compared with other tissues similarly placed. Mason et al. (1986) recently demonstrated the rapid rejection of histoincompatible neural tissues transplanted beneath the kidney capsule, a nonprivileged site. Furthermore, the simultaneous placement of allogeneic neural sue in the third ventricle and under the kidney capsule led to the rejection of both transplants, although the intra-CNS tissue was rejected more slowly than that placed under the kidney capsule. This demonstrates that peripherally placed allogeneic neural tissues can effectively immunize the host and casts doubt on the speculation that CNS tissue might itself be immunologically privileged. Freed et al. (1988), using numerous strain and species combinations, recently demonstrated the same phenomenon. Allogeneic and xenogeneic intra-CNS transplants were rapidly rejected if neural tissue was placed both in a subcutaneous site and intraventricularly at the same time.

The experiments outlined above indicate that allogeneic neural tissues are highly immunogenic when placed in nonprivileged sites. In addition, it appears that host sensitization is delayed but not precluded by the placement of allogeneic neural tissues in immunologically privileged sites.

In intra-CNS allogeneic neural transplants are capable of sensitizing the host, one would expect the same to hold for intra-CNS xenografts. This is, indeed, the case. Brundin et al. (1988) have demonstrated sensitization of rats to antigens on human T cells following the placement of human fetal neural tissue in the rat brain. Antibodies that bound human T cells were detected in the serum of all rats 19–21 weeks after placement of intracerebral human fetal transplants. In contrast, little if any binding of antibodies from control rats to human T cells was observed. Interestingly, antibody levels were as high in those rats that received chronic immunosuppression with cyclosporin as they were in rats that were not immunosuppressed.

Cellular Infiltrates in Intra-CNS Allografts and Xenografts

One way to study the mechanisms underlying graft rejection is to evaluate the inflammatory infiltrate in the grafted tissue itself (Hall, 1987). Tissue sections can be examined using either routine or immunohistochemical techniques. Alternatively, if invading cells are isolated from the graft, both their phenotypic (i.e., expression of surface molecules) and functional properties can be studied. Because lymphatic drainage in the CNS differs from that in other organs, evidence of systemic sensitization may be delayed or substantially diminished, as already discussed. Therefore the characterization of lymphocytes isolated directly from CNS tissue may aid in understanding the nature of the response. To date, few studies have been conducted to evaluate the phenotypes of cellular infiltrates in allografts or xenografts to the CNS. To our knowledge, no immunohistochemical evaluations of inflammatory cells in nonneural tissues transplanted to the CNS have been made. Additionally, no studies of the functional properties of graft-invading cells obtained from intra-CNS transplants have been reported.

ALLOGRAFTS

As mentioned earlier, many investigators have reported success with the transplantation of allogeneic neural tissues to the brain. Freed, for example, has had considerable success in transplants between several strains of inbred

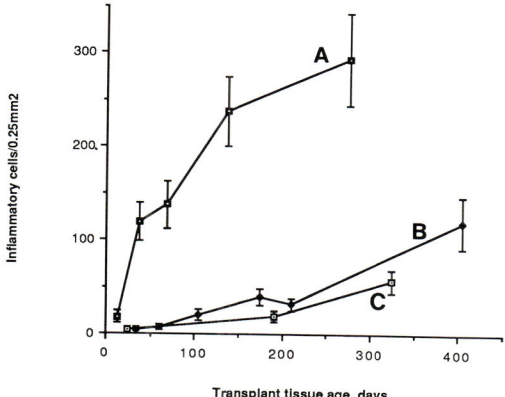

Figure 15–7. Quantitation of inflammatory cells in intraventricular fetal spinal cord allografts in the rat as a function of time. The numbers of inflammatory cells per 0.25 mm^2 area of grafted spinal cord were compared in three donor-host combinations. The tissue was evaluated 20–410 days after transplantation. Tissue from three to five animals was evaluated at each time point indicated. As seen in the figure, considerable variability in the degree of inflammation exists between groups. The greatest numbers of inflammatory cells were seen in transplants between outbred Hotzmann rats (A). Tissues exchanged between inbred rats [Brown Norway into Lewis (B) and Lewis into Brown Norway (C)], had considerably fewer inflammatory cells at all time points analyzed. Holtmann rats are routinely outbred; thus genetic disparities between donor and host cannot be determined. Outbreeding will, however, promote considerable histoincompatibility at both MHC and mH loci. Brown Norway and Lewis rats are inbred strains. They differ from one another at the MHC and at many mH loci. (Data courtesy of R.C. Yu).

rats. Yu has experienced similar success with some donor-host combinations. He has had considerably less success, however, with transplants between outbred rats (R.C. Yu, personal communication). As shown in Fig. 15–7, the numbers of inflammatory cells per unit area within fetal spinal cord implants to the lateral ventricle of adult rat hosts differed markedly from one donor-host strain combination to another. The reasons for these differences are, at the moment, unclear.

Mason et al. (1986) and Sloan and Charlton (1988) have used immunohistochemical markers to characterize the cellular infiltrates in fetal neocortical allografts to the third ventricle of adult rat hosts. The majority of the grafts were found to be rejected if the transplanted tissue differed from the host at both MHC and mH loci. Early after implanting, NK cells were detected in the allografts. This infiltrate was transient, and a comparable early NK infiltrate was seen in syngeneic grafts. A major role for NK cells in brain allograft rejection seems improbable based on these observations. Within 2 weeks of grafting, macrophages and T cells were found in all transplants. A heavy cellular infiltrate was present in most grafts evaluated 20–30 days after transplantation. By day 60, many grafts could not be found at all. Tissue was not rejected when donor-host combinations involved either MHC disparities alone (both class I and II) or mH disparities alone. Interestingly, Mason et al. (1988) observed diffuse patches of inflammatory cells in those transplants involving only mH donor-host disparities, but no cellular infiltrates were reported in the transplants involving MHC donor-host disparities alone. The data suggests that MHC disparities alone, unlike the situation with other tissues undergoing rejection, may not suffice for rejection of CNS implants to brain. CNS tissue fully compatible at the MHC but differing from the host at multiple mH loci may be similarly unaffected.

In the studies detailed above, T cells were identified by antibodies directed against determinants present on all mature T cells. The relative proportions of CD4 + and CD8 + cells in the infiltrates were not determined. Mason, et al. (1986) did compare the composition of the cellular infiltrates in the intraventricular transplants to transplants of the same tissue placed under the kidney capsule. Mast cells were often observed at the graft-host interface in transplants placed under the kidney capsule, whereas none were observed in the intraventricular grafts. This observation underscores that mechanisms of rejection may differ when the same tissue is transplanted to different anatomic sites. It is known that the CNS excludes mast cells (Olsson, 1968).

We (Nicholas et al., 1987a) have conducted a phenotypic analysis of the cells infiltrating fetal neocortical allografts in the mouse. In the experiments described below, fetal neocortex was transplanted to the lateral ventricle of mice that differed from one another at all class I and II MHC loci as well as at multiple mH loci. Using immunohistochemical techniques, we found cellular infiltrates composed of CD4 + and CD8 + T cells, macrophages, and B cells in all transplants evaluated 1–2 months after transplantation. This inflammation increased over time, and gross tissue destruction was evident in large areas of the transplants 4 months after transplantation. CD4 + cells were found to predominate when serial sections of transplant tissue obtained from allograft-bearing mice were alternately stained with monoclonal antibodies directed against CD4 + or CD8 + cells. No immunocytes were found in isografts evaluated at these time points.

We (Nicholas et al., 1988) also isolated lymphocytes from the brains of mice receiving intraventricular fetal neocortical allografts, donors and hosts again differing at both class I and II of the MHC and at multiple mH loci. The CD4:CD8 ratios of cells obtained by this method were determined by flow cytometry 1, 2, and 4 months after transplantation. As suggested by the immunohistochemical data, we found a much larger proportion of CD4 + cells than of CD8 + cells in all allografts evaluated within the first 2 months of transplantation. Similar findings were obtained when cells were evaluated 4 months after transplantation, although the relative number of CD8 + cells was sometimes increased over that observed at 1 and 2 months. No T cells were obtained in isolates of cells from the brains of isograft-bearing animals, regardless of the time at which they were evaluated. If animals were allowed to reject orthotopic skin allografts (the skin being syngeneic with the brain implants) prior to lymphocyte isolation and analysis, the proportion of CD8 + cells within the intra-CNS graft increased dramatically. These findings are shown in Figure 15–8.

It is unclear why CD4 + cells should so markedly predominate in the cellular infiltrates of neural allografts within the first months of transplantation. Graft rejection, as emphasized earlier, is a complex process involving interactions between numerous cell types. Nevertheless, depending upon the donor-host disparities and the transplant scheme involved, a particular cell or cell sub-

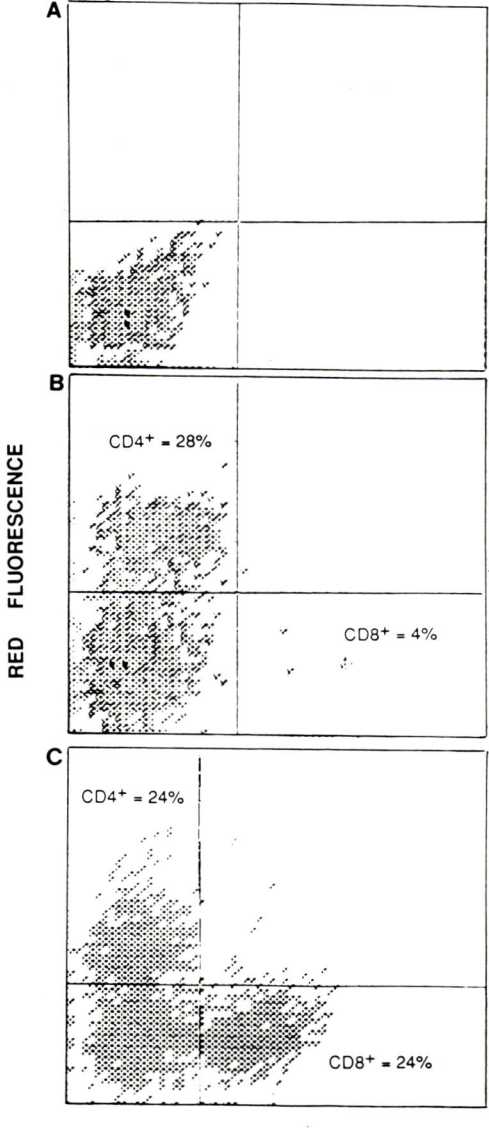

GREEN FLUORESCENCE

Figure 15–8. Analysis by flow cytometry of lymphocytes isolated from the CNS of mice with intraventricular fetal neural allografts and stained with monoclonal antibodies directed against CD4 + and CD8 + cells. The antibodies are conjugated to fluorescent markers, CD4 + cells fluorescing red upon excitation (axis) and CD8 + cells fluorescing green upon excitation (x axis). **A:** The profile obtained by unstained cells. **B:** The profile obtained when lymphocytes are isolated 4 weeks after transplantation. Note the marked CD4 + predominance. **C:** The profile obtained if cells are isolated from the intra-CNS allograft 10 days after the placement of an orthotopic skin graft. Both the grafted skin and neural tissue were obtained from an animal of the same strain. Note the marked increase in CD8 + cells. No lymphocytes are isolated from the brains on animals with isogeneic neural implants.

set alone may be sufficient to effect graft rejection. As mentioned before, both CD4 + and CD8 + cells have been shown capable of effecting skin graft rejection: CD4 + cells mediating the rejection of class II MHC disparate grafts and CD8 + cells mediating the rejection of class I MHC disparate grafts. Immunohistochemical analysis of T cell subsets in renal, hepatic, and heart allografts has revealed a spectrum of CD4:CD8 ratios, ranging from CD4 to CD8 predominances. In most allografts in which donor-host disparities include both class I and class II MHC loci, CD8 + cells are found to outnumber CD4 + cells, but some interesting exceptions have been observed. In one study, serial analyses of T cell subsets in biopsies of human hepatic allografts were made (Perkins et al., 1987). Several distinct patterns of inflammation were seen. One involved lobular infiltrates of CD8 + cells, another portal infiltrates of CD4 + cells. A third pattern, also found in the portal tracts, involved a mixture of CD4 + and CD8 + cells. Livers from which biopsies revealed portal CD4 + cells either alone or with CD8 + cells were usually undergoing rejection. Those with lobular CD8 + cells were not. It should be borne in mind that study and interpretation of graft rejection events in man is complicated by the fact that graft recipients are invariably receiving immunosuppressive agents.

CD4 + cells have been shown to play a pivotal role in the rejection of kidney allografts even when donor-host disparities include both class I and II MHC molecules (von Willebrand, 1983). von Willebrand reported that rejection episodes in renal allograft recipients could be successfully reversed with vigorous immunosuppressive therapy if a biopsy taken at the time of rejection crisis indicated a CD8 + T cell predominance. Graft rejection could seldom be reversed when CD4 + cells predominated. The preponderance of CD4 + T cells in neural allografts in which donor and host differ at both class I and II MHC loci may, we suggest, indicate a critical role for CD4 + cells in the rejection of neural allografts. It has been reported that rejection of allogeneic skin grafted to rat brain is dependent upon differences at the A locus (class I) of the rat MHC, which would suggest that rejection of allogeneic skin in brain,

unlike allogeneic brain in brain, is a function of CD8 + effector cells.

The reasons for the relatively low percentage of CD8 + cells in rejecting neural allografts remain unknown. It is possible that the methods used to isolate and detect these cells preferentially yielded CD4 + cells. This is not likely, because relatively large numbers of CD8 + cells were isolated from the brains of animals with both neural allografts and orthotopic skin grafts. A predominance of CD8 + cells has also been noted under other circumstances, such as in MS plaques (Klein, 1978). As mentioned earlier, CD8 + cells are the primary effectors of antigen-specific cytotoxicity, and a surprisingly large percentage of these cells appear to recognize MHC alloantigens. It is possible that the increase in CD8 + cells within the grafts late in the rejection process (4 months after transplantation) represent allograft-specific cytotoxic activity. This hypothesis remains to be tested.

As mentioned earlier, the effector cells involved in the rejection of skin grafts exchanged between mice that differ at either class I or class II MHC loci only (not both) appear to be largely MHC-restricted. This is, CD4 + cells are found to be both neccessary and sufficient to effect the rejection of class II MHC disparate skin grafts, while CD8 + cells are found to mediate rejection of class I MHC disparate grafts. As a means of evaluating the relative importance of these cells in the rejection of neural transplants, we have been conducting studies to determine the effect of donor-host disparities *within* the MHC on the survival of intra-CNS neural transplants (unpublished data). Donors in this model are the B6.C-H-2^bm11 and B6.C-H-2^bm12 mice. Both were derived from C57BL/6 mice and are known to differ from the parental line at only class I (bm11) or class (bm12) MHC loci (Klein, 1978). The differences between these mutants and the C57BL/6 parental line from which they were derived are small, consisting of one to several point mutations within a single MHC molecule. These small differences are sufficient, however, to cause the rapid rejection of skin grafted from either bm11 or bm12 mice to the C57BL/6 mouse. As mentioned earlier, tissues exchanged between mice that differ from one another only by point mutations within the MHC are often rejected (Isakov and Bach, 1983).

We have evaluated the inflammatory infiltrates in grafts of fetal neocortex transplanted from these class II and class I mutant mice to the lateral ventricle of the C57BL/6 mouse. When examined 8 weeks after transplantation, some inflammation was seen in all transplants. When MHC class I mutant grafts were compared with MHC class II mutant grafts, substantial differences were found in both the degree and the pattern of inflammation. In grafts in which the donor-host disparity involved only a class I MHC molecule, large areas of the transplant were completely free of infiltrating cells. Occasional discrete inflammatory foci were observed. In contrast, when the donor-host disparity involved the class II MHC molecule, multiple perivascular inflammatory infiltrates were found throughout the grafts. Diffuse intraparenchymal mononuclear cells were also observed. These findings suggest that the immune response directed against intra-CNS neural allografts may depend more upon host response to class II MHC molecules than upon host response to class I MHC molecules. These findings are also consistent with our earlier observation that CD4+ cells predominate in intraventricular allografts in which donor-host disparities involve both class I and II MHC loci as well as multiple mH loci. Note that the degree of inflammation observed is less than that found when donor-host disparities involve both class I and II MHC loci and multiple mH loci.

XENOGRAFTS

Several years ago, Björklund et al. (1982) reported the successful transplantation of fetal neural tissues across species barriers. In this study, fetal mouse tissue containing dopaminergic neurons was placed into cavities overlying the neostriatum of dopaminergically denervated rats. Surviving neurons in the transplanted tissue were later identified using catecholamine fluorescence histochemistry. No surviving tissue was found in 44% of the animals. In the remainder, surviving neurons were found as either small nonvascularized clusters near the site of transplantation or as individual cells within the host caudate-putamen. Functional recovery of dopaminergi-

cally mediated activity correlated with the degree of neuronal survival in the transplanted tissue. The investigators hypothesized that transplanted cells that migrated shortly after transplantation to an area protected by the blood-brain barrier were spared, while those exposed to the host circulation were rejected. This important report demonstrated that xenogeneic tissues were capable of restoring function. It also served as a reminder that the immunologic privilege enjoyed by the CNS is limited and poorly understood.

Other investigators have also reported success with intra-CNS xenografts. Most, however, have found rejection to be the rule. Fetal neural tissues obtained from humans, mice, and pigs have all been reported to undergo rejection following transplantation to the CNS of imunocompetent rats. In addition to the allograft studies mentioned above, Mason et al., (1986), Freed et al. (1988), and Sloan and Charlton (1988) have all studied the immunologic fates of intraventricular fetal neural xenografts in rodents. Most grafts were heavily infiltrated with mononuclear cells within 10 days of transplantation, and little or no surviving tissue could be found 30 days after transplantation.

To demonstrate the T cell dependence of this response, Mason's group (1986) transplanted fetal xenogeneic neocortex to the third ventricle of both nude mice and T cell-deficient rats. Graft survival was the rule in both cases, although cellular infiltrates were seen in some transplants of mouse neocortex to T cell-deficient rats. The rats were depleted of their T cells by thymectomy and irradiation. The cellular infiltrates observed in transplants placed in some T cell-deficient rats was probably due to incomplete T cell depletion prior to transplantation.

Finsen et al. (1988) have conducted a time course study of the cellular infiltrates in mouse to rat intraparenchymal xenografts. They found mononuclear infiltrates consisting of T cells, B cells, and macrophages within the first week of transplantation. Inflammation increased with time, reaching maximal levels within 3 weeks in most cases. Little or no surviving tissue could be found 5 weeks after transplantation. At the peak of the inflammatory response, CD8+ cells were found to outnumber CD4 + cells. The findings suggest a significant role for class I-restricted cytotoxic T cells in neural xenograft rejection. In neural allografts evaluated at comparable time points, we demonstrated a CD4 + predominance. Comparing the two sets of results suggests that the mechanisms underlying rejection of neural allografts and xenografts may differ. Faster rejection of xenografts than of allografts also suggests different mechanisms.

It is not surprising that inherent differences might exist in the processes by which allo- and xenogeneic transplants are rejected. As already discussed, MHC-encoded cell surface molecules are the major transplantation antigens in allograft rejection. The MHC molecules comprise the most polymorphic cell surface proteins within a species. The number of potential antigens increases dramatically when one crosses species boundaries. In most cases, MHC-encoded xenoantigens remain potent imunogens. In addition, small structural differences in any number of other cell surface proteins may invoke immune responses. That is to say, proteins that are identical on the cells of animals within the same species may differ slightly in amino acid sequence in more distantly related animals. Structural differences resulting from these changes in amino acid sequence may lead to the generation of immune responses, both cellular and humoral. In fact, humoral immune responses to xenogeneic neural proteins following the intra-CNS transplantation of human fetal neurons to the rat brain have been reported by several investigators (Brundin et al., 1988; Seiger et al., 1988).

What is the Role of Antibody in Rejection of Intra-CNS Transplants?

Antibody responses to intracerebral grafts have seldom been measured, despite their potential relevance to graft acceptance or rejection. As already noted, antibody can favor graft rejection or, alternatively, can enhance graft survival. Under yet other circumstances, antibodies directed against grafted tissue seem not to influence graft survival one way or the other.

One theoretical explanation for the privileged survival of grafts within the CNS would be that the grafts somehow lead to the synthesis of enhancing (i.e., protective) antibodies.

Were this the case, then the previous placing of an allogeneic transplant to the brain should be followed by the slowed rejection of a subsequently placed skin graft from a donor genetically identical to the brain graft donor. This process has not been seen (Freed, 1983; Nicholas et al., 1987b), and we conclude that production of quantities of enhancing antibodies sufficient to impede skin allograft rejection does not occur following placement of transplants in the CNS.

Such a finding is perhaps surprising, since it has been reported that injection of particulate antigens such as xenogeneic red blood cells into the subarachnoid space is followed by a brisk systemic antibody response (Panda et al., 1965; Quirico Santos and Valdimarsson, 1982). The antibody response is said to be T cell-dependent and to be in large measure abrogated by splenectomy. Clearly, antigen injected into the subarachnoid space reaches the periphery. The response seen after subarachnoid injection compares favorably with that which follows intravenous antigen administration. Since the bulk of the spinal fluid flows into the venous circulation, the result is not altogether unexpected. It is widely accepted in transplantation biology that transportation of antigen by vascular routes favors the production of: 1) suppressor T cells; 2) serum blocking factors; and 3) graft survival (Waksman, 1980).

In published reports, antigens such as xenogeneic red blood cells placed within the brain parenchyma, rather than in the subarachnoid space, have provoked only low-level antibody responses, comparable to those seen after subcutaneous injection of antigen (Panda et al., 1965; Quirico Santos and Valdimarsson, 1982). Subcutaneously injected antigen drains to the regional nodes, where it is sequestered before it can reach the circulation. The data hint, perhaps, that drainage of antigen placed intraparenchymally in brain may also make its way, in part, to lymph nodes rather than to the circulation. In any case, the data given above might suggest that intraventricular transplants would be more likely to elicit a vigorous antibody response than intraparenchymally placed ones. Murphy and Sturm (1923) thought that xenogeneic sarcoma grafts in mice fared poorly if they were in contact with the CSF. Since such contact might favor antibody production and since antibody may have a greater role in xenograft rejection than in rejection of allografts, it is possible that a site that is more favorable for an allograft may be less favorable for a xenograft and vice versa.

Direct measurements of antibody levels after brain transplantation are few, the data are fragmentary, and no clear picture emerges. Freed (1983) measured anti-MHC cytotoxic antibodies after implanting Brown Norway rat brain into the ventricle of Fischer 344 rats. The strains differ at all MHC and at several mH loci. No cytotoxic antibodies could be detected. Orthotopic Brown Norway skin grafts were then placed onto Fischer 344 animals with Brown Norway brain implants. Skin and brain were both rejected by most rats, and cytotoxic antibodies appeared. A few rats rejected their skin grafts but did not totally reject their brain grafts. These rats had higher cytotoxic antibody titers than the others. The data suggest that the antibodies, although cytotoxic by in vitro testing, were not harmful to the brain grafts.

As mentioned earlier, Brundin et al. (1988) detected antibodies directed against human T cells in the serum of rats that had received intraparenchymal transplants of human fetal neural tissue. The authors suggest that these antibodies did not play a major role in the observed graft rejection. Until proven, however, the possibility that they might contribute to the rejection process cannot be discounted.

Head and Griffin (1988) studied serum alloantibody responses after intracerebral grafting of parathyroids or skin. In agreement with the work of Freed, no antibodies were detected. Raju and Grogan (1977) placed Brown Norway rat skin into the brains of Lewis rat recipients. Hemagglutinating anti-Brown Norway antibodies were demonstrable at 20 days, although the grafts survived beyond 100 days. Titers of the antibody were very low—at the limits of detection of the assay system used. Lodin et al. (1977) studied cytotoxic antibodies in rats injected intracerebrally with sarcoma cells. Cytotoxic antibody titer was higher after intracerebral inoculation than after inoculation into the leg. Despite this finding, tumors grew better in the brain than in the leg. The role of antibodies in brain implant acceptance or rejection has been inadequately studied, and no firm conclusion can be drawn.

HOST IMMUNOSUPPRESSION TO CONTROL INTRA-CNS GRAFT REJECTION

If neural transplants prove to be feasible in the treatment of human disorders, the source of tissues for transplantation will pose a significant problem. As mentioned above, several investigators have suggested the use of xenogeneic tissues. Others have suggested the use of allogeneic human fetal tissues. In either case, to ensure the long-term survival of most allogeneic and all xenogeneic tissues transplanted to the CNS of man, some degree of host immunosuppression will probably be necessary. While immunosuppression makes possible the survival of transplanted tissues, it carries with it substantial risks and side effects of its own. Because of the brain's immunologically privileged status, it may be possible to control intra-CNS graft rejection with lower doses of immunosuppressive drugs, given for shorter periods of time, than are required to prevent rejection of other tissues. On the other hand, entirely new ways of approaching immunosuppressive therapy may need to be developed.

Several methods exist for suppressing immune responses directed against transplanted tissues. As noted earlier, Zalewski et al. (1978) demonstrated the enhanced survival of allogeneic vagal nodose ganglia transplanted to the spinal cord of rats rendered unresponsive at birth to donor histocompatibility antigens. While the method of tolerance induction used in these experiments remains a valuable laboratory tool, it has little, if any, practical application to clinical transplantation. Tolerance induction is poorly understood, and a further consideration of its complexities lies beyond the scope of this discussion. Suffice it to say that allogeneic histocompatibility barriers to intra-CNS transplantation of peripheral nervous tissue can be overcome by this method.

Cyclosporin A (CsA), a compound with profound immunosuppressive effects, has been used by several investigators to control the rejection of both intra-CNS allografts and xenografts. CsA is thought to work by inhibiting the production of lymphokines by T cells following activation of them by antigen. Among lymphokines inhibited are Il-2 and γ-interferon (Autenreid and Halloran, 1985; Ferrini et al., 1986). Il-2 plays a critical role in the initiation and maintenance of an immune response through its effects on T cell proliferation, as already mentioned, and γ-interferon is known to induce MHC antigen expression on susceptible cells, including those of the CNS, as previously discussed. Down-regulation of both the host immune response (by inhibition of Il-2 production) and of donor MHC-encoded antigens (by inhibition of γ-interferon production) are the most likely ways by which CsA promotes the survival of foreign tissue grafts. In the one published report concerning intra-CNS allografts and CsA, Tulipan et al. (1986) found that pituitary allografts were rejected when placed in the median eminence of host rats that differed from the donor at only mH loci. Treatment with CsA prevented rejection. Interestingly, pituitary transplants across MHC barriers failed even in the presence of host immunosuppression with CsA.

The degree to which CsA will protect grafts across species barriers is unpredictable. In studies in which peripheral nodose ganglia were transplanted to the sternocleidomastoid muscles in several xenogeneic donor-host combinations, Azzam et al. (1986) found CsA beneficial in some instances (hamster or mouse ganglia into rat muscle) but not others (rat ganglia into hamster muscle and hamster ganglia into mouse muscle). In the same study, they found that xenografts of hamster sensory ganglia to the spinal cords of rat hosts were protected as long as CsA levels were maintained. Removal of the drug resulted in acute rejection. Similarly, Inoue et al. (1985a,b) found that CsA prevented the rejection of mouse to rat intraventricular neonatal neural xenografts. In the latter studies, stopping the drug after a 2-week treatment period was not followed by graft rejection. The tissue was evaluated only 2 weeks after stopping CsA administration, however.

At least two groups have reported that CsA prevents the rejection of intra-CNS xenografts of human fetal dopaminergic neurons to the brain of the rat (Brundin et al., 1985, 1988; Seiger et al., 1988). In at least one case, however, removal of CsA after transplantation was followed by rapid rejection, suggesting the need for long-term immunosuppression.

Freeman et al. (1988) have reported similar success with the transplanting of fetal swine dopaminergic neurons to the striatum of CsA-treated rats. In their study, high levels of CsA were used to ensure graft survival. They elected to use high doses of CsA because previous experience had shown that low doses of CsA were ineffective in preventing rejection of rabbit to rat xenografts (Freeman et al., 1987). Surviving transplant tissue was found in all cases when high-dose CsA was used. Many animals experienced side effects of high-dose CsA, including systemic infections and fatal seizures following methamphetamine administration. In the experimental model employed by Freeman and coworkers, rotational behavior induced by methamphetamine was used to evaluate functional recovery following transplantation. Because the first few animals challenged with this drug died, most were not tested. Thus no objective assessment of functional recovery could be made in this study.

Sloan and Charlton (1988) transplanted mouse neural tissue to the ventricle of Brattleboro rats. These rats are deficient in antidiuretic hormone (ADH) and, as such, are an excellent animal model of diabetes insipidus in man. In prior work, intra-CNS transplantation of allogeneic neural tissue containing cells from the supraoptic and paraventricular nuclei of fetal rats had been shown to alleviate the symptoms of ADH deficiency (increased water consumption and urinary output) in these rats (reviewed in Azmitia and Björklund, 1987). In the present study, the transplantation of *mouse* neural tissue to the ventricle of Brattleboro rats resulted in, at best, transient reductions in water intake and urinary output in some animals. No surviving mouse tissue could be found in any rats 30 days after transplantation, however, even those treated daily with CsA. In contrast, surviving mouse tissue was found in CsA-treated Wistar rats evaluated 30 days after transplantation, suggesting differences in the host response to the xenogeneic challenge depending on the strain of the host. Thus, not only is there unpredictability in the survival of xenogeneic tissues transplanted across species barriers, but between members of a species as well.

A Caveat

Extreme caution should be taken in the application of xenogeneic neural transplantation models to the therapy of human disorders, for several reasons. First, the effectiveness of CsA in preventing rejection of xenografts appears to be both species- and strain-dependent, and which species will be accepted or rejected cannot be predicted a priori. Second, xenogeneic neural tissues, when transplanted outside the CNS, can cause neuroparalytic accidents (see opening paragraphs). The experience of an additional group of investigators merits discussion in this context. Kinutani, et al. (1986) described the development of a demyelinating disease in quail-chick spinal cord chimeras. The chimeras are created by transplanting small pieces of quail embryonic neural crest tissue into chicken embryos. These chimeras have been used extensively to study early CNS development, but until the study conducted by Kinutani et al., none of the birds had been followed to maturity. While the chimeras behaved normally for the first few weeks of life, most developed a severe neurologic disorder characterized by paralysis of the wings and legs within 2 months. Histologic evaluation of their spinal cords and brains revealed a lymphocytic infiltrate that appeared first in the quail tissue and subsequently spilled over to involve the chicken CNS as well. The observation was surprising, because in other models (as discussed above) injection of fetal and neonatal animals with immunocytes usually leads to the induction of tolerance in the recipient animal. In the case of quail-chick spinal cord chimeras, tolerance, if established at all, appears to be overridden early in the life of the animal, resulting in a fatal CNS disease.

CONCLUSIONS

The brain's status as an immunologically privileged site is well established and is supported by most of the evidence presented in this chapter. Immunologic privilege as it pertains to brain is, however, a relative term and is not unconditional. For example, immunologic privilege does not eliminate the need for immune surveillance in guarding against CNS infection, nor does it preclude the occurrence of immune-mediated diseases in brain. The mul-

titude of CNS infections encountered by persons with AIDS and the occurrence of diseases such as postvaccinal encephalomyelitis bear ample witness to these effects. In keeping with some functional interaction between the CNS and immune system, considerable evidence supports the view that foreign tissues transplanted to the brain are recognized and responded to by the immune system of the host, albeit in ways that differ from recognition of and response to the same tissues transplanted to other sites. In this review we have attempted to address those issues that might bear upon the fate of tissues transplanted to the CNS. Many of the questions raised are still matters for speculation. The need for extensive study of brain-immune system interactions as they pertain to intra-CNS transplantation is amply demonstrated by the unanswered questions and equivocal findings presented here. The success experienced by many investigators with neural transplant models in experimental animals has generated considerable enthusiasm for the extension of these applications to man. In the context of these encouraging findings, some readers may find our position overly conservative and skeptical. So be it.

ACKNOWLEDGMENTS

The authors gratefully acknowledge the generous support of The Markey Charitable Trust, The Spinal Cord Research Foundation, The Brain Research Foundation, and The James and Ruth Glasgow Parkinson's Disease Research Fund.

REFERENCES

Allen P (1987): Antigen processing at the molecular level. Immunol Today 8:270–273.

Anderson ND, Wyllie RG, Shaker IJ (1977): Pathogenesis of vascular injury in rejecting rat renal allografts. Johns Hopkins Med J 141:135–147.

Arnason BGW (1987): Neuroimmunology. New Engl J Med 316:406–408.

Ausprunk DH, Folkman J (1976): Vascular injury in transplanted tissues: Fine structural changes in tumor, adult, and embryonic blood vessels. Virchows Arch [Cell Pathol] 21:31–44.

Autenried P, Halloran P (1985): Cyclosporine blocks the induction of class I and class II MHC products in mouse kidney by graft-vs-host disease. J Immunol 135:3922–3928.

Azmitia EC, Björklund A (eds)(1987): "Cell and Tissue Transplantation Into the Adult Brain." New York: The New York Academy of Sciences.

Azzam NA, Zalewski AA, Goshgarian HG, Kadota Y (1986): Unpredictability of cyclosporin-A immunosuppression in promoting neuronal survival in xenografts. Anat Rec 215:6A.

Barker CF, Billingham RE (1977): Immunologically privileged sites. Adv Immunol 25:1–54.

Bauer HJ (1983): Umschrittene MS therapie. Nervenarzt 54:400–405.

Bevan MJ (1975): Interaction antigens detected by cytotoxic T cells with the major histocompatibility complex as modifier. Nature 256:419–421.

Binz H, Wigzell H, Hayry P (1976): Correlation between specific cytolysis and expression of idiotypic receptors of allograft-infiltrating cells. Nature 259:401–403.

Björklund A, Stenevi U (eds) (1985): "Neural Grafting in the Mammalian CNS" Fernstrom Foundation Series, vol 5. Amsterdam: Elsevier.

Björklund A, Stenevi U, Dunnett SB, Gage FH (1982): Cross-species neural grafting in a rat model of Parkinson's disease. Nature 298:652–654.

Bohn MC, Cupit L, Marciano F, Gash DM (1987): Adrenal medulla grafts enhance recovery of striatal dopaminergic fibers. Science 237:913–916.

Bradbury MWB, Cserr HF, Westrop RJ (1981): Drainage of cerebral interstitial fluid into deep cervical lymph of the rabbit. Am J Physiol 240:329–336.

Brundin P, Nilsson OG, Gage FH, Björklund A (1985): Cyclosporin A increases survival of cross-species intrastriatal grafts of embryonic dopamine-containing neurons. Exp Brain Res 60:204–208.

Brundin P, Strecker RE, Widner H, Clarke DJ, Nilsson OG, Åstedt O, Björklund A (1989): Human fetal dopamine neurons grafted in a rat model of Parkinson's disease: Immunological aspects, spontaneous and drug-induced behavior, and dopamine release. In: Progress in Brain Research," vol 78. Amsterdam: Elsevier, in press.

Cutler RWP, Lorenzo AV, Barlow CF (1967):Brain vascular permeability to I^{125}-g-globulin and leukocytes in allergic encephalomyelitis. J Neuropathol Exp Neurol 26:558–571.

Das GD (1983): Neural transplantation in mammalian brain: Some conceptual and technical considerations. In Wallace RB, Das GD (eds): "Neural Tissue Transplantation Research." New York: Springer-Verlag.

Dernouchamps JP, Michiels J (1977): Molecular sieve properties of the blood-aqueous barrier in uveitis. Exp Eye Res 25:25–31.

DeTolla LJ, Passmore HR, Palczuk NC (1977): Cardiac allografts in mice congenic at non-H-2 histocompatibility loci. Immunogenetics 5:553–560.

De Tribolet N, Hamou MF (1984): Demonstration of HLA-DR antigens in normal human brain. J Neurosurg Psychiatr 47:417–418.

Duncan WR, Stepkowski SM (1986): Role of T cell subpopulations in the acceptance or rejection of allografts. Transplant Proc 18:202–206.

Dunn EH (1917): Primary and secondary findings in a series of attempts to transplant cerebral cortex in the albino rat. J Comp Neurol 27:565–582.

Dunnett SB, Björklund A, Stenevi U, Iversen SD (1981a):

Grafts of embryonic substantia nigra reinnervating the ventrolateral striatum ameliorate sensorimotor impairments and akinesia in rats with 6-OHDA lesions of the nigrostriatal pathway. Brain Res 229:209–217.

Dunnett SB, Björklund A, Stenevi U, Iversen S (1981b): Behavioural recovery following transplantation of substantia nigra in rats subjected to 6-OHDA lesions of the nigro striatal pathway. II. Bilateral lesions. Brain Res 229:457–470.

Dvorak HF, Mihm MC, Dvorak AM, Barnes BA, Galli SJ (1980): The microvasculature is the critical target of the immune response in vascularized skin allograft rejection. J Invest Dermatol 74:280–284.

Ebeling E (1914): Experimentelle Gehirntumoren bei mausen. Z Krebsforsch 14:151–156.

Erlich SS, McComb JG, Hyman S, Weiss MH (1986): Ultrastructural morphology of the olfactory pathway for cerebrospinal fluid drainage in the rabbit. J Neurosurg 64:466–473.

Fabre JW, Milton AD, Spencer S, Settaf A, Houssin D (1987): Regulation of alloantigen expression in different tissues. Transplant Proc 19:45–49.

Faustman DL, Steinman RM, Gebel HM, Hauptfeld V, Davie JM, Lacy PE (1984): Prevention of rejection of murine islet allografts by pretreatment with anti-dendritic cell antibody. Proc Natl Acad Sci USA 81:3864–3868.

Ferrini S, Moretta A, Biassoni R, Nicolin A, Moretta L (1986): Cyclosporin-A inhibits II-2 production by all human T-cell clones having this function, independent of the T4/T8 phenotype or the coexpression of cytotoxic activity. Clin Immunol Immunopathol 38:79–84.

Ferry B, Halttunen, Laszczynski D, Schelleknes H, V.D. Meide PH, Hayry P (1987): Impact of class II major histocompatibility complex antigen expression on the immunogenic potential of isolated rat vascular endothelial cells. Transplantation 44:499–503.

Finsen B, Oteruelo F, Zimmer J (1989): Immunocytochemical characterization of the cellular immune response to intracerebral xenografts of brain tissue. In: "Progress in Brain Research," vol 78. Amsterdam: Elsevier, in press.

Fleming HL, Silvers WK (1981): An immunogenetic analysis of skn antigens in mice. Immunogenetics 14:517–526.

Foldi M (1969): Lymphogenous encephalopathy. In Kugelmass NI (ed): "Diseases of Lymphatics and Lymph Circulation." Springfield: Charles C. Thomas.

Foldi M (1977): Prelymphatic-lymphatic drainage of the brain. Am Heart J 93:121–124.

Fontana A, Fierz W, Wekerle H (1984): Astrocytes present myelin basic protein to encephalitogenic T cell lines. Nature 307:273–276.

Freed WJ (1983): Functional brain tissue transplantation: Reversal of lesion-induced rotation by intraventricular substantia nigra and adrenal medulla grafts, with a note on intracranial retinal grafts. Bio Psychiatry 18:1205–1266.

Freed WJ, Dymecki J, Poltorak M, Rodgers C (1989): Survival and rejection of intraventricular brain isografts, homografts, allografts, and heterografts. In: "Progress in Brain Research," vol 78. Amsterdam: Elsevier, in press.

Freeman TB, Brandeis L, Pearson J, Flamm ES (1987): Cross-species grafts of embryonic rabbit mesencephalic tissue survive and cause behavioral recovery in the presence of chronic immunosuppression. In Azmitia EC, Björklund A (eds): "Cell and Tissue Transplantation into the Adult Brain." New York: New York Academy of Sciences, pp 699–702.

Freeman TB, Wojak JC, Brandeis L, Michel JP, Pearson J, Flamm ES (1989): Cross-species intracerebral grafting of embryonic swine dopaminergic neurons. In: "Progress in Brain Research," vol 78. Amsterdam: Elsevier, in press.

Gailiunes P, Suthanthiran A, Person A, Strom TB, Carpenter CB, Garavoy MR (1978): Post transplant immunologic monitoring of the renal allograft recipient. Transplant Proc 10:609–611.

Galkin WS (1930): Uber die bedeutung der "nasenbahn" fur den abfluss aus subarachniodalraum. Z Gesamte Exp Med 72:65–71.

Geyer SJ, Gill TJ (1979): Immunogenetic aspects of intracerebral skin transplantation in inbred rats. Am J Pathol 3:569–579.

Geyer SJ, Gill TJ, Kunz HW, Moody E (1985): Immunogenetic aspects of transplantation in the rat brain. Transplantation 39:244–247.

Giulian D, Baker TJ, Shih LN, Lachman LB (1986): Interleukin-1 of the central nervous system is produced by ameboid microglia J Exp Med 164:594–604.

Gorer PA (1936): The detection of antigenic differences in mouse erythrocytes by employment of immune sera. Br J Exp Pathol 17:42–50.

Grounewoud AR (1987): The impact pf HLA-DR incompatibilities on kidney graft function and on the number of rejection treatments. Transplant Proc 19:683–684.

Hall BM (1987): Cellular infiltrates in allografts. Transplant Proc 19:50–56.

Hall BM, Bishop GA, Duggin GG, Horvath HS, Philips J, Tiller DJ (1984): Increased expression of HLA-DR antigens on renal tubular cells in renal transplants: Relevance to the rejection response. Lancet 2:247–251.

Halloran PF, Wadgymar A, Autenried P (1986): The regulation of expression of major histocompatibility complex products. Transplantation 41:413–420.

Hart DNJ, Fabre JW (1981): Demonstration and characterization of Ia-positive dendritic cells in the interstitial connective tissue of rat heart and other tissues, but not brain. J Exp Med 154:347–361.

Hart MN, Waldschmidt MN, Hanley-Hyde JM, Moore SA, Kemp JD, Schelper RL (1987): Brain microvascular smooth muscle expresses class II antigens. J Immunol 138:2960–2963.

Hasek M, Chutna J, Sladecek M, Lodin A (1977): Immunological tolerance and tumor allografts in the brain. Nature 268:68–69.

Hauser SL, Bhan AK, Gilles CJ, Hoban EL, Reinherz EL, Schlossman SF, Weiner HL (1983): Immunohistochemical staining of human brain with monoclonal antibodies that identify lymphocytes, monocytes, and the Ia antigen. J Neuroimmunol 5:197–205.

Hayes GM, Woodroofe MN, Cuzner ML (1987): Microglia are the major cell type expressing MHC class II in human white matter. J Neurol Sci 80:25–37.

Head JR, Billingham RE (1985): Immunologically privileged sites in transplantation immunology and oncology. Perspect Biol Med 29:115–131.

Head JR, Griffin ST (1984): Functional capacity of solid tissue transplants in the brain: Evidence for immunological privilege. Proc R Soc Lond [Biol] 224:375–387.

Hemachudha T, Griffin DE, Giffels JJ, Johnson RT, Moser AB, Phanupak P (1987): Myelin basic protein as an encephalitogen in encephalomyelitis and polyneuritis following rabies vaccination. New Engl J Med 316:369–374.

Hunig TR, Bevan MJ (1982): Antigen recognition by cloned cytolytic T lymphocytes follows rules predicted by the altered-self hypothesis. J Exp Med 155:111–125.

Inoue H, Kohsaka S, Yoshida K, Ohtani M, Toya S, Tsukada Y (1985a): Cyclosporin A enhances the survivability of mouse cerebral cortex grafted into the third ventricle of rat brain. Neurosci Lett 54:85–90.

Inoue H, Kohsaka S, Yoshida K, Otani M, Toya S, Tsukada Y (1985b): Immunohistochemical studies on mouse cerebral cortex grafted into the third ventricle of rats treated with cyclosporin A. Neurosci Lett 57:289–294.

Isakov N, Bach FH (1983): Thyroid graft rejection between C57BL/6 and H-2K^b mutant mice. Transplantation 36:571–577.

Isakov N, Yankelevich B, Segal S, Feldman M (1979): Differential immunogeneic expression of an H-2-linked histocompatibility antigen on different tissues. Transplantation 28:31–35.

Jerne NK (1985): The generative grammar of the immune system. Science 229:1057–1059.

Kamada N, Brons G, Davies HS (1980): Fully allogeneic liver grafting in rats induces a state of systemic nonreactivity to donor transplantation antigens. Transplantation 29:429–431.

Kaplan DR, Griffith R, Braciale VL, Braciale TJ (1984): Influenza virus-specific human cyctotoxic T cell clones: Heterogeneity in antigenic specificity and restriction by class II MHC products. Cell Immunol 88:193–206.

Key EAH, Retzius MG (1875): "Studien in der Anatomie des Nervensystems und des Bindgewebes." Stockholm: Samson und Wallin.

Kinutani M, Coltey M, LeDouarin NM (1986): Postnatal development of a demyelinating disease in avian spinal cord chimeras. Cell 45:307–314.

Klein J (1978): H-2 mutations: Their genetics and effect on immune functions. Adv Immunol 26:55–146.

Klein J (1986): "The Natural History of the Major Histocompatibility Complex." New York: John Wiley and Sons.

Knorr-Held S, Brendel W, Kiefer H, Paal G, von Sprecht BU (1986): Sensitization against brain gangliosides after therapeutic swine brain implantation in a multiple sclerosis patient. J Neurol 233:54–56.

Krum JM, Rosenstein JM (1987): Patterns of angiogenesis in neural transplant models: I. Autonomic tissue transplants. J Comp Neurol 258:420–434.

Krum JM, Rosenstein JM (1988): Patterns of angiogenesis in neural transplant models: II. Fetal neocortical transplants. J Comp Neurol, 271:331–345.

Lampson L, Hickey WF (1986): Monoclonal antibody analysis of MHC expression in human brain biopsies: Tissue ranging from "histologically normal" to that showing different levels of glial tumor involvement. J Immunol 135:4054–4062.

Lampson LA, Siegel G (1989): Defining the mechanisms that govern immune acceptance or rejection of neural tissue. In: "Progress in Brain Research," vol 78. Amsterdam: Elsevier, in press.

Lance EM (1967): A functional and morphologic study of intracranial thyroid allografts in the dog. Surg Gynecol Obstet 125:529–539.

Landsteiner K (1931): Individual differences in human blood. Science 75:403–409.

LaRosa FG, Talmage DW (1985): Synergism between minor and major histocompatibility antigens in the rejection of cultured allografts. Transplantation 39:480–485.

Lassmann H (1983): "Comparative Neuropathology of Chronic Experimental Allergic Encephalomyelitis and Multiple Sclerosis." Berlin: Springer-Verlag.

Lechler RI, Batchelor JR (1982): Restoration of immunogenicity to passenger cell-depleted kidney allografts by the addition of donor strain dendritic cells. J Exp Med 155:31–41.

Lindahl KF, Wilson DB (1977): Histocompatibility antigen-activated cytotoxic T lymphocytes II. Estimates of the frequency and specificity of precursors. J Exp Med 145:508–522.

Lindsay RM, Raisman G (1984): An autoradiographic study of neuronal development, vascularization and glial cell migration from hippocampal transplants labelled in intermediate explant culture. Neuroscience 12:513–530.

Lindsay RM, Emmett C, Raisman G, Seely PJ (1987): Application of tissue culture and cell-marking techniques to the study of neural transplants. In Azmitia EC, Björklund A (eds): "Cell and Tissue Transplantation into the Adult Brain." New York: The New York Academy of Sciences, pp. 35–52.

Littman DR (1987): The structure of the CD4 and CD8 genes. Annu Rev Immunol 5:561–584.

Lodin Z, Hasek M, Chutna J, Sladecek M, Holan V (1977): Transplantation immunity in the brain. J Neurosci Res 3:275–280.

Lopez-Lozano JJ, Gash DM, Leary JF, Notter MFD (1987): Survival and integration of transplanted hypothalamic cells in the rat CNS after sorting by flow cytometry. Azmitia EC, Björklund A (eds): "Cell and Tissue Transplantation into the Adult Brain." New York: New York of Academy of Sciences, pp. 736–739.

Loveland B, Simpson E (1986): The non-MHC transplantation antigens: Neither weak nor minor. Immunol Today 7:223–229.

Lowry RP, Forbes RCD, Hruby Z (1986): Immune effector mechanisms in organ allograft rejection. VII: Graft rejection must be viewed as the product of a complex immune/inflammatory process. Transplant Proc 18:198–201.

Madrazo I, Druckler-Colin R, Diaz V, Marinez-Mata J, Torres C, Becerril JJ (1987): Open microsurgical autograft of adrenal medulla to the right caudate nucleus in two patients with intractable Parkinson's disease. New Engl J Med 316:831–834.

Madrazo I, Leon V, Torres C, et al (1988): Transplantation of fetal substantia nigra and adrenal medulla to the caudate nucleus in two patients with Parkinson's disease. New Engl J Med 318:51.

Marrack P, Kappler J (1987): The T cell receptor. Science 238:1073–1079.

Mason DW, Charlton HM, Jones AJ, Lavy CBD, Puklavec M, Simmonds SJ (1986): The fate of allogeneic and xenogeneic neuronal tissue transplanted into the third ventricle of rodents. Neuroscience 19:685–694.

Massa PT, Ter Meulen V, Fontana A (1987): Hyperinducibility of Ia antigen on astrocytes correlates with strain-specific susceptibility to experimental autoimmune encephalomyelitis. Proc Natl Acad Sci USA 84:4219–4223.

Matis LA, Glimcher LH, Paul WE, Schwartz RH (1983): Magnitude of response to histocompatibility-restricted T-cell clones is a function of the produce of the concentrations of antigen and Ia molecules. Proc Natl Acad Sci USA 80:6019–6023.

Mato M, Aikawa E, Mato T, Kurihara K (1986): Tridimensional observation of fluorescent granular perithelial (FGP) cells in rat cerebral blood vessels. Anat Rec 215:413–419.

McCarron RM, Spatz M, Kempski O, Hogan RN, Muehl L, McFarlin DE (1986): Interaction between myelin basic protein-sensitized T lymphocytes and murine cerebrovacular endothelial cells. J Immunol 137:3428–3435.

Medawar PB (1948): Immunity to homologous grafted skin. III. The fate of skin homografts transplanted to the brain, to subcutaneous tissue, and to the anterior chamber of the eye. Br J Exp Pathol 29:58–69.

Morris PJ (1980): Suppression of rejection of organ allografts by alloantibody. Immunol Rev 29:93–125.

Morris R (1985): Thy-1 in developing nervous tissue. Dev Neurosci 7:133–160.

Murphy JB, Sturm E (1923): Conditions determining the transplantability of tissue in the brain. J Exp Med 38:183–197.

Nicholas MK, Antel JP, Stefansson K, Arnason BGW (1987a): Rejection of fetal neocortical neural transplants by H-2 incompatible mice. J Immunol 139:2275–2283.

Nicholas MK, Stefansson K, Antel JP, Arnason BGW (1987b): An in vivo and in vitro analysis of systemic immune function in mice with histologic evidence of neural transplant rejection. J Neurosci Res 18:245–257.

Nicholas MK, Sagher O, Hartley JP, Stefansson K, Arnason BGW (1989): A phenotypic analysis of T lymphocytes isolated from the brains of mice with allogeneic neural transplants. In: "Progress in Brain Research," vol 78. Amsterdam: Elsevier, in press.

Nieto-Sampedro, M, Cotman, CW (1985): Growth factor induction and temporal order in CNS repair. In Cotman, CW (ed): "Synaptic Plasticity and Remodeling." New York: Guilford Press, pp. 407–455.

Nixon DR, Ting JPY, Frelinger JA (1982): Ia antigens on non-lymphoid tissues: Their origins and functions. Immunol Today 3:339–342.

Nottenbohm F (ed) (1985): "Hope for a New Neurology." New York: The New York Academy of Sciences.

Oettgen HC, Terhorst C (1987): The T-cell receptor-T3 complex and T-lymphocyte activation. Hum Immunol 18:187–204.

Olsson Y (1968): Mast cells in the nervous system. Int Rev Cytol 24:27–70.

Opelz G (1987): Effect of HLA matching in 10,000 cyclosporine-treated cadaver kidney transplants. Transplant Proc 19:641–646.

Panda JN, Dale HE, Loan RW, Davis LE (1965): Immunologic response to subarachnoid and intracereberal injection of antigens. J Immunol 94:760–764.

Perkins JD, Wiesner RH, Banks PM, LaRusso, NF, Ludwig J, Krom RA (1987): Immunohistologic labelling as an indicator of liver allograft rejection. Transplantation 43:105–108.

Perry VH, Hume DA, Gordon S (1985): Immunohistochemical localization of macrophages and microglia in the adult and developing mouse brain. Neuroscience 15:315–326.

Pfeffer PF, Foerster A, Frøysaker T, Thorsby E (1987): Correlation between HLA-DR mismatch and rejection episodes in cardiac transplantation. Transplant Proc 19:691–692.

Pichler WJ, Walker C, Wolff-Vorbeck G, Koponen M, Tax WJM, deWeck AL (1985) Characterization of T8 epitopes by enzymatic digestion, cross-blocking, and involvement in cell-mediated lympholysis. Cell Immunol 96:398–408.

Pomerat CM, Breckenridge CG, Gordon L (1944): Homeoplastic adrenal grafts to the cerbral cortex of the rat. Endocrinology 34:60–68.

Prineas JW (1979): Multiple sclerosis: Presence of lymphatic capillaries and lymphoid tissue in the brain and spinal cord. Science 203:1123–1125.

Quirico Santos T, Valdimarsson H (1982): T-dependent antigens are more imunogeneic in the subarachnoid space than in other sites. J Neuroimmunol 2:215–222.

Raju S, Grogan JB (1977): Immunologic study of the brain as a privileged site. Transplant Proc 9:1187–1191.

Rammensee HG, Robinson PJ, Crisanti A, et al. (1986): Restricted recognition of β_2-microglobulin by cytolytic T lymphocytes. Nature 319:502–504.

Rao K, Lund RD, Kunz HW, Gill TJ III (1988): Conditions leading to rejection of neural xenografts transplanted to neonatal rats. In "Progress in Brain Research," vol 74. Amsterdam: Elsevier, in press.

Rosenberg AS, Mizuochi T, Singer A (1986) Analysis of T-cell subsets in rejection of K^b mutant skin allografts differing at class I MHC. Nature 322:829–831.

Rosenstein JM (1987): Neocortical transplants in the mammalian brain lack a blood-brain barrier to macromolecules. Science 235:772–774.

Rosenstein JM, Brightman MW (1983): Circumventing the blood-brain barrier with autonomic ganglion transplants. Science 221:879–881.

Scheid M, Boyse EA, Carswell EA, Old LJ (1972): Serologically demonstrable alloantigens of mouse epidermal cells. J Exp Med 135:938–955.

Scheinberg LC, Edelman FA, Levy WA (1964): Is the brain an "immunologically privileged site?" I. Studies based on intercerebral tumor homotransplantation and isotranplantation to sensitized hosts. Arch Neurol 11:248–264.

Scheinberg LC, Kotsilimbas DG, Karpf R, Mayer N (1966): Is the brain an "immunologically privileged site?" Arch Neurol 15:62–67.

Seiger Å, Stromgerg I, Bygdeman M, Goldstein M, Hoffer B, Olson L (1988): Human fetal catecholamine-containing tissues grafted intraocularly and intracranially to immunocompromised rodent hosts. In: "Progress in Brain Research," vol 74. Amsterdam: Elsevier, in press.

Shirai Y (1921): On the transplantation of the rat sarcoma in adult heterogeneous animals. Jpn Med World 1:14–15.

Skias DD, Kim D, Reder AT, Antel JP, Lancki DW, Fitch FW (1987): Susceptibility of astrocytes to class I MHC antigen restricted cytotoxicity. J Immunol 138:3254–3258.

Skoskiewicz MJ, Colvin RC, Scheenberger EE, Russell PS (1985): Widespread and selective distribution of major histocompatibility complex-determined antigens in vivo by interferon. J Exp Med 152:1645–1664.

Sladek JR, Gash DM (eds) (1984): "Neural Tranplants: Development and Function." New York: Plenum Press.

Sloan DJ, Charlton HM (1989): Survival of allogeneic and xenogeneic grafts in rodents. In: "Progress in Brain Research," vol 78. Amsterdam: Elsevier, in press.

So SKS, Platt JL, Ascher NL, Snover DC (1987): Increased expression of class I major histocompatibility complex antigens on hepatocytes in rejecting human liver allografts. Transplantation 43:79–85.

Sprent J, Schaefer M (1986): Capacity of purified lyt-2$^+$ T cells to mount primary proliferative and cytotoxic responses to Ia^{ms} tumor cells. Nature 322:541–544.

Sprent J, Schaefer M (1985): Properties of purified T cell subsets. I. in vitro responses to class I and class II H-2 alloantigens. J Exp Med 162:2068–2088.

Sprent J, Schaefer M, Lo D, Korngold R (1986): Properties of purified T cell subsets II. In vivo responses to class I vs. class II H-2 differences. J Exp Med 163:998–1011.

Steiniger B, Klempnauer J, Wonigeit K (1985): Effect of the rejection process on class I and class II major histocompatibility complex antigen expression in the rat pancreas. Transplant Proc 17:407–411.

Steinmuller D (1983): Skin-specific histocompatibility antigens. In Ninneman JL (ed): "Traumatic Injury, Infection, and Other Immunologic Sequelae." Baltimore: University Park Press., pp. 181–196

Stewart PA, Wiley MJ (1981): Developing nervous tissue induces formation of blood-brain barrier characteristics in invading endothelial cells: A study using quail-chick transplantation chimeras. Dev Biol 84:183–192.

Stewart PA, Clements LG, Wiley MJ (1984): Revascularization of skin transplanted into the brain: Source of the graft endothelium. Microvasc Res 28:113–124.

Svendgaard N-A, Björklund A, Stenevi U (1975a): Regenerative properties of central monoamine neurons. Studies in the adult rat using cerebral iris implants as targets. Adv Anat Embryol Cell Biol 51:7–77

Svengaard N-A, Björklund A, Hardebo J-E, Stenevi U (1975b): Axonal degeneration associated with a defective blood-brain barrier in cerebral implants. Nature 255:334–337.

Ting JPY, Nixon DR, Weiner LP, Frelinger JA (1983): Brain Ia antigens have a bone marrow origin. Immunogenetics 17:295–301.

Traugott U, Reinhert L, Raine CS (1983): Multiple sclerosis: Distribution of T cells, T cell subsets and Ia-positive macrophages in lesions of different ages. J Neuroimmunol 4:201–203.

Tulipan NB, Huang S, Allen GS (1986): Pituitary transplantation: Cyclosporine enables transplantation across a minor histocompatibility barrier. Neurosurgery 18:316–320.

Tze WJ, Tai J (1984): Intracerebral allotransplantation of purified pancreatic endocrine cells and pancreatic islets in diabetic rats. Transplantation 38:107–111.

Uchimura I, Shiraki H (1957): A contribution to the classification and the pathogenesis of demyelinating encephalomyelitis. J Neuropathol Exp Neurol 16:139–208.

von Willebrand E (1983): OKT4/8 ratio in the blood and in the graft during episodes of human renal allograft rejection. Cell Immunol 77:196–201.

Wagner CR, Vetto MR, Burger DR (1985): Expression of I-region-associated (Ia) and interleukin 1 by subcultured human endothelial cells. Cell Immunol 93:91–104.

Waksman BH (1980): Cellular hypersensitivity and immunity: Inflammation and cytotoxicity. In Parker CW (ed): "Clinical Immunology." Philadelphia: WB Saunders, pp 173–218.

Wekerle H, Linington C, Lassmann H, Mayerman R (1986) Cellular reactivity within the CNS. Trends Neurosci 6:271–277.

Whelan JP, Eriksson U, Lampson LA (1986): Expression of mouse β_2-microglobulin in frozen and formaldehyde-fixed central nervous tissue: Comparison of tissue behind the blood-brain barrier and tissue in a barrier-free region. J Immunol 137:2561–2566.

Widner H, Johansson BB, Moller G (1985): Qualitative demonstration of a link between brain parenchyma and the lymphatic system after intracerebral antigen deposition. J Cereb Blood Flow Metab 5:88–89.

Widner H, Brundin P, Björklund A, Moller E (1989): Immunological aspects of neural grafting in the mammalian central nervous system. In: "Progress in Brain Research," vol 78. Amsterdam: Elsevier, in press.

Willams AF (1982): Surface molecules and cell interactions. J Theor Biol 98:221–234.

Willams AF (1987): A year in the life of the immunoglobulin gene superfamily. Immunol Today 8:296–303.

Williams GM, Hume DM, Hudson RP, Morris PJ, Kano K, Milgrom F (1968) Hyperacute renal homograft rejection in man. New Engl J Med 279:611–618.

Williams KA, Hart DNJ, Fabre JW, Morris PJ (1980): Distribution and quantitation of HLA-ABC and DR (Ia) antigens on human kidney and other tissues. Transplantation 29:274–279.

Wong GHW, Bartlett PF, Clark-Lewis I, Battye F, Schrader JW (1984): Inducible expression of H-2 and Ia antigens on brain cells. Nature 310:688–691.

Wong GHW, Bartlett PF, Clark-Lewis I, MCKimm-Breschkin JL, Schrader JW (1985): Interferon-γ induces the expression of H-2 and Ia antigens on brain cells. J Neuroimmunol 7:255–278.

Woodruff MFA (1960): "The Transplantation of Tissues and Organs." Springfield, IL: Thomas.

Woolsey D, Minckler J, Rezende N, Klemme R (1944): Human spinal cord transplant. Exp Med Surg 2:93–102.

Zalewski AA, Goshgarian HG, Silvers WK (1978): The fate of neurons and neurilemmal cells in allografts of ganglia in the spinal cord of normal and immunologically tolerant rats. Exp Neurol 59:322–330.

Zinkernagel RM, Doherty PC (1974): Restriction of in vitro T cell-mediated cytotoxicity in lymphocytic choriomeningitis within a syngeneic or semiallogeneic system. Nature 248:701–702.

Index